KINESIOLOGY

Application to Pathological Motion

SECOND EDITION

KINESIOLOGY

Application to Pathological Motion

SECOND EDITION

GARY L. SODERBERG, PhD, PT, FAPTA

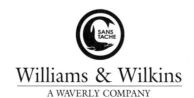

Williams & Wilkins
A WAVERLY COMPANY

BALTIMORE • PHILADELPHIA • LONDON • PARIS • BANGKOK
BUENOS AIRES • HONG KONG • MUNICH • SYDNEY • TOKYO • WROCLAW

Editor: John P. Butler
Managing Editor: Linda S. Napora
Production Coordinator: Anne Stewart Seitz
Copy Editor: Bonnie Montgomery
Designer: Dan Pfisterer
Illustration Planner: Ray Lowman
Typesetter: Bi-Comp, Inc.
Manufacturer: Maple Press

Concrete Carving on the cover by Ralph Prata, Box 317, Bloomingdale, New York 12913.

Printed in the United States of America

Library of Congress Cataloging-in-Publication Data

Soderberg, Gary L.
　　Kinesiology: application to pathological motion / Gary L.
　Soderberg.—2nd ed.
　　　　p.　cm.
　　Includes bibliographical references and index.
　　ISBN 0-683-07851-8
　　1. Movement disorders.　2. Kinesiology.　3. Human mechanics.
　I.　Title.
　　[DNLM: 1. Biomechanics.　2. Movement.　3. Movement Disorders.　　WE
　103 S679k 1996]
　RC925.5.S63　1996
　616.7′4—dc20
　DNLM/DLC
　for Library of Congress　　　　　　　　　　　　　　　　　　96-21426
　　　　　　　　　　　　　　　　　　　　　　　　　　　　　　　　CIP

Call our customer service department at **(800) 638-0672** for catalog information or fax orders to **(800) 447-8438.** For other book services, including chapter reprints and large quantity sales, ask for the Special Sales department.

To purchase additional copies of this book or for information concerning American College of Sports Medicine certification and suggested preparatory materials, call **(800) 486-5643.**

Canadian customers should call **(800) 268-4178,** or fax **(905) 470-6780.** For all other calls originating outside of the United States, please call **(410) 528-4223** or fax us at **(410) 528-8550.**

Visit Williams & Wilkins on the Internet: **http://www.wwilkins.com** or contact our customer service department at **custserv@wwilkins.com.** Williams & Wilkins customer service representatives are available from 8:30 am to 6:00 pm, EST, Monday through Friday, for telephone access.

　　　　　　　　　　　　　　　　　　　　　　　　97 98 99 00 01
　　　　　　　　　　　　　　　　　　　　　　　　1 2 3 4 5 6 7 8 9 10

Preface

This second edition has evolved from numerous years of teaching, clinical practice, and research associated with normal and pathological motion. The work assimilates materials fundamental to both kinesiology and pathokinesiology so that professional program entry-level students in health or related fields may achieve an understanding of principles applied to normal and pathological movement. The work is primarily intended for physical therapists but has broad application across any discipline that incorporates movement science.

The primary objective of this volume is to present knowledge in sufficient depth to provide a true understanding of factors that predispose abnormal motion. This text assumes prerequisite knowledge in physics, pathology, gross and applied anatomy, and physiology. No intention exists of reviewing fundamentals in the physiology of muscle contraction related to human movement. Serious attempts have been made to include applications of basic principles and sciences to movement dysfunction. The reader and student will also find an abundance of references that may be used to further enhance the understanding of kinesiology and pathokinesiology.

The content of the work is broken into three major sections. The first includes fundamentals of evaluating movement, muscle mechanics and applied neurology, articular function, and a chapter on material properties of biological tissues. The second and major section deals with articular kinesiology and pathokinesiology. The third section discusses posture, balance, gait, and ergonomics. Included with each of the latter two sections will be reiterations of the principles presented and discussed in the first section. Many examples are provided for the application of the fundamentals attended to in the early chapter. The material here is intended to encourage students to establish adequate competencies for provision of patient care and serve as a precursor for further study and a greater understanding of pathological motion.

G. L. Soderberg, PhD, PT, FAPTA

Acknowledgments

The preparation of this work would not have been possible without the diligent effort of many friends and colleagues. For the first edition Don Neumann and David Johnson provided many comments and suggestions for the content and the delivery of the material. Chapter reviewers for the first edition included Bob Lamb, Bruce Miller, Jim Andrews, Tom Cook, Don Shurr, and Carolyn Wadsworth. Since much of the original work is still included in this second edition, my continuing thanks is extended to these people. This second edition has been formulated with the assistance of three others who have had a profound impact on the inclusiveness and quality of the manuscript. Thanks are expressed to Darren Averett for his insight, positive attitude, and very nature; Gina Diaz for her thoroughness and commitment; and Lynn Schmitz for his high-quality efforts in modifying many of the original illustrations and inventing many of the new ones. Further, thanks is expressed to Cheri Annin for her advice and counsel on many formatting and preparation questions. Finally, my profound thanks to Loretta Knutson for her encouragement and support in pursuit of excellence and truth in all that we do.

Contents

1

Principles Applied to Movement

The study of kinesiology and pathological motion necessarily begins with an understanding of the terms and units used to describe motion and the forces producing or resulting from motion. While these topics are not particularly interesting or enjoyable to study, appropriate use of the fundamentals and accurate use of terminology is basic to the study of human function. Also essential is an overview of factors that influence motion. The reader then should be able to relate these factors to an understanding of normal and abnormal movement. This chapter focuses on an overview of the factors most pertinent to the description of motion, factors that will be referred to and elaborated on in later chapters, primarily those discussing the individual joints.

TERMINOLOGY
Systems and Units

While there is a great amount of information directly related to kinesiology and the description of pathological motion, most of the literature does not use consistent units or terminology. Therefore, the student of normal and pathologic motion must have a working understanding of the meaning of the fundamental units as well as the ability to convert various measurement systems. Without this level of comprehension, a student or practitioner will have difficulty reading and effectively comparing results presented in relevant journals.

The **International System of Units**, known as SI, has become widely preferred. The SI, a modern version of MKSA (metre, kilogram, second, ampere), is based on seven fundamental units that by convention are regarded as dimensionally independent. Of most importance to the study of movement are length (metre), mass (kilogram), and time (second) because they are base units in the system (Fig. 1.1) (20). From these units other quantities are derived. Note that with few exceptions, such as joules/sec for power, the units are all derived from the base units. The following systems of measurement are in use but are to be avoided:

English absolute (foot, pound mass, second, and poundal)
Metric gravitational (metre, metric slug, second, kilogram-force)
English gravitational (foot, slug, second, pound force)

Note that the principal departure of SI from the gravimetric system of metric engineering units is the use of explicitly distinct units for mass and force. In SI, the name kilogram is restricted to the unit of mass. The kilogram-force, from which the suffix *-force* was in practice often erroneously dropped, should not be used. In its place is the SI unit of force, the **newton** (N), which is defined as the force when applied to a mass of 1 kilogram gives it an acceleration of one meter/s² ($1 kgm/s^2$). Likewise, the newton rather than the kilogram-force is used to form derived units

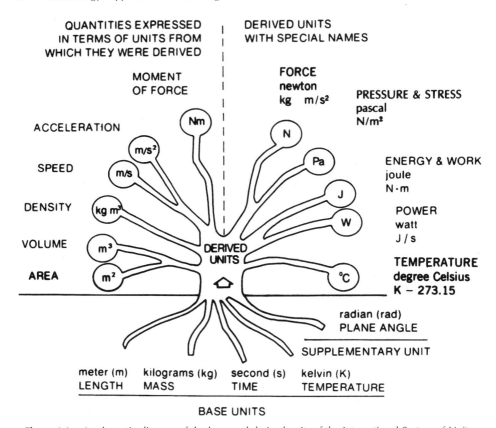

Figure 1.1. A schematic diagram of the base and derived units of the International System of Units.

that include force. For example, pressure or stress (N/m² = pascals), energy and work (N × m = joules), and power (N × m/s = watts) are all commonly used (26).

Considerable confusion exists from use of the term *weight* as a quantity to mean either force or mass. In commercial and everyday use, the term *weight* often means *mass*. Thus, when one speaks of a person's weight, the quantity often referred to is mass. This technically incorrect use of the term *weight* in everyday life will probably persist. In science and technology, the term weight of a body means the force that, if applied to the body, would give it an acceleration equal to the local acceleration of a free falling body. The adjective *local* in the phrase *local acceleration of a freely falling body* refers to that particular location on the surface of the earth. In this context the local acceleration of gravity is designated by the symbol g, with observed values of g differing by over .5% at various points on the earth's surface. The use of *gravity force* (mass × acceleration of gravity) is recommended instead of weight with this meaning. Because of the dual use of the term *weight* as a quantity, this term should be avoided in technical practice except under circumstances in which its meaning is completely clear. When the term is used, it is important to know whether mass or force is intended. Preferably, use SI units such as kilograms for mass or newtons for force (2, 3).

The use of the same name for units of force and mass causes confusion. When the non-SI units are used, a distinction should be made between force and mass: for example, lbf to denote force in gravimetric engineering units and lbm for mass (3). Table 1.1 gives conversion factors for entities specified in the presently used inch-pound system and the new SI system proposed for use in the United States. To obtain the measurement unit when the SI unit is given, multiply the SI quantity by the numerator factor X. Use the denominator factor Y as the multiplier to convert from the right hand column to the SI system. The latter is much preferred (25).

An example of using conversions occurs if one uses the foot-pound output of an isokinetic dynamometer, a device frequently used in clinical settings. Assume that the patient generates 80 ft lbf (same as foot-pounds) of torque during isometric knee

Table 1.1. Conversions

Entity	SI	→X→ ←Y←	Misc. Units
Acceleration	m/sec^2	3.2808 0.3048	ft/sec^2
Angle	rad	57.296 0.0175	degree
Area	m^2	10.763 0.0929	ft^2
	m^2	1550.0 0.000645	inch^2
Density	kg/m^3	0.0624 16.018	lbm/ft^3
	kg/m^3	0.0000361 27680.	lbm/inch^3
Energy, work	N·m = J^a	0.7376 1.3558	ft lbf
Force	N	0.2248 4.4482	lbf
	N	$\frac{X}{9.81}$	kgf
Length	m	3.2808 0.3048	ft
	m	39.370 0.0254	inch
Mass	kg	2.2046 0.4536	lbm
Mass moment of inertia	kg m^2	23.730 0.0421	lbm ft^2
Moment, torque	Nm	0.7376 1.3558	lbf ft
	Nm	$\frac{X}{9.81}$	kgf m
Pressure, stress	N/m^2 = Pa^a	$\frac{X}{98,066}$	kgf/cm^2
	N/m^2 = Pa^a	0.000145 6895.6	lbf/inch^2
Stiffness	N/m	5.667 0.177	lbf/inch
Velocity	m/sec	3.2808 0.3048	ft/sec
Volume	m^3	35.313 0.0283	ft^3
	m^3	61023. 0.0000164	inch^3

[a] Official recommended units of SI.

extension. To convert to SI multiply by 1.3558 (see Table 1.1). The Nm of torque should equal 108.46. Other conversion tables exist and the student or practitioner should either select one or generate commonly used measures that are most consistent with his or her needs (11, 25).

In addition to the entities described and quantified above, there are other terms to which a specific meaning is attached. Each is basic to understanding kinesiology and each will be used later in this volume. The discussion that ensues presents the most important and useful concepts. A complete list of terms can be found in White and Panjabi (25).

Reference Frames

In order to adequately describe motion, a reference frame is required. This reference frame, often arbitrarily located, is used so that displacement data adequately represent the motion or motions occurring. Often, human motion is described relative to the location of the body in a given room or location. Clinically, however, therapists will register motion with respect to the perceived axis of a given joint or from the anatomical position in standing. Although these techniques are prone to inaccuracies, these clinical methods are not likely to be significantly altered.

Degrees of Freedom

Degrees of freedom are the number of independent coordinates (usually x, y, and z) in a system that are necessary to accurately specify the position of an object in space. For example, a pure hinge joint would have one degree of freedom because only one coordinate exists around which motion will take place. Anatomical joints are said to have one to three degrees of freedom, depending on the structure. However, later in this volume we will argue that all joints have six degrees of freedom because of how the bones move relative to one another.

Kinematics and Kinetics

Kinematics is the description of motion without regard to the forces. Systems commonly in use include filming techniques and goniometry, i.e., any method that collects displacement data. Kinetics is the study of force or forces applied to the body. These forces can be internally generated forces (muscular tensions or restraint forces produced by tensions in ligaments) or external forces (gravity and segmental masses). The application and magnitude of all the forces determines whether motion does or does not take place, forming the basis for isometric and isotonic exercise forms. The forces, of both internal and external generation, produce the resultant effects at joints. It is these joint forces that are often of ultimate interest to the clinician.

Other factors, such as inertia and body segment parameters, are common to the motion of the human body. How these and other quantities influence and interact during motion will be elucidated throughout the remainder of this volume.

REPRESENTATION OF MUSCLE FORCES
Vectors

As you recall from physics, scalar quantities have magnitude only. Temperature is an example. We are more interested in **vector representations** of muscle, however, as tensile forces can be represented by a vector that has magnitude (length), a line of application (in this case the action line of the muscle), a direction, and a point of application. Although vectors will be used to represent displacement, velocity, and accelerations, we are most interested in muscle forces.

Figure 1.2A shows the arrangement of two segments with a muscle attached. In Figure 1.2B the muscle has been replaced with a vector that fulfills the four requirements in the definition provided in the previous paragraph. In this simple hinge joint we are interested in how the muscle will control the turning of one segment about the other. For the sake of example, assume that the upper, more vertical segment is fixed to other segments of the body. The lower, more horizontal segment will move in a counter-clockwise direction on the page if enough tension is generated in the muscle to cause movement.

Resolution and Composition

In Figure 1.2C the vector representation has been divided into two components perpendicular to each other. One component will exert a force along the lower segment that will go directly into the joint. The other is perpendicular to the segment and is the component that is responsible for the turning of the lower segment on the upper segment during a muscle contraction. What has been done is to resolve the force in the muscle into two components, a rotary (or turning) and a stabilizing (or joint compressive) force. Further, if the joint configuration is altered, as in Figure 1.2D, the effect is different. Note that a rotary component remains, but that the other force has a distractive (or destabilizing) effect. The result is that as a joint goes through a range of motion the effect of the muscle on the joint and the magnitude of turning effect will change continuously. To picture the effects sketch a simple segment, in many positions, similar to the one shown. Then add the rotatory and stabilizing or

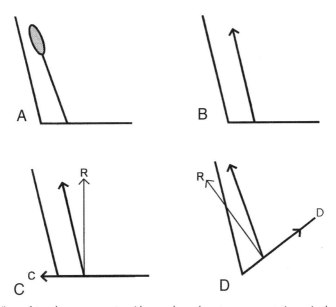

Figure 1.2.   View of two bone segments with muscle and vector representations. **A**, the segment with the muscle in situ. **B**, the muscle replaced with a vector representation for the force that can be generated in the muscle. **C** resolves the muscle force into two components, a rotatory (*R*), and a compressive (*C*). **D**, the joint in a different position, which maintains a rotatory effect (*R*), but changes the compressive component to a distractive (*D*) component.

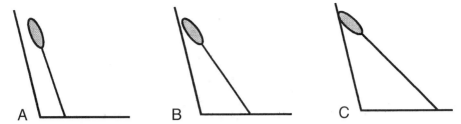

Figure 1.3. Schematic views of two bone segments with muscle attachment sites that vary relative to the joint axis. If the assumption is made that the force in the muscle is the same, the rotation and compressive forces will change from *A* to *C*: the rotation in *A* will be greater than that in *B* and *C*, while the compressive effect in *C* will be greater than in *A* and *B*.

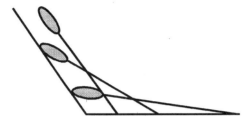

Figure 1.4. Schematic view of three muscles that would have the same actions at a joint. The rotation and compressive components from each of the muscles can be summed.

destabilizing vectors. Make sure that when the vectors are **resolved** into the two components that they are not of such magnitude that they would exceed the force in the muscle. In this example the location of the muscle attachment to the lower segment was kept constant. However, if the attachment is at a different site, as shown in Figure 1.3, the magnitude of the rotary and compressive forces will be different, even though the magnitude of the force in the vector representing the muscle is the same in each case.

The antithesis is the **composition** of forces, again which can be represented as vectors. This is appropriate when more than one muscle contributes to rotation at the joint, such as shown in Figure 1.4. In these situations the vector sums for joint compression and rotation can be computed to attain the effect. Classical methods of solution for composition are the parallelogram and the trigonometric method, discussed later in this chapter.

Torque

The effects of both the rotary and compressive (or distractive) forces are of interest to physical therapists because the effects at the joint are determined by these forces. For example, if a joint is positioned such that all the surrounding muscles are small angles of pull as they contract, the magnitude of the compression (or distraction) may increase markedly because all of the force from the muscle is along the shaft of the bone and into the joint (Fig. 1.5A). Conversely, if the joint is positioned at 90° a muscle may exert only rotation and neither a compression nor distraction effect (Fig. 1.5B). This rotation effect is known as **torque** (or **moment**), defined as the magnitude of the force multiplied by the perpendicular distance to the axis of rotation ($\mathbf{M} = \mathbf{F} \times \mathbf{d}$). In Figure 1.5B the moment would be equal to the force in the muscle times the distance (d) from the muscle attachment site to the joint axis around which the one segment is moving. As both a force and a distance are included, the measurement is in newton-meters. Often, however, units will be in pound-feet, but as noted above a pound and a kilogram is a mass, not a force. Thus, if pound is used, it should be specified as a force. Often this will need to be an assumption. Conversion factors are provided in Table 1.1.

The moment or torque is described as positive or negative, clockwise or counter-clockwise, or by some other convention. Any are acceptable, as long as the user clearly, operationally defines the usage. From the definition and the diagrams one can appreciate that the rotation, or torque, can be increased by (a) altering the angle of attachment of the muscle to the bone, or by (b) altering the amount of tension available in the muscle or muscles responsible. Altering the angle of attachment may be done in certain surgical procedures. The therapist can create an effect by position-ing the joint so that the angle of muscle attachment is at 90°. However, in virtually all situations, multiple muscles are responsible for the production of the joint moment; thus, the joint position becomes specific to the muscle of interest. In actuality, while joint torque curves are specific to the circumstances, some general configurations are shown in Figure 1.6.

The use of moment or torque is very important for a number of reasons. Use of these principles essentially replaces the applications of levers. While examples of the three classes of levers can be found in the human body to explain movements, the type of lever is irrelevant since the matter of importance is the resultant moment at the joint of interest. The net effect is the sum of the moments produced, not because some are first, second, or third class levers.

The use of torques also allows for comparison across conditions or multiple examin-ers. Consider the assessment of "strength" by means of conventional manual muscle testing. To perform a test the patient may be asked to hold a segment in a certain

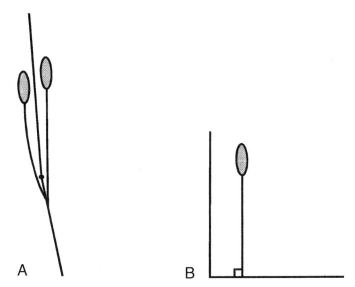

Figure 1.5. Schematic view of two bone segments with muscles attached on opposite sides of the distal segment. **A,** the compressive forces will be high if both muscles contract simultaneously. In **B** there is neither a compressive nor distractive force at the joint.

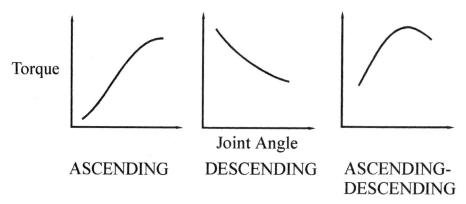

Torque

Joint Angle

ASCENDING   DESCENDING   ASCENDING-
                                        DESCENDING

Figure 1.6.   Torque curves as the joint angle changes are dependent on a number of factors.

position while the therapist provides a resistance. In this situation the internal moment generated by the patient is being matched by the therapist producing a resistive moment of equal intensity. If another therapist were to assess "strength" by resisting this patient at a different location on the extremity, the result may be different than the initial assessment because the resistive requirements were different during the two tests. If, in both of the cases of measurement, the force was monitored and the distance at which the measurement was recorded, a moment could be calculated for purposes of comparison. Another practical issue is how the therapist chooses to apply resistive loads for muscle testing. Applying resistance at the distal portion of the segment is done because less resistance is required by the therapist. The patient also perceives less force at the interface of the therapist's hand with the patient's body part.

Couples

Muscles may also be configured to act in synergy (together) to carry out a function or motion. Two muscles may form what is known as a force couple, defined as two parallel forces equal in magnitude but opposite in direction. When these forces are aligned on opposite sides of a joint axis the result will be an effective turning of the segment. Figure 1.7 shows the pelvis during the typical relaxed standing posture, the abdominal and gluteal muscles depicted by force vectors. As the person simultaneously contracts these two muscle groups the pelvis is rotated posteriorly. Later chapters will discuss other examples of this phenomenon as it occurs in each of the joints.

Contraction Types

The amount of tension generated in muscle will vary for a number of reasons, including intensity of activation and type of muscle contraction performed. How the magnitudes of these muscle tensions vary will be discussed in subsequent chapters. Before they are presented it is important to agree on terminology; however, definitions have not been commonly accepted. The student or clinician must use this as an observandum against indiscriminate use because the same term may be interpreted differently.

The most consistently used term is **isometric**. In this contraction type, constant muscle length is implied because segments remain fixed. However, since there is considerable shortening at the protein filament level in any condition of tension generation, no contraction appears to satisfy isometric conditions (9).

Isotonic contractions, literally translated as same tension or force, are typically broken down into two subcategories. O'Connel and Gowitzke (21) use these definitions:

> **isotonic**—sometimes called concentric or shortening contraction; a muscle contraction in which the internal force produced by the muscle exceeds the external force of the resistance, the muscle shortens and movement is produced.
>
> **eccentric**—a muscle contraction, in an already shortened muscle, to which an external force greater than the internal force is added and the muscle lengthens while continuing to maintain tension.

Bouisset provides another set of definitions (5):

> **isometric**—external resistance is equal to the internal force developed by the muscle and there is no external movement.

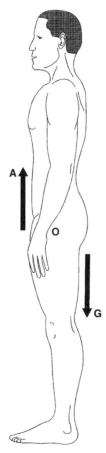

Figure 1.7.   Subject standing demonstrates the action of a force couple when contracting the abdominal (*A*) and gluteus maximus (*G*) muscles to move the pelvis into posterior tilt. The axis of rotation is marked with *o*.

isotonic—a muscle contraction when the external force is constant.
anisotonic—a contraction during periods of increasing or decreasing external force.
anisometric—a muscle contraction resulting when external resistance is smaller or greater than the internal muscle force—if smaller, muscle shortens (concentric or positive work); if greater, muscle lengthens (eccentric or negative work).

It is readily recognized that there are some commonalities in definitions. Although Bouisset's (5) definitions may make more sense, the most frequently used terms are isotonic or concentric, eccentric and isometric. Usually, concentric and eccentric contractions are both considered forms of isotonic exercise.

More recently, **isokinetic** contractions have become a popular exercise mode. A literal interpretation of the term isokinetic means constant or same force. In actuality these electromechanical or hydraulic systems enable exercise through a range of motion at a constant angular velocity. However, patients and/or normal subjects will typically not have the constant force output implied in the definition. In reality the device allows individuals to perform at constant velocity, thus making constant force a possibility but not a requirement. In fact, as will be described in subsequent chapters, changes in the forces and resulting torques may be indicative of pathology. Finally, although concentric and eccentric forms of isokinetic exercise may be performed clinically, the latter is limited by loading requirements and concerns for patient safety in terms of the ability to control load.

Functional Roles

Muscle function frequently will be classified by its functional role in movement. Such classification systems are frequently arbitrary, exclusionary, and less than meaningful. What is important is to have a working knowledge of the various terminology that is used both clinically and in the literature. By understanding the most frequently used terms one can then adopt operational definitions so that a specific meaning is attached to the use of the word or phrase.

When a muscle is labeled as a **prime mover**, the intention is that the muscle is the single most important force creating a particular torque. An **assistant mover** is a servile muscle or one that can aid the prime mover to act as an "emergency" muscle either when great force is required or when paralysis has occurred. An **agonist** simply means a muscle that performs a similar action while an antagonist means a muscle that has an opposite action. For example, the biceps brachii and brachialis muscles are agonists while the triceps brachii muscle is their antagonist. A **stabilizer** is classically considered a muscle that will steady or support so that another muscle may act effectively. Wrist extensors commonly perform this function for the hand. This contraction is generally an isometric one. Finally, a muscle can assume the role of a **synergist**. In this case the muscle will control or neutralize undesired actions produced by other active muscles. Earlier editions of Brunnstrom's text further defined two categories of synergists (15). The helping synergist is two muscles with a common joint action but each with an action antagonistic to each other. The anterior gluteus medius muscle internal rotation and abduction function compared to the posterior gluteus medius muscle external rotation and abduction function provides a useful example. Pure or true synergy is identified as the condition when a muscle that contracts statically to prevent an action in one of the joints traversed by two or more joint muscles. An example at the hand and wrist can be used. To make an effective closure of the fingers, long flexors originating in the forearm will be active. Because during the grasp there would be a tendency for the wrist to flex, the wrist extensors become active for purposes of maintaining the wrist in a neutral position. Thus, the extensors have neutralized the tendency for flexion.

The student should note that there are many other classification systems and terms available; for example, postural, impulse, slow or rapid tension, ballistic and cocontraction. In addition, the terms fast, slow, and intermediate are assuming a more precise definition and role in considerations applied to human movement. None of the classification systems enjoys any advantages over the others, and they should be considered only as descriptors of the functional ability or capability of muscle.

While the locations of the attachment sites are considered important to function, the reader should be reminded that in human function the sites identified by anatomists as the origin and insertion are frequently reversed. In general this would happen when the distal part of the extremity is fixed. Specifically, when rising from a chair or during gait the foot is fixed and the more proximal segments of the leg move about the foot. Thus the "origin" is the part attached to the moving segment, contrary to the usual definition. Similar events occur commonly during walking in that the foot is fixed and the proximal portion of the extremity moves over the foot-floor interface. Other examples occur in the upper extremity when the hand is fixed to an object. This fixation of the distal portion of the extremity is now commonly known as closing the kinetic chain, and thus the use of the term encountered in exercise, the closed kinetic chain. Thus, therapists are advised to attend to the attachment sites relative to the motion being performed rather than to a known but arbitrary definition of origin and insertion.

MacConaill, in 1949, proposed that muscles be labeled as **spurt** or **shunt** depending on the characteristics of the muscle location (17). For example, muscles that insert most distal in relationship to the joint on which they act tend to compress the joint rather than produce a turning effect (Fig. 1.8). Therefore, this muscle would be labeled as a shunt muscle since most of the generated tension is shunted into the joint. The most commonly cited example is the brachioradialis muscle. Another good example is the coracobrachialis muscle because glenohumeral joint compression tends to occur instead of flexion. Conversely, muscles such as the biceps, with a great turning or moment effect, would be identified as spurt muscles. In this case attachments are close to the joint axis around which motion is occurring. Others have criticized the spurt and shunt classification system on the basis of mechanical principles (11). They point out that if in fact a muscle would be considered a shunt muscle according to MacConaill's criteria, the muscle would have the opposite function if considered to act on the proximal rather than the distal segment. Consider,

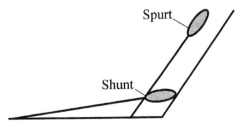

Figure 1.8. Schematic view of two bone segments with a spurt and a shunt muscle.

for example, the brachioradialis muscle. In the case where the hand and wrist were fixed and the upper arm allowed to move, the muscle would be a spurt muscle (elbow flexion) rather than a shunt muscle. So, in the common case where muscles act on the proximal segments (i.e., reverse functions) the muscle also changes classification as having a spurt or shunt function.

When considering human motion, which usually occurs three dimensionally, there are two useful laws that have been cited by MacConaill (18). The first, the **law of approximation**, states that when a muscle contracts the muscle tends to bring its attachments together. This is a straightforward concept, but the point can again be made that the standard anatomy textbook identification of muscle origin or insertion should not be used.

The second law is known as the **law of detorsion**. This law states that when a muscle contracts the tendency will be to bring the origin and insertion into one and the same plane. This law, demonstrated in Figure 1.9, particularly applies to muscles that are twisted prior to contraction. Examples include the sternocleidomastoid, the hip adductors, and pectoralis major. This law is important because it stresses that motion is three dimensional and that origin and insertion will in effect be brought into one and the same plane.

Other terms that are encountered are active and passive insufficiency. In **active insufficiency** the patient is not able to generate tension in the muscle because the muscle is too short. A specific explanation will be offered when the length-tension relationship is discussed in the next chapter. To demonstrate, stand so that only your right anterior thigh is against the corner of a table. Weight bear on the left leg and actively bend the right knee, bringing the heel towards the buttock. When you have reached the maximum approximation reach back with your right hand, grasp the foot and pull the foot closer to the buttock. That the knee flexors are not able to achieve this range of motion is active insufficiency. **Passive insufficiency** is a decrease in the range of motion due to lack of extensibility of the muscles or muscle groups that are antagonistic to the motions being performed. The most commonly used

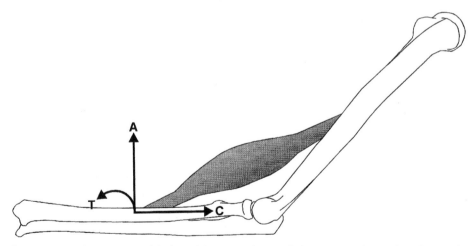

Figure 1.9. A schematic view of the law of detorsion. The muscle force vector, shown along the muscle, will tend to generate force into the joint (c) as well as create a moment (A). If the muscle attachment on the mobile segment is broad or not located in the midline of the segment a twisting (T) effect will also occur or tend to occur, depending on the degrees of freedom in the joint.

example is "hamstring tightness" tested via the straight leg raise (hip flexion and knee extension). The range of motion is inhibited by the hamstring muscles, which when they contract are responsible for the motions of hip extension and knee flexion. Other examples will be presented in subsequent chapters on each of the joints.

Some have used tissue constituency to enhance tension output. **Stretch-shortening** contractions are an example in that a movement that causes a lengthening contraction precedes a shortening or concentric contraction. In effect the lengthening of the musculotendinous unit stretches the elastic element in muscle. The energy is stored until the unit is released during motion in the opposite direction produced by an accompanying concentric contraction. This contraction allows the stored elastic energy to be recovered and contributes to the shortening contraction (8, 13). Variables that determine the magnitude of the effect are the degree of joint motion and the velocity of the stretch imposed. This preload has been produced in certain activities, for example in the squat jump (10). Applications of these principles in physical therapy practice may be more limited to the later stages of rehabilitation because of the dependence on velocity of stretch. Many patients will not be able to tolerate high velocity movements due to capability of the tissues or because of potentially injurious effects.

In summary, there are multiple factors that influence muscle function. Figure 1.10 demonstrates the interactive environment in which the musculotendinous unit functions. Some factors have now been discussed. The remainder will be covered in subsequent sections.

SYSTEMS AND THE APPLICATION OF FORCES
General Configurations and Operation

In human motion the turning effect at the joint will be the result of the sum of the moments produced by the variety of forces and their point of attachment. Figure 1.11 shows one muscle force represented by F, the weight of the forearm and hand G, and the weight of the mass held in the hand, W. The force in the muscle (F) would be multiplied by the distance a since this is the appropriate perpendicular distance to the axis O. Likewise b would be used for G and c would be used for W. The sum of these three respective moments would be represented in an equation by $(F)(a) - (G)(b) - (W)(c) = 0$. In such an equation if the sum of the three terms were zero, static equilibrium would be demonstrated. If not equal to zero the segment would rotate according to the direction of the greatest moment application. In the case shown in Figure 1.11 the mass of the weight in the hand (W) and the weight of the forearm and hand (G) produce the tendency for a clockwise moment while the muscle force F produces the opposite effect. Note that positive and negative signs are given to the respective terms. Thus, the direction that the arm will turn depends on the magnitudes of the forces and their respective distances from O. These moments may be called an **external or resistive moment** that is opposed or controlled by the **internal or muscular moment**.

A simple configuration for a single plane motion is shown as an example in Figure 1.12. Rarely, if ever, are forces applied to the segment perpendicularly. This is particularly true of muscle insertions. In cases where the forces are applied at an angle other than 90°, trigonometric functions can be used to calculate the component of the force that will have a turning effect. Consider Figure 1.12 to analyze the effect of the application of the muscle force at an angle of insertion of 45°. Clearly not all

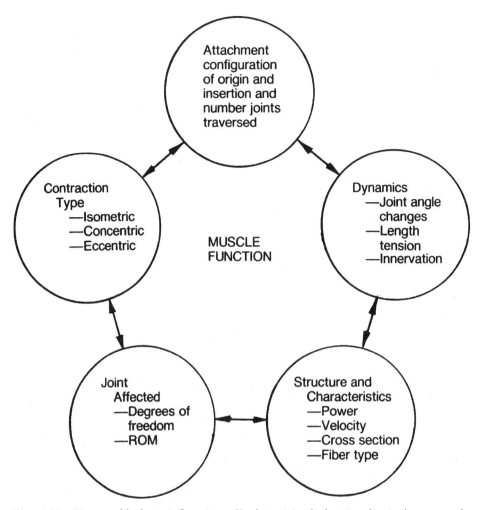

Figure 1.10.   Diagram of the factors influencing and/or determining the function of in vivo human muscle.

of the tensile force generated in muscle can have a rotation (R) effect. Rather, significant force is shunted (S) into the joint itself. The magnitude of the force that will have a turning effect will vary with the magnitude of the trigonometric function associated with the angle of insertion of the muscle producing the moment. This example and Table 1.2 provide an index of the magnitude of the effect of the change in angle of insertion. Specifically, in this example, only .7071 of the force in the tendon will have a turning effect on the mobile segment. Further discussion of this factor is provided in the next chapter; a review of trigonometry and a complete table of functions is found in Appendix A.

For a practical example of a situation that uses moments assume the configuration in Figure 1.13. A therapist pushing against the patient's arm with a force F_1 will tend to move the patient sideways but will not cause rotation about the glenohumeral joint (S) since the line of force passes through S. A weight F_2, held in the hand, however, would produce a clockwise moment equal to $F_2 \times d$ (Fig. 1.13A). Now, after removing the weight, if the therapist exerts an upward force F_3 at an angle A with the vertical (Fig. 1.13B), it will create a counterclockwise moment equal to $F_3 \times d$ or $F_3 \times cosine \, A \times D$ (i.e., the component of the force through H perpendicular to S). Either solution, $F_3 \times d$ or $F_3 \, cosine \, A \times D$, yields the same answer. In the former method the force F_3 remained the same and the distance was modified. In the latter, note two things. One, that D remained constant but the force was modified, and two, that the other component of F_3, ($F_3 \, sine \, A$) has no moment about S because

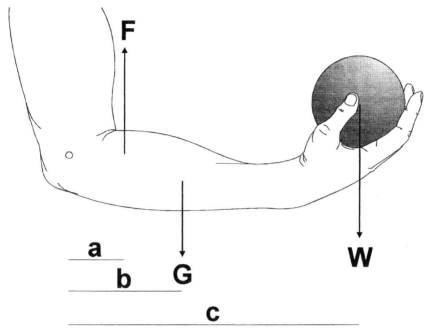

Figure 1.11.   A lateral view of the arm with a mass held in the hand. *F* is muscle force, *G* is the weight of the forearm and hand, and *W* is the weight of the mass held in the hand. The letters *a*, *b*, and *c* represent the perpendicular distance to the axis *O*.

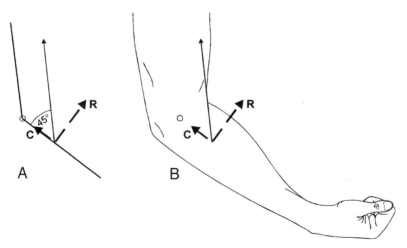

Figure 1.12.   Diagrammatic mechanical (**A**) and anatomical (**B**) representation of two body segments with a musculotendinous unit spanning a joint with a specified axis of rotation (*O*). Muscle force is shown with the solid vector. The respective force into the joint (*C*) and the rotary effect (*R*) are shown as dashed vectors.

Table 1.2.   Angle of Insertion—Trigonometric Functions

Degrees	Cosine Function
10	0.9848
20	0.9397
30	0.8660
40	0.7660
45	0.7071

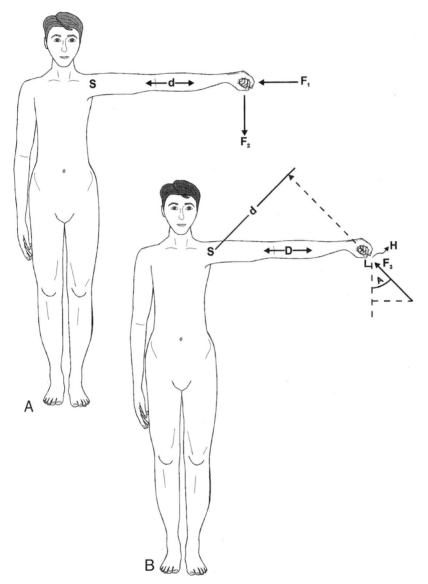

Figure 1.13.   Diagrammatic representation of the effect of forces on the glenohumeral joint (*S*).

$F_3 \times$ sine A $\times$ 0 = 0. While the moment of a force can be represented by the sum of the moments of its two components, in application to practice what is of concern is the magnitude of the turning, or moment, at the joint.

Each of the examples provided thus far have been systems that are predominantly coplanar. For thorough analyses, however, there are usually coplanar force systems that require three dimensional solutions. As a result, an understanding of the fundamentals of vector algebra is required. For those interested an overview of the topic is presented in Appendix B. Further discussion and applications of the topic, considered outside of the scope of this volume, can be found in Miller and Nelson (19) and Winter (26).

In analyzing various exercises and assessing their relative difficulty, the clinician should consider the point of rotation; the proportion of the body weight being supported, raised, or lowered; and whether or not there are any external resistances. In addition, it is necessary to consider what muscles are acting to produce the desired movement. More sophisticated analyses include the moments created by the nonmuscular forces (such as ligaments or other tissues that may be under tension) about the point of rotation. No matter the movement or whether it is planar or multiplanar, the muscles must create appropriate moments of force to produce the desired movements.

FRICTION

The role of frictional force in kinesiological problems or in clinical practice is frequently ignored. However, in many instances the presence or lack of friction will determine the degree of success of the applied therapy. In gait, for example, friction is necessary between the foot and the supporting surface so that force can be transmitted up the leg in contact with the floor. The same is true for patients using crutches. Witness how the use of extremely worn crutch tips invites a potentially disastrous slipping of the crutch on the floor. Exercise equipment also has frictional characteristics, whether they be in pulley devices or in the mechanical bearings of resistive equipment. Friction during administration of traction, usually considered as negligible, may be considerable. Further, frictions within the body are important to normal function. Primary examples are increased friction associated with degenerative joint diseases or in cases of inflammatory conditions of tendons such as tenosynovitis.

Other examples are available from a study of joint motion. Because the bony surfaces are bathed in a fluid medium, friction between the surfaces is minimized. Further discussion of this factor will follow in Chapter 4. In addition, muscles contain fluids. Thus, in treatment, consideration must be given to the influence of high and low loads and the impact of velocity, particularly when viscosity of the fluid affects the friction present in joints. Other types of friction include dry, rolling, and internal friction.

Coefficient of Friction

Friction is described by means of a **coefficient of friction**. This coefficient is a ratio of forces, the force required for motion divided by the compressive (normal) force between the two bodies. The coefficient of friction is unitless because it is the ratio of two forces. Consider the situation in Figure 1.14 where an object rests on a surface. In this free body diagram the N or normal force is equal to the load of 100 newtons. Now, if a push (P) of 5 newtons is applied to the load, a force parallel to the surface

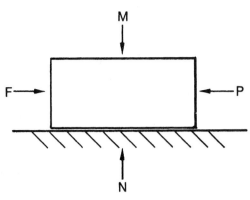

Figure 1.14. A mass (*M*) resting on a surface. *N* represents the normal force, *P* a pushing force, and *F* the frictional force.

is developed that is called F, the frictional force. This value may be any value up to a maximum value, and, based on Fmax = u N, will depend upon u and the normal force. u, as known from practical experiences, depends upon the materials of the surfaces of the two objects as well as the degree of lubrication. For example, certainly two surfaces of sandpaper provide greater friction than two teflon surfaces, given the same amount of compression between the two surfaces and the same pushing force. Returning to our example, assume that we push harder, so that 50 newtons of force are required to start the object moving. Substitution into the equation yields 50 = u 100. Division shows that the coefficient of friction is .5. Conversely, if u is known and N is known the force needed to move the object can be calculated by simple multiplication. Note that the area of the surface is not a factor in considering the friction. Further, if frictional force is plotted against the pushing force we note that the static friction will always be greater than the kinetic friction. In other words getting the object in motion will be more difficult than keeping the object in motion (19).

Clinical Relevance

Seldom will clinicians need to calculate the specific u or be concerned with the amount of force required to produce motion. However, if a patient of large mass is supine on a table during pelvic traction the therapist must be cognizant that the force required to produce distraction is dependent on the mass (normal force) and the coefficient of friction.

Brand states that the coefficient of friction in joints is in the range of .005 to .01. Such a finding is interesting when considered in view of u values of .05 in mechanical systems (4). Even skating on ice lubricated by water produces a u of only .03. Walker has produced a table of values that shows coefficients that range from .142 to .163 for cobalt-chrome hip replacements sliding on themselves for different lubricants and different concentrations of albumin, globulin, and hyaluronic acid (24). That joint lubrication is superior to man-made systems points out the effectiveness of the human body in controlling factors critical to efficient performance. More specific discussion of lubrication in joints is included in Chapter 4 on articular mechanics and function.

FREE BODY DIAGRAMS

In many instances analytic or descriptive approaches will be based upon forces applied to a given body or segment of a body. An accurate representation of all the forces is called a **free body diagram** because an artificial boundary or limit of any structure or segment can be made at any location, depending on the problem that needs to be solved. In actuality the correct placement of the external forces acting on the body is essential for the correct interpretation or solution of any system on which forces are acting. The forces are represented by vectors and typically include muscle forces, gravity, friction, wind resistance, ground reaction forces, and fluid forces. They are graphically represented by the magnitude, direction, and angle at which the force is applied. Therefore a correct quantitative graphical solution to the problem or configuration is implied (Fig. 1.15). Identification or use of incorrect free body diagrams result primarily from lack of inclusion of all the forces or from adding unnecessary forces. Application of the principles of free body diagrams will be stressed in several of the chapters on joints.

BODY SEGMENT PARAMETERS

In the process of analyzing normal and abnormal human motion, there are various measures that are pertinent when motion is quantified. Length, mass, volume, density, center of mass, and moment of inertia are known as body segment parameters because they provide the data needed in kinematic analyses and in formulae required to complete kinetic analyses. Practically, these data have been used in comprehensive analyses of pathological motion, in the design of industrial tools and seating devices, and for development of prostheses. In actuality, little work has been completed

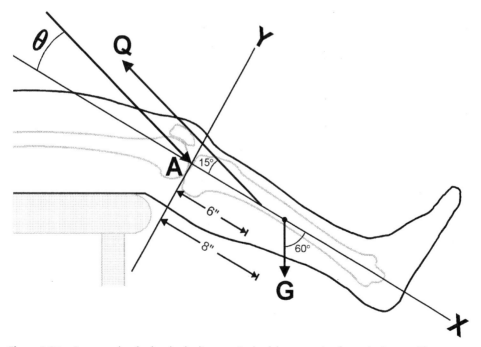

Figure 1.15.   An example of a free body diagram. Each of the respective forces is shown with a vector.

on body segment parameters because the work is tedious and difficult. Accurate techniques are probably available but frequently the expense or degree of complexity prevents the completion of comprehensive studies. The texts of Miller and Nelson (19) and Winter (26) provide discussions of these parameters. Williams and Lissner also thoroughly discuss their importance (16). Most will use data from the work of Dempster (7). The following material will provide an overview of the parameters and stress their importance in the study of kinesiology and pathokinesiology.

Segment **length**, or link, data are important from the standpoint of allowing the determination of end points for each body part. Identification of these points, usually at specific anatomical landmarks, enables the definition of segment displacement, yielding the ultimate data of interest, the velocities and accelerations. Although identification of specific landmarks are difficult to accurately reproduce, these methods appear to produce reliable data.

Mass, defined as weight/gravity, is a function of two other parameters, the volume and the **density** of a particular segment. Keeping in mind the earlier discussion under the terminology section of this chapter, the concept becomes important because mass is distributed differently in each segment of the body. Further, each body segment, or link, has a specific mass and location of the center of mass (the location where mass is centered). Table 1.3 provides a compilation of the percentages of weights for each of the segments of the body (26).

Table 1.3. Anthropometric Data

Segment	Definition	Seg Weight/ Tot Body wt[a]	Center of Mass Segment Length[a]		Radius of Gyration/ Segment Length[a]			Density
			Proximal	Distal	C of G	Proximal	Distal	
Hand	Wrist axis/knuckle II middle finger	0.006	0.506	0.494	0.297	0.587	0.577	1.16
Forearm	Elbow axis/ulnar styloid	0.016	0.430	0.570	0.303	0.526	0.647	1.13
Upper arm	Glenohumeral axis/ elbow axis	0.028	0.436	0.564	0.322	0.542	0.645	1.07
Total arm	Glenohumeral joint/ ulnar styloid	0.050	0.530	0.470	0.368	0.645	0.596	1.11
Foot	Lateral malleolus/ head metatarsal II	0.0145	0.50	0.50	0.475	0.690	0.690	1.10
Shank	Femoral condyles/ medial malleolus	0.0465	0.433	0.567	0.302	0.528	0.643	1.09
Thigh	Greater trochanter/ femoral condyles	0.100	0.433	0.567	0.323	0.540	0.653	1.05
Total leg	Greater trochanter/ medial malleolus	0.161	0.447	0.553	0.326	0.560	0.650	1.06
Head and neck	C7-T1 and 1st rib/ ear canal	0.081	1.000		0.495	1.116[b]		1.11
Thorax and abdomen	C7–T1/L4–L5[c]	0.355[b]	0.63	0.37				
Trunk head neck	Greater trochanter/ glenohumeral joint[c]	0.578[b]	0.66	0.34	0.503	0.830	0.607	

[a] Data from Dempster W. *Space Requirements of the Seated Operator.* Washington DC: Office of Technical Services, US Dept of Commerce; 1955. WADC Technical Report 55-159.

[b] Calculations required.

[c] These segments are presented relative to the length between the greater trochanter and the glenohumeral joint.

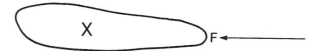

Figure 1.16. An isolated segment with an identified center of mass (*X*). *F* represents the application of a force.

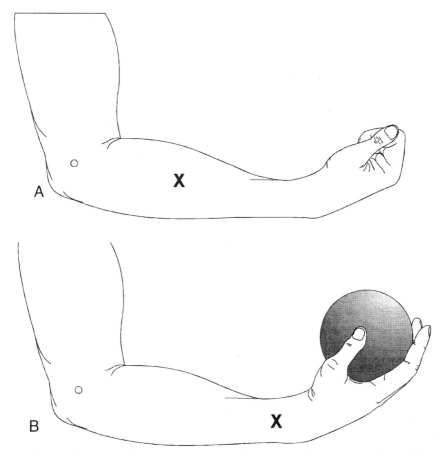

Figure 1.17. **A**, a forearm and hand segment with an axis of rotation *O* and a center of mass *X*. **B**, when a mass (*M*) is added to the hand the mass moment of inertia is larger, making movement more difficult.

Of particular relevance is the location of the **center of mass**, also shown in Table 1.3, of each of the body segments. This is because the location of the center of mass determines the relative ease, or difficulty, with which the segment will turn. Consider the free body diagram in Figure 1.16, an isolated link with an identified center of mass x. If a force (F) is applied such that the force passes through the center of mass, no rotation will occur. Rather the segment would move linearly across the surface of the page. A more realistic view is shown in Figure 1.17. With no load the center of mass will be located more proximal to the axis of rotation (Fig. 1.17A) than in the instance when a 10-pound mass is held in the hand (Fig. 1.17B). Thus, if an attempt is being made to move the arm from this position, more difficulty will be encountered in the latter case because the mass **moment of inertia** is larger. This is due to the fact that both the mass and the distance from the axis of rotation to the center of the mass have increased. Note that this increased mass and the distribution of the mass are both factors because the moment of inertia (I) = mass × the radius of gyration. This "special" average of the distribution of all of the mass particles from the point of rotation (i.e., the radius of gyration) is necessary for the calculation of the mass moment of inertia (I). Additional discussion of this topic will be presented in Chapter 15 on posture and gait.

The factors of volume and density, mentioned as constituents of mass, are less important because they are accounted for in the mass quantity. Density is a function of the type of tissue(s) that make up the segment. For example, fat is less dense that muscle. Volume is contingent upon the quantity of the tissue. Differences in body types result from the degree of each tissue present in the individual.

When are body segment parameters important in practice? Actually, they are a factor in every motion that is completed. Segment mass provides a resistive effect when the motion is completed against gravity, as do the masses of any devices to which a patient's body segment may be attached. In some clinical cases, for example in recovering from a surgical procedure, the patient who is obese may have difficulty performing exercises because of the mass of the segment, and/or the inclusion of any additional mass added by the therapist. As another example, while individuals who are unable to completely extend the knee could have disrupted osteokinematics or arthrokinematics, the cause may also be that the resistive effect caused by the body segment is too great for the internal moment to overcome. Finally, when using dynamometers the option of "gravity correction" is available. In this instance the segment mass is determined and accounted for in the software's calculation of the recorded joint torque. Therefore, body segment parameters are most important in cases where patients are weak and/or the segment masses are significant, such as in the case of obesity. In cases of high torque generation the use of these parameters seems less important in clinical practice.

LAWS OF MECHANICS GOVERNING MOTION

To completely analyze human motion in a clinical sense or with sophisticated techniques both kinematics and kinetics are involved. The need for this information results in the necessity to collect information that will describe the motion and the forces producing the motion. Simon et al. has suggested a clinical method to analyze four dimensional motion (22) while Soderberg and Gabel (23) have proposed a method for sagittal plane analysis. More sophisticated approaches have been used in many laboratories, common examples being found in a variety of sources (1, 6).

Displacement, Velocity, and Acceleration

There are several concepts related to kinematics that are important to clarify. Although the basic constituents of the description of motion are the same, the derivation of the quantities differs depending upon whether the motion is angular or linear. Table 1.4 shows the derivation of each of the three quantities and provides the symbol and terminology for each. Therapists will have interest in both. During gait, for example, the patient must move from one location to another and, considering the total body, a displacement per time period would enable the calculation of the patient's velocity. However, individual segment displacements are responsible for

Table 1.4. Displacement, Velocity, and Acceleration

Formulas	Units
Linear	
Displacement d	Meters
Velocity d/t = v	Meters/sec
Acceleration $\dfrac{v_2 - v_1}{t_2 - t_1} = a$	Meters/sec/sec
Angular	
Displacement θ	Radians or degrees
Velocity $\dfrac{\theta}{t} = \omega$	Radians/sec
Acceleration $\dfrac{\omega_2 - \omega_1}{t_2 - t_1} = \alpha$	Degrees/sec/sec

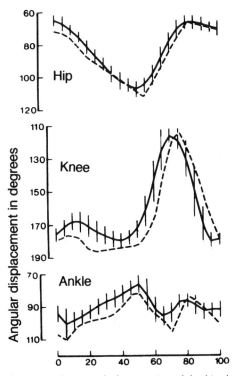

Figure 1.18. Angular displacements for sagittal plane motion of the hip, knee, and ankle for normal subjects (*solid line*) and for patients (*dashed line*) during a gait cycle.

the walking, a graph of which is shown in Figure 1.18. Once the **displacement** and time is known, velocities and accelerations can also be determined (Table 1.4). Note that high quality displacement data are essential because these quantities are also used in the **velocity and acceleration** calculations. Average velocity may also be used by adding the appropriate quantities and dividing by the number of values included in the numerator. Instantaneous linear or angular velocity is calculated by division of the difference of two displacements by the difference in the time interval.

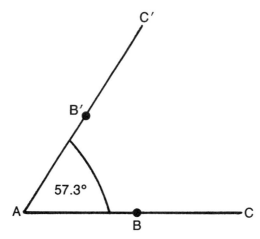

Figure 1.19. Segment *AC* with an intermediate point *B* identified. The segment is then displaced to a new location, indicated by *B'* and *C'*.

The closer that time approximates zero the better the representation of instantaneous velocity.

Use of an example will clarify differences associated with the kinematics of linear and angular motion. Shown in Figure 1.19 is segment AC that has been displaced through one radian, 57.3 degrees, to position AC'. Given that the segment moved through the range in one second the angular velocity would be 57.3 degrees/second. However, the linear velocity of point B to B' on the segment would be considerably different than point C to C'. This can be clearly demonstrated by connecting B to B' and C to C' using a straight line, noting the respective lengths. Because both displacements were completed in the same amount of time due to the fixed location of the points, C would have a greater linear velocity because of the larger displacement. To generalize then, every part of a rigid body has the same angular displacement, velocity, and acceleration but the linear values for any part are a function of the distance from the point of rotation. Maximum angular velocities for human performance are approximately 18 radians/sec, but in most functional activities the value is usually less that 1 radian/sec.

There are a number of specific laws that govern motion. A complete treatise is not intended for incorporation into this volume. However, the fundamentals as applied to movement will be discussed so that some understanding of the limitations and applications presented in later chapters will be more readily understood.

Force, Mass, and Acceleration

Newton's law of F = m × a (force equals mass times acceleration) is of most importance. Applied to linear motion the mass portion is considered to be the segment mass previously described. The acceleration, determined by a number of available kinematic techniques, would be used in producing the appropriate product in newtons of force. However, for angular motion of the segment consider that the torque, or turning effect, results from the product of the moment of inertia and the angular acceleration (T = Iα). In turn, as noted above, moment of inertia is dependent on the product of the mass times the square of the radius of gyration (rho). Therefore, the determining equation becomes moment equals mass times ρ^2 times the angular acceleration $(T = m\rho^2\alpha)$.

Impulse and Momentum

The $F = m \times a$ relationship is also of import in other applications to human motion. Substituting v/t for a yields $F = m \times v/t$. Multiplication of both sides by t produces $F \times t = m \times v$, or the impulse-momentum relationship. The implications will be specifically discussed in later chapters. Similarly, for angular motion $M \times t = I \times \alpha$ (angular acceleration). Note that momentum is dependent on velocity and that inertia always exists, regardless of velocity.

Work, Energy, and Power

Other laws are applied to work, energy, and power. Simply put, the amount of work is the product of the force in the direction of movement times the distance the body supplying the resistance is moved. For angular motion the work is equal to the moment times the angular displacement. Units are, therefore, newton-meters (not to be confused with torque), or the preferred term, joules (Fig. 1.1). When time becomes a consideration power is the preferred quantity. Power is the rate of doing work (force times distance divided by time). The measurement unit is watts. Energy, or the capacity to do work, occurs in many different forms. Of primary interest is mechanical energy, consisting in turn of potential energy or kinetic energy. Potential energy is equal to the product of mass, gravity, and height, yielding a quantity in joules. Kinetic energy is equal to ½ mass $\times$ velocity^2 for linear motion and ½ Iω for angular motion. Since work and kinetic energy calculations produce the same units it can easily be shown that for a given kinetic energy so much work can be done. Clarification of these concepts has been presented by Knuttgen as they apply to exercise science (12). Laird and Rozier have discussed the implications of these mechanical principles as applied to exercise as a modality (14). An in-depth discussion of mechanical work, energy, and power is also presented in Winter (26). Applications of these principles will be included in Chapter 15 on posture and gait.

Statics and Dynamics

Under any given set of circumstances it is possible for any given link or system of links to be stationary (static) or in motion (dynamics). Equations governing the system are equilibrium equations that will determine whether or not the system is in equilibrium or undergoing motion. Williams and Lissner thoroughly develop the rationale for these equations and apply them to a number of situations applicable to therapeutics (16).

Solution of Problems

In practical circumstances there is a reasonable protocol to follow in the solution of link segment problems. However, detailed descriptions of the necessary procedures are beyond the scope of this volume. In brief, first complete an accurate free body diagram. Then, kinematic data must be gathered so that velocities and accelerations of the various body parts are available for use in equations of motion. Data on body segment parameters are also necessary for inclusion into equations demanding either mass or the mass moment of inertia. Information on associated kinetics is also required and is usually obtained by a force transducing device. These techniques range in sophistication from the multidimensional force plate to a simple hand held dynamometer. Once all these data are available it would be possible to arrive at the joint reaction forces and the net muscle moments responsible for creating or controlling the motion. Problems analyzing three dimensional motion become elaborate and a true appreciation of the complexities requires study of engineering mechanics and the appropriate mathematics necessary for solution. Those that desire more complete information on this topic are referred to the texts by Miller and Nelson (19) and Winter (26).

SUMMARY

The information in this chapter presents concepts related to the description of human motion. The material is fundamental to the following chapters and thorough understanding is recommended. However, the information presented in this chapter should be used as a reference if review is needed. Each of the concepts presented in this chapter will be reinforced in some subsequent chapter so that specific applications are made to both normal and pathological human motion.

References

1. Allard P, Stokes IAF, Blanchi JP. *Three-Dimensional Analysis of Human Movement*. Champaign, IL: Human Kinetics; 1995.
2. Andrews J. College of Engineering, University of Iowa, personal communication; 1982.
3. *ASTM Standard for Metric Practice (E 380-79)*. Philadelphia: American Society for Testing and Materials; 1980.
4. Brand RA. Joint lubrication. In: Albright JA, Brand RA, eds. *The Scientific Basis of Orthopedics*. New York: Appleton-Century-Crofts; 1987:373–386.
5. Bouisset S. EMG and muscle force in normal motor activities. In: Desmedt JE, ed. *New Developments in Electromyography and Clinical Neurophysiology*. Basel, Switzerland: Karger; 1973;1:547–583.
6. Crowninshield RD, Johnston RC, Andrews JG, et al. A biomechanical investigation of the human hip. *J Biomech*. 1978;11:75–85.
7. Dempster W. *Space Requirements of the Seated Operator*. Washington DC: Office of Technical Services, US Dept of Commerce; 1955. WADC Technical Report 55-159.
8. Enoka RM. *Neuromechanical Basis of Kinesiology*. Champaign, IL: Human Kinetics; 1988.
9. Gordon AM, Huxley AF, Julian FT. The variation in isometric tension with sarcomere length in vertebrate muscle fibers. *J Physiol (Lond)*. 1966;184:170–192.
10. Hubley CL, Wells RP. A work-energy approach to determine individual joint contributions to vertical jump performance. *Eur J Appl Physiol*. 1983;50:247–254.
11. Jackson KM, Joseph J, Wyard SJ. Sequential muscular contraction. *J Biomech*. 1977;10:97–106.
12. Knuttgen HG. Force, work, power, and exercise. *Med Sci Sports Exerc*. 1978;10:227–228.
13. Komi PV, Bosco C. Utilization of stored elastic energy in leg extensor muscles by men and women. *Med Sci Sports Exerc*. 1978;10:261–265.
14. Laird CE, Rozier CK. Toward understanding the terminology of exercise mechanics. *Phys Ther*. 1979;59:287–292.
15. Lehmkuhl LD, Smith LK. *Brunnstrom's Clinical Kinesiology*. 4th ed. Philadelphia: FA Davis; 1983.
16. LeVeau B. *Williams and Lissner's Biomechanics of Human Motion*. 3rd ed. Philadelphia: WB Saunders; 1992.
17. MacConaill MA. The movement of bones and joints. 2. Function of the musculature. *J Bone Joint Surg Br*. 1949;31:100–104.
18. MacConaill MA, Basmajian JV. *Muscles and Movements: A Basis for Human Kinesiology*. New York: Krieger; 1977.
19. Miller DI, Nelson RC. *Biomechanics of Sport*. Philadelphia: Lea & Febiger; 1973.
20. Nordin M, Frankel VH. *Basic Biomechanics of the Musculoskeletal System*. 2nd ed. Philadelphia: Lea & Febiger; 1980.
21. O'Connel AL, Gowitzke B. *Understanding the Scientific Bases of Human Movement*. Baltimore: Williams & Wilkins; 1972.
22. Simon SR, Nuzzo RM, Koskinen MM. A comprehensive clinical system for four dimensional motion analysis. *Bull Hosp Jt Dis*. 1977;38:41–44.

23. Soderberg GL, Gabel R. A light emitting diode system for the analysis of gait: a method and selected clinical examples. *Phys Ther.* 1978;58:426–432.
24. Walker PS. *Human Joints and Their Artificial Replacements.* Springfield, IL: Charles C Thomas; 1977.
25. White AA, Panjabi MM. *Clinical Biomechanics of the Spine.* Philadelphia: JB Lippincott; 1990.
26. Winter DA. *The Biomechanics and Motor Control of Human Movement.* New York: John Wiley & Sons; 1990.

2

Tissue Structure and Function: Normal and Disrupted Muscle Mechanics

Diverse muscular function is required for efficient and effective human motion. This chapter includes discussion of several physiological aspects that allow for a wide range of muscular functions. For example, important relationships in muscle mechanics are the length-tension and force-velocity features. However, force-time characteristics and an understanding of tension resulting from eccentric and concentric contractions are also critical to the topic of muscle mechanics. The second major portion of this chapter deals with the effects of immobilization, exercise, and the response to injury on muscle, connective tissue, collagen, and ligament. An understanding of these effects is important for appropriate clinical practice.

MUSCLE MECHANICS
Muscle Morphology

The obvious purpose of muscle is to contract so as to produce efficient and smooth movement of the body. In general, muscle form has been arranged according to location and specific function. Although muscles have been identified as fusiform and pennate, some have taken triangular, cruciate, spiral, and other forms (50). Muscle varies greatly in length: compare the 30 cm long sartorius to the 1.4 cm long dorsal interossei. Similarly, fiber organization appears to be based on function.

If muscle is considered according to two pure forms, fusiform and pennate, a number of comparisons can be made. **Fusiform** typically means spindle-shaped or spindle-like in form. An example is the sartorius muscle with parallel muscle fibers that extend from the anterior rim of the pelvis to the medial aspect of the knee. **Pennate** means feather shaped; a typical bipennate muscle is the gastrocnemius, while an example of a multipennate muscle would be the deltoid. Fusiform fibers can shorten by 30% of their initial length, achieving a relatively great range of motion. Fusiform muscles have been credited with the ability to contract through three times as great a distance as pennate muscles. In contrast, the configuration of the pennate muscle influences the actual distance through which the muscle can contract. For example, a pennate muscle whose fibers are quite parallel to a central tendon would come close to simulating the shortening ability of the fusiform muscle. Compare this to a pennate muscle whose fibers are more perpendicular to the central tendon; it has a relatively limited ability to shorten and exert tension via the insertional tendon.

Figure 2.1 provides a demonstration by use of the cosine of the angle of attachment (48). Note that as the angle between the central tendon approaches 45° the effective amount of force in the direction of muscle pull would be only 70.71% of the force generated by fiber contraction (see Table 1.2). At 60° the effective force would be

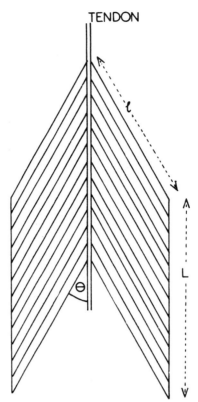

Figure 2.1. A typical arrangement of pennate muscle fibers relative to the central tendon of attachment. *L* is total muscle length and *l* is the length of a single fiber. The force exerted equals $LAx/l \times f$ cosine θ, where *A* is the total cross-sectional area, *f* is the force, and *x* is the number of fibers per unit area measured perpendicularly to the fibers.

only 50% of the tension generated by muscle contraction. Thus the fusiform muscle has been credited with the ability to contract through a great range of motion while the pennate muscle generally shortens a much lesser total distance. The cross-sectional area of the pennate muscle is, however, usually much greater than that of the fusiform fiber. Therefore, muscles of pennate structure have the potential for creating the greatest amount of tension since there is a rather direct relationship between cross-sectional area and muscular tension generated.

There are other differences if the purest form of fiber arrangement remains under consideration. Typically, the fusiform muscles attach at a distance closest to the joint while the pennate muscles have a tendency to attach a greater distance from the axis of rotation of a particular joint. The importance of this will be brought out in subsequent chapters. Before discussing other features of muscle suffice it to say that in general mechanical terms, the fusiform muscle has the capability to lift a lesser load through a greater range of motion, therefore yielding generally less power at perhaps a greater velocity. Conversely, the pennate structure can typically lift a greater load through a lesser range of motion and, therefore, has generally high power capabilities but velocities that are significantly slower than the fusiform structure.

While this morphology is of some significance, it should be pointed out that these considerations have been developed with the purest forms of fiber arrangement. In actuality, muscles in the human are a compromise between the fusiform and the pennate type of structure. According to Alexander (2), the angles of pennation are usually 30° or less. Another piece of investigative work, although done on the cat hind limb, provides supporting data. In this case the angles of pennation were all relatively small, all being less than the medial gastrocnemius angle of 21°. The effect, in terms of the percentage of maximum potential tension and velocity, can be determined by converting the angle of pennation to the cosine of the angle. The effect of the angle of pennation by muscle is seen in Figure 2.2 (37). Because these attachment angles produce cosine function values of .866 (30°) or greater, the result may be that muscle length or cross-sectional area is far more important than angle of pennation in the production of muscle tension.

The effects of **sarcomere arrangement** within muscle can be demonstrated effectively, but we must assume that the two muscles have identical masses and share the same biochemical features (see Chapter 3). Figure 2.3 shows two arrangements that satisfy these criteria. Note first that if each muscle is stimulated the contraction times (Fig. 2.3A) and subsequently the time to reach peak tension (Fig. 2.3B) are the same. However, note that the muscle arranged in series (S) develops only half the tension in the same time interval. Observation of the shortening behavior reveals

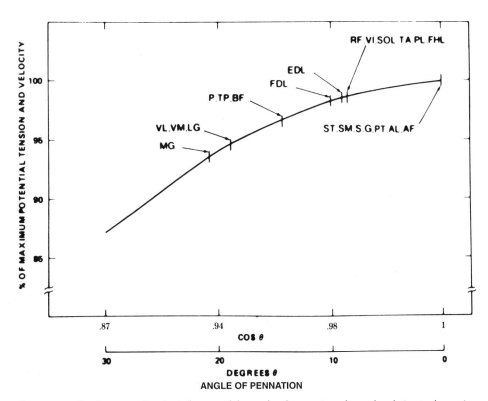

Figure 2.2.   Plot demonstrating the influence of the angle of pennation of muscle relative to the cosine function and the resultant effect on the percentage of the maximum potential tension and velocity available in muscle. Note as the angle increases there is an exponential decrease in the maximum potential with respect to the force.

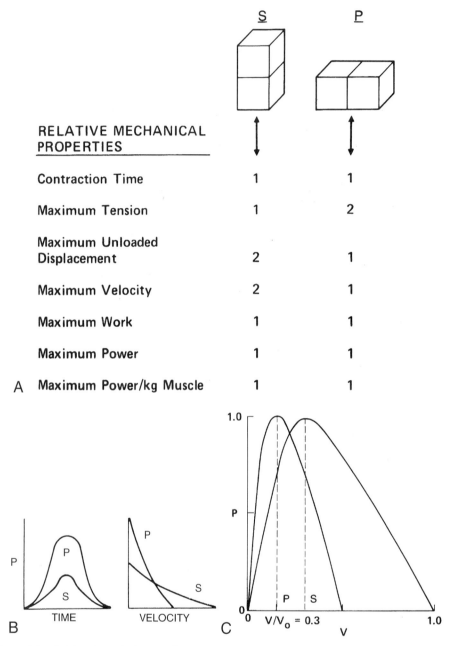

RELATIVE MECHANICAL PROPERTIES

	S	P
Contraction Time	1	1
Maximum Tension	1	2
Maximum Unloaded Displacement	2	1
Maximum Velocity	2	1
Maximum Work	1	1
Maximum Power	1	1
Maximum Power/kg Muscle	1	1

Figure 2.3. **A.** Two theoretical ways of arranging sarcomeres, in series (S) and in parallel (P). **B.** The time to peak force (*left*) and the force-velocity relationship for S and P fiber configurations. **C.** The theoretical power from the two muscle configurations shown. Dashed lines show the velocity at which peak power occurs relative to maximum velocity of shortening.

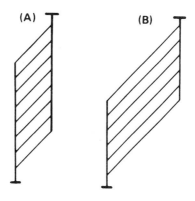

RELATIVE VALUES

MUSCLE WEIGHT	1	1
X - SECTIONAL AREA	2	1
TENSION	2	1
MUSCLE LENGTH	1	1
FIBER LENGTH	1	2
MUSCLE DISPLACEMENT	1	2
VELOCITY PER MUSCLE FIBER	1	2
ISOMETRIC CONTRACTION TIME	1	1

Figure 2.4. A schematic view of a different representation than that shown in Figure 2.3. In this case the muscle is shown as the same length.

that when stimulated maximally in the unloaded state the sarcomeres arranged in series will shorten twice as much as the parallel arrangement of fibers. As a result the maximal velocity of shortening of the parallel arrangement will be twice as high as in the parallel form as in the series configuration. Because of the relationship between force and velocity there are implications for the muscle power, applications of which will be discussed in the next sections (Fig. 2.3C) (12). Sacks and Roy have developed a similar explanation of the effect of the muscle's geometry (37). In this scenario (Fig. 2.4) two muscles are illustrated that differ in fiber length and number. Fiber angle, muscle mass, and fiber type are assumed to be identical. Note that fiber length is different between the two muscles. Extensions of this work have been accomplished, showing that at different lengths shortening speeds of fibers and aponeurosis are quite different. It has been noted by some that the geometrical aspects of muscle architecture should include both pennation angle and aponeurosis angle (56).

There are a host of other factors that play a role in muscle function. For example, consideration must be given to two joint muscles and their ability to maintain appropriate length during the course of a contraction. Another factor is that many muscles attach only after significant modification of the angle of insertion. One example occurs as the quadriceps tendon uses the patella to increase the angle of insertion. Other examples include the volar carpal groove and the tendon of the flexor digitorum profundus lifting the superficialis tendon at the terminal digits of the fingers. The

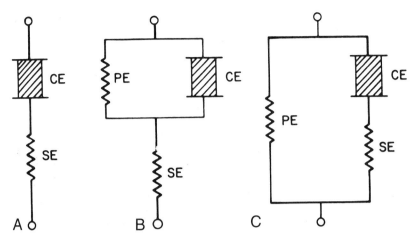

Figure 2.5. Several examples of models of human muscles. **A.** According to the Hill model the series elastic (*SE*) and the contractile element (*CE*) are in series. **B.** In the Voight model a parallel element (*PE*) has been added in parallel to *CE*. **C.** In the Maxwell model note that the *PE* is in parallel with both *CE* and *SE*.

significance of these length and insertion factors will be detailed in the following chapters on each joint.

Structural Models

Numerous models of the musculotendinous unit as a functional unit have been described and presented in the literature (Fig. 2.5) (35). Hill was among the most prolific original workers in this area, successfully describing the force velocity relationship over 40 years ago (23). Others have produced results that closely parallel in vivo responses of muscle (40, 47). Although the model used makes some difference, the relationship of the elements within the muscle, in addition to viscosity, is primarily responsible for the mechanical properties described in the following sections.

Length-Tension

The models in Figure 2.5 show the basic elements responsible for producing the **length-tension** relationship. CE designates the **contractile component** or the overlap of actin and myosin filaments. The PE or **parallel elastic component** is made up of the connective tissues surrounding the muscle filaments. The **series elastic component** is labeled as the SE portion of the model and can be considered to be the tendinous portion of the neuromuscular unit. These components exist in every muscle, but exactly how these various elements relate to each other determines the length-tension relationship for a given muscle.

To explain the length-tension relationship the contribution of each of the elements must be evaluated. Consider the results when an attempt is made to lengthen muscle (Fig. 2.6). To do so, move to the right on the abscissa. When this is done, passive tension, indicated by the *r* curve, arises within the muscle. The total tension (*a*) is available under conditions of contraction of muscle and represents the combined effect of the passive and the contractile (*d*) elements. Note that the curve generated by the contractile element is the tension achieved under different lengths by the contractile component, i.e., the actin and myosin filaments. However, the right hand portion of the contractile element curve is not totally discernible to us functionally because as contractions are performed at different lengths we must account for the contribution of the passive elements. Thus the tension shown by curve *a* is the result of the passive plus the contractile components, or $a = d + r$.

On review of the length-tension relationships for the three different muscles in Figure 2.6, one readily notes the difference in configuration. Differences in the shape of the curve are accounted for by the location of the passive element. Moving from the model shown in C to A, or to the left, passive tension becomes a factor earlier in the lengthening process. Since the total tension *a* is a result of $r + d$ there are concurrent changes in *a* that are reflective of the shifting of the passive element to the left. Thus the gastrocnemius muscle would have a much greater total tension generating capability than semitendinosus at equivalent lengths of the respective muscles (52).

Configuration of the length-tension curve also varies between animals. Goldspink (21) and White (51) have respectively presented length-tension (Fig. 2.7) and resting tension (Fig. 2.8) diagrams for the bumblebee, locust, frog, and snail. Two things are apparent from these figures. First, the net voluntary tension curve is contained along a very short length axis (Fig. 2.7). Second, the passive elements have varying degrees of slope (Fig. 2.8). Consider these two factors, the active component and the passive element, in relationship to each other. For the bumblebee, the steep slopes for both of these portions of the muscle match. Also compare the characteristics of the snail and note that the slopes are not nearly so steep. Knowing the functions performed by each animal it is not remarkable that the bumblebee is capable of sustaining wing motions upwards of 600 Hz while the snail moves at such a slow pace (21).

These characteristics vary across muscles, not only in lower animal forms but also in humans. For example, cardiac muscle will more closely simulate the frog gastrocnemius than the semitendinosus because of functional requirements related to cardiac output. Intact human muscle has been difficult to evaluate in vivo for obvious reasons, but work published by Ralston (36) indicates that characteristics identified in animals have similar features in humans. Subjects in their experiments

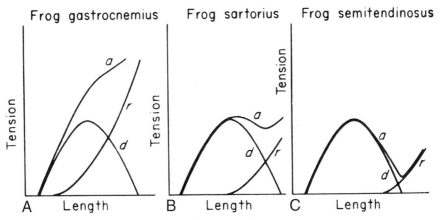

Figure 2.6. Length-tension curves for three different muscles: **A.** Frog gastrocnemius. **B.** Frog sartorius. **C.** Frog semiteninosus. *Legend*: *r*, passive tension; *a*, total tension; *d,* contractile tension.

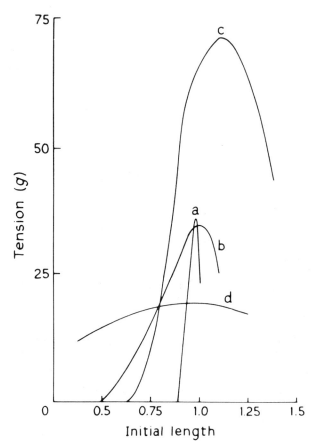

Figure 2.7.   The length/active tension curves are shown for a variety of muscles. The tensions cannot be directly compared because they are not in grams per unit cross section. *Legend*: *a*, bumblebee flight muscle; *b*, locust flight muscle; *c*, frog sartorius muscle; *d*, snail pharynx retractor muscle.

were amputees who had undergone a "cineplastic" procedure. In this instance surgeons placed a tunnel through the muscle tendon so that a cable or other mechanical mechanism can be permanently and directly attached to muscle. Subsequently, the passive component and other features associated with tension development at various biceps brachii muscle lengths were evaluated. That the passive components for human muscles vary has been demonstrated and graphically displayed by Yamada (Fig. 2.9) (55).

Length-tension factors must also be considered in surgical procedures and in therapeutic programs. Outright **releases, tenodeses** (surgical fixation of tendons), and **transfers** of muscles offer primary examples. The pes anserine transfer serves as a good example of the importance of appropriate length. In this case the common tendon is adjusted for the express purpose of limiting external tibial rotation and providing stability to the medial aspect of the knee. Thus, the success of transfers are very dependent on correct length; otherwise, the patient may not have sufficient active or passive tension because the muscle is too short. In all cases therapists need to be cognizant of lengthening muscle for the purpose of eliminating contracture yet

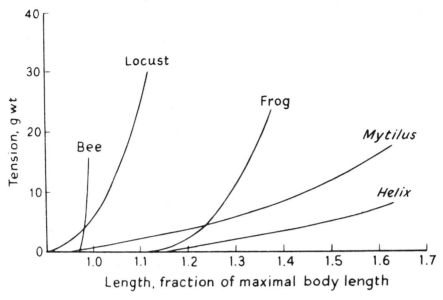

Figure 2.8.   Resting length/passive tension curves for the muscles shown in Figure 2.7 and the mytilus. The combined curves of Figure 2.7 and Figure 2.8 would form similar active and resting tension curves as for those shown in Figure 2.6 accounting for the mechanics of each of the muscles.

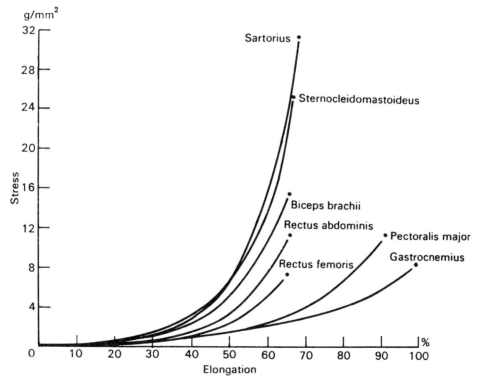

Figure 2.9.   Stress-elongation curves for tension of skeletal muscle in 29 year olds. Practically, stress is equivalent to tension and elongation equal to length. Note the variation between muscles.

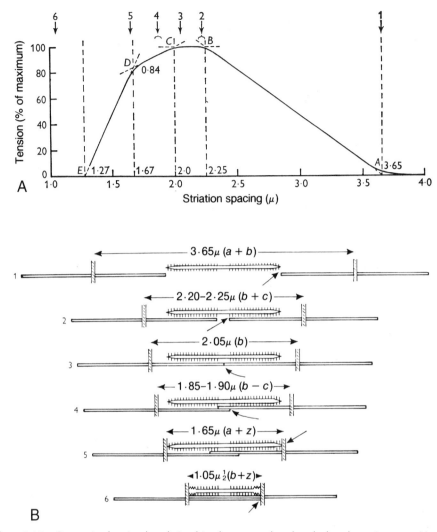

Figure 2.10. Composite showing the relationship of sarcomere length to the length-tension curve. Vertical arrows in **A** show the various stages of overlap portrayed in **B** at the corresponding number. Lengths in microns (μ): a = 1.60, b = 2.05, c = .15−2, z = .05.

conversely avoiding excessive shortening that may remove the musculotendinous unit from the tension generating range. Specific examples as applied to joints will be presented in later chapters.

Confirming evidence of the length-tension phenomenon has been provided via the study of the length-tension curve at the sarcomere level (22). A schematic summary of result is shown in Figure 2.10. Assuming similar findings hold true for all other sarcomeres a large population of such curves would produce the dome-shaped configuration of the contractile component of the length-tension relationship for a total muscle, as seen earlier in Figure 2.6.

There are several specific applications and implications arising from the length-tension relationship. The first is the influence of **precontraction stretch**. Figure 2.11 shows the effect of the passive or elastic element on muscle action and ultimate tension output. Note, however, that the figure ignores the concept of viscosity that really exists because of the fluid elements within the muscle. This viscosity, influenced by factors such as temperature and amount of body fluids, is difficult to determine. However, for the sake of a more complete model of muscle, inclusion is well warranted. Note that in Figure 2.11B the contractile component has shortened and stretched the series elastic component, producing the tension shown on the dial. In Figure 2.11C a quick stretch has been applied to the muscular unit while at the same time the contractile component is shortening the same degree as shown in B. The ultimate result is an increase in total tension output. Thus, by applying stretch or by lengthening the muscle during the course of the contraction a greater amount of tension can be generated. The matter of stretch applied to muscle in a contractile state is applied in many therapeutic situations and will be elucidated in later chapters.

It is well known that **elastic energy** can, in fact, be stored and transformed into kinetic energy. Such was the case in Figure 2.11 when stretch was applied as the contraction occurred. Other examples can be located. Goldspink (21) has noted that fleas have a substance known as resilin. This near perfect rubber material, when stretched or deformed, can rapidly return to its original state. Thus, muscle is used to develop tension over a long period of time. Then, with a quick tension release the flea performs a tremendous leap.

Similar characteristics have been evaluated in humans. The squat jump has been compared to a jump preceded by a rapid counter movement to stretch the muscle and to a jump from a height. Findings showed that the counter movement jump was 22% higher than the jump from a static position. Likewise, the jump from a height was 3–13% higher (6). In other work these same investigators have calculated that

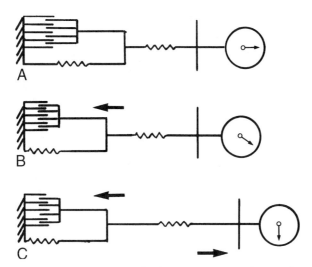

Figure 2.11.   Influence of elongation upon the ultimate tension generated in muscle. **A.** Model of resting muscle. **B.** Generation of isometric tension. Note that the two attachments of the muscle have not been separated. **C.** Contraction of the contractile component with simultaneous lengthening of the muscle increases the tension available.

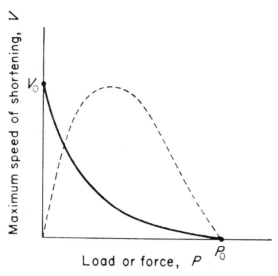

Figure 2.12.   Force-velocity and power curves for muscle. V_0 stands for the maximum velocity of shortening while P_0 signifies the maximum load or force. The dotted line represents the mechanical power produced.

in humans 35–53% of the energy absorbed during the negative phase is reused during positive work (5). Most recently Bosco et al. (10) have shown that concentric contraction performance can be attributed to a combination of elastic energy and myoelectric potentiation of muscle activation. Thus, these factors become important any time motion causes the muscle to undergo lengthening prior to contraction.

Force-Velocity

The basic **force-velocity** relationship uncovered by Hill is shown in Figure 2.12. At maximum velocity (V_0), muscle is capable of lifting the lightest load while as the velocity approaches zero the maximum load (P_0) can be lifted. At P_0 there is zero velocity, and thus the condition of isometric contraction. The mechanical **power** produced is derived by substituting the formula velocity = d/t into the power = fd/t relationship so that P = FV. Note that the maximum mechanical power is available at approximately ⅓ maximum velocity and ⅓ maximum load or force.

As an example, because the cross section of the gastrocnemius is greater than that of the semitendinosus muscle, the gastrocnemius would produce greater force than the semitendinosus. If velocity of contraction (d/t) was held constant clearly the greater power would be generated by the gastrocnemius muscle because the force would be greater. Recall also, that the degree of shortening is influenced by angle of fiber insertion and that the pennate muscle shortens less per unit time than does the fusiform muscle. The result is a tendency for velocity of pennate muscles to be somewhat less than that for the fusiform type of muscle. The specific power capabilities of any muscle are therefore determined by the contractile properties and mechanisms that are responsible for the force and the velocity. The product of the force multiplied by the respective velocity produces the power or dashed curve shown in Figure 2.12.

A practical example of how this force-velocity relationship is manifested in performance is during bicycle riding. If an individual attempts to initiate pedaling on a steep upgrade it is usually impossible to turn the crank because sufficient tension cannot be generated at the velocity of pedal revolution. Conversely, when descending a steep grade the bicycle is shifted into a higher gear so that the velocity of the extremities can exert an effective force on the crank. Other examples of this fundamental relationship can be established for isokinetic testing, whereby the clinician has an opportunity to control or adjust the velocity of the angular movement. In most instances, however, velocities for patient care circumstances are slow, thus tending to produce far less than optimal power. This loss of ability to exert power is manifested in their clinical behavior as weakness, both in activities requiring specific performances and in functional activities.

Thus far, we have discussed the force-velocity relationship for the shortening or concentric type of contraction. Figure 2.13 shows the force-velocity relationship for elbow flexor musculature for concentric and eccentric contractions. Observe that at the highest velocity of concentric work the lowest possible tension is achieved. During the eccentric contraction the highest tension available is at the highest velocity while the isometric value is recorded at approximately 31 kg(f). In retrospect, these data are as expected since eccentric work is, in fact, stretching the muscle concurrently while a contractile component is attempting to shorten the entire musculotendi-

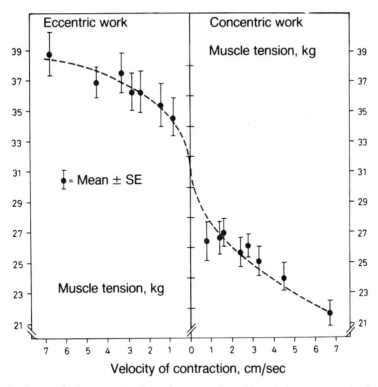

Figure 2.13. Force-velocity curve for elbow flexor muscles. Although the tension and velocity scales are reversed compared to Figure 2.12, the relationship is unaltered. The vertical line in the center of the graph indicates an isometric condition. Concentric work, when the muscle shortens, is on the right side of the graph. Conversely, eccentric contraction is to the left.

nous unit. Since it has been established that humans can move at over 1000°/sec, the 7 cm/sec velocity (corresponding to approximately 120°/sec) represents only a limited range of the velocity available to human muscle (26).

Some attention should be paid to particular characteristics of the curve. First, note that the changes in the available tension are most dramatic for a small change in velocity. For example, when the muscle rate of shortening falls by 1% the tension falls 5%. At 10% of maximum the tension drops by 35% (28). Conversely the tension in the direction of lengthening increases to a maximum with a rather small change in velocity, essentially reaching a plateau at a velocity of under 100°/second. Second, while the tension is increased in eccentric contractions the magnitude of increase is not comparable to the decrease in tension in the concentric contraction. Specifically, from Figure 2.13, the isometric value is 32, the maximum eccentric approximately 39 while the concentric will essentially fall to 0 at the highest velocities.

Other exercise physiology studies have shown that the energy required by eccentric contractions is far less than those created by concentric exercise (1). For example, it is well known to be easier to descend stairs than to ascend a similar flight of stairs or to control a specific therapeutic load while lengthening muscle as opposed to shortening the muscle. These specific examples demonstrate the ability of muscle to utilize the elastic components during lengthening contractions. More specifics about eccentric contractions and their effect on muscle will be given in later sections of this chapter.

Force-Time

The fundamental relationship of force and time for the isometric contraction is demonstrated in Figure 2.14 (42). Shown on the figure are several measures used in evaluating **force-time** curves. The overall shape of the curve can be explained on the basis of muscle structure. As the contraction is initiated the contractile component proceeds to stretch the elastic components within the muscle. During that phase there is an upward, nonlinear increase in the creation of the force production. Once the elastic components have been "pulled out" the development of force will reach an essentially linear stage around the point of inflection through which the slope or tangent line has been drawn. Toward the end of the contraction the maximum tension is reached as the contractile component can generate no greater tension through the series elastic component. Studies involving training have indicated that maximum tension can be generated in approximately 300 ms (43).

The rapid development of force is important in at least selected circumstances of pathological movement or in recovery of normal movement capabilities. And, although not a primary factor in low velocity activities such as gait the development of adequate amounts of tension becomes an important consideration when relating temporal events to injury or reinjury prevention. Specific rapid tension development associated with athletic requirements may also be pertinent when patients attempt to complete an effective rehabilitation program that will allow return to competition.

Finally, realize that as the joint angle is varied the force-time curve will vary in the magnitude of the P_{100} (maximum tension) reached. Recall that at angles of muscle insertion less than 90° a component of the force will be transmitted to compress the joint. Consequently, less tension can go toward creating the turning moment, thus resulting in a lower maximum value that is measured. It is for this additional reason that moments should be used as the standard and comparative measure within and

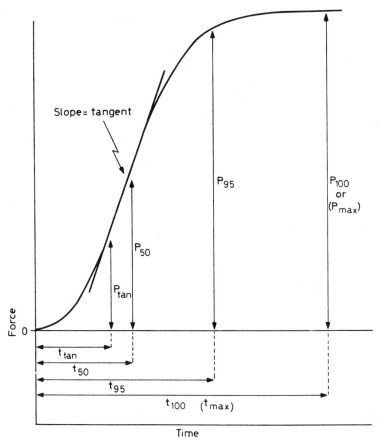

Figure 2.14.   Force-time curve for human muscle and several common measures used to evaluate tension generation and maintenance.

between patients. Also recall that at greater than 90° a component of the muscular tension is distracting the joint and, therefore, changes the features of the force-time curve.

Interaction of Factors in Muscle Mechanics

Production of effective and appropriate joint moments depends, then, on a number of factors. In addition to the physiological features and the structural arrangement of the fibers within muscle, tension available is highly dependent upon the length at which muscle is required to contract as well as the type (i.e., concentric, isometric, or eccentric) of contraction. Velocity is another prime variable that clinicians must take into account in applying knowledge to patient care situations (27). How these factors interact will determine the ultimate or final torque produced in the temporal sequence allowed. In the case of any of the joint torque curves, note that the force output varies significantly throughout the range of motion, recognizing that the mechanical curve is dependent on the angle of insertion and the joint angle at every given point in the range of motion. While only the effective or resultant force and subsequent moment is what ultimately matters, an understanding of how these factors interact is essential to understand normal human motion and how this motion may be ultimately disturbed in pathology (29).

EFFECTS OF IMMOBILIZATION

This section of the chapter presents information relative to changes in tissue as a result of immobilization. Primary focus will be on muscle, but the effects on extra-articular tissues, collagen, ligament, connective tissue, and the myotendinous junction will also be discussed. The results of both short and long-term immobilization on these tissues are profound (38). The effects on the tissues lead to an alteration of the mechanical properties of the tissue, manifested as a change in functional state. The effect of these alterations will be discussed in Chapter 5 on material properties of biological tissues. A model depicting some of the factors associated with immobilization and the effect on tissues is shown in Figure 2.15.

Muscle

Changes within muscle have been demonstrated to exist as early as 2 days post-immobilization (7). The earliest changes include a swelling of the terminal cisternae of the sarcoplasmic reticulum. Compared to normal muscle (Fig. 2.16) mitochondria appeared more electron dense and by day 5, many of the Z-disks were wavy. Figure 2.17 shows a typical appearance of muscle 5 days post immobilization: the sarcomeres are extremely distorted. I bands may be almost impossible to detect. In some cases, fibers near the proximal and distal end regions of the muscle demonstrated greater changes than those seen in the mid-belly region. An increased number of macrophages in other connective tissue between adjacent fibers have also been noted (7). Four weeks post immobilization there is considerable distance between contractile elements and adjacent fibers, irregularity, and changes in fiber size and shape. There is considerable loss of muscle mass. Z-disks within the muscle are distorted and located obliquely or even longitudinally. After 8 weeks of immobilization, Z-disks appear to be randomly oriented. By the end of 14 weeks, the muscle is significantly altered in comparison in normal (Fig. 2.18) (11). Thus, muscle has

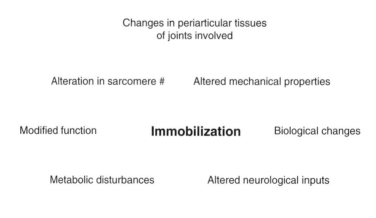

Changes in periarticular tissues
of joints involved

Alteration in sarcomere #   Altered mechanical properties

Modified function   **Immobilization**   Biological changes

Metabolic disturbances   Altered neurological inputs

Adaptation of connective tissue

Figure 2.15. Injuries or insults lead to immobilization, which in turn results in tissue changes. Specific examples include fractures, sprains, strains, lesions of the neuraxis, and surgical procedures.

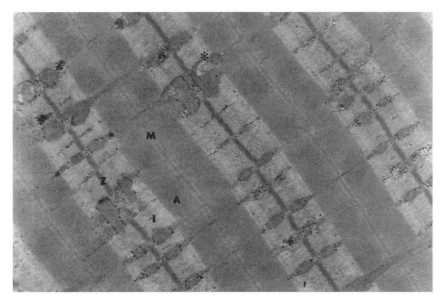

Figure 2.16. Longitudinal sections of normal human muscle fibers. *Legend*: *A*, A-band; *I*, I-band; *Z*, Z-disk; *M*, M-band; *T*, transverse tubule; *arrows*, junctional sarcoplasmic reticulum.

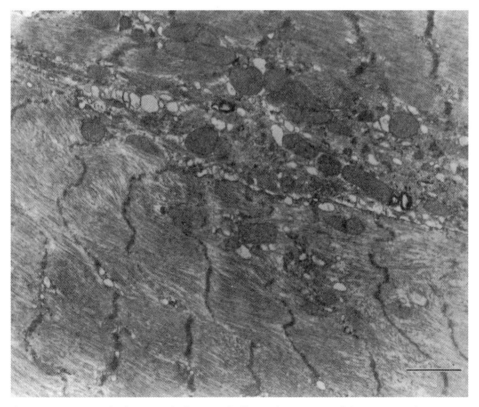

Figure 2.17. Longitudinal section of soleus muscle fibers 5 days post immobilization. Note the streaming of the Z-disks and the myofibrillar contraction and disruption.

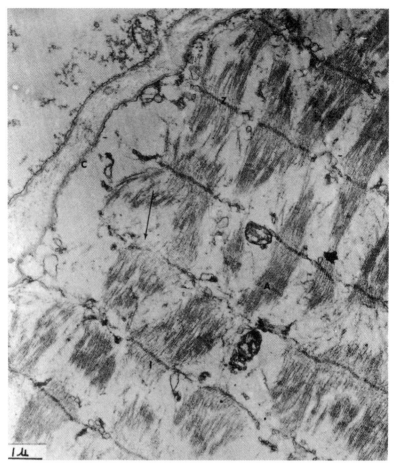

Figure 2.18. Cat toe flexor muscle 14 weeks post immobilization. Sarcomeres are fragmented while some Z-disks remain. Some thin I filaments persist in selected locations. *Legend*: *A*, A-band myofilaments; *I*, I filaments (thin); *c*, fragmented cell membrane; *z*, Z-disks; *arrow*, loss of Z-disks and thin filaments.

become extremely disorganized with significant loss of fiber mass and a decrease in dry weight. As has been observed clinically, there is concurrent loss in tension generating capabilities.

Interestingly, Lieber and coworkers (28) have studied the effect of immobilization on several different muscles in the dog. As a result of their work, they predict that those muscles most vulnerable to immobilization-induced atrophy are those that function as antigravity muscles, cross a single joint, and contain a relatively large proportion of slow fibers. Examples are the soleus, vastus intermedius, and vastus medialis muscles. The next most susceptible muscles would be antigravity muscles that are predominately slow and that cross multiple joints, such as the erector spinae, gastrocnemius, and rectus femoris muscles. Finally, phasically activated, predominantly fast muscles are lesser affected (28). While this work is somewhat supported by other investigations, the specific applications to human function and dysfunction are yet to be specifically evaluated. The fact that most human muscles have relatively equal proportions of slow and fast twitch fibers may mean that there is a more generalizable effect of immobilization.

Changes in muscle are also documented in that the number of **sarcomeres** significantly decreases in muscles that are immobilized in a shortened position (44). In a classic study of the cat soleus muscle, the ankle joint was immobilized at different lengths. In the muscles that were immobilized in a shortened position the sarcomere number decreased by almost 40%. In the muscle which was immobilized in a lengthened position, there was an increase in sarcomeres by almost 20%. That the changes in sarcomere number can influence the overall length of the muscle and its subsequent mechanical properties is a well-known fact. Also of interest is other work that demonstrates that when a muscle is stimulated for 12 hours, there is a decrease in sarcomeres by as much as 25%, concurrent with subsequent hypoextensibility. However, when the muscle is not allowed to shorten, the sarcomere number and hypoextensibility remain the same (45). While this investigative work included passive shortening that showed no effect in 12 hours, the implication is that, for those with lesions of the nervous system, excessive stimulation of the muscle (i.e., spasticity and hypertonicity) could lead to increased motor neuron drive, muscle contraction, and in turn muscle shortening and loss of sarcomeres. The subsequent decrease in extensibility would be measured as a loss of range of motion by the therapist evaluating the patient.

There is also evidence that the number of sarcomeres significantly decreases in young developing muscles that are immobilized in a shortened position. However, very young muscles immobilized in a shortened position do not add sarcomeres. These nuances have been offered as explanations for changes in the shape of the curve generated by the contractile element in the length-tension relationship (53).

In summary, changes in muscle are apparent histologically and manifested functionally. Loss of muscle mass and changes in the number of sarcomeres significantly decreases a muscle's functional ability in terms of generation of tension. Strong evidence exists that changes in sarcomere number can be significantly influenced by maintaining tension and/or elongating muscle tissue. Prolonged immobilization will continue to negatively affect any muscle's normal capability and may produce irreversible changes within the muscle, leading to permanent dysfunction.

Connective Tissue

Immobilization also has an effect upon **connective tissue**. An increased fibrosis of periarticular tissues, cartilage proliferation at joint edges, and atrophy of weight-bearing areas have all been reported (49). In addition, there is regional bony sclerosis and resorption after 2 weeks of immobilization, a change in load bearing characteristics, and an increase in synthesis of collagen. Prolonged immobilization can result in formation of fibro-fatty tissue that encroaches on joint clefts and envelops the ligaments. There is resorption of the articular cartilage and further replacement by fibro-fatty tissue. Degenerative changes, including inhibition of synovial fluid into the articular cartilage, have also been noted. The synovial membrane gradually adheres to the cartilage and newly synthesized collagen is laid down haphazardly. Further, ligaments have been noted to be weakened significantly due to alterations in the glycosaminoglycans and the collagen's fiber relationship (49).

Immobilization has also been known to affect the passive element within muscle. Experiments have been performed while immobilizing tissue in both a lengthened and shortened position. One experiment, performed on cat soleus muscle, indicated that the passive element of muscle immobilized in a shortened position shifted to

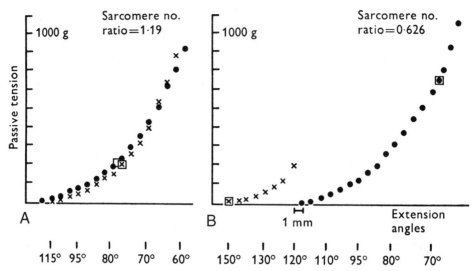

Figure 2.19. Plots of passive tension and joint extension. Results from immobilized muscle are shown with an *x* and contralateral controls with an •. Larger angles produced shorter muscles. **A.** Muscles immobilized in the lengthened position. **B.** Muscles immobilized in the shortened position.

the left (Fig. 2.19). Such a shift in this passive element could potentially eliminate extensibility of tissue, resulting in a decrease in range of motion. That is, as the therapist attempts to elongate muscle, the change in the length-tension relationship is due to the shifting of the passive element to the left, the small x's as shown in Figure 2.19B. Immobilization in the lengthened position shows virtually no change in the passive element (Fig. 2.19A), and thus there would be no effect on the length-tension relationship and/or the subsequent tension that could be generated in the musculotendinous unit.

Collagen

Specific studies have also been completed on the effects of immobilization on **collagen** (13). Immobilized collagen fibers are usually profoundly disorganized. Some areas are devoid of collagen while other areas are relatively well organized. Eight weeks post immobilization, the cross-sectional area of collagen had declined to 50% of the control areas. Thus, tendons as well as muscle are also weakened. In addition, changes in the collagen can impair tendon gliding. Further, a shortening of ligaments and an increase in articular adhesions occur (13).

Ligament

Most of the information relative to the changes in **ligament** with immobility have focused on the biochemistry and biomechanical characteristics. Woo and others (3) have shown that osteoclasts do resorb subperiosteal bone and disrupt the ligament's attachment site to the bone (Fig. 2.20). Overall, the tissue is disorganized on a gross scale with large bundles of poorly organized matrix after 1–2 weeks of immobilization. Large defects were present between bundles and the substance of the ligament (34).

Myotendinous Junction

The myotendinous junction is of particular interest because it is a very common site of injury. Specific evaluations have been done of the tissue associated with this junction.

Two types of insertion sites have been described, the direct and the indirect (54). In the case of the **direct insertion**, most fibers are deep fibers meeting the bone at a right angle. Superficial fibers, at both the proximal and distal end of the structure, continue with the periosteum of the bone surface. With the direct insertion, the deep fibers insert in four distinct zones. In the case of the **indirect insertion**, the superficial fibers predominate and the insertion to the bone is mainly the fibers blending with the periosteum. The deeper fibers attach with little or none of the transitional zone of fibrocartilage seen in the direct insertions. In general, however, the collagen fibers insert into the deep recesses or insert into deep recesses that are formed between the finger-like processes of the muscle cells (Fig. 2.21). This serves to increase the area of contact between the muscle fibers and the tendon collagen; thus, the force per unit area is reduced.

Immobilization has been shown to affect the insertion sites of slow (Type I) and fast (Type II) muscle fibers in different ways. In one study the contact area at the junction was reduced by 48% for Type I fibers and 46% for Type II fibers. Structurally, during immobilization the terminal processes of the muscle cells became "bulky and shallow" (25). No differences in collagen fibrils at the tendinous end of the junction were noted. There were some minor changes in the type of collagen in that

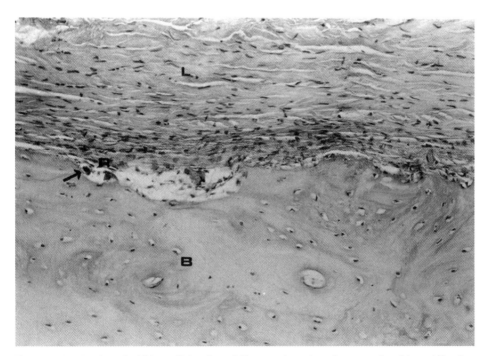

Figure 2.20. Section of rabbit medial collateral ligament insertion after 9 weeks of immobilization. Osteoclasts (*at arrow*) have resorbed subperiosteal bone (*B*) and altered the ligament's attachment to bone (*R*). Superficial ligament fibrils (*L*) are also shown.

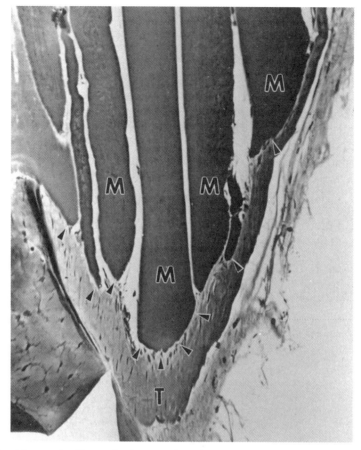

Figure 2.21. Micrograph of longitudinal section through attachment of muscle cells (*M*) to the tendon of insertion (*T*).

Type III was increased. The authors speculated that the changes at the musculotendinous junction assist in protecting the contractile component.

EFFECTS OF EXERCISE

Certain exercises can create injurious effect in muscle, particularly lengthening contractions (17). Isometric, isotonic, or shortening contractions have not been reported to produce injury during normal use. This would suggest that the contractility of the tissue is not capable of damaging those elements that limit extensibility. That is, the contractile components cannot extend the passive elements beyond the constraints of the tissue. However, when additional tension is added into the system by means of an eccentric or lengthening contraction the potential for injury appears to exist (4).

Post-exercise soreness, or **delayed onset of muscle soreness**, has been reported as a consequence of eccentric muscle loading. The symptoms, including dull pain of variable intensity, have been reported to occur usually 24–48 hours after the exercise bout. Signs of muscle swelling, loss of active range of motion, and decreased tension generating capability are all reported signs. While five general theories have been advanced, the build-up of lactic acid and tonic muscle spasm theories have little supportive evidence, allowing the discounting of these two theories. The tearing of either connective or muscle tissue, or both, have been advanced as theories relative to the mechanism for creating the delayed onset of muscle soreness. There is selective support that damage occurs to the series elastic component as a result of the eccentric exercise. However, little of this evidence is experimental in nature (14).

There is, however, extensive evidence indicating damage to the components of muscle as a result of exercise (18, 19, 31, 32). Using a 20 inch step test in which one leg performed a concentric contraction and the other leg performed the eccentric contraction, Newham was able to show changes in the quadriceps muscles. The tissue samples, obtained from needle biopsies, showed that changes were most marked 1–2 days after the exercise. Immediately after exercise, 6–16% of the total fibers in the muscle showed focal changes, 16% of the total fibers showed extensive changes, and 8–28% showed very extensive changes. For the very extensive changes, the myofilaments are in disarray and the Z-disks are distorted or even absent (Fig. 2.22). The investigator concluded that the damage is considerable in the post-exercise period and even though there was no muscle pain, the force generation capability was decreased (32). Another study in which participants descended 10 flights of stairs showed similar focal defects in Z-disk streaming (18). Thirty-two percent of the sections biopsied 1 hour after exercise showed abnormality at the myofibril level. Fifty-two percent of the sections showed abnormalities at the 3 day interval. The tissue samples showed disrupted Z-disks, formation of protein components, and a

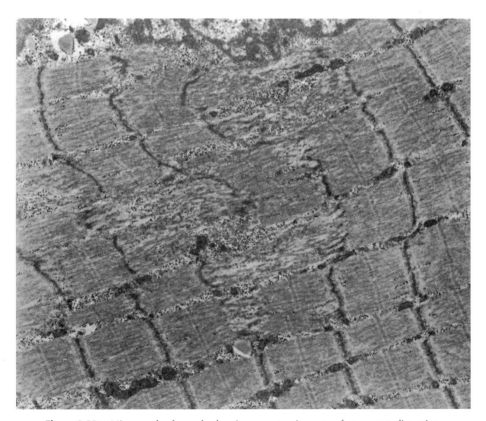

Figure 2.22. Micrograph of muscle showing an extensive area of sarcomere disruption.

release of protein bound ions. Another study using downhill walking until exhaustion also has shown that changes occur, including verifying that force is decreased after the exercise when maximal exertion is attempted via electrical stimulation (39).

All this evidence from human muscles verifies some of the work completed evaluating shortening, isometric, and lengthening contractions on the extensor digitorum longus muscle in mice. The lengthening force used was 160% of the isometric force. This work showed the most significant decrease in force, 33% of the isometric value, for lengthening contractions within approximately 10 minutes of the completion of the contraction. One day after these lengthening contractions, many of the fibers appear abnormal and, followed serially, the fibers showed signs of disruption and sometimes disappeared entirely. Some fibers had multiple areas of disruption with normal areas in between. Overall, the changes in degeneration peaked within 3 days (31).

Lieber has advanced an explanation for these changes in muscle based on findings that only fast glycolytic fibers demonstrated histological abnormalities. If, in fact, muscle fiber oxidative capacity is a determining factor in fiber damage, then the suggestion is made that the fast glycolytic fibers fatigue. A state of rigor or high stiffness is reached and then the stretch of the stiff fibers mechanically disrupts fibers resulting in the cytoskeletal and myofibril damage (28).

One additional theory that has been advanced as an explanation for the delayed onset of muscle soreness is that enzyme efflux occurs. As a result of the torn muscle or connective tissue, cellular damage produces pronounced enzyme protein degradation product release into the extracellular spaces. This efflux of collagen and protein metabolites establishes a diffusion gradient for fluid across the cellular membrane into extracellular spaces that leads to swelling and edema (41).

Which one of these theories will eventually lead to a true explanation is open to speculation. In fact, each of these effects may be participating to cause the syndrome of delayed onset of muscle soreness. For the ordinary clinical situation, these issues are not a factor since patients will not generally be training at such high levels of intensity. However, practitioners need to be aware of the implications of what could be considered relatively light intensity eccentric exercise with regard to the risk of muscle damage and the subsequent repair that could be required.

RESPONSE TO INJURY

In general, soft tissues respond in similar fashion as a result of injury. Inflammation and repair occur in a logical sequence while the time course may vary depending upon a variety of different factors, such as age, general health, nutritional status, and related injuries. The remainder of the section of this chapter will discuss the healing of various tissues, including muscle, tendon, musculotendinous junction, and ligament (30).

Muscle

Immobilized muscle will generally begin a reparative process somewhere around 3 or 4 weeks. Fibers will demonstrate regenerative changes including a straightening of the I bands and a reappearance of normal sarcoplasm for reticulum and t-tubules. Other signs of recovery indicate increased protein synthesis (7).

Cooper noted that 1 week after release from immobilization, many fibers displayed regenerative activity. As time progressed, more and more fibers in each muscle exhibited regeneration. For those interested in specific histological changes, study of the articles by Cooper (11) and Baker and Matsumoto (7) is recommended. Cooper, in particular, noted splitting of fibers longitudinally (11). This splitting phenomenon has also been noted by others and demonstrated with electron microscopy. Apparently, regeneration and creation of tension in the system is responsible for the splitting of the myofibrils (12).

Considering that sarcomeres are lost if the muscle is immobilized in a short position, some relevance can be attached to recovery time. In general, based upon a variety of different data sources, recovery and sarcomere number take approximately twice as long as the period of immobilization (53). Further evidence is available from studies of myofibrillar content, which showed that immobilization in a shortened position caused the greatest degree of atrophy (24). In general, the least changes occurred in the lengthened position. Assuming that Sargent's data can be related to patient care situations would mean that, by 6 weeks after removal from immobilization, the mean fiber area of the leg recovering post-injury would be at approximately 75% of the area of the uninjured leg. And, since Booth has shown differences in mechanical and physiological characteristics in fiber numbers between slow and fast twitch muscle fibers as a result of immobilization, implication may well be that therapists need to rehabilitate muscles using training programs that offer higher degrees of specificity and/or variations in restrictive load, duration of contraction, and velocity of contraction (9). Virtually no studies have been completed as to the effects of these training programs on patients.

Tendon

Studies of the effects of immobilization on tendon have typically followed surgical transection. In these cases, the tendon or the accompanying joint is immobilized for a period of days and then the effect on the tissues for biochemical, biomechanical, and histological changes are analyzed. In general, these studies are pertinent because at least part of the effect is due to the immobilization required post-injury. In effect, these studies show that the collagen fibrils are not uniformly oriented longitudinally with a long axis of the typical collagen fibers in tissue that has not been injured or undergone surgery. In some cases, fibrils are shortened, assembled in patches, and oriented at diverse angles. Over the post-injury period, the area between the cut ends of the tendon initially is filled with loose connective tissue. As healing occurs, the collagenous tissue becomes more organized. Investigators have also noted a wider range of collagen fiber diameters in post-injury or immobilized tissue (Fig. 2.23) (8, 20).

Myotendinous Junction

There is little documentation of the types of tissue injury that occur at the myotendinous junction. Some evidence does indicate that immediately, or within 48 hours after injury, there is inflammation with limited muscle fiber necrosis, presence of leukocytes, tissue edema, and hemorrhage (33, 46). However, within 48 hours, there is evidence of complete breakdown of damaged fibers. After 7 days, there is a marked decrease in inflammation and immaturation of fibroblasts into elongated fiber sites and localized fibrosis. These results imply that changes at the myotendinous junction occur rather quickly. Virtually no information is available as to the toleration of these sites for tension development as may occur during rehabilitation processes (33).

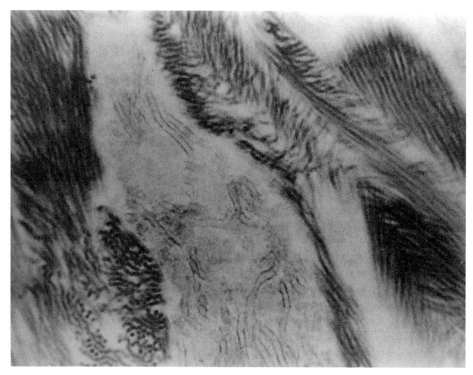

Figure 2.23. Orientation of collagen fibrils at divergent angles in repaired canine flexor tendon repaired 7 days after injury.

Ligament

After injury, blood clots form in the space between the retracted ends of the ligament (3). Within a period of 3 days fibrinous scar fills in the gap and the overlying fascia becomes adherent to the ligament. Matrix reconstitution begins within a week and new fibrils provide additional strength by 10 days (16). Cellularity and vascularity decrease between 6 and 24 weeks en route to a normal histological appearance sometime between 24 and 52 weeks after injury (30). In the scars the fibril diameter is less than in the contralateral, unoperated ligaments. Alignment of collagen fibrils is also changing during the healing process, becoming more parallel as time proceeds (15).

Also of interest are the additional effects. For example, the bone-ligament complex changes substantially, resulting in the histological changes and the mechanical effects that are addressed in Chapter 5. In addition, properties are regained at a much slower rate. In one study 12 months of reconditioning was required for "strength" lost during 8 weeks of immobilization (30).

General Therapy Considerations

The effects on soft tissue due to exercise or injury often are profound. The magnitude of the injury and the time course associated with the healing of the insulted tissue should be taken into account by the therapist in the management of joint and soft tissue injuries so that the treatment of choice is selected on a sound basis and progressed in a logical fashion. Without the most appropriate interventions recovery may be delayed or incomplete.

References

1. Abbott BC, Bigland B, Ritchie JM. The physiological cost of negative work. *J Physiol.* 1953;117:380–390.
2. Alexander RM. Mechanics of skeleton and tendons. In: Brooks VB, ed. *Handbook of Physiology.* Bethesda, MD: American Physiological Society; 1981;4:17.
3. Andriacchi T, Sabiston P, DeHaven K, et al. Ligament: injury and repair. In: Woo SL-Y, Buckwalter JA, eds. *Injury and Repair of the Musculoskeletal Soft Tissues.* Park Ridge, IL: American Academy of Orthopaedic Surgeons; 1988.
4. Armstrong RB, Warren GL, Lowe DA. Mechanisms in the initiation of contraction-induced skeletal muscle injury. In: Gordon SL, Fine SI, Blair LJ, eds. *Repetitive Motion Disorders of the Upper Extremity.* Park Ridge, IL: American Academy of Orthopaedic Surgeons; 1995.
5. Asmussen E, Bonde-Petersen F. Apparent efficiency and storage of elastic energy in human muscles during exercise. *Acta Physiol Scand.* 1974;92:537–545.
6. Asmussen E, Bonde-Petersen F. Storage of elastic energy in skeletal muscles in man. *Acta Physiol Scand.* 1972;91:385–392.
7. Baker JH, Matsumoto DE. Adaptation of skeletal muscle to immobilization in a shortened position. *Muscle Nerve.* 1988;11:231–244.
8. Best TM, Collins A, Lilly EG, et al. Achilles tendon healing: a correlation between functional and mechanical performance in the rat. *J Bone Joint Surg.* 1993;11:897–906.
9. Booth FW, Seider MJ. Effects of disuse by limb immobilization on different muscle fiber types. In: Pette D, ed. *Plasticity of Muscle.* New York: de Gruyter; 1980:373–383.
10. Bosco C, Tarkka I, Komi PV. Effect of elastic energy and myoelectrical potentiation of triceps surae during stretch-shortening cycle exercise. *Int J Sports Med.* 1982;3:137–140.
11. Cooper RR. Alterations during immobilization and regeneration of skeletal muscle in cats. *J Bone Joint Surg Am.* 1972;54A:919–953.
12. Edgerton VR, Roy RR, Gregor RJ, et al. Morphological basis of skeletal muscle power output. In: Jones NL, McCartney N, McComas AJ, eds. *Human Muscle Power.* Champaign, IL: Human Kinetics; 1986.
13. Enwemeka CS. Connective tissue plasticity: ultrastructural, biomechanical, and morphometric effects of physical factors on intact and regenerating tendons. *J Orthop Sports Phys Ther.* 1991;14:198–212.
14. Francis, KT. Delayed muscle soreness: a review. *J Orthop Sports Phys Ther.* 1983;5:10–13.
15. Frank C, MacFarlane B, Edwards P, et al. A quantitative analysis of matrix alignment in ligament scars: a comparison of movement versus immobilization in an immature rabbit model. *J Orthop Res.* 1991;9:219–227.
16. Frank C, Schachar N, Dittrich D. Natural history of healing in the repaired medial collateral ligament. *J Orthop Res.* 1983;1:179–188.
17. Fridén J. Biomechanical injury to skeletal muscle from repetitive loading: eccentric contractions and vibrations. In: Gordon SL, Blair SI, Fine LJ, eds. *Repetitive Motion Disorders of the Upper Extremity.* Park Ridge, IL: American Academy of Orthopaedic Surgeons; 1995.
18. Fridén J, Sjöström M, Ekblom B. A morphological study of delayed muscle soreness. *Experientia.* 1981;37:506–507.
19. Fridén J, Sjöström M, Ekblom B. Myofibrillar damage following intense eccentric exercise in man. *Int J Sports Med.* 1983;4:170–176.
20. Gelberman RH, Siegel DB, Woo SL-Y, et al. Healing of digital flexor tendons: importance of the interval from injury to repair. *J Bone Joint Surg Am.* 1991;73A:66–75.
21. Goldspink G. Design of muscles in relation to location. In: Alexander RMcN, Goldspink G, eds. *Mechanics and Energetics of Animal Locomotion.* London, England: Chapman & Hall; 1977.
22. Gordon AM, Huxley AF, Julian FT. The variation in isometric tension with sarcomere length in vertebrate muscle fibers. *J Physiol (Lond).* 1966;184:170–192.
23. Hill AV. Heat and shortening and the dynamic constants of muscle. *Proc R Soc Lond [Biol].* 1938;126:136–195.
24. Jokl P, Konstadt S. The effect of limb immobilization on muscle function and protein composition. Presented at 28th Annual Orthopedic Research Society; January 19–21, 1982; New Orleans, LA.
25. Kannus P, Jozsa L, Kvist M, et al. The effect of immobilization on myotendinous junction:

an ultrastructural, histochemical and immunohistochemical study. *Acta Physiol Scand.* 1992; 144:387–394.

26. Komi PV. Measurement of the force-velocity relationship in human muscle under concentric and eccentric contractions. In: Cerquiglini S, ed. *Biomechanics III.* Basel, Switzerland: Karger; 1973:224–229.
27. Komi PV. Neuromuscular performance: factors influencing force and speed production. *Scand J Sports Sci.* 1979;1:2–15.
28. Lieber RL. *Skeletal Muscle Structure and Function: Implications for Rehabilitation and Sports Medicine.* Baltimore: Williams & Wilkins; 1992.
29. Lieber RL, Bodine-Fowler SC. Skeletal muscle mechanics: implications for rehabilitation. *Phys Ther.* 1993;73:844–856.
30. Loitz, BJ, Frank CB. Biology and mechanics of ligament and ligament healing. In: Holloszy JO, ed. *Exerc Sports Sci Rev.* Baltimore: Williams & Wilkins; 1993:33–64.
31. McCully KK, Faulkner JA. Injury to skeletal muscle fibers of mice following lengthening contractions. *J Appl Physiol.* 1985;59:119–126.
32. Newham DJ. Ultrastructural changes after concentric and eccentric contractions of human muscle. *J Neurosci.* 1983;61:109–122.
33. Nikolaou PK, Macdonald BL, Glisson RR, et al. Biomechanical and histological evaluation of muscle after controlled strain injury. *Am J Sports Med.* 1987;15:9–14.
34. Padgett LR, Dahners LE. Rigid immobilization alters matrix organization in the injured rat medial collateral ligament. *J Orthop Res.* 1992;10:895–900.
35. Phillips CA, Petrofsky JS. The passive elastic force-velocity relationship of cat skeletal muscle: influence upon the maximal contractile element velocity. *J Biomech.* 1981;14:399–404.
36. Ralston HJ, Inman VT, Strait LA, et al. Mechanics of human isolated voluntary muscle. *Am J Physiol.* 1947;151:612–620.
37. Sacks RD, Roy RR. Architecture of the hind limb muscles of cats: functional significance. *J Morphol.* 1982;173:185–195.
38. Sargent AJ, Davies CTM, Edwards RHT, et al. Functional and structural changes after disuse of human muscle. *Clin Sci Mol Med.* 1977;52:337–342.
39. Sargeant AJ, Dolan P. Human muscle function following prolonged eccentric exercise. *Eur J Appl Physiol.* 1987;56:704–711.
40. Spector SA, Simard CP, Fournier M, et al. Architectural alterations of rat hind-limb skeletal muscles immobilized at different lengths. *Exp Neurol.* 1982;76:94–110.
41. Stauber WT. Eccentric action of muscles: physiology, injury and adaptation. *Exerc Sports Sci Rev.* 1989;19:157.
42. Stothart JP. Relationship between selected biomechanical parameters of static and dynamic muscle performance. In: Cerquigliani S, ed. *Biomechanics III.* Basel, Switzerland: Karger; 1973:210–217.
43. Sukop J, Nelson RC. Effects of isometrical training in the force-time characteristics of muscle contractions. In: Nelson RC, Morehouse CA, eds. *Biomechanics IV.* Baltimore: University Park Press; 1974:440–447.
44. Tabary JC, Tabary C, Tardieu C, et al. Physiological and structural changes in the cat's soleus muscle due to immobilization at different lengths by plaster casts. *J Physiol (Lond).* 1972;224:231—244.
45. Tabary JC, Tardieu C, Tardieu G, et al. Experimental rapid sarcomere loss with concomitant hypoextensibility. *Muscle Nerve.* 1981;4:198–203.
46. Taylor DC, Dalton JD, Seaber AV, et al. Experimental muscle strain injury: early functional and structural deficits and the increased risk for reinjury. *Am J Sports Med.* 1993;21:190–194.
47. Thorsten IH, Halkjaer-Kristensen J. Force-velocity relationships in the human quadriceps muscle. *Scand J Rehabil Med.* 1979;11:85–89.
48. Tricker RAR, Tricker BJK. *The Science of Human Movement.* New York: Elsevier; 1967.
49. Videman T. Connective tissue and immobilization: key factors in musculoskeletal degeneration? *Clin Orthop.* 1987;221:26–32.
50. Warwick R, Williams PL, eds. *Gray's Anatomy.* 36th British ed. Philadelphia: WB Saunders; 1980.
51. White DCS. Muscle mechanics. In: Alexander RMcN, Goldspink G, eds. *Mechanics and Energetics of Animal Locomotion.* London, England: Chapman & Hall; 1977.
52. Wilkie DR. *Muscle.* New York: St. Martins Press; 1968.
53. Williams PE, Goldspink G. The effect of immobilization on the longitudinal growth of striated muscle fibres. *J Anat.* 1973;116:45–55.
54. Woo SL-Y, Maynard J, Butler D, et al. Ligament, tendon, and joint capsule insertions to bone. In:

Woo SL-Y, Buckwalter JA, eds. *Injury and Repair of the Musculoskeletal Soft Tissues.* Park Ridge, IL: American Academy of Orthopaedic Surgeons; 1988.

55. Yamada H. Mechanical properties of locomotor organs and tissues. In: Evans FG, ed. *Strength of Biological Materials.* Baltimore: Williams & Wilkins; 1970.

56. Zuurbier CJ, Juijing PA. Influence of muscle geometry on shortening speed of fibre, aponeurosis and muscle. *J Biomech.* 1994;25:1017–1026.

3

Neural Regulation, Control, and Electromyography

Essential to movement is the excitation of nerve and muscle. Excitation alone is not sufficient: the excitation also must be correct in onset, magnitude, and duration. These factors, coupled with a musculotendinous unit that can generate sufficient levels of tension, produce the desired tension over the correct interval. Practitioners risk the possibility of minimizing the full therapeutic effect of their treatment when they emphasize the amount of tension development or torque without attending to the capability of the nervous system to "drive" the muscle.

NEURAL REGULATION
Motor Unit

To produce muscle tension by active contraction, the muscle must receive the appropriate stimulus from the central nervous system. The mechanism to do this is through the **motor unit**, composed of a motor neuron, its axon, and all the muscle fibers innervated by that neuron (Fig. 3.1). The discharge of the motor neuron at the level of the spinal cord transmits a depolarization down the axon and across the neuromuscular junction, resulting in a depolarization of the muscle fibers innervated by the motor neuron. (The actual generation of the motor unit potential will be discussed in a later section of this chapter.) How many muscle fibers are included is dependent on several factors, including size of the neuron, type of muscle being innervated (i.e., fast, slow, intermediate), and such factors as the muscle's cross sectional area. Variation in the number of muscle fibers innervated per motor unit is large, as indicated by the following list (7):

Laryngeal, 2–3	Lateral eye rectus, 9
Platysma, 25	First lumbrical, 108
First dorsal interosseus, 340	Anterior tibialis, 562
Lateral head of gastrocnemius, >1000	Masseter, 640

How the fibers in each motor unit are distributed in each muscle is not necessarily consequential to the kinesiologist, except those with interest in motor control or study of the motor unit. In those cases it may be important to know that motor unit fibers are distributed over 12–26% of the cross section of a muscle, with a mean distribution of 17% (5).

Some have suggested that the type of fiber innervated by the motor unit may be a more appropriate means for understanding human movement. The rationale for this approach is that the fibers differ in mechanical, metabolic, and histochemical properties. For example, the **type I (SO) fibers** generate tension slowly and have a high resistance to fatigue, while the **type IIA (FOG)** and **IIB (FG) muscle fibers** generate tension quicker but are susceptible to fatigue (6, 17). Burke (4) created still

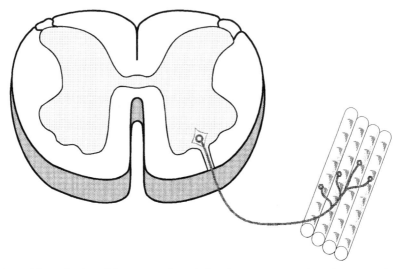

Figure 3.1.   Schematic view of the motor unit, including the motor neuron from the anterior horn of the spinal cord, the accompanying axon, and all the muscle fibers innervated by the neuron.

another system that classified motor units as slow twitch (S) with type I fibers; FR as fast twitch, fatigue resistant type IIA fibers; and FF, containing type IIB muscle fibers. While the extremes of motor unit behaviors create possibilities for great functional discrepancy, the homogeneity of fibers in humans implies that these differences are likely not that important in human function. Some features of these unit types, however, have an impact not only on the recruitment and rate coding of motor units, but also on the tension generated in muscle.

Recruitment, Rate Coding, and Segmental Innervation

Active contraction of muscle, no matter the type of contraction, is dependent on two factors for the generation of tension: (*a*) the recruitment of the motor units and (*b*) rate coding, the rate at which these motor units are discharged. Which of these mechanisms predominates the control of muscular tension, or do these two elements coexist to produce the required output? This is controversial. No matter which strategy holds relative to human performance, the neuromuscular system is known to use each.

Recruitment is defined as the initial activity of inactive motor units as the demand for muscular tension increases. **Rate coding** is an increase in the frequency of discharge of active motor units when increased tension output is required from muscle (17). These rates generally range from 5 to 50 discharges per second (Hz) (14). Rates can increase dramatically, however, in high velocity contractions. Variance also exists between muscles (6).

Figure 3.2 shows a recording of potentials from human motor units. Generally each motor unit has a "usual firing rate," a frequency at which the unit will "run" given the tension needed in the musculotendinous unit to perform the task. Rates are also dependent on muscle type, the slow units firing at lower average rates, and the fast and larger units firing at higher average rates.

Recruitment order has also been thoroughly studied, both in animals and humans. Evidence shows that the orderly recruitment of motor units depends on the variation in motor neuron size, called the **size principle** (8). At least under specified conditions motor units are recruited and derecruited in order. Smaller, slow units are recruited first; large units are recruited later or when greater tensions or fast movements are needed. Enoka (6) also points out that once a motor unit is recruited the firing of that unit will continue until the force declines. Derecruitment of units seems likely to follow the reverse order in which they are recruited.

Another factor to consider is **segmental innervation**. As techniques to assess motor unit function have improved, we have discovered that many muscles thought to operate as a unit now appear to function as many muscles or segments within a muscle. Selective activity in separate sections of the muscle (and occasionally sections of muscles divided by fascia or other tissue layers) is evidence to support this view. Muscles in the lower extremity, such as the gluteus medius (19), the lateral gastrocnemius (23), and other muscles (16) have all shown this compartmentalization. What is at least implied is that parts of muscles function to complete or participate in the task required. Thus, a higher degree of specificity of function may exist than has yet been realized. With more analyses we can anticipate that other muscles will be evaluated for the demonstration of the same phenomenon.

The clinical implications of motor unit structure and function can be either broad or limited, depending on the practitioner. On the limited side, one can say that these factors only determine the output from the system and only the output matters. For example, therapists need not know which units are being recruited first or in what order. Rather, they need to know the total output so that any necessary gross adjustments in these levels may be made. Conversely, others would say that these factors form the basis for practice, and without them therapists will lack pertinent understanding of the operational principles of the neuromuscular system. Neither view should be considered right or wrong but the information provided here can give the student a framework for evaluating movement dysfunctions, assessing the literature, and improving understanding of the pathophysiology of disorders.

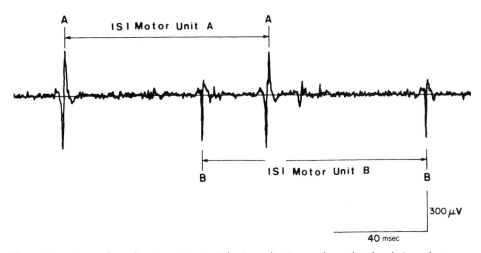

Figure 3.2. A recording of motor unit potentials. Several units are shown but for clarity only two are labeled. The interspike interval (ISI) for motor unit B is 95 msec, which converts to a frequency in Hz of 10.5 firings per second. A larger unit (A) discharges at approximately the same rate as B. While possible that this is a larger unit, in terms of number of fibers innervated by the neuron, it is also feasible that this unit is closer to the electrode recording the activity.

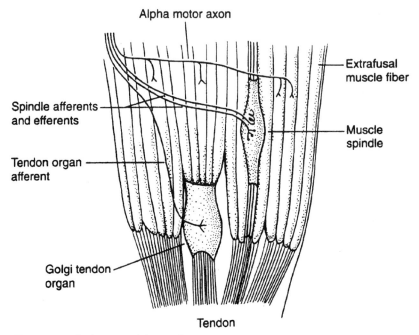

Figure 3.3.   The location of the regulatory structures in gross muscle (extrafusal fibers).

Regulation

As motor units respond during shortening, lengthening, and isometric contraction, the net effect is a product of the neural input or regulation combined with the mechanical effect associated with the state of the tissue in the musculotendinous unit. **Central and peripheral influences** exist, however, that modify or have some responsibility in movement and its control. Central influences would include visual and vestibular systems, while peripheral influences would include free nerve endings, ligaments, capsules, and Pacinian corpuscles. Golgi tendon organs, found primarily at musculotendinous junctions, in the aponeurosis, and in tendons, appear to be primarily tension-sensitive (Fig. 3.3). They are less affected by passive stretch because they are in inelastic tendons that lengthen little in comparison to muscle. Also central to the control of movement are the flexion, withdrawal, and cutaneous reflexes.

Very important is the **stretch reflex**, also known as the **myotatic reflex**. Apparently the reflex continuously activates extensor and axial muscles and results in counteraction of the force of gravity. The reflex may also contribute to maintenance of upright posture. The primary organ responsible for effecting this reflex appears to be the muscle spindle (10).

Muscle Spindle Anatomy

The spindle perceives length or change in length of muscle. Distribution of spindles has been studied extensively, revealing that high populations appear in the hand and back extensors as compared to few in the diaphragm and shoulder area (4).

The muscle spindle (Fig. 3.3) is found within the muscle in parallel to the gross muscle fibers (10). Within the capsule of the spindle are a small number (usually about 7) **"intrafusal" muscle fibers** composed of two fiber types—**nuclear chain** and **nuclear bag** fibers. Both are contractile at either pole and noncontractile in the nucleated central region. Two types of sensory fibers originate from the intrafusal muscles. The Ia afferents, also called primary, annulospiral, or nuclear bag, have endings that terminate on both chain and bag fibers and project to the spinal cord through very large diameter fibers (Fig. 3.4). The II or secondary afferents, also called flower spray or myotube, terminate on the chain fibers and on selected bag fibers called "static" because the discharge of the neuron comes under static conditions (10). These fibers project to the cord through medium sized fibers.

The intrafusal fibers receive motor innervation from small γ **motoneurons** (also called fusimotor, γ efferent) interspersed among the large α **motoneurons** of the spinal cord ventral horn. The γ fibers terminate on the striated polar regions of the intrafusal muscle fibers, and discharge of these motoneurons produces intrafusal muscle contraction; the gammas cause no direct change in the gross muscle tension.

Muscle Spindle Function

Sensory discharge from the spindle is produced by gross muscle stretch (increased muscle length), which also stretches the spindle intrafusal fibers, depolarizes the terminal endings of the spindle afferents, and causes action potentials to be transmit-

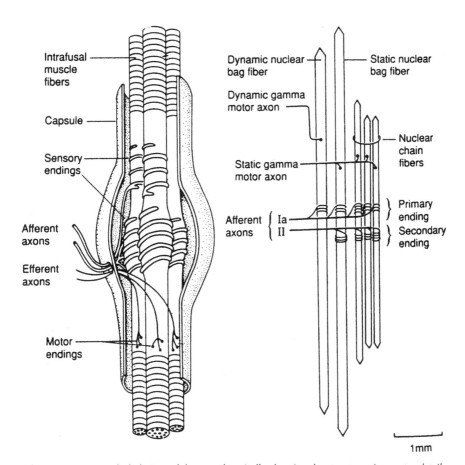

Figure 3.4.   An exploded view of the muscle spindle showing the structures in greater detail.

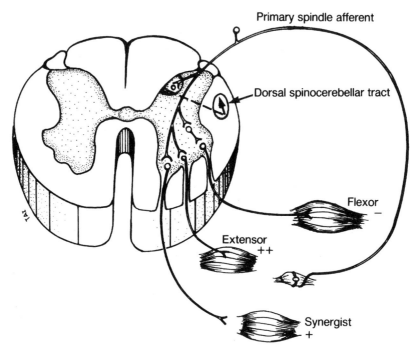

Figure 3.5. Schematic view of the circuit used in the stretch reflex.

ted centrally along the afferent fibers. The primary afferents discharge to stretch at a lower threshold than do the secondary afferents and show both an initial burst of rapid discharge (dynamic component) and a somewhat less rapid sustained increase in discharge (static component) (4).

The stretch reflex is elicited by muscle stretch sufficient to discharge the primary spindle afferents. The large myelinated primary afferent fibers enter the dorsomedial portion of the spinal cord dorsal horn and project directly, or monosynaptically, onto homonymous α motoneurons (neurons innervating the muscle from which the spindle discharge originated) to produce contraction of the homonymous muscle. Concurrent monosynaptic reflex activation of the synergist muscle also occurs, which results in stabilization of the joint across which the synergists attach. Contralateral influences have also more recently been recognized. Many extensor and axial muscles are continuously activated by this stretch reflex circuit (Fig. 3.5). The group IIs have been shown to contribute a monosynaptic excitation to homonymous (synergistic) muscle (20). Functional implications will continue to be debated. Another form of innervation has been demonstrated in a variety of mammalian muscles. β fibers distribute branches of a given fiber to both intrafusal and extrafusal muscle fibers. For more comprehensive descriptions current neurophysiology texts should be consulted.

During contraction of the gross muscle, the musculotendinous unit shortens and the muscle spindles go slack. As a result, the intrafusal fibers are no longer stretched, and the spindle afferent discharge ceases. Following contraction, the muscle returns to precontraction length, as do the intrafusal fibers. When the intrafusal fiber stretch is sufficient to depolarize the afferent terminals, the spindle sensory discharge resumes.

Gamma Regulation of Spindle Discharge

Another mechanism is the discharge of the γ motoneurons. They produce contraction of the striated polar regions of the intrafusal muscle fibers, which, in turn, stretches the central noncontractile region and depolarizes the afferent terminals. The resultant spindle discharge is thus a direct effect of γ motoneuron excitation of the intrafusal fibers. If the γ motoneurons are very active, the resultant intrafusal fiber contractions may be sufficient to overcome the slack resulting from gross muscle contraction and thus prevent spindle discharge cessation. The amount of spindle discharge that is due to γ motoneuron activation of the intrafusal fibers is called the gamma bias of the spindle (12, 13).

The small γ motoneurons, interspersed with the α motoneurons throughout the motor pools of the spinal cord, have control connections similar to the α motoneurons, except for the primary spindle afferents that do not project to the γ motoneurons. Cutaneous stimuli, for example, produce reflex discharge of the γ motoneurons, and descending projections from higher centers produce excitation or inhibition of gamma discharge. In general, γ and α motoneurons innervating the same muscle are activated in the same direction of excitation or inhibition by an incoming stimulus (alpha-gamma linkage), but the γ motoneurons respond at lower thresholds than do the α motoneurons.

Clinical Correlations

Practical examples of spindle-modulated effects are seen in the assumption of postures. In the lower leg during standing, spindles in the anterior compartment perceive stretch as the body sways posteriorly. Muscle contraction of the dorsiflexors follows, bringing the body more anteriorly over the supporting foot. Because the same mechanism operates in the triceps surae, the constant sagittal plane sway is closely monitored and controlled. Another example is spindle control in head posture when people fall asleep in the seated position, say in a lecture hall. As sleep (and relaxation) ensues, posterior cervical muscles lengthen, allowing the head to drop forward. When the spindles are sufficiently stretched, the posterior neck muscles contract and the head abruptly returns to the upright position.

A phasically induced stretch reflex is a common neurological test of motor function and is called a **tendon jerk** or **knee jerk**. A tap on the tendon of the tested muscle stretches the muscle and produces a phasic, synchronous discharge of primary spindle afferents that in turn triggers the monosynaptic stretch reflex. A hyperactive tendon jerk (hyperactive stretch reflexes) on one side of the body is generally indicative of damage in the motor pathways descending from the cortex. The increased resistance to passive movement due to hyperactive stretch reflexes is termed spasticity. In the hyperreflexic patient, if a constant stretch is applied to the muscle and a tendon tap is superimposed, not one, but a series of tendon jerk reflexes results. This repetitive jerking is called clonus and reflects the highly sensitive state of the motoneurons to synchronous afferent volleys.

Modulation by the spindle is also responsible for other features of interest to the clinician. For example, muscle stiffness, defined as a change in force divided by the corresponding change in length, will determine the effect of both external and internal disturbances on motion production. Because muscle contains elastic elements, viscous elements, and spindle control, the behavior of muscle is fundamentally nonlinear but under restricted experimental conditions. To predict the movement resulting

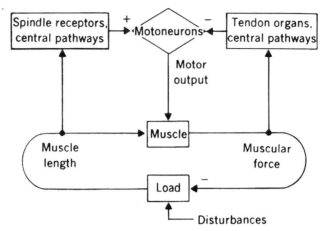

Figure 3.6. Schematic view of the role of muscle length and force in regulating muscle stiffness.

from a given contraction, conditions such as level of motor unit activation and firing rate, as well as initial length and contraction velocity, must be taken into account. Further, the action of antagonistic muscle must also be considered. Thus, a combination of length and force feedback would tend to regulate stiffness (since these are the two factors involved). One example of a model used to describe the interactions is presented in Figure 3.6 (3).

ELECTROMYOGRAPHY
Utility in Practice

Since the 18th century discovery that electrical potentials were derived from muscle, the role of electromyography (EMG) in the study of function has expanded significantly. Inman and coworkers (9) completed in 1944 the first major comprehensive EMG study by evaluating function of the shoulder. Since then, there has been exponential growth in EMG studies of human motion. Rudimentary knowledge of EMG, how it can be applied and interpreted, is fundamental to understanding kinesiology and pathokinesiology. Commonly used as a form of biofeedback for patients, this technique offers a readily available method for monitoring muscle function to assist with discrimination of movement dysfunction or effects of treatment protocols. Further, EMG is commonly used in analyzing motion or making inferences about the forces responsible for the motion.

The uses of EMG may be placed into several broad categories: (*a*) delineation of the nature, scope, and prognosis of diseases involving the neuromuscular system; (*b*) pre- and postsurgical evaluations of phasic muscle function to facilitate effective surgical results (to be discussed more fully in chapters covering the lower extremity and gait); (*c*) myoelectrics, in which action potentials derived from muscle are electronically modified to control another body part, segment, prosthesis, or orthosis; and (*d*) biofeedback for such applications as headache control, reeducation following muscle transfers, and stroke rehabilitation. Finally, EMG has been used to study kinesiological function of muscle. Reviews have been provided by Soderberg and Cook (18) and Turker (21). Use of the electromyogram has clarified pure functions of muscles and furthered the understanding of the relationship between concentric and eccentric contractions. EMG is of interest to the biomechanician to attempt to establish a relationship between EMG and tension level.

Physiological Basis

The electromyograph records the electrical activity of a muscle, the fundamental contractile unit of which is the motor unit. The electrical activity can be evaluated both visually and aurally with signal amplification. How the **potential** is derived from the fibers within each unit is shown in Figure 3.7. Several features should be noted. The first is that the potential from each fiber, labeled as 1, 2, i, and n, has a different amplitude. To explain the differences in magnitude note the position of the two electrodes at the recording site. They are closest to the fibers that have the largest amplitudes. As the distance from the recording site to the remaining muscle fibers is increased, note that the amplitude is decreased. This is a natural phenomenon, in that the closer the electrical potential to the electrode, the larger will be the amplitude of the EMG derived from that fiber. Second, observe that the potential from each fiber is initiated at a different time due to the distance of the axon as it divides and courses to each fiber. The shorter distances allow for the signal to be recorded earlier. This factor, combined with the distance to the recording site from each fiber, accounts for the differences in the onset of fiber depolarization. As all of the fibers shown in this figure are from the same motor unit each fiber will contribute to the motor unit potential, shown as h(t). Summing all the voltages at every point in time yields the shape and amplitude of the potential.

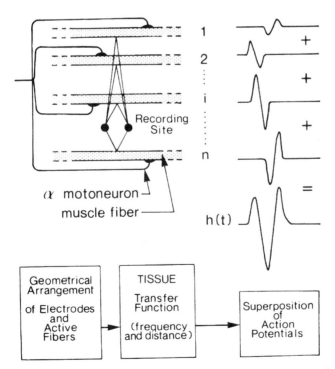

Figure 3.7.   Diagram of the generation of the motor unit action potential. Note that each fiber generates a potential summated to produce h(t). The summation of the temporal and voltage characteristics are responsible for the features that produce the unique shape of each motor unit.

Each motor unit has a specific size, shape, and sound. The former two are usually unique to a motor unit since the geometry of the recording electrodes relative to the fibers will be unique for each motor unit. The sound is dependent on the shape, and thus units are distinguishable on this basis. Amplitudes of motor unit potentials thus have various amplitudes, and may in fact range from 300 microvolts to 5 millivolts. Variation is due to location of the recording electrodes, the distance of the electrode from the motor unit, the age of the subject, and the muscle studied. The duration of the motor unit action potential ranges from 3 to 16 msec with a mean time of 9 msec (17).

Recording Methods

To record these small myoelectric potentials, an amplifier is necessary. A display device such as an oscilloscope or computer is suggested. To record the myopotentials, **surface electrodes** are most frequently used. The size, shape, and configuration of the attachment of the surface electrodes are at the discretion of the user. These electrodes have advantages; i.e., they can be easily applied, and the technique is standardized and relatively pain free. Disadvantages of using surface recording electrodes are the area recorded from is relatively large and recordings only represent superficial muscle activity. Biofeedback systems commonly used in clinical settings use a surface electrode, usually of the disposable type. While practical in a clinical setting, the instrumentation associated with these systems often does not contain the most desirable settings to record the signal: most instruments have a low frequency cutoff that does not record an important portion of the electromyographic signal of interest (21). Thus, caution must be exerted in using these instruments.

Partly from these limitations, some have used needle or implanted fine wire electrodes. For kinesiological study, needle electrodes are seldom used. Rather, **fine wires** are threaded through a hollow core needle and cut off at each end. At the end of the needle the wires are bent back along the shaft of the needle. After the needle is inserted and withdrawn, the wires remain in the muscle and the ends protruding through the skin are used to connect to an amplifier for purposes of recording the action potentials. This technique was used to generate the potentials shown in Figure 3.2. One advantage is considered, by some, to be ease of this technique. Disadvantages include the puncture of skin required by the needle. In addition, the wires tend to migrate within the muscle. The degree of migration is dependent upon the type of contraction and the strength of the contraction. A thorough discussion of the uses and advantages of each of these techniques is covered comprehensively in a manual on electromyography for ergonomists (17) or in the classic texts on electromyography (1). Uses of clinically relevant systems are found in many journal articles and in textbooks.

The first and most important feature of EMG display is to evaluate the **raw signal**. A sample is shown in Figure 3.8. After evaluation for quality, the signal may be electrically managed in many fashions. Some hardware instruments and nearly all worthwhile software will produce a linear envelope after the raw EMG has been full wave rectified. Another name typically applied to these linear envelopes is averaged. Others prefer to integrate the signal. Figure 3.9 shows several modes of integration available. Other forms of analysis include envelopes and procedures that create "off-on" data. No matter which signal modifications is used, the user or interpreter must be aware of the potential for artifacts: 60 cycle current, mechanical movement of lead wires, and other extraneous signals. Hence the need to first evaluate the raw EMG signal.

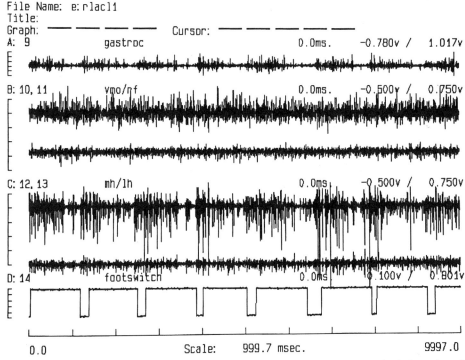

Figure 3.8. A sample record of multiple channels of raw EMG during rotation of a balance board. Muscles, from top to bottom, are gastrocnemius (*gastroc*), vastus medialis oblique (*vmo*), rectus femoris (*rf*), medial hamstrings (*mh*), lateral hamstrings (*lh*). Voltage range is provided for each signal channel and the footswitch indicates when the posteriormost point on the board contacts the supporting surface. Time is shown in milliseconds (msec).

Relationships to Muscular Tension

EMG has been most frequently used to evaluate muscle activity occurring in any given muscle. Many have attempted to relate EMG activity to muscle tension. It is generally accepted that as muscle shortens the electromyographic output increases. Although this may be due in part to an increase in fibers below the recording electrodes, the relationship generally holds. Figure 3.10 shows the EMG derived from three lengths of muscle. Note the change as the length is altered.

Because, as already introduced in Chapter 2, the total tension increases at longer muscle lengths, it is speculated that the contractile component (and subsequent EMG) is effectively reduced. Less activity from the contractile component would in fact decrease the tension so that a potentially damaging tension can be avoided.

Most evaluation of the **muscle tension-EMG relationship** has occurred during isometric contractions. Considerable evidence supports a linear relationship between electromyography and isometric contraction. However, many have shown a nonlinear relationship, depending upon the circumstances attendant to the study of isometric contractions. Representative examples are shown in Figure 3.11 (22). This between muscle difference is likely due to the type of motor units in any given muscle. As the proportion between the types of motor units vary, some effect is likely to be seen in the electromyographic record.

Of even more interest is the relationship of the EMG to muscle under dynamic conditions, such as the concentric and eccentric contraction. The general rule for these contractions is that there will be less EMG activity in eccentric than concentric contractions, when comparisons are made under similar mechanical conditions. A primary reason that activity from eccentric contractions is less is that the muscle can effectively use the elastic elements to generate tension. Refer to Chapter 2 as necessary for the relevant discussion of muscle mechanics. Thus, for the eccentric contraction to have the same amount of tension as concentric contractions, there will be less activity in the contractile component during an eccentric contraction. Others have also evaluated the relationship under conditions of constant velocity and constant tension. Figure 3.12 shows those conditions (2). This work provides a good example in that the mechanical conditions have been held constant, allowing the comparability.

Interpretation and Clinical Correlations

Anyone interpreting EMG records or data included in either the clinic or laboratory must exercise discretion in analyses of the information. Because recordings from different muscles are influenced by the amount of subcutaneous tissue, electrode configuration, orientation of muscle fibers, and other factors, extreme limitations are imposed on across channel comparisons. Comparisons between subjects are also

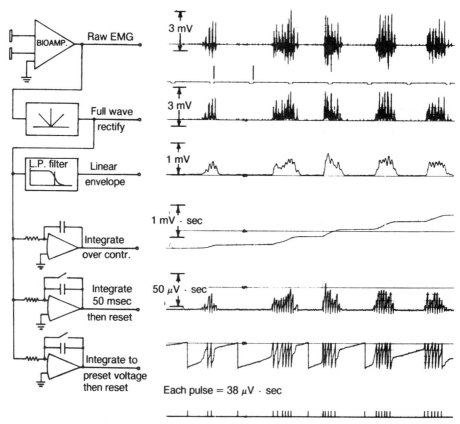

Figure 3.9. Description of the raw electromyogram and the mode of processing used to provide the output shown. The raw EMG used in the top line was used for all processing represented in the figure.

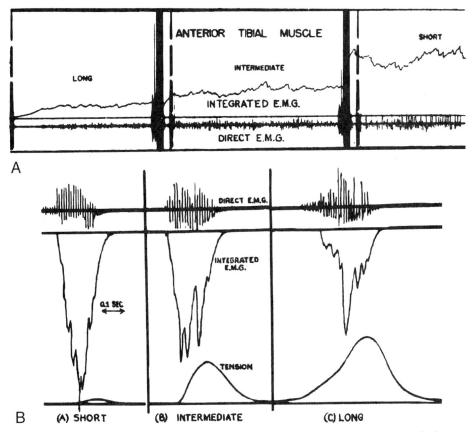

Figure 3.10.   A. Maximal voluntary isometric contractions for a normal subject. As the muscle shortens, the EMG dramatically increases. Note that the integrated EMG is really a linear envelope. **B.** The same relationship holds for the triceps muscle of the cineplastic amputee. Isometric tension is also shown.

dangerous, for similar reasons, unless care is taken in the technique and study methodology. The most common method to allow for comparisons is the normalization process where the subject performs a maximum voluntary contraction while EMG is recorded. Then, data collected during subsequent trials can be related to this quantity (for example, percentage of activity evoked during the maximum contraction). Quantified data can then be compared across subject and muscle. In pathological cases, other forms of normalization should be considered (11, 22).

The most common use of the EMG is for assessing the intensity of contraction effort. As inferred above, consideration must be given to the contraction type, the velocity of the movement, and other factors before comparisons can be made. For example, a concentric contraction versus an eccentric contraction can have the same amount of EMG but quite different levels of tension because of the role of the parallel and series elastic components in muscle. In EMG biofeedback, audio and/or light arrays indicate intensity of contraction. As the intensity of contraction increases, the sound level or the light array increases. Since the contraction level is valid only for the muscle from which the recording is being made during a single evaluation or treatment session, the between contraction comparisons can be made legitimately.

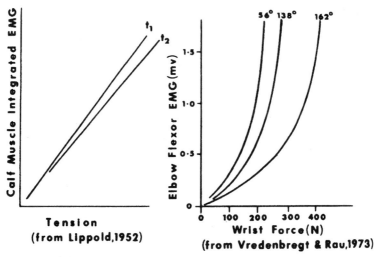

Figure 3.11. Linear (*left*) and nonlinear (*right*) relationships between amplitude of EMG and muscle tension under conditions of isometric contraction.

Thus, EMG biofeedback has great utility where patients are being trained (*a*) to vary the intensity of contraction (usually increasing), (*b*) to activate muscles or parts of muscles selectively, or (*c*) to balance the intensity of contractions of muscles acting to produce the same effect at a joint.

Another characteristic of interest is the timing, or "on-off," of the muscle or muscles of interest. This, like intensity of contraction, is also key in returning the patient to normal function: if the intensity is appropriate but ill-timed, the joint torques required to achieve normal motion will not be achieved. Perry (15) labels these temporal disturbances as premature, prolonged, continuous, curtailed, delayed, or out of phase, each representing an alteration in the timing of the contractions relative to the activity being performed. Many clinicians will be interested in the timing of muscular contractions in patients who are seen postoperatively. In at least some cases, the patient probably cannot use the proper sequence. The patient with more than mild involvement due to cerebral palsy is one example. Those who have undergone surgical transfers of muscles are another obvious example. With biofeedback patients who cannot contract during part of a range of motion may cause a limitation in joint range achieved or exacerbate a pathology (Fig. 3.13).

Once again the importance of the raw EMG signal is stressed. In interpreting data, always remember that processing can mask unwanted or inappropriate signals, including artifacts that could enter the recording system from many sources. Thus, in evaluating the literature or using EMG data be sure to validate the quality of the recording to assure of the quality of the derived signal.

SUMMARY

The neural input from the muscle is a constant factor in determining the state of responsiveness or (what some may call) muscle tone. That these neural influences play a primary role in normal and pathological motion cannot be overemphasized. The electromyographic recording can assist us with analyzing human motion but some caution must be exerted in both applications and interpretations.

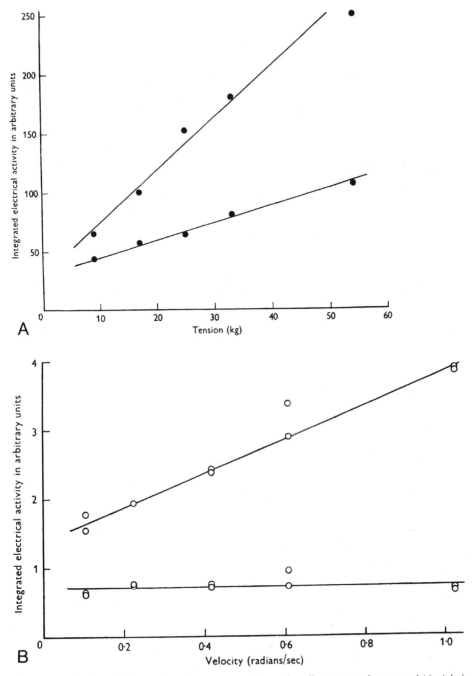

Figure 3.12. Surface EMG recordings from human calf muscle. All points are the mean of 10 trials for one subject. **A.** Integrated EMG is plotted versus tension. Concentric contraction (steeper slope) and eccentric contraction were performed at constant velocity. **B.** Integrated EMG plotted versus shortening (*above*) and lengthening at the same tension.

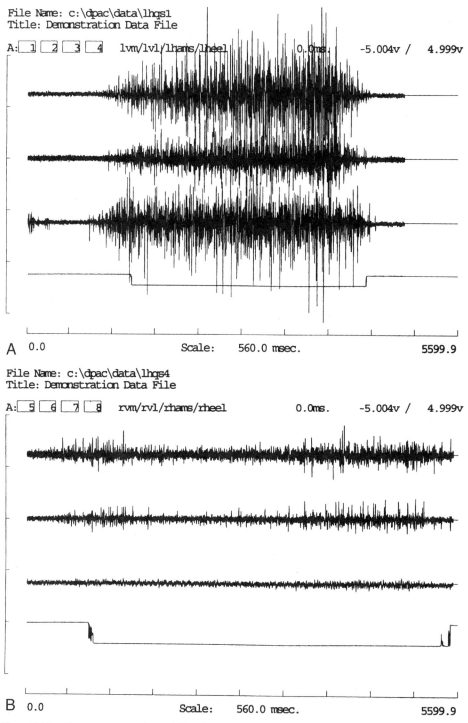

Figure 3.13. Electromyograms for (**A**) left and (**B**) right leg musculature. A marker indicates the duration of the exercise, here a quadriceps set. While comparisons across channels have limitations, note the differences during the performance of the same exercise with each leg. The right leg was symptomatic. *Legend*: *vm*, vastus medialis; *vl*, vastus lateralis; *hams*, hamstrings.

References

1. Basmajian JV. *Muscles Alive: Their Function Revealed by Electromyography*. Baltimore: Williams & Wilkins; 1979.
2. Bigland B, Lippold OCJ. The relation between force, velocity and integrated electrical activity in human muscles. *J Physiol (Lond)*. 1954;123:214–224.
3. Binder MD, Houk JC, Nichols TR, et al. Properties and segmental actions of mammalian muscle receptors: an update. *Fed Proc*. 1982;41:2907–2918.
4. Burke RE. Motor units: anatomy, physiology and functional organization. In: *Handbook of Physiology: Section 1. The Nervous System: Motor Control*. Bethesda, MD: American Physiological Society; 1981;2:345–422.
5. Edstrom L, Kugelberg E. Histochemical composition, distribution of fibres and fatiguability of single motor units. *J Neurol Neurosurg Psychiatry*. 1968;31:424–433.
6. Enoka, RM. *Neuromechanical Basis of Kinesiology*. Champaign, IL: Human Kinetics; 1988.
7. Feinstein B, Lindegard B, Nyman E, Wohlfart G. Morphological studies of motor units in normal human muscles. *Acta Anat*. 1955;23:127–142.
8. Henneman E. Functional organization of motoneuron pools: the size-principle. In: Asanuma H, Wilson VJ, eds. *Integration in the Nervous System*. Tokyo: Igaku-Shoin; 1979:13–25.
9. Inman VT, Ralston HJ, Saunders JB, et al. Relation of human electromyogram to muscular tension. *EEG Clin Neurophysiol*. 1952;4:187–194.
10. Kandel ER, Schwartz JH, Jessell TM, eds. *Principles of Neural Science*. 3rd ed. Norwalk, CT: Appleton and Lange; 1991.
11. Knutson LM, Soderberg GL, Ballantyne BT, et al. A study of various normalization procedures for within day electromyographic data. *J Electromyogr Kinesiol*. 1994;4:47–60.
12. Matthews PBC. *Mammalian Muscle Receptors and Their Central Actions*. London: Arnold; 1972.
13. Matthews PBC. Muscle spindles; their messages and their fusimotor supply. In: Brooks VB, ed. *Handbook of Physiology*. Bethesda, MD: American Physiological Society; 1981;1:189–228.
14. Milner-Brown HS, Stein RB, Yemm R. The orderly recruitment of human motor units during voluntary isometric contractions. *J Physiol (Lond)*. 1973;230:359–370.
15. Perry J. *Gait Analysis: Normal and Pathological Function*. Thorofare, NJ: Slack; 1992.
16. Segal RL, Wolf SL, DeCamp MJ, et al. Anatomical partitioning of three multiarticular human muscles. *Acta Anat*. 1991;142:261–266.
17. Soderberg GL, ed. *Selected Topics in Surface Electromyography for Use in the Occupational Setting: Expert Perspectives*. U.S. Department of Health and Human Services, Publication No. 91–100; 1992.
18. Soderberg GL, Cook TM. Electromyography in biomechanics. *Phys Ther*. 1984;64:1813–1820.
19. Soderberg GL, Dostal WF. Electromyographic study of three parts of the gluteus medius muscle during functional activities. *Phys Ther*. 1978;691–696.
20. Stauffer EK, Watt DGD, Taylor A, et al. Analysis of muscle receptor connections by spike-triggered averaging. 2. Spindle group II afferents. *J Neurophysiol*. 1976;39:1393–1402.
21. Turker KS. Electromyography: some methodological problems and issues. *Phys Ther*. 1993;73:26–37.
22. Winter DA. *Biomechanics and Motor Control of Human Movement*. 2nd ed. New York: John Wiley & Sons; 1990.
23. Wolf SL, Segal RL, English AW. Task oriented electromyographic activity from the human lateral gastrocnemius muscle. *J Electromyogr Kinesiol*. 1993;3:87–94.

4

Articular Mechanics and Function

The function of individual joints and the collective actions of many joints are responsible for the array of human motions possible. Although often appearing as remarkably simple in both form and function, any joint is a complex structure with a specific set of surfaces, all of which contribute to gross or finite movements. This chapter will focus on the structure of the typical diarthrosis and thoroughly discuss the mechanics associated with the movements of the articular surfaces of the joint. The concept of the instant center of rotation will be elucidated and theories of lubrication will be presented in terms of their impact on function. Representative pathologies and their influence upon joint function and dysfunction will also be included.

CLASSIFICATION SYSTEMS
General Terminology

Various classification systems for the description of joints have been used for many years, all for purposes of clarifying joint function. The most frequently considered factors taken into account in adoption of any of the current systems in use have included (a) the complexity and number of structures, (b) number and distribution of the axes, (c) geometric form, and (d) movements permitted. Using these factors Steindler (28) classified joints as simple and composite, discussing simple cylindrical joints such as the ankle, or screw surfaces whereby one bone moves in a progressive direction while also moving circularly. Steindler also discusses the oval surface, semicircles rotating about an axis as in the shoulder, and the saddle-like surfaces as found in the carpometacarpal joint of the thumb. In presenting another view MacConaill (19) has stated that joints should be classified as simple (two articulating surfaces), compound (three articulating surfaces), and complex (not only surfaces but also an intercapsular disc, meniscus, or fibrocartilage).

The most frequent designation of joint type is based on the form and function as they occur in the human body. Seven basic types have been identified:

plane variety—consists of flat or fairly flat surfaces such as the intermetatarsal or some of the intercarpal joints.

hinge joint or ginglymus—a uniaxial joint with strong collateral ligaments. Examples appear in the interphalangeal and ulnohumeral joints.

pivot joint—these are limited to rotation, but also have an osteoligamentous ring. These joints are usually uniaxial, such as the radioulnar joint.

condylar joint—the principal movement is in one plane but the motion also includes a small amount of rotation. The knee and temporomandibular joint are frequently used as examples.

ellipsoid or biaxial joint—joint between one convex articular surface and one concave articular surface with motion possible in two planes. Typically the rotation is limited. Examples are the radiocarpal and the metacarpal-phalangeal joints.

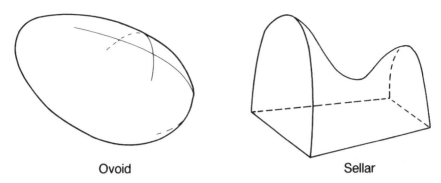

Ovoid   Sellar

Figure 4.1. General form and shape of ovoid and sellar surfaces.

saddle or sellar joints—biaxial joints with surfaces that are concavo-convex. Either surface has a convexity, but 90° to it a concave surface exists. Motions are primarily in two directions, but with some rotation existing as a by-product motion.
ball and socket, or spheroidal joint—this type is a multi-axial, egg-shaped joint such as the hip or shoulder (32).

Other terms occasionally used include **synchondrosis**, meaning that cartilaginous structures are included within the joint. A **schindylesis** means that there is one bone with a long process that fits into a groove, for example, the vomer bone in the nose. A **gomphosis** means that there is a peg inserted into a socket such as for the teeth. Of some interest to therapists are the types of **amphiarthroses**. In general, the amphiarthrosis is a limited motion articulation connected by fibrocartilage or, in the case of the synarthrosis, by ligaments. This amphiarthrosis has two varieties, **symphysis** and **syndesmosis**, the former being a joint with an all cartilaginous junction and no capsular or synovial membrane. They all lie in the midline of the body. Examples are the sternomanubrium joint and the pubic symphysis. The syndesmosis is defined as a closely interposed joint attached by ligaments (32).

Any of these classification systems contribute little to our understanding of the function of joints. Each system serves as a description of the surfaces and leads to a discussion of how the surface characteristics influence the motion.

Geometry and Mechanics

MacConaill (19) would maintain that virtually all joints have a convex and a concave surface. The **ovoid**, or egg shape, adequately describes the contours. In addition, he would state that there are **sellar**, or saddle shaped, surfaces which are concavo-convex (Fig. 4.1). Although the surfaces may vary in degree of curvature, there are no true flat or other kind of joint existing in the human body.

Kaltenborn (14) provides a somewhat different classification scheme. In classifying bony connections into synarthroses and diarthroses he further subdivides the diarthrosis into full joints or synovial joints and half joints or symphyses with a partial joint space. Articulations are further divided according to whether the range of motion exceeds 10°. The full joints, i.e., those with a range greater than 10°, are subclassified into anatomically and mechanically simple or compound joints. Table 4.1 shows a schematic view of the system (16). Another system, shown in Table 4.2, has been proposed by Wadsworth (31).

A purely mechanical approach may also be taken when considering joint function.

Table 4.1 Classification of Joints According to Kaltenborn

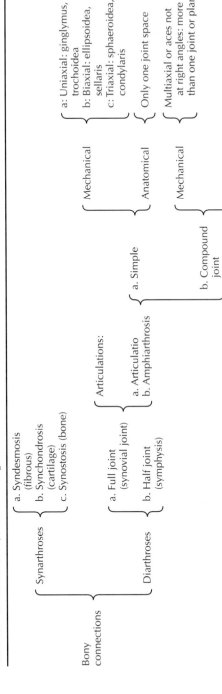

Table 4.2. Classification of Joints According to Wadsworth

Synarthroses	Fibrous
	    Suture—allows no movement
	    Syndesmosis—permits minimal movement
	Cartilaginous
	    Synchrondrosis—temporary (epiphyseal plate)
	    Symphysis—fibrocartilage

Diarthroses	Uniaxial
	    Ginglymus (hinge)
	    Trochoid (pivot)
	    Condylar
	Biaxial
	    Ellipsoid
	    Sellar (saddle)
	Multiaxial
	    Spheroid (ball and socket)
	Plane

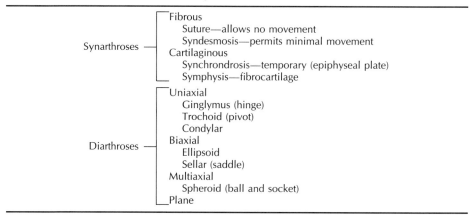

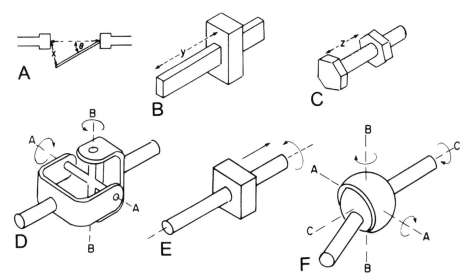

Figure 4.2. Mechanical systems with varying degrees of freedom. Distances are labeled with *x*, *y*, and *z*. **A–C.** Single degree of freedom systems. Although **C** may be interpreted to have more than a single degree, in effect the motion of the nut can be described by either the distance moved (*z*) or the number of revolutions needed to perform the excursion. **D.** Two degrees of freedom: a double hinge mechanism such as in automobile transmission systems. **E.** Two degrees of freedom: the block can both rotate or slide along it; therefore, two quantities are needed to specify the position. **F.** The ball-and-socket joint requires three quantities to specify the position of the joint.

Mechanical configurations simulating joints are shown in Figure 4.2. In these cases the motions allowed (either one, two, or three degrees of freedom) are perfectly described based on the motion allowed in the mechanical system. However, the diarthrosis is clearly the joint of most interest to practitioners. Because the features of these synovial joints are critical to the understanding of joint function, key characteristics will be described in the next section.

STRUCTURE OF SYNOVIAL JOINTS

The diarthrosis or typical synovial joint has several components fundamental to structure (Fig. 4.3) (24). In general this joint is between two bony surfaces with attached specialized hyaline cartilage. Between the two surfaces is synovial fluid, a lubricating and nutritive substance in a cavity that extends to the synovial membrane lining the fibrous capsule. These structures may influence mechanics, leading to the production of pathology as manifested in abnormal kinematics and/or kinetics. A primary structure, the articular cartilage, will be dealt with extensively in this chapter. Other components, including the synovial fluid, the meniscus or disc, the capsule, and the synovial membrane and fluid, will be dealt with less extensively but discussed in terms of importance to the understanding of pathological motion.

Articular Cartilage

Many functions have been ascribed to this aneural, alymphatic, and avascular mass nourished by synovial fluid. The main functions are to distribute loads over the joint surfaces so that the contact stresses are decreased and to allow movement with minimum friction and wear (27). Durability is exceptional. At least indirectly this specialized **hyaline cartilage** prevents damage to bone that might occur because of excessively large stress or energy inputs or from abrasive wear (15). In effect, cartilage, because of its constituents, can distribute stress more uniformly and increase the contact area across a joint. In fact, it has been shown that the elastic modulus is less for cartilage than for bone, ranging from 2 to 15 MN/m^2 as compared to 300 MN/m^2 (15). Weightman and Kempson (34) demonstrated in 1979 that cartilage can effectively reduce the maximum contact stress in a joint by 50% or more. Such findings are critical to the appreciation of the joint surfaces' ability to tolerate incessant loading: during the common weight bearing activities of walking and running, joint compression forces typically exceed five times body weight.

   The constituents of articular cartilage are responsible for adequately serving the designated functions. Included among the key features is that 60–80% of the tissue is water (3). This high water content contributes to the material properties of the tissues and participates in joint lubrication. Of the 20–40% of the wet weight made up by solid matrix, collagen fibers compose 60% and proteoglycan gel 40% of the

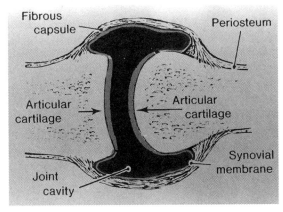

Figure 4.3.   Schematic view of a typical synovial joint. The actual joint space and the capsule are enlarged. Synovial fluid, contained in the joint cavity, serves the purposes of nutrition and lubrication.

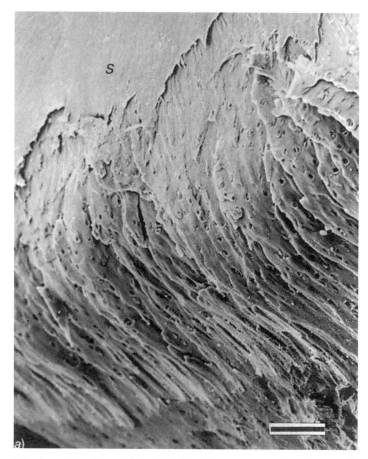

Figure 4.4.   Articular cartilage from rabbit patella. S is the intact surface. Curve is due to fibers that curve in a common direction through the transitional zone. Fibers flatten and overlap as they turn and reach a tangential orientation.

volume (3). The collagen fibers, having important tensile, stiffness, and strength properties, provide a fibrous ultrastructure for the articular cartilage.

Thickness may vary from 1 to 7 mm (32). Edwards and Chrisman thoroughly describe four zones based upon cellular arrangement (7), collagen fibril diameter and orientation matrix, water content, and proteoglycan content (3). Outermost on the articular surface, the **superficial**, or **gliding**, zone is made up of two layers, the superficial and the tangential (Fig. 4.4) (5). The superficial layer contains fine fibrils (3) and is only 200 microns thick. Principally, the collagen is randomly oriented in flat bundles of very fine fibrils. The **tangential layer**, comprising between 10 and 20% of the total cartilaginous thickness, is densely packed fibrils running parallel to the joint surface (3). One of the primary purposes of this arrangement appears to be for protection of the cartilage surface. The next deepest layer, the **transitional zone**, demonstrates an oblique orientation of the collagen bundles. This section makes up approximately 40–60% of the total depth of the cartilage. The **deep zone**, previously called the radial zone by some, contains more vertical orientation of the collagen bundles and a columnar arrangement of cartilage cells that are larger than those found in the superficial zone. Thus, in moving from superficial to deep we have noted that the water content has decreased and the proteoglycan content has increased (26). The zone of calcified cartilage, separating the softer hyaline cartilage from the stiffer subchondral bone, is the precursor to the subchondral end plate composed of dense cortical bone.

Whether or not the differences in the different zones reflect mechanical function is difficult to establish. For example, the superficial zone resists shearing forces, the transitional zone change in fibril orientation allows for the transmission of vertical loads, and the radial zone resists and distributes compressive loads. Then, the calcified cartilage provides for the transition to bone and anchors the hyaline cartilage to the bone (3). Certainly the histological data appear to support the functions desired for effective load transmission and joint function, as is discussed in the following paragraphs.

The other major constituent besides water is the **proteoglycan gel**, which has a high affinity for water. Because of the negative charge associated with these long flexible chains of disaccharides there is an apparent affinity for an osmotic swelling pressure that in effect produces a "preload" in the cartilage. Because of this property the tissue is attempting to expand outwardly, such as when a closed container has been filled under pressure. Just how the proteoglycans and collagen fibers interact has really not been absolutely determined (26). It is known, however, that even when no stress is applied to the cartilage the collagen fibers are in tension. The relatively complex interaction between these two constituents is beyond the scope of this volume and the reader is referred to the work of Maroudas (21). The swelling pressures, gradients, and permeability factors allow, however, viewing of the cartilage as a fluid filled porous medium. The mechanical features of this medium, which can be likened to a water saturated sponge, become difficult to analyze on a mechanical basis.

The primary features determining the biomechanical properties are the structure of the collagen and the permeability of the tissues. Edwards and Chrisman (7), citing the Simon et al. work from 1973, have stated that the thickness of the cartilage is related to the degree of congruence in the joint surfaces. Subsequently, the ankle and ulnohumeral articular cartilage is thin as compared to the hip and knee. Cell configuration also appears to play a role since it has been shown that the tensile stiffness in the superficial layers of cartilage were 20 times greater than in the deepest zones (16). Studies of the late 1800s as cited by Kempson (17) showed a **split line pattern** of collagen fiber alignment in the superficial layers. In verifying this work, the tensile stress-strain features in directions parallel and perpendicular to the split line pattern were evaluated (Fig. 4.5). Those specimens tested with parallel orientation had increased stiffness while the perpendicularly oriented specimens were less stiff. Thus, fiber orientation represents the ability of the cartilage to resist the maximum tensile strain produced by the compression and friction produced at the joint. Perhaps this most superficial layer of dense collagen serves as a tough, protective surface for the remainder of the tissue. While the more random orientation of the deeper fibers resists compressive loading there is still some allowance for resiliency (7).

Capsule

Generalized white collagen fibers make up the continuous series of attachments connecting the bony segments contributing to the joint. Hettinga states that the capsule consists of two parts. The outer layer, blending into the periosteum and

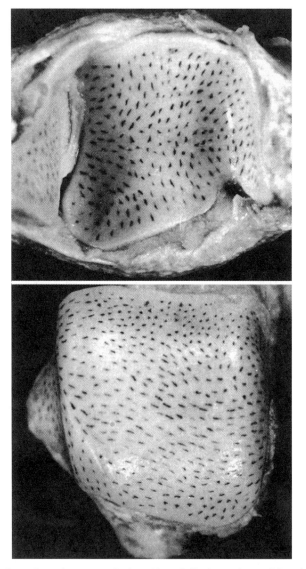

Figure 4.5. Articular surface of superior (tibial) and lateral (fibular) surfaces of the talus. These patterns are produced by multiple insertions of a needle previously immersed in India ink.

perichondrium, does not extend over the articular cartilage. Serving a protective function while enclosing the **synovial membrane**, this portion is often reinforced by tendons or slips from tendons (12). Thickenings of the capsule are frequently encountered and located for purposes of providing increased support and/or stability to the joint. Because these thickenings, known as **ligaments**, are important to joint kinematics and kinetics by virtue of inherent tensile properties, their function will be discussed in subsequent chapters discussing each joint. Accessory ligaments, however, are considered separated from capsules and may be either intracapsular or extracapsular (32).

Synovial Membrane and Fluid

This capsular lining consists of loose, highly vascularized connective tissue. The membrane encloses any bony surfaces, ligaments, or tendons that are intercapsular. The membrane is nonexistent, however, over the surfaces of discs or menisci and stops at the margins of the articular cartilage. In addition, the cellular substructure allows for location of fat pads and vascular connective tissues that are important for joint function and nutrition. Of rather specific interest is the **synovial intima**, because the cells that produce and absorb the synovial fluid are located here. The fluid, essential to joint function, is clear or pale yellow, slightly alkaline, and viscous in nature. These features are a result of the fluid being a dialysate of blood plasma with mucin added (32). The physical properties, as evaluated by a number of studies, have shown the fluid to be non-Newtonian. That is, fluids may demonstrate increasing viscosity with increasing **shear rate** or decreasing viscosity with increasing shear rate. The former, known as a dilatant fluid, is best represented by putty. At low shear rates, completed by hand molding the putty, the material is pliable, while thrown at high speeds the material has high viscosity, i.e., is hard. Conversely, a fluid such as catsup is **thixotropic**, demonstrating decreasing viscosity with increasing shear rates. Features of this fluid are best remembered by recalling that the initial flow of catsup from the bottle is far more difficult than the continuation of the flow. Because synovial fluid behaves like a thixotropic fluid the behavior is described as non-Newtonian. Figure 4.6 shows the effects of shear rate on shear stress and viscosity (2). Functions of the synovial fluid are believed to be provision of a liquid environment, maintenance of nutrition for the articular cartilage, discs, or menisci, and provision of a lubricant (32).

Disc

Contained within many synovial joints are fibrocartilaginous structures known as discs or menisci. According to *Gray's Anatomy* the latter term should be applied only to incomplete discs such as those found in the knee joint (32). At any rate these largely avascular, aneural structures are composed largely of fibrous tissue with interconnections to the fibrous capsule. Based on a comprehensive review of available literature Ghadially (10) states that few studies on the fine structure of discs and menisci have been reported. The precise functional role is as yet unclear, in spite of numerous suggestions. Among the possible functions are load absorption and distribution, improvement of fit of surfaces, limitations of joint translatory motions, and protection of the edges of articular surfaces and lubrication (32). Regardless of their exact role these structures play an intimate part in both joint kinetics and joint kinematics. Further discussion of their influence on pathology will be provided later in this chapter.

LUBRICATION

In an excellent chapter on joint lubrication Brand (2) points out the efficiency of animal joints. In the best, well-oiled metal surfaces the **coefficient of friction** is of the order of .05, and for a skate on ice about .03. Joints, however, are capable of coefficients in the range of .005–.01. Maintenance of these low coefficients is contingent upon synovial fluid, smooth articular surfaces, and appropriate mechanisms for effective lubrication. These considerations require the study of deformation of surfaces

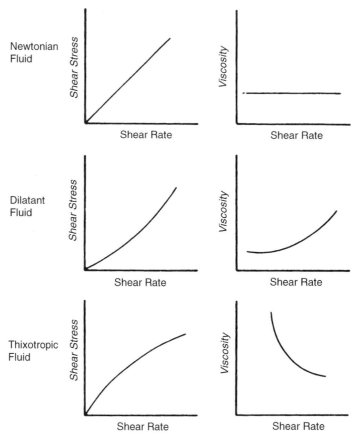

Figure 4.6.   Effects of shear rate on shear stress and viscosity for various fluids.

and flow of matter (rheology) and the study of friction, lubrication, and wear (tribology).

Many types of lubrication mechanisms exist, although Mow and colleagues (27) maintain that two fundamental types exist. One type, boundary lubrication, occurs when a synovial fluid constituent exists between the two surfaces. During motion the **lubricating glycoprotein** (lubricin) that is adsorbed onto the articular surfaces slide over each other, preventing adhesion and abrasion (Fig. 4.7) (26, 29, 30). **Fluid film lubrication** occurs when there is a thin film of lubricant between the surfaces, causing a much greater separation of the joint surfaces. Still, the distance is probably less than 25 microns (26). The pressure in the fluid thus supports the load bearing, and under stationary conditions may be known as hydrostatic lubrication. In dynamic circumstances fluid creates a lifting effect as it is pulled between the two surfaces (**hydrodynamic lubrication**). However, if the surfaces are being compressed together, such as in the knee during standing posture, fluid is squeezed out from the area between the two surfaces (**squeeze film**) (Fig. 4.8). In these latter two cases, the thickness, extent, and load bearing abilities of the fluid film are determined by viscosity, the shape of the joint surfaces, and the velocity of the relative motion of the joint surfaces. But, because the articular cartilage is relatively soft, deformation may occur, therefore changing the contact area and geometry and subsequently altering the fluid conditions. These circumstances produce **elastohydrodynamic lubrication**, enabling the surfaces to increase their load-carrying capacity (26, 27, 36).

When certain conditions of load and velocity prevail then fluid film and boundary lubrication may occur concurrently in different parts of the joint. This is mixed lubrication. Even another type, **boosted lubrication**, has been proposed, which relies

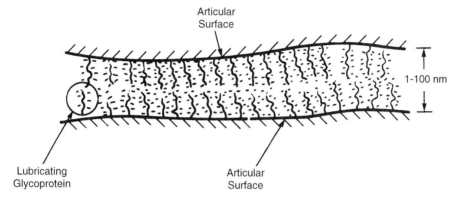

Figure 4.7. Structures relevant to boundary lubrication of the articular cartilage. The monolayer of lubricating glycoprotein adsorbed onto the articular surfaces carries the load.

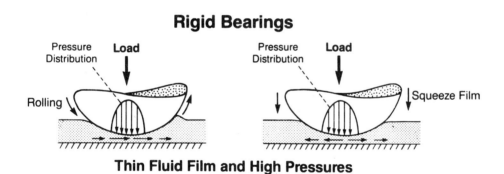

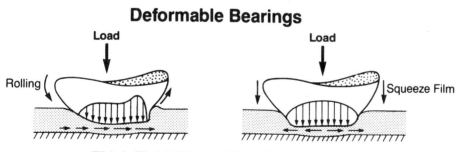

Figure 4.8. Comparison of rolling (hydrodynamic) (*top left*) and squeeze film lubrication (*top right*) of rigid surfaces, and elastohydrodynamic lubrication of deformable bearing surfaces under a roll (hydrodynamic) (*bottom left*) and a squeeze film action (*bottom right*).

on the passing of components of the synovial fluid into the articular cartilage (22). Brand points out that **boundary lubrication** may be augmented by this boosted lubrication due to cartilage porosity. This may also be governed by molecular size. The effect is to increase the viscosity of the fluid. Brand (2) also points out that during high shear the boundary level may be destroyed and, therefore, convert the lubrication mechanism back to the **hydrostatic** version that is characteristic of low speed and heavy load bearings.

In summary, mechanical transport of fluids, from a time perspective, is reasonable. However, the molecular restrictions are questionable. It seems unlikely that a single mode of lubrication can effectively respond to the large number of variables, such as load, velocity, viscosity, and geometry of bony surfaces, for which we must account. These mechanisms do, however, play a role in normal and abnormal joint kinetics and kinematics (25, 26). Demonstration of these concepts will follow in subsequent chapters.

STRUCTURE AND FUNCTIONAL JOINT MECHANICS
General Considerations

Accurate description of joint arthrokinematics has been difficult to achieve. Because of variance in surface geometry among joints, different degrees of motions are known to occur. Steindler (28) addressed several types of motion, including subfactoring of gliding motion into surface and linear types. To fit his criterion for rocking or rolling motion, equidistant points were required to touch each other in the course of the motion. Further, Steindler classified rocking combined with gliding. Axial rotation was also listed under types of joint movement.

Angular movement or rotations are also frequently used both clinically and in the literature to describe range of motion in degrees. The term circumduction is also used, conceded to be motion accomplished by a combination of motions in the three cardinal planes. Now, based on strong clinical and experimental evidence, there is consensus that both translatory and angular motions occur during virtually all joint motions. The evidence for this statement will be presented in each respective joint chapter, but for the present consider the geometry of the articular surfaces and their impact upon joint motion.

Surface Geometry and Motion

The most extensive student and author of joint geometry and resultant mechanics has been MacConaill (19, 20). He maintains, with sound anatomic and geometric data, that articular surfaces are never flat. Rather, surfaces are ovoids or compounded by more than one ovoid surface. If convex in all one direction they are referred to as male surfaces. Likewise, concave shapes are referred to as female surfaces. The other type of surface is the sellar or saddle shaped surface, described as being concave in one direction and convex in another plane (see Fig. 4.1). Although the surfaces may vary in degree of curvature, there are no true flat or other kinds of joints existing in the human body.

Movements of the bones upon each other are then described by ovoids of motion, and MacConaill uses a specific set of terminology to describe the motion. In essence, specific paths are described upon the articular surface, and, because the surface is not flat, the displacements follow a curved path, labeled as a chord or an arc. Further, all motions are classified around a "true" mechanical axis. Motions around this axis are labeled as spins while all other motions are swings. The spins that accompany certain varieties of swings are called conjunct rotations (19, 20). These rotations are inherent to the joint surfaces and a result of the concave and convex surfaces interacting as the motion is completed.

There are several key points that should be made when considering joint geometry. The first is that joint geometry is responsible for the available motions. Positioning the joint, or surfaces, in different configurations has a definite effect. Considering two ovoid surfaces one readily discovers that there is only one single position of best fit of the two surfaces. In this configuration, known as the **close-packed position**, the bones are in maximum congruence, implying that the area of contact is at a maximum. The joint is compressed by virtue of the fact that the capsule and ligaments are spiralized and tense. In this situation the surface cannot be separated by distractive force, but the position does subject the joint to possible damage. Typically, the close-packed position occurs at one extreme of most habitual movements of the joint. While there is some disagreement among the sources the following are close-packed positions for the joints most commonly involved in injury:

Shoulder	Abduction and External Rotation
Ulnohumeral	Extension
Radiohumeral	Semiflexion and Semipronation
Wrist	Dorsiflexion
Metacarpophalangeal (2–5)	Full flexion
Interphalangeal (fingers)	Extension
First carpometacarpal	Full opposition
Hip	Extension and Internal Rotation
Knee	Extension
Ankle	Dorsiflexion
Tarsal joints	Full supination
Metatarsophalangeal	Dorsiflexion
Interphalangeal (toes)	Dorsiflexion
Intervertebral	Dorsiflexion (20)

All other positions of the joint are known as the **loose-packed position**, allowing for motions referred to as spin, roll, and glide. Compared to the close-packed position this loose-packed configuration has decreased the contact area of the articular surfaces. Frequent changes in contact areas serve to decrease friction and minimize the possibility of cartilaginous erosion. The loose-packed position also provides for efficient joint lubrication and increases the available range of motion.

Because joints are maintained in the loose-packed position during most of the range of motion as conventionally known there are motions known as joint play or intrinsic motions (32). A simple demonstration of these motions can be provided by considering two ovoid surfaces (Fig. 4.9). These motions, although shown to exist through application of external forces, are part of the natural arthrokinematics of the articular surfaces. These intrinsic, or joint play movements, give yet three more degrees of freedom to the joints. Added to the three primary motions available in the cardinal planes shown to exist in virtually every joint (see Chapter 2 and subsequent chapters), a total of six degrees of freedom are available. That each of these degrees of freedom is therapeutically important has been shown by Mennell and other clinicians and will be emphasized throughout this volume (18, 23).

A second consideration relates directly to movement. Strong clinical implications also result from findings as to how one surface moves on the other. To consider the events, move the female, or concave, surface over the stationary male surface. When this motion is performed the female surface will roll and slide in the same direction as the distal end of the extremity. When the male surface is moved upon the female surface slide and roll will occur in opposite directions. The direct result is that there is an increase in the amount of angular motion possible without increasing the size of the articular surfaces. A specific example of how these mechanisms work is shown in Figure 4.10 for the knee (32). The best demonstration of this concept comes

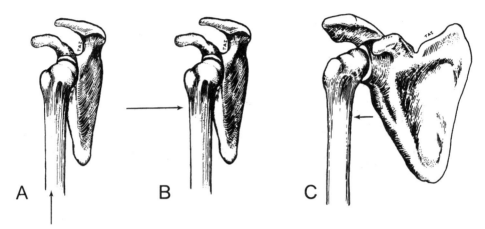

Figure 4.9. Three views of a joint consisting of one ovoid and one sellar surface. **A.** A force applied in the direction of the shaft of the bone creates a shear force, or superior glide, at the articular surface. **B.** The humerus being driven posteriorly on the glenoid creates a shear force or glide in a direction perpendicular to that in **A**. **C.** The humeral head is being distracted from the glenoid through the application of a force applied to the inner, proximal surface of the humerus.

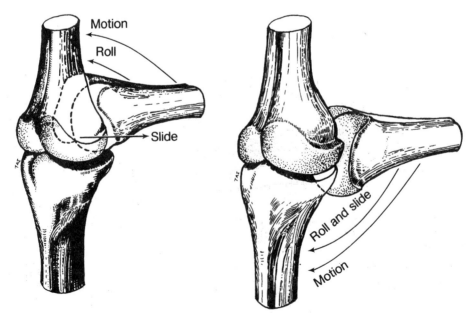

Figure 4.10. Representation of the dependency of the nature of the joint surfaces upon the motions that occur between bony surfaces. See text for a complete description.

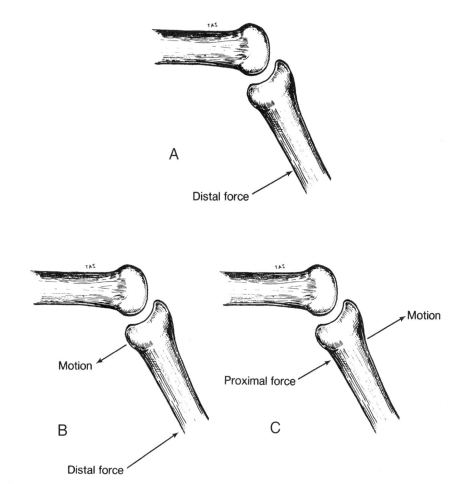

Figure 4.11. Schematic representation of the effects of incorrect and correct applications of forces when considering the arthrokinematics. **A.** Passive motion is manually applied to the bone containing the concave (female) surface. **B.** If the force is applied on the distal aspect of this segment and the joint motion is firmly restricted, say by collagenous structures in or surrounding the joint, the effect can be a levering of the female surface in a direction opposite to that desired in normal arthrokinematics. **C.** Where the force application is close to the joint, the segment can only move in the same direction as the required rolling.

through example by obtaining a femur and a tibia as independent bone segments. Place the joint in a normal congruence in the position of knee extension. Keeping the tibia fixed, flex the joint but do not accommodate for the sliding that should occur in the anterior direction. Watch as the joint dislocates when the femur falls off the posterior aspect of the tibial plateau at approximately 90° of flexion. Repeat the exercise with the anterior slide that will depict the normal mechanics, allowing the two surfaces to remain in contact.

Therapeutic Implications

For therapeutic purposes, therapists must be aware of the mechanics because the technique of application will determine the resultant motions between two articular surfaces. Use, as an example, a joint limited to 60° of flexion as shown in Figure 4.11. When passive motion is manually applied to the distal aspect of the bone

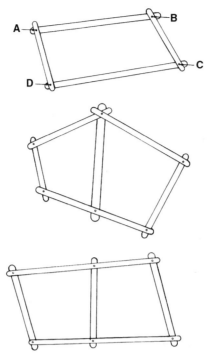

Figure 4.12. Examples of types of closed kinematic chains in which the joints shown are pinned and freely movable. The joints fixed, i.e., A, A and D, or other combinations, determine the resultant ranges of motion.

containing the concave (female) surface and the joint motion is firmly restricted (say by collagenous structures in or surrounding the joint), the effect can be a levering of the female surface in a direction opposite to that desired in normal arthrokinematics. Where the force application is close to the joint, the segment can only move in the same direction as the required rolling. The latter situation is much preferred because therapeutic effort produces the normal arthrokinematics.

Numerous examples are available in clinical situations that have the potential for producing deleterious effects at the joint and the joint surfaces. Joints that have been subjected to prolonged immobilization are commonly constrained from normal motion. Incorrect hand location to apply forces to encourage passive or actively assisted range of motion may invoke the situation seen in Figure 4.11B. Similar scenarios can be created when therapists use manual techniques to apply resistance for purposes of muscle testing. While location of the resistive force is easier on the therapist, consideration should be given to location of resistance in view of the joint arthrokinematics. Finally, in exercises performed for therapeutic purposes the location of the resistance should be monitored. One example is for knee extension exercises. If the resistance is placed distally on the lower leg segment and a strong contraction of the quadriceps is elicited, the tibia can be displaced anteriorly on the femur. Excessive motion in this direction may create unnecessary loads on the anterior cruciate ligament, which is attempting to control this displacement. Moving the resistance more proximal will provide the same therapeutic effect and allow for proper control of the joint arthrokinematics.

LINKS AND CHAINS

Use of the terms **link** and **chain** has arisen from descriptions of collective joint actions. In most practical situations multiple segments move and the joints are considered to be the centers for the connections of the various links. Therefore this concept serves a useful purpose in describing the kinematics of a multi-segment model. Certain assumptions, however, are necessary for effective use of the link segment model (11). The technique detailed by Dempster (6) and discussed in Chapter 1 is considered useful and can be important to the clinician in dealing with clinical problems. Examples specific to particular segments will be provided in the subsequent chapters on each of the joints. Gowitzke (11) and Milner and Steindler (28) discuss chains, differentiating between the closed and open systems. The closed system is operational when one link moves, which in turn causes all the other links to move in a predictable pattern (Fig. 4.12). Conversely, open systems result when the segment is not fixed, i.e., as the leg moves during the swing phase of gait. Thus, open systems are the rule for the upper extremity. In gait the lower extremities operate with **closed kinetic** and kinematic chains only to produce **open chains** during the swing phase of the extremity. In effect then, rotatory motion at the joints turns into translatory motion of the whole body. How these chains affect the practitioner will be discussed in the following chapters.

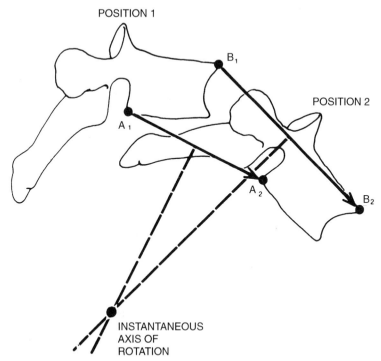

Figure 4.13. The method for construction of the instantaneous axis of rotation, also called the instant center of rotation. The same vertebrae has been moved from one position to the other. Note that the location, in this case, is not contained within the motion segment being considered.

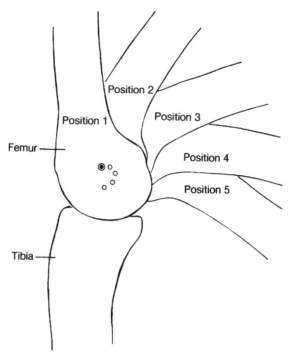

Figure 4.14. Location of the instant centers for the knee with respect to both and tibia and femur. The solid circle is the instant center for position 1.

INSTANT CENTER OF ROTATION

In practice therapists commonly measure the range of the joint motion available. To do so the concept of the instant center of rotation is important to include in the principles of measurement. This is because as a joint goes through a range of motion the location of the axis changes. The center of rotation at any point in time is considered to be the instant center of rotation, defined as the location of a point resulting from the construction of an intersection of two axes perpendicular to the plane of motion. Because the axes do change use of the instant center of rotation (**ICR**) is valuable in the correct determination of the axis around which to consider motion at any point in time. There are a number of techniques available for determining the ICR. Figure 4.13 shows a graphic technique when a segment has been moved from one location to another. Note that the landmarks selected must be readily identifiable in both positions, thus placing constraints on the ICR determinations. ICRs relative to other bony segments may also be determined. As White and Panjabi (35) point out, the ICR of any kind of plane motion, translation, rotation, or combinations of the two can be described. For other planes, similar procedures are followed. Frankel and Burstein present an excellent discussion of the procedures involved in determining the joint ICRs (8). One illustration for the knee is shown in Figure 4.14.

PATHOLOGY AS AFFECTING JOINTS

There are several reasons why pathology frequently affects joints or the materials responsible for maintaining the integrity of the joint. Articular cartilage, by virtue of location on the ends of the bones, is subject to wear because of the cyclic loading that must be tolerated to accomplish the normal activities of daily living. Alterations in the synovium will also profoundly affect the frictional factors, while trauma effectively stresses the collagenous tissues in and around the synovial joint. Each of these pathological effects will be discussed in this chapter and many will be elaborated on in subsequent chapters on the individual joints.

Ligament is the most commonly injured structure associated with the joint. The nature of the material provides protection against excessive and unwanted motion, but when excessive elongation takes place this inelastic structure is damaged. The ankle sprain and now infamous tear of the anterior cruciate ligament are perfect examples of how damage can result in abnormal function, even in spite of prolonged rehabilitation. Changes within ligament due to immobilization are discussed in Chapter 2, and relevant material properties are discussed in Chapter 5. In view of the changes that occur with injury and recovery extreme care should be given to avoid repetitive incidences of injury since chronicity will lead to further dysfunction and likely degenerative changes.

According to Mow et al. (27) wear is the removal of material from solid surfaces by means of mechanical action. Interfascial wear can take place either by adhesion or by abrasion. The former takes place when fragments are torn from one surface and adhere to another. Abrasion can occur if a soft surface is scraped by a harder surface, be it from loose particles or from an opposing surface. There is evidence that once there is destruction of the surface further softening of deeper layers of the cartilage will occur. Thus fluid movement may be altered, destroying the normal relationships and further exacerbating the abrasion process. The other type of wear, fatigue, is due to repetitive loading of the cartilage. Most injuries of this type are thought to be due to the solid matrix and/or to the fluid flow mechanisms (27). Two investigators have hypothesized that the cartilaginous failure is due to tensile failure of the collagen framework (9, 32). Defects frequently seen are splitting (or fibrillation) and erosion. There is little evidence that one type of wear is the cause of cartilaginous injury. Perhaps all mechanisms exist but that they are specific to the features of any given joint (3, 27).

There have been numerous factors identified as playing a role in joint wear. Among these factors are stress magnitude, number of applied stresses, and the molecular and microscopic structure of the solid matrix (33). For example, diminished joint contact areas often produce increased stresses at particular locations in the joint such as produced following simple meniscectomies of the knee. These increased stresses also make maintenance of the fluid film barrier more difficult, therefore increasing the chances for wear. Occupations requiring repetitive loadings may also contribute to wear mechanisms, there being some evidence among certain types of workers and athletic performers. Finally, rheumatoid arthritis may predispose patients to alterations in the matrix, leading to ultimate degeneration of the cartilage (27).

Some evidence exists that cartilage is capable, under certain circumstances, of healing by formation of fibrocartilage. Even in cases of complete fracture, fibrous tissue with an overlay of polysaccharides may closely resemble the original hyaline cartilage. Hettinga (13) details many of the gross and cellular changes that occur due to injury of the cartilage. Caution must be exercised in dealing with these injuries so that the regeneration process may proceed without sacrificing joint mobility.

Interarticular discs are frequently injured, primarily in the knee. As to be expected, most injuries result from the application of greater stresses than the tissue can tolerate. Rotation and/or medial-lateral stress applied to this joint while bearing body weight is the classic position for the production of the torn meniscus. And, because of the avascular nature of the fibrocartilage, primarily in the central portions, healing does not occur. Peripheral displacements are complicated by concurrent injury of the synovium, leading to effusion. Healing of the peripheral portion of the meniscus is accomplished by infiltration of fibrous tissue (4).

Injuries to the capsule are of importance because involvement of the synovial membrane can potentially produce chronic effusions and long-term disabilities of considerable magnitude. Hettinga (12) summarizes the inflammatory responses to be a proliferation of surface cells, an increase in the vascularity, and a gradual fibrosis of the subsynovial tissue. Posttraumatic synovitis may also be differentiated from other inflammatory and degenerative changes. In this case the synovial membrane has become thicker. Synovial fluid changes also appear, as do changes in the blood vessels. Fibrosis of the synovial membrane was concurrently noted as mature, densely packed collagen fibers formed up to the synovial surface. Continuation of the symptoms also has been blamed for other cellular and functional changes.

Lubrication of artificial joint surfaces has also been of some interest. Brand (2) discusses the work relative to the findings and their influence on joint mechanics. Although indicating that lubrication problems are of less magnitude than other changes that occur, considerable work has been done on polyvinylpyrrolidone and silicone oil. Each has been demonstrated to be less effective than synovial fluid, however, indicating that further work needs to be done before fruitful results are available.

SUMMARY

Diarthrodial joints are of importance because of the dependency of the human body upon their delivering normal motion. Normal mechanics are frequently negated by traumatic or degenerative processes, thereby creating pathological motion that must be treated with anticipation of correction. While many pathologies are specific to individual joints, this chapter has discussed the basic structure and function of joints so that each can be more thoroughly discussed in subsequent chapters.

References

1. Alexander RM. Mechanics of skeleton and tendons. In: Brooks VB, ed. *Handbook of Physiology, Section 1: The Nervous System.* Bethesda, MD: American Physiology Society; 1981;2:17.
2. Brand RA. Joint lubrication. In: Albright JA, Brand RA, eds. *The Scientific Basis of Orthopedics.* New York: Appleton Century Crofts; 1987:373–386.
3. Buckwalter J, Hunziker E, Rosenberg L, et al. Articular cartilage: composition and structure. In: Woo SL-Y, Buckwalter JA, eds. *Injury and Repair of the Musculoskeletal Soft Tissues.* Park Ridge, IL: American Academy of Orthopaedic Surgeons; 1988:405–425.
4. Calliet R. *Soft Tissue Pain and Disability.* Philadelphia: FA Davis; 1977.
5. Clark, JM. The organisation of collagen fibrils in the superficial zones of articular cartilage. *J Anat.* 1990;171:117–130.
6. Dempster W. *Space Requirements of the Seated Operator.* Washington, DC: Office of Technical Services, US Dept of Commerce; 1955. WADC Technical Report 55-159.
7. Edwards CC, Chrisman OD. Articular cartilage. In: Albright JA, Brand RA, eds. *The Scientific Basis of Orthopedics.* New York: Appleton-Century-Crofts; 1979:313–348.
8. Frankel VH, Burstein AH. *Orthopedic Biomechanics.* Philadelphia: Lea & Febiger; 1970.
9. Freeman MAR. The fatigue of cartilage in the pathogenesis of osteoarthritis. *Acta Orthop Scand.* 1975;46:323–328.
10. Ghadially FN. Fine structure of joints. In: Sokoloff L, ed. *The Joints and Synovial Fluid.* New York: Academic Press; 1978;1:105–176.

11. Gowitzke BA, Milner M. *Understanding the Scientific Bases of Human Movement.* 3rd ed. Baltimore: Williams & Wilkins; 1988.

12. Hettinga DL. II. Normal joint structure and their reaction to injury. *J Ortho Sports Phys Ther.* 1979;1:83–88.

13. Hettinga DL. III. Normal joint structure and their reaction to injury. *J Ortho Sports Phys Ther.* 1980;2:178–185.

14. Kaltenborn FM. *Manual Therapy for the Extremity Joints.* Oslo, Norway: Olaf Norlis Bokhandel; 1976.

15. Kempson GE. The mechanical properties of articular cartilage. In: Sokoloff L, ed. *The Joints and Synovial Fluid.* New York: Academic Press; 1978;2:177–239.

16. Kempson GE, Freeman MAR, Swanson SAV. Tensile properties of articular cartilage. *Nature.* 1968;220:1127–1128.

17. Kempson GE, Spivery CJ, Swanson SAV, et al. Patterns of cartilage stiffness on normal and degenerate human femoral heads. *J Biomech.* 1971;4:597–609.

18. Kessler RM, Hertling D. *Management of Musculoskeletal Disorders.* Philadelphia: Harper & Row; 1983.

19. MacConaill MA. The movements of bones and joints: 5. The significance of shape. *J Bone Joint Surg.* 1953;35(B):290–297.

20. MacConaill MA, Basmajian JV. *Muscles and Movements: A Basis for Human Kinesiology.* Baltimore: Williams & Wilkins; 1977.

21. Maroudas A. Balance between swelling pressure and collagen tension in normal and degenerate cartilage. *Nature.* 1976;260:808–809.

22. Maroudas A. Hyaluronic acid film. *Proc Inst Mech Eng.* 1967;181:122.

23. Mennell JMc. *Joint Pain.* London, England: Churchill-Livingstone; 1964.

24. Moore KL. *Clinically Oriented Anatomy.* Baltimore: Williams & Wilkins; 1985.

25. Mow VC, Ateshian GA, Spilker RL. Biomechanics of diarthrodial joints: a review of twenty years of progress. *J Biomed Eng.* 1993;115:460–467.

26. Mow VC, Rosenwasser M. Articular cartilage: biomechanics. In: Woo SL-Y, Buckwalter JA, eds. *Injury and Repair of the Musculoskeletal Soft Tissues.* Park Ridge, IL: American Academy of Orthopaedic Surgeons; 1988:427–463.

27. Mow VC, Roth V, Armstrong CG. Biomechanics of joint cartilage. In: Frankel VH, Nordin M. *Basic Biomechanics of the Skeletal System.* Philadelphia: Lea & Febiger; 1980:61–86.

28. Steindler A. *Kinesiology of the Human Body under Normal and Pathological Conditions.* Springfield, IL: Charles C Thomas; 1955.

29. Swann DA, Radin EL, Hendren RB. The lubrication of articular cartilage by synovial fluid glycoproteins. *Arthritis Rheum.* 1979;22:665–666. Abstract.

30. Swann DA, Silver FH, Slayter HS, et al. The molecular structure and lubricating activity of lubricin isolated from bovine and human synovial fluids. *Biochem J.* 1985;225:195–201.

31. Wadsworth C. *Manual Examination and Treatment of the Spine and Extremities.* Baltimore: Williams & Wilkins; 1988.

32. Warwick R, Williams PL, Dyson M, et al., eds. *Gray's Anatomy.* 37th British ed. Philadelphia: WB Saunders; 1989.

33. Weightman B. Tensile fatigue of human articular cartilage. *J Biomech.* 1976;9:193–200.

34. Weightman BO, Kempson GE. Load carriage. In: Freeman MAR, ed. *Adult Articular Cartilage.* London, England: Pitman; 1979.

35. White AA, Panjabi MM. *Clinical Biomechanics of the Spine.* 2nd ed. Philadelphia: JB Lippincott; 1990.

36. Wright V, Radin EL. *Mechanics of Human Joints: Physiology, Pathophysiology, and Treatment.* New York: Marcel Dekker; 1993.

5

Material Properties of Biological Tissues

An understanding of materials and their properties is important because therapists will deal with many pathologies produced by acute loading. Other tissue failures will result from repetitive loading that creates stresses within tissues. Material properties are also a factor in joint prostheses and their retention in the human body. The properties of tissue are also very significant in cases of burns and in such common afflictions as capsulitis. Lumbar discs, in particular, are known to have material properties altered because of degenerative processes. Further, fracture repair and the management of scoliosis are both significantly affected by applied forces. This chapter will present basic definitions necessary to understand the reactions of biological tissues to applied forces. Properties of tissues, including bone, muscle, ligament, and cartilage, will be discussed. Finally, how the properties affect normal and pathological motion will be presented. While the content of this chapter may seem beyond the limits of the student's precept of professional practice, applications abound. These applications will come forth in each chapter on the joints. Reference back to and diligent pursuit of the concepts in this chapter may be required during reading of subsequent chapters. Only when applications are made to the pathologies associated with total movement or specific joints will these concepts become solidified.

FORCES, LOADS, AND STRESS
Definitions

Biological materials are constantly subjected to contact or remote forces. By definition, a **force** is the action or effect of one body on another. Because, as noted in Chapter 1, these forces are vector quantities, they have magnitude, a point and line of application, and direction. Recall also from Chapter 1 that where the force is applied will determine whether rotational or linear movement will potentially or actually occur. While one may think that we are interested primarily in force created by muscle, the forces created by muscles on other tissues can reach surprising levels. For example, muscle contractions add significantly to forces at joint surfaces. Further, forces from outside the body, such as another person falling on the outside of a knee, can cause considerable trauma because the tissues cannot withstand the forces applied. Even more examples come from the work environment, where repetitive motion, often of a high frequency, creates stress in tissue, resulting in an overuse syndrome that creates pathological effects.

Usually, and for purposes associated with management of patients, forces can be a push or pull, a tendency to compress, or an application of tension to a structure. Five types of forces have been identified:

Compression—the act of pressing together
Tension—the normal force tending to stretch or pull a body apart
Bending—deformation due to loading of a structure when load is applied at an area where no direct support exists

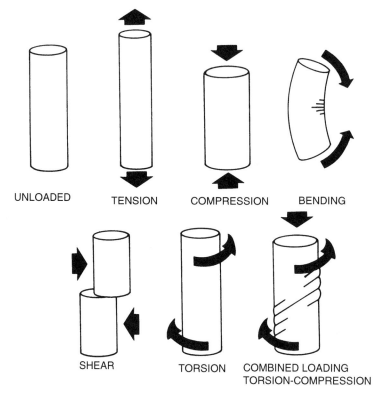

UNLOADED   TENSION   COMPRESSION   BENDING

SHEAR   TORSION   COMBINED LOADING
TORSION-COMPRESSION

Figure 5.1.   Representation of various loading modes.

Torsion—the force tending to twist a body
Shear—forces that act like the cutting action of a scissors. That is, the force is applied parallel to the surface or plane within an object.

Representations of these forces are shown in Figure 5.1 (8).

Two other terms are commonly encountered when forces are described. The first, **normal**, means that force is applied perpendicular to a surface or a plane within an object. An example of normal loads is shown in the tension and compression modes in Figure 5.1. An **axial** force is one applied along the long axis of the body or object being considered. In Figure 5.1 both the tension and compression modes are also axial since they are applied along the long axis.

Applications

Examples of ways these forces are applied to biological tissues may be helpful in understanding the effect of the force. Before doing so, however, some understanding of stress and strain is necessary. One may define **stress** as the intermolecular resistance within a body to the deforming actions of an outside force or as a "uniformly distributed force acting on a particular small surface of a defined block of material" (2). Stress is measured in units of newtons/meter^2 because its intensity is a result of the magnitude of the force divided by the surface area over which the force acts. Note that in the international system of units 1 newton/meter^2 is a **pascal** (Pa) (see Table 1.1). The symbol used for identification is the Greek letter sigma (σ). The other measure of import is **strain**, the measure of deformation, describing the change in the dimensions of a body because of load application. Designation is by means of the epsilon (ε). For both stress and strain two types are possible. By definition, recall that normal stress or strain occurs perpendicular to the plane of the cross section of the loaded object. Shear stress or strain occurs parallel to the plane of the applied load (Fig. 5.2).

Loading, defined as the application of a force and/or moment to a structure, can be applied to produce **compression**, causing the structure to shorten and widen. Both compressive stress and strain occur within the structure, and according to Frankel and Nordin (8), maximal compressive stress occurs on a plane perpendicular to the applied load. The skeletal system is commonly loaded in compression during weight bearing by the lower extremities, but note that any time a structure is undergoing bending, compression must always occur on the concave surface (Fig. 5.3). Muscle contractions across joints that are fully extended also are responsible for increasing compressive load across joints. Specific examples of the effect of this mechanism will be discussed in the chapters on each joint.

In **tension**, stress and strain also occur in materials. Maximal tensile stress occurs, as for compression, in a plane perpendicular to the applied load as the structure

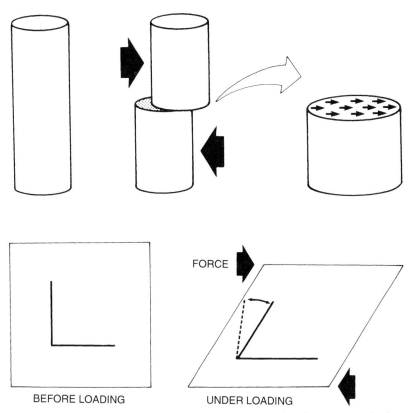

Figure 5.2. Shear loading and the stress and strain occurring within the structure. The bottom two structures show that when loading occurs in shear, lines change their orientation, the angle formed becoming obtuse or acute. This change indicates shear.

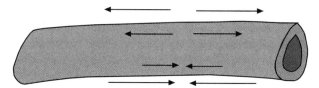

Figure 5.3.   Bone undergoing bending.

now narrows and elongates. Tensile force occurs in the convex side of a long bone undergoing bending (see Fig. 5.3). Muscles also generate tensile forces within the muscle proper and into the tendon. Thus, a normal stress is created. The elasticity of the tissue reacts to the strain imposed by the elongation created by contraction. During shearing internal deformation causes the tissue to change internally. This demonstrable shear, shown in Figure 5.2, is also shown in Figure 5.4. In the latter case note that tension and compression also produce shear strain. Most human tissues are subjected to shear forces. Menisci of the knee are very vulnerable and must accommodate the twisting of the femur on the tibia. Anterior or posterior displacement of the tibia on the femur would have a similar effect (8, 9, 37).

   Bending, as indicated above, creates both compression and tension forces. However, at the neutral or central axis there are no stresses or strains. Moving away from the central axis, the stresses increase in proportion to the distance moved (see Fig. 5.3). Throughout the body bending forces are regularly produced. This bending motion is resisted by the very nature of the structure and is usually not readily discernible as gross motion. Individual bones are continually subjected to bending forces but only in extreme cases would a fracture result.

   Torsional forces, by nature of application, cause shear stress distribution over the

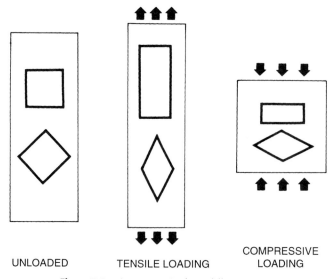

UNLOADED   TENSILE LOADING   COMPRESSIVE LOADING

Figure 5.4.   A structure in three different states.

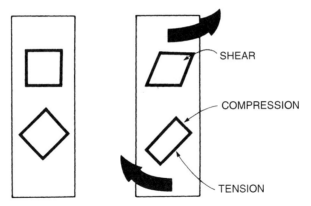

Figure 5.5. Segment of bone unloaded (*left*) and then loaded (*right*) in torsion.

entire material. Similar to bending, stresses are increased as the distance from the axis of rotation is increased. With the application of torsional forces the maximal shear stress is on the plane perpendicular to the axis of rotation (Fig. 5.5). Also note in Figure 5.5 that the tensile and compressive stresses are on a plane diagonal to the neutral axis. These forces are commonly seen in compound fractures, classic examples being provided by the lower extremity fractures in downhill skiers. Any of these five types of forces can occur in a pure sense, but most frequently they occur in combinations (see Fig. 5.1), particularly in producing pathological situations (8, 9, 37).

Forces and Loads

The distinction between forces and loads is often confusing. Forces are any action that changes the shape, size, or state of inertia or the motion of a body (37). A load is a force or moment applied to the material. In a strict sense, loads should be considered as torsional, bending, normal, or shear. **Buckling loads** are sometimes also mentioned. The application of muscle tension to a bone in fact applies a load to the bone. Units are total load, such as 1000 lbf, or unit load, such as 200 psi. More typical units are newtons/meters^2. No matter the specific classification system used, the terminology should be consistently applied in relation to the human tissues being discussed.

Interaction of Forces, Loads, and Stress

Normal forces are force components directed perpendicular to the surface upon which they act. Shear forces are force components directed parallel to the surface on which they act. Bending moments are moment components directed parallel to the surface on which they act. Torsional moments or torques are moment components directed perpendicular to the surface on which they act. Stress and strain produce the resultant configuration of the tissues and are dependent on how the forces are applied.

LOAD-DEFORMATION AND STRESS-STRAIN

Behavior of materials is often described by means of relating an applied load to the amount of deformation that occurs in the material or tissue (**load deformation** or **elongation**). From the resulting plot shown in Figure 5.6 several key characteristics

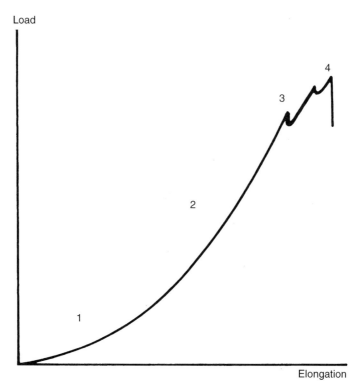

Figure 5.6. Load-elongation curve. 1, toe region; 2, linear region; 3, failure of fiber bundles; and 4, failure point.

may be evaluated. One is the degree of tissue **stiffness**, defined as the resistance offered to external loads by a specimen or structure as it deforms. The degree of stiffness is indicated by the slope of the line of the early part of the curve. Note that if the load is increased and decreased the deformation is linear. This results in the classification of the material as "**elastic**." If too great a load is applied, however, the tissue becomes permanently deformed and the **elastic limit** is said to have been exceeded. Even further loading will cause the **failure point** (strength) of the material to be reached (8, 9).

Using standardized techniques, i.e., such as during a clinical tension or compression test, the load per unit area and the amount of deformation can be determined. Recognize that loading is the manner of force application and that stress is obtained by dividing the load by the cross-sectional area (37). Thus, stress is not directly measured but derived. Elongation in tissue is used to derive strain in that the deformation, or change in length, is divided by the value of the original length of the material.

The derivation and plotting of these stress and strain values produces a **stress-strain curve**. The resulting relationship, stress divided by strain, represents the mechanical behavior of a material. Samples of stress-strain curves are shown in Figure 5.7, displaying configurations similar to those of the load-deformation curve. The differences in stiffness are readily shown by the differences in the slopes during the portion of the curve demonstrating elasticity. That is, the slope of the linear elastic part of the stress-strain diagram (Modulus of Elasticity or Young's Modulus) varies with the material being tested (2). On each of the plots the yield point also occurs at a location specific to the material being tested. The **yield point** is that point where progressive deformation occurs without increasing the load on the material. The soft metal has a great deal of deformation, whereas glass would be considered a **brittle** material since little deformation occurs before failure. While many examples of stress-strain curves abound in the literature, specific applications to each joint will be presented in subsequent chapters.

Two other measures should be noted. One is **Poisson's ratio** (or **effect**). This measure is the ratio of transverse to axial strain. An example is how a rubber band changes upon stretch, becoming thinner, yet longer. In orthopaedic practice when a screw is used to secure a fracture, the bone is compressed and the screw is lengthened as the screw is tightened. Simultaneously the thread diameter in the bone expands and the screw diameter decreases. The resulting unitless ratio quantifies the behavior of the material (37). The other measure is the **modulus of rigidity** (or **shear modulus**), defined as the ratio of shear stress to shear strain. The resulting quantity can be used as a "measure of the resistance of a material to distortion when placed under load" (2). For therapists the uses of these latter two quantities are neither common nor of much practical consequence.

OTHER PROPERTIES

Other terms that may be used in describing stress-strain properties include **plastic**, essentially meaning non-elastic, and **ductility**, meaning that the material has the capacity to absorb large amounts of plastic deformation energy before failure. Two other properties of significance to normal and pathological motion are the concepts of creep and relaxation. **Creep**, the increase in strain with time under constant load, is applicable in cases where tissue elongation is attempted. Cases of serial cast application for clubfoot or for treatment of scoliosis are excellent examples of the direct application of methods used to alter tissue properties. Principles of **relaxation**

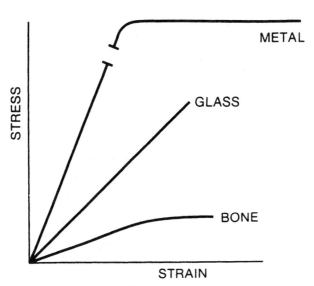

Figure 5.7. Stress-strain curves for metal, glass, and bone. Note that bone is not linearly elastic in behavior. The soft metal, being ductile, has a long plastic region. Glass, having no plastic region, is brittle.

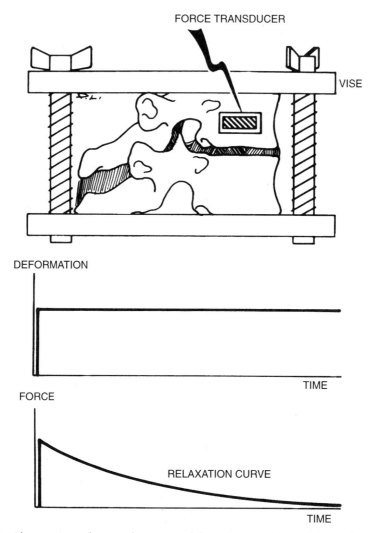

Figure 5.8. The experimental set up, the constant deformation over time, and the resulting relaxation curve are shown from top to bottom.

can also be demonstrated by means of evaluating the effects of stress on tissues. White and Panjabi, defining relaxation as the decrease in stress in a deformed structure with time when the deformation is held constant, use the stress diminution in a vertebral body as an example. Figure 5.8 shows the experimental conditions, showing the constant deformation with time. Concurrently, the force in the specimen, as revealed by the force transducer, diminishes with time. The resulting decrease in stress with time shows relaxation (37). Both connective and muscle tissue demonstrate considerable amounts of creep and relaxation (24). Specific illustrations and their associations with pathologies will be forthcoming in subsequent chapters.

Resilience, damping, and viscosity are also important. **Resilience** is the ability of an object to rebound from a surface or another object. Tennis balls demonstrate much greater resilience than do nylon, foam, or plastic materials. Lead would be considered nonresilient. Examples of different states of resiliency are shown in Figure 5.9. In damping, the opposite of resiliency, the material would return to original shape slowly.

Also shown in Figure 5.9 is hysteresis, an important characteristic because many human tissues of interest to therapists are viscoelastic materials. **Viscoelasticity** means that the behavior of the material is time dependent compared with loading and unloading. Muscle is clearly a viscoelastic substance, as are other tissues in the body. By definition **hysteresis** is the phenomenon associated with energy loss exhibited by viscoelastic materials when subjected to loading and unloading cycles. The actual energy loss is from the differences in the strain energy stored and released during the loading and unloading cycles, respectively. This dissipation of energy is believed to be from mechanical damage to the tissue and from internal friction (see Fig. 5.9) (2).

Each of the material properties that exist in human tissues affects human motion, particularly when the tissue is impaired from injury or response to a pathology. The concepts presented in this section will be discussed further in the applications section of this chapter, and how the principles are applied to each joint will be discussed within each respective chapter.

PROPERTIES OF HUMAN TISSUES

The properties of tissues vary depending on the available collagen, elastin, and other constituents, as well as on the structural arrangement and proportion of these

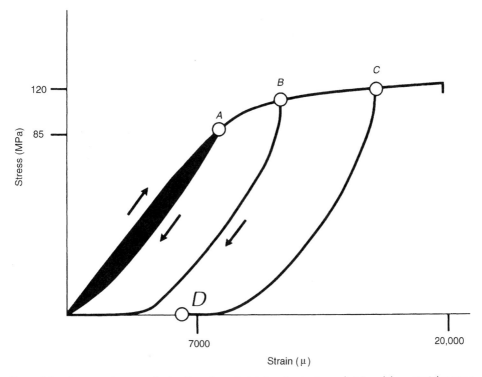

Figure 5.9.   Stress-strain curves for loading of a material. Loading is stopped at *A* and the material returns to the original configuration. After loading to *B* the material returns in a different pattern. When loaded to *C* the material only returns to point *D*. Shading for the load to *A* and release represents hysteresis.

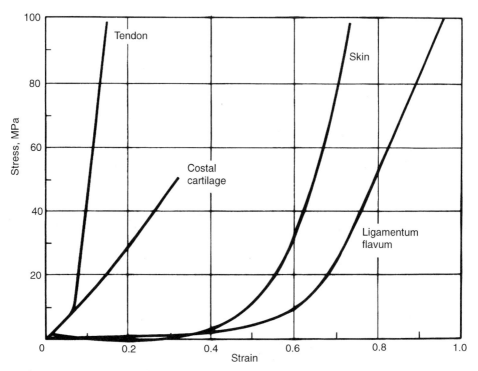

Figure 5.10.   Stress-strain plots for various human connective tissues tested in uniaxial tensions.

elements. Each tissue's material properties can be examined by applying specific tests to the tissue of interest. For example, stress-strain tests applied to various structures produce the forms shown in Figure 5.10 (8). The properties of the most common types of tissue are discussed in the following sections.

Bone

Bone is a specialized connective tissue of which collagen makes up approximately 95% of the extracellular matrix. Mineral content is made up primarily of calcium and phosphate (23). The mechanical properties of bone differ between cortical bone and cancellous bone, the former being stiffer than the latter (3). In actuality bone is subjected to forces and moments from various directions, resulting in a variety of changes in the structure; usually a fracture results if a great enough force or moment has been applied. Cortical bone responds differently depending on the direction of the force applied. This is called **anisotropic** behavior; that is, the mechanical properties vary with different spatial orientations. Frost (9) has suggested that for bone the proportional limit and rupture strength are approximately equal. Because the proportional limit is the greatest stress at which stress is still proportional to strain, bone is classified as a brittle material. Caution must be exercised, however, because strength will depend upon the loading mechanism. For example, shear strength is approximately 4,000 psi, tensile strength 12,000 psi, and compressive strength 15,000 psi. Further, bone is also viscoelastic. Thus, the biomechanical behavior varies depending on the rate of loading. In turn, the rate of loading influences both the fracture pattern and the amount of soft tissue damage.

Because of existing material properties, bone is seldom deformed greater than 3% and the tensile forces to fracture are generally less than the compressive forces. Age, sex, wetness, and other elements are also factors in influencing the material properties. Yamada (38) provides a thorough presentation of mechanical test data on all types of bone. Many investigators have established that cellular structure has adjusted to accommodate for the needs of the bone to bear loads. Trabecular structure through the femoral neck is configured in a pattern that will effectively resist the large bending moments. Further, that bone responds by adaptive remodeling has been shown (4).

Finally, because of intrinsic properties bone is also subject to failures from fatigue (24). Most common are those that occur in bones of the foot, but some evidence exists that these fractures are responsible for painful syndromes of the lower leg resulting from fractures of the tibia and fibula. Fatigue failure is also of interest because some pathologies are directly related to stresses and strains resulting from activities requiring the performance of cyclic loading.

Cartilage

Articular cartilage has a large amount of water retained within the tissue, up to 75% in the hyaline form (6, 9). Thus, cartilage can respond to loads as a viscoelastic material. The proteoglycans are largely responsible for holding water, but are also a key factor in holding the water osmotically and through controlling matrix permeability. This control of "swelling pressure" amounts to restrictions associated with fluid flow (21). Therefore, by controlling this flow the mechanical characteristics are influenced. For example, during a prolonged mechanical load, fluid will move within the tissue and be exuded by the tissue (17). So, as the rate of exudation varies over time the creep characteristics of the articular cartilage present different features than those of other viscoelastic materials (20).

Further, because of the low permeability the behavior is also dependent upon the rate at which loads are applied and removed. In rapid loading little time is available for exchange of fluid, so the cartilage acts as an elastic material. Some creep follows this elastic phase. Because the cartilage has properties of a viscoelastic material, the response is time dependent. That is, when rapidly loaded, the initial stiffness is high, followed by deformation over a longer interval of time (8). Conversely, during prolonged loading such as standing, deformation will occur with time, squeezing fluid out. In either case, as the load is removed, the cartilage will return to the original configuration. Nordin and Frankel (24) presents a comprehensive evaluation of the behavior of this tissue under a variety of loading conditions.

Cartilaginous tissue is also important in pathologies because the tissue is subjected to wear and degenerative changes. Cellular makeup of articular cartilage was discussed in Chapter 4. While the peripheral cellular orientation is adeptly suited to resist shear forces of articular surfaces, circumstances arise that are not controllable by the tissue. For example, for almost 40 years evidence has accumulated that suggests that articular cartilage deforms almost instantaneously upon application of loads. However, if loads are applied so quickly that there is inadequate time for internal fluid redistribution to relieve the compacted region, then the high stresses could cause damage (24). In addition, **adhesive or abrasive wear** can occur due to surface fragments or a harder surface coming into contact with the other.

Degeneration of cartilage is also a significant clinical problem, and as the number of persons who are aged increases, the incidence of the arthritides is highly likely to increase. The magnitude of stress in cartilage is determined by the total load on

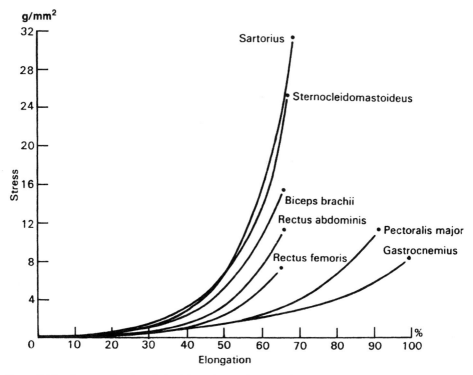

Figure 5.11. Stress-strain plots derived from the application of tension to skeletal muscle in 29-year-old subjects.

the joint and how the load is distributed over the joint contact area. Thus, any change in these two factors would lead to increased stress in the cartilage. Examples would include poor joint congruity, loss of menisci, dysplasia, and such things as fractures that result in disrupted arthrokinematics (24). Add to these possibilities those who are subjected to particularly high loads or increased loading frequency. Based on these factors interest in the segment of the population that has taken up running during the last decade will surely increase.

Muscle

Mechanical properties of muscle have also been determined. The features attendant to behavior of muscle have been thoroughly addressed in Chapter 2. As for other tissues the specifics of the properties will depend on the muscle evaluated and on age. Yamada (38) has evaluated the stress-strain features of several muscles of humans (Fig. 5.11). Further, since muscle is essentially a viscous structure surrounded by an elastic membrane, the properties are therefore similar to other viscoelastic materials. The difficulty in arriving at precise properties for muscle is due to tendinous attachments at one or both ends of the muscle. Of the muscles tested the sartorius appears to have the greatest ultimate strength while the gastrocnemius and the rectus femoris have the least. Further, ultimate strength is greatest in thin muscle than in thick as well as in extensor muscles as opposed to flexor muscles (38).

Collagen

Common to ligament, tendon, and skin is collagenous tissue. Incorporated within these tissues are three types of fibers, collagen for strength, elastic for elastic properties, and reticulin for bulk (36). A fourth, but less important, component is the ground substance.

According to Frankel and Nordin (24) the behavior of collagen is affected by three factors. First is the fiber orientation. The organization of collagen in tendon, ligament, and skin is remarkably different (Fig. 5.12). Because of the parallel fiber orientation, tendon can bear the highest tensile loads. The skin, with a more diverse arrangement of fibers, is more extensible for the allowance of tension, compression, and shear. Ligamentous behavior would be somewhere between tendon and skin although certainly designed to tolerate tensile loading.

The second factor important to tissue behavior is the properties of the individual collagen and elastic fibers. These two factors make up approximately 90% of the tissue. The collagen is ductile while the elastic fibers are brittle. This can be shown in plots of stress-strain behavior, from which grossly different features are readily discernible (Fig. 5.13). Besides the overall shape of the curves, note also that the percentage of strain axes for the two tissues is of extremely different magnitude.

The third factor that determines behavior is the relative proportion of the collagen and elastic fibers. The proportion is usually according to function. For example, tendons are nearly all collagen. Thus, great loads can be tolerated without a large degree of tendon deformation as tension is developed within the muscle. According to some, the percentage of elastic recovery in certain ligaments is as high as 99% (38). Fielding and colleagues, as cited by Frankel and Nordin (8), have shown that ligaments are also mainly collagen while the ligamentum nuchae and ligamentum flavum are made up of more than 60% elastic fibers. As a result, ligamentous strength is directly related to the number of fibers and the thickness and width of the fibers. During testing, and probably during function and/or injury, note that the elastic limit approximately equals the ultimate strength.

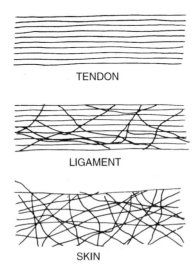

TENDON

LIGAMENT

SKIN

Figure 5.12. Orientation of collagen fibers in tendon, ligament, and skin.

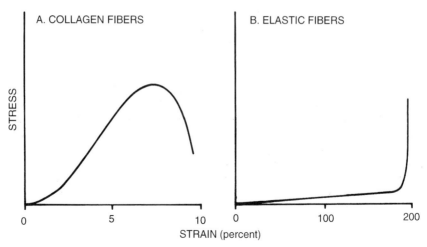

Figure 5.13. Stress-strain curves for collagen and elastic fibers when tested to failure in tension. Note the remarkable differences in the shape of the curve and the scale of the abscissa.

Given what is known about collagen and the makeup of various tissue types, assessments can be made by applying loads and determining the resulting deformation. Figure 5.14 shows a typical curve for the testing of ligament. Several portions of the curve have been given descriptors. The earliest portion is the **toe region**, a nonlinear segment due to a straightening of the collagen fibers. Little force is necessary in this early stage, but as the force increases the response is usually quite **linear**. At the end of this region the curve levels off and when the **failure** of fibers or fiber bundles occurs the maximum load has been reached (16). This maximum load reflects the **ultimate tensile strength** and complete failure usually follows rapidly. Note the similarity of this figure to that of Figure 5.6.

Applications can be made to clinical testing in that manual loading can produce displacements at the joint. Typical examples can be found when evaluating the integrity of the medial collateral or anterior cruciate ligaments of the knee. The latter can be done with an instrumented arthrometer. In the **clinical test** the loading may extend through the toe region and into the linear range, causing **physiological loading**. **Microfailure** can occur in the later stages of the linear range, for which the corollary in function is ligament injury. **Complete failure** would correspond to ligament rupture. In most situations the clinician would not achieve the load at which micro or complete failure could occur. However, in certain instances, for example, in evaluating a severe acute injury that has resulted in a rupture or avulsion, caution may need to be exerted compared with the rate or total load applied (24).

The mechanical properties of ligament can be assessed by a variety of experimental means. These techniques could include the clamping and subsequent elongation of isolated tissue segments or whole joints subjected to a full complement of loads and moments. While results of some of these tests will be presented in subsequent chapters, examples of how patient evaluation and treatment may be effected should help with clarifying why clinicians should understand these material properties (29). For example, evaluation of carbon fiber ligament replacement for the knee has shown that when subjected to continuous passive motion (CPM) the load required to failure is higher. Thus, the ligament can probably tolerate more stress (39). The results of this work, considered with a host of other sources in the literature suggests that tension is a major factor in the facilitation of the healing process. What remains is to study the effects of tension adequately so that the frequency and magnitude of the applied loads can be appropriate and clinically applicable.

Also known is that immobilization alters maturation of ligament, inhibiting growth and maturation and true structural "degradation" (35). Further, there is mounting evidence that ligaments from contralateral limbs of the same specimen also have altered mechanical properties when compared with age-matched normals from an external group. While the contralateral ligaments may be bigger, they are weaker and not as stiff as normal controls. That the values range between 50 and 66% of the external normals implies that treatments may need to be applied to the contralateral limb as well (35). Similar results have also been noted for torque generation by the quadriceps muscles in a group of patients who had sustained a below knee amputation (30).

Tendon

Tendon, with collagen fibers arranged largely in parallel, can tolerate high loads. For example the estimated tensile breaking strength of human calcaneal tendon is approximately 5.6 kg(f)/mm² (38). Several studies have determined in vivo loading of tendon. Results suggest that in normal activities the tendon be subjected to less than 25% of the ultimate stress that the tissue can withstand (23). Some differences

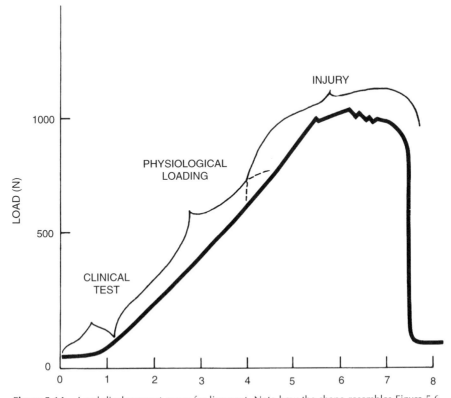

Figure 5.14. Load-displacement curve for ligament. Note how the shape resembles Figure 5.6.

have been noted, however, in patellar tendons of middle-aged versus older persons (14). Readily observed is that the larger muscle masses are accompanied by larger tendons that can effectively manage increased loads. Because the major component of the tendon is collagen, the shape of the load-deformation curve is similar to that shown in Figure 5.14.

As for ligament, tension has also been found a positive factor in tendon repair. The increased fibroblast proliferation, protein synthesis, the amount of newly synthesized collagen, and the alignment of collagen fibrils parallel to the applied force are all helpful in restoring tissue integrity and more normal mechanical properties. Because of loading, tendons have been shown to have increased strength values. The loaded tendons (here rabbit flexor tendons) were not significantly different from unloaded tendons; however, the increase in strength and other material properties lends additional evidence that tension is likely an important factor in assisting with repair and a return to more normal function (19).

Skin

Skin as a tissue is often ignored by therapists, but because scarring can cause limitations of movement during gross joint motions, considerable attention should be paid to the material properties. Gibson (11) discussed the biomechanical aspects of plastic surgery, specifically noting the material properties of the skin. The collagen and elastin fiber makeup accounts for the tension that normally exists in skin, mostly in retraction. Generally the crease lines parallel maximum tension, the minimum being at right angles. Therefore, wounds across tension lines produce hypertrophic scarring. Gibson also points out four effects of increased tension:

1. blanching and necrosis
2. rupture of the dermis (for example the striae in the abdomen during pregnancy)
3. permanent stretching
4. no effect on surrounding normal skin (i.e., scar contractures do not induce surrounding skin to stretch)

As will be further emphasized in later sections the response of skin to pressure and the tissue's natural creep with deformation over time is an important consideration. Overall, interest is being revived in the material properties of the skin since the mid-1800 work of Langer. For example, a work by Potts and colleagues (26) has evaluated the dynamic in vivo properties of human skin in response to applications of shear waves over a frequency from near zero to 1000 Hz. Implications for pressure sores resulting from sitting postures and prostheses and orthoses would be a natural topic for study by therapists.

APPLICATIONS TO PRACTICE

There are many effects of material properties of biological tissues on human performance, in injury, and in treatment procedures (5). Physical therapists frequently treat patients with fatigue failures and fractures. The pathology has been caused by repetitive loading and unloading within the design limits. In other words, the number of cycles through which the material is loaded is critical. For example, a glass rod, manufactured to fail at 200,000 psi will fail at 10,000 psi after a thimble full of sand has fallen on the rod (9). Often, material properties are modified by means of providing greater strength than actually needed to function effectively. Bone, as an example,

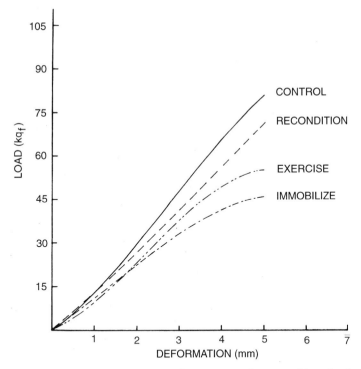

Figure 5.15. Calculated load-deformation curves for experimental groups subjected to immobilization and rehabilitation.

can tolerate loads of 8,000 psi in shear parallel to the long axis but up to 12,000 psi across the long axis (9).

More generalized uses of properties are also in use and of practical value. For example, the influence of the magnitude of loading the spine in compression and distraction on the torsion stiffness gives us practical information about how the purposes of the spine are served by the soft tissue (12). Even the role of insulin therapy on tissue properties has been studied in an attempt to establish how injuries such as contracture, tenosynovitis, joint stiffness, and osteoporosis are thwarted (15).

Soft Tissue Injuries

An area where material properties are particularly important is in soft tissue ruptures or avulsions. These injuries can occur at virtually any site but are frequently seen as avulsion fractures. In other words tensile strength of a given material may not be sufficient to prevent the fracture.

For ligamentous tissue the lowest strength has been reported to occur in immobilized animals. The highest values appeared in trained animals. These animals also have higher collagen content with increased thicknesses and diameters. Junctional strength also increased with training (34). As an example, Figure 5.15 shows a load-deformation curve for the anterior cruciate ligament in the tension mode. All these animals' ligaments were immobilized for 8 weeks. Note the minimal effect of local exercise: the tissue response post immobilization might not be the same as the reconditioned curve that included ambulation and free activity for 5 months. One question that yet remains to be answered is whether or not an increase in ligament strength, above the normal, is created by exercise. The study by Noyes et al. (25) seems to lend credence to that possibility.

Material properties are important in plastic surgery and in the formation of scar tissue resulting from burns. Barbanel (1) has, in fact, shown that excised skin that has undergone repeated cycling causing extension displayed progressive alteration of response in uniaxial tension. That is, the strain curve shifted to the right for equivocal stresses applied over different periods. The concept of creep may also become very important in treating these tissue injuries caused by burns. Further, pressure sores are the result of reaction forces at the skin and the support surface interface. The site is usually over bony prominences. Many other examples will be provided concerning joint forces and their distribution to show how tissue properties play a role in the pathology and the rehabilitative treatment that physical therapists will provide.

Specific studies have also been completed to evaluate the strength of tendon. Investigators have found that tendons are weakest 3–14 days post surgery because the collagen remains soft. The ability of these tissues to resist the shearing at the suture area that occurs during tensile loading is markedly diminished (18). Although clinical experience shows that 3 weeks of immobilization is necessary to prevent rupturing, anything greater than 3 weeks yields adhesions between the tendon and the sheath and the surrounding soft tissues. Approximately 40–50 weeks is necessary to regain normal strength post surgery (23). Work by Steiner (31) may give the clinician some guidelines. His study on the biomechanics of tendon healing has shown that after 4 weeks' healing, unsutured rat tendon exhibited 70% of the normal stiffness and only 40% of the normal muscle rupture strength. About 25% of the normal tendon strength had returned at 4 weeks. These relatively low values show that high loading in the early stages of recovery must be avoided.

Treatment Implications

Because therapists frequently encounter different surgical techniques and apply loads to these tissues, evaluations have been completed on various surgical methods associated with tendon suturing. Interrupted sutures provide tensile load directly on the tendon ends, while the Kessler technique provides mostly tensile and some compressive force through the adjacent tendon ends. Bunnell's technique uses both compression and tensile forces, while the fishmouth or endweave creates some shearing at the anastomosis sites as well as compressive loads. This latter technique has been shown to provide the greatest immediate strength but the problem is that the resultant site is relatively bulky (8). Other work has evaluated the biomechanical properties of tendon repairs because knowing the characteristics associated with tendon gliding and tensile strength is important. In assessing the multiple surgical techniques, results show that the joint motion and ultimate load vary depending on the procedure. Therapists need to be aware of the type of repair used by the surgeon and familiar with the biomechanical properties to decide how much loading can be tolerated by exercise protocols (22).

In a review article Soderberg (30) has detailed some work concerning alterations in the morphological and physiological features of biological tissues resulting from immobilization and treatment procedures. Studies have shown a significant decrease in the available number of sarcomeres resulting from immobilization (32, 33). These results are of significance because they show that elongation tension is apparently

Table 5.1 Comparison of the Stress, Stiffness, and Weight of Materials

Material	Maximum Permissible Stress (Tensile)	E (Stiffness)	Weight
High tensile steel	45–85 ton/inch^2 (70–130 × 10^7 N/m^2)	30 × 10^6 lb/inch^2 (2.1 × 10^{11} N/m^2)	0.283 lb/inch^3 (0.0078 kg/cm^3)
Mild steel	30 ton/inch^2 (46 × 10^7 N/m^2)	30 × 10^6 lb/inch^2 (2.1 × 10^{11} N/m^2)	0.283 lb/inch^3 (0.0078 kg/cm^3)
Titanium	70 ton/inch^2 (108 × 10^7 N/m^2)	16 × 10^6 lb/inch^2 (1.10 × 10^{11} N/m^2)	0.16 lb/inch^3 (0.0044 kg/cm^3)
Plastics (unreinforced)	3–7 ton/inch^2 (5–11 × 10^7 N/m^2)	0.35 × 10^6 lb/inch^2 (approx.) 0.024 × 10^{11} N/m^2)	0.03–0.07 lb/inch^3 (0.0008–0.0019 kg/cm^3)
Plastics (carbon fiber reinforced) High strength	Up to 200 ton/inch^2 (309 × 10^7 N/m^2)	33 × 10^6 lb/inch^2 (2.3 × 10^{11} N/m^2)	0.06–0.07 lb/inch^3 (0.00166–0.00194 kg/cm^3)

needed to facilitate the return of sarcomeres and the subsequent length-tension relationship required for normal function of the musculotendinous unit.

Other work relates to the effect of immobilization and passive motion techniques upon tendon. These investigative works have shown that mobilized animals had greater increases in strength and stiffness and more callous formation than the caged or immobilized groups (10, 28). Material properties have also been a factor in the production of soft tissue pathology. Excessive elongation, particularly at high rates, is conceded to produce either strains or complete ruptures of soft tissues. That muscle rupture is far more common than tendon rupture is substantiated by work showing the maximum stress to failure for tendon to be twice that for muscle (7).

Orthotics and Prosthetics

Properties of materials used in orthotic and prosthetic appliances are also important. Of main concern is that consideration be given to the material's maximum permitted stress, stiffness, weight, and fatigue life. Materials available include metals, plastics, wood, and leather. Primary support, however, needs to be offered by metals and plastics. Table 5.1 contains a contrast of the stress, stiffness, and weight. Redford and Licht (27) state that of the metals, steel and aluminum alloys are most suitable for orthotic appliances. Henshaw (13) discusses the use of reinforced plastics and states that although the latter have excellent tensile strength, stiffness, and other features, other qualities are often not satisfactory. Consider also that the materials are subjected to bending loads. Because the thin metals or alloys do not resist these loads well, the materials may be unsatisfactory for use, at least in certain situations. Further, aluminum alloys have a much higher incidence of fatigue failures than do the steels. They are also relatively corrosion resistant and of high strength. Magnesium alloys are now appearing as a major component of wheelchair fabrication because of their light weight and amenability to welding and brazing (27).

The more than 30 major families of plastics have revolutionized the practice of orthotics. Splinting has been dramatically simplified. Two major categories of plastics are thermoplastics and thermosetting plastics. Thermoplastics soften with heat and harden when cooled. They can be remolded with additional heating. Thermosetting plastics develop a permanent set when heat and pressure are applied and cannot be softened or reshaped when heated. As an example, polypropylene is a rigid material with high impact strength. The material is also able to withstand several million repetitive flexures before showing signs of failure. The molecular structure of this and other plastics provide the properties necessary for functional use. Important considerations in orthotic materials are resistance to bending, impact, and fatigue, while affording the patient a lightweight structure (27).

SUMMARY

This chapter has covered material properties of biological tissues. Examples of how the basic concepts of load, stress, and strain apply to humans have also been provided through representative examples. Further applications to specific tissues will be included in subsequent chapters and related to meaning in clinical practices.

References

1. Barbenel JC, Evans JH, Jordan MM. Tissue mechanics. *Engineering in Medicine.* 1978;7:5–9.
2. Burstein AH, Wright TM. *Fundamentals of Orthopedic Biomechanics.* Baltimore: Williams & Wilkins; 1994.
3. Carter DR, Hayes WC. Bone compressive strength: the influence of density and strain rate. *Science.* 1976;194:1174–1176.
4. Churches AE, Howlett CR, Waldron KJ, et al. The response of living bone to controlled time-varying loading: method and preliminary results. *J Biomech.* 1979;12:35–45.
5. Cochran GVB. *A Primer of Orthopedic Biomechanics.* New York: Churchill Livingstone; 1982.
6. Edwards CC, Chrisman OD. Articular cartilage. In: Albright JA, Brand RA, eds. *The Scientific Basis of Orthopedics.* New York: Appleton-Century-Crofts; 1979:313–348.
7. Elliott DH. The biomechanical properties of tendon in relation to muscular strength. *Ann Med.* 1967;9:1–7.
8. Frankel VJ, Nordin M. *Basic Biomechanics of the Musculoskeletal System.* Philadelphia: Lea & Febiger; 1980.
9. Frost HM. *An Introduction to Biomechanics.* Springfield, IL: Charles C Thomas; 1967.
10. Gelberman RH, Woo SL-Y, Cobb N, et al. Flexor tendon healing: the effects of early passive mobilization. In: *Proceedings of the 27th Annual Orthopedic Research Society.* Chicago: Dependable Publishing; 1981:81.
11. Gibson T. Biomechanical aspects of plastic surgery. In: Akkas N, ed. *Progress in Biomechanics.* The Netherlands: Sitjhoff and Noordhoff; 1979.
12. Goodwin RR, James KS, Daniels U, et al. Distraction and compression loads enhance spine torsional stiffness. *J Biomech.* 1994;27:1049–1057.
13. Henshaw JT. The design of orthotic appliances. In: Murdoch G, ed. *The Advance in Orthotics.* Baltimore: Williams & Wilkins; 1976.
14. Johnson GA, Tramaglini DM, Levine RE, et al. Tensile and viscoelastic properties of human patellar tendon. *J Orthop Res.* 1994;12:796–803.
15. Lancaster RL, Haut RC, DeCamp CE. Changes in the mechanical properties of patellar tendon preparations of spontaneously diabetic dogs under long-term insulin therapy. *J Biomech.* 1994;27:1105–1108.
16. Loitz, BJ, Frank CB. Biology and mechanics of ligament and ligament healing. In: Holloszy JO, ed. *Exercise and Sports Science Reviews.* Baltimore: Williams & Wilkins; 1993:33–64.
17. Maroudas A. Physico-chemical properties of articular cartilage. In: Freeman MAR, ed. *Adult Articular Cartilage.* London, England: Pitman; 1973.
18. Mason ML, Allen HS. The rate of healing of tendons: an experimental study of tensile strength. *Ann Surg.* 1941;113:424–459.
19. Mass DP, Tuel RJ, Labarbera M, et al. Effects of constant mechanical tension on the healing of rabbit flexor tendons. *Clin Orthop.* 1993;296:301–306.
20. Mow VC, Roth V, Armstrong CG. Biomechanics of joint cartilage. In: Frankel VH, Nordin M, eds. *Basic Biomechanics of the Skeletal System.* Philadelphia: Lea & Febiger; 1980.
21. Mulholland R. Lateral hydraulic permeability and morphology of articular cartilage in normal and osteoarthrotic cartilage. In: *Proceedings of the Symposium of the Institute of Orthopaedics.* London, 1974.
22. Noguchi M, Seiler JG, Gelberman RH, et al. In vitro biomechanical analysis of suture methods for flexor tendon repair. *J Orthop Res.* 1993;11:603–611.

23. Nordin M, Frankel VH. Biomechanics of whole bones and bone tissue. In: Frankel VH, Nordin M, eds. *Basic Biomechanics of the Skeletal System*. Philadelphia: Lea & Febiger; 1980.

24. Nordin M, Frankel VH. *Basic Biomechanics of the Musculoskeletal System*. Philadelphia: Lea & Febiger; 1989.

25. Noyes FR, Torvik PJ, Hyde WB, et al. Biomechanics of ligament failure: II an analysis of immobilization, exercise, and reconditioning effects in primates. *J Bone Joint Surg*. 1974;56(A):1406–1418.

26. Potts RO, Chrisman DA, Buras EM. The dynamic mechanical properties of human skin in vivo. *J Biomech*. 1983;16:365–372.

27. Redford RL, Licht S. Materials for orthotics. In: Licht S, ed. *Orthotics etc*. New Haven, CT: E. Licht, 1980.

28. Salter RB, Bell RS. The effect of continuous passive motion on the healing of partial thickness lacerations of the patellar tendon of the rabbit. In: *Proceedings of the 27th Annual Orthopedic Research Society*. Chicago: Dependable Publishing; 1981:82.

29. Soderberg GL. Below-knee amputee knee extension force-time and moment characteristics. *Phys Ther*. 1978;58:966–971.

30. Soderberg GL. Muscle mechanics: their clinical relevance. *Phys Ther*. 1983;63:216–220.

31. Steiner M. Biomechanics of tendon healing. *J Biomech*. 1982;15:951–958.

32. Tabary JC, Tabary C, Tardieu C, et al. Physiological and structural changes in the cat's soleus muscle due to immobilization at different lengths by plaster casts. *J Physiol (Lond)*. 1972;224:231–244.

33. Tabary JC, Tardieu C, Tardieu G, et al. Experimental rapid sarcomere loss with concomitant hypoextensibility. *Muscle Nerve*. 1981;4:198–203.

34. Tipton CM, James SL, Mergner W, et al. Influence of exercise on strength of medial collateral knee ligaments of dogs. *Am J Physiol*. 1970;218:894–902.

35. Walsh S, Frank C, Shrive N, et al. Knee immobilization inhibits biomechanical maturation of the rabbit medial collateral ligament. *Clin Orthop*. 1993;297:253–261.

36. Warwick R, Williams PL, eds. *Gray's Anatomy*. 36th British ed. Philadelphia: WB Saunders; 1980.

37. White AA, Panjabi MM. *Clinical Biomechanics of the Spine*. Philadelphia: JB Lippincott; 1978.

38. Yamada H. *Strength of Biological Materials*. In: Evans FG, ed. Baltimore: Williams & Wilkins; 1970.

39. Zarnett R, Velazquez R, Salter RB. The effect of continuous passive motion on knee ligament reconstruction with carbon fibre. *J Bone Joint Surg*. 1991;73(B):47–52.

6

Analytical Methods for Normal and Pathological Motion

Kinesiologic evaluation requires skills fundamental to the collection of kinematic and kinetic information that pertains to human motion. These skills are important in initial and serial evaluations whether the patient attempts a fundamental task of raising the arm overhead or a more complicated one such as gait. In addition, clinicians will constantly be exposed to literature that uses motion analysis techniques. Reliable measurements, the ability to accurately record motion, are important both within and between day and across different persons making the measurements. It is essentially a precursor to validity—a necessary but not sufficient condition for validity. Validity means that the tool, system, or device measures what it purports to measure. Another concern in analyzing motion is objectivity. In all cases, the quantifiable measure should not suffer from prejudice. This chapter will focus on available methods used to gather objective and reliable information as related to normal and pathological motion. Emphasis will be placed on improving the ability to interpret literature and apply the information to pathological motion.

COORDINATE SYSTEMS

Fundamental to motion analysis is the method adopted. In all circumstances the technique should be designed and tested to describe adequately the position that the human body and individual body segments can assume. This task is relatively easy when we make a measure of how much the elbow flexes during a clinical assessment procedure. Our analysis is far more complicated, however, when we evaluate a more complex function such as walking. The factor of time also has been added, which in effect adds a valuable parameter of interest. Measurement error can significantly distort the quality of the information in most methods. With any of the methods described below a system should be adopted by which the motion can be precisely determined.

Clinical

Joint range of motion, whether static or dynamic, is usually measured according to three planes and given the standard labels of movement that occurs in flexion/extension, abduction/adduction, and internal/external rotation. However, other motions occur within the joints, such as rolling and gliding, and are not included in the **triplanar analyses** that assess this gross motion. In Chapter 4 these osteokinematic motions were described and discussed compared with the arthrokinematic motions. These latter motions are much smaller but are likely critical to normal joint motion. To integrate these concepts, consider an example at the glenohumeral joint. First raise the entire arm, with the palm of the hand starting against your side, into forward flexion of 90° at the glenohumeral joint. Direct the arm laterally for 90° while maintaining the arm in the horizontal position, then lower the arm to the starting position. If conscious effort is taken not to rotate the radio-ulnar joints during this series of motions the hand will be in a position rotated 90° from the original position. Known as **Codman's paradox**, the rotation is due to the geometry and the interaction of the male and female surfaces of the respective humeral head and glenoid. What is difficult for the clinician is to recognize the type and measure the magnitude of motion in any joint.

Note that clinical systems would have usually described this sequence as motion, ignoring the rotation that has occurred. Several methods have been proposed to address this difficulty, but none appear likely to be widely adopted. A system developed by Roebuck (38) is one example. Applicable for description of total body or link motion, Roebuck's method is a triplanar angular coordinate system and a notation system that completely and adequately describes motion. However, the method was never adopted by either the clinical or research community and is no longer in use. Albert's perimeter, detailed in Steindler, is another example of a little used motion analysis system (44).

Despite the advances in technology the clinical methods and terminology used for describing and quantifying motion will not likely be replaced. Although suffering from weaknesses in reliability and objectivity the clinically applicable techniques are the most widely used. As indicated, one of the most acute limitations of the clinical system is the inability to describe certain movements adequately, therefore limiting validity. Yet, ease of application, efficiency, and understanding, coupled with widespread and longstanding use, shows that clinical techniques will necessarily thrive. Perhaps as a more thorough understanding of arthrokinematics becomes available, the intrinsic joint movements can be incorporated into the methods currently used.

Reference Frames

Spatial reference frames may be relative or absolute. The former method requires the anatomical coordinates to be reported compared with a fixed anatomical landmark. Thus, this method is used to describe the position of one limb compared with the other. Using the absolute system means that coordinates are in relation to an external reference frame in space. Here motion is described in relation to the ground or the direction of gravity. The study of gait frequently uses this method. Use of either system is dependent on the means of data collection; either system will provide sufficient information for the determination of the kinematic data. However, the absolute method is seldom used in the clinical setting.

Cartesian

Another method frequently used in motion analysis is the **Cartesian coordinate system**. Using this method the therapist has a choice of use of one, two, or three dimensions depending on the type of movement being studied. Polar coordinate technique limits the analysis to one or two planes, the latter allowing the determination of three-dimensional motion. Most studies analyzing complex motions will use the Cartesian system because virtually any movement characteristic can be derived.

KINEMATICS

Recall that kinematics is the description of motion no matter the forces causing the movement. Inherent to this description are **time and displacement** parameters. In the clinic, temporal events may be estimated from a watch's second hand. In the laboratory, several decimal places may be required to provide adequate resolution. The same may be said about angular or linear displacement data. Sometimes millimeters of displacement cannot satisfy the rigors necessary to comply with laboratory accuracy. Yet, in docking great ocean liners meters of displacement are satisfactory to accomplish the task. Instruments are available to quantify and highly resolve these parameters if the purpose of the technique can be justified as to the expense and sophistication involved.

Many techniques are available for collecting kinematic information, but the one chosen is usually determined by the purpose for which the data are being gathered. Laboratory systems are frequently dependent upon computer control and/or interpretation of the data derived. Although simple systems are available for use in the clinical setting, their use is limited by such factors as interest, expense, or time.

Kinematic data collection systems can be either direct and indirect. Each system's technique, its advantages and disadvantages, its output, and its interpretation will be discussed below.

Direct

The direct recording techniques include goniometers, accelerometers, polgons, electromagnetic and acoustic systems, and intracortical pins. The latter three will not be discussed because of their limited use and application, particularly in the clinical environment. Other hybrid systems have also been developed, but generally their use is limited to temporal and distance factors (17) or is dependent on computerized techniques for specific pathologies (12).

Goniometry

Clinical goniometers have been widely used for decades in the assessment of joint motion. Available in multiple sizes and shapes for the measurement of any joint movement the standard form has been reliable, at least when used under controlled circumstances (9, 36). Although these measurements suffer from various sources of error, such as poor inter rater reliability and landmark locations, their use will continue in the clinical setting.

More complex forms of collecting angular displacement data have been in use for many years. In practice, the **electrogoniometer** is an electrical potentiometer attached to a mechanical arrangement (or exoskeleton) (Fig. 6.1). In turn, it is attached to body segments so that displacement changes the voltage through the potentiometer. As an inexpensive means of collecting data this technique also provides an output signal in relative angles. Applicability is high in instructional settings and the manufacture of simple, single plane goniometry can be accomplished without much effort. For coordination with electromyographic and even force measures these goniometers are useful; however, it is sometimes difficult to fit and adapt the mechanical systems to a wide range of body types. As might be expected from the previous discussion on arthrokinematics and osteokinematics, these systems would also have difficulty with assessing all the relevant motions. Accuracy, however, even given an adequately designed system, is regarded to be good. Patient encumbrances may also become significant if multiple joints or multiple axis goniometers are used. An example of a multi-axis goniometer has been provided, and the device has been used for studying patterns of hip motion in patients with hip pathology (Figs. 6.2 and 6.3) (27, 49).

Others have used a triaxial goniometer in studying elbow motion during a variety

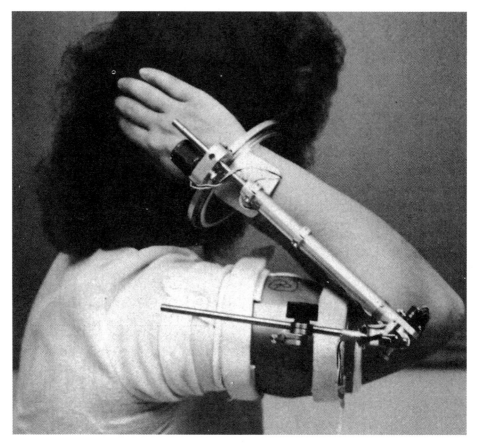

Figure 6.1.   A triaxial goniometer applied to the right elbow.

of functional activities (29). Chao has thoroughly discussed the triaxial goniometer, pointing out that although the spatial goniometer can measure both rotary and translatory motion in joints the current system does not provide a direct joint motion measurement (13).

Electrogoniometers have also been used to produce angle-angle plots that yield useful information about the interaction of two joints (Fig. 6.4) (21). These plots have been useful in providing clinically relevant data regarding the interaction of two joints, and display the angular changes over time for the segments of interest. Some will use these plots analytically to detect degree of pathology present, but applications are limited because the data are usually derived with the assistance of digital computers. These manipulations of the data offer potential as a meaningful tool in the diagnosis of type and size of movement dysfunction. Examples of applications are in their earliest stages and how they will be applied to the clinic is still unclear.

One more interesting application of a series of planar goniometers has also been suggested. The system proposes use of simple trigonometric calculations for measuring step length. The 3% average error makes the method attractive, in spite of the need for a computer (5).

In summary, the standard goniometer has many applications. The electrogoniometer has limitations and requires instrumentation and a recording device to capture the data. Given these constraints and the expansive development of video techniques that lead to three-dimensional plots of movement, any further expansion of techniques to derive displacement data by means of a clinical goniometry system is unlikely.

Accelerometry

The use of accelerometers is another direct technique used in motion studies. These devices are simple electrical circuits that measure accelerations of the segment or segments to which it is attached. Morris (30) describes the technique, how it may be extended to other body segments, and how the signals from six accelerometers can be used to define the movement of a body in space completely.

Other accounts have shown the utility of such a technique in discriminating among normal subjects, those using assistive devices, and those suffering from pathology. Figure 6.5 shows the **accelerographic patterns** for fore-aft and vertical directions for a normal and a postoperative hip surgery patient who walked with a crutch (40). Although triaxial accelerometers are available, problems still arise because of difficulties associated with attaching the device to the body. Encumbrance also becomes a problem if many devices are used. Offsetting the disadvantage that the acceleration is relative to the position on the limb segment is the advantage that output is readily available for direct recording or additional processing. In practice accelerometers are little used. Most commonly high accuracy displacement data are wanted so that acceleration and velocity can be derived. However, use of the acceleration data directly into the $\mathbf{F} = \mathbf{M} \times \mathbf{A}$ equation is a desirable feature of this method.

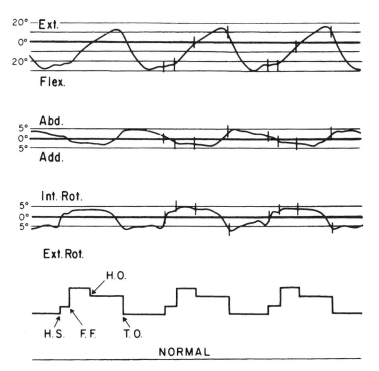

Figure 6.2. Electrogoniometric pattern in degrees of motion for the hip joint in a normal subject. For the foot switch pattern shown at the bottom *HS* indicates heel strike, *FF* is flat foot, *HO* is heel off, and *TO* is toe off.

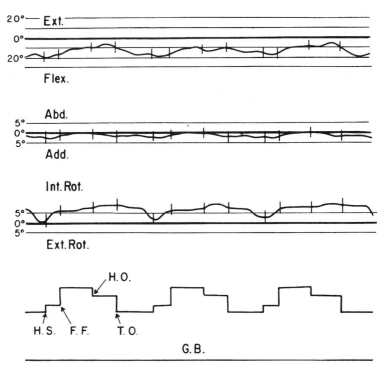

Figure 6.3. Electrogoniometric pattern for a patient with degenerative arthritis of the hip and accompanying pain. Note the marked limitation of motion compared to Figure 6.2.

Indirect

The indirect or imaging methods are the most widely used for collecting information about human movement. The techniques include **cinematography** and **videotape**. By far photography is the most common technique used, be it still, low, or high speed. Since the early moving picture days of Muybridge, use of cinematography has expanded to great proportions (32). His works of animal and human motion are considered classics, particularly when considering the state of the art in the 1800s.

More recently, a strong case has been made for video recording systems. Other more sophisticated devices have also been developed that promise to simplify (but likely increase the cost of) the technique of collecting highly accurate kinematic data. Generally these photographic techniques are moderate in cost and provide minimal encumbrance on patients and subjects. Data may also be permanently stored for later use. However, reduction time for photographic methods can be increased unless automated systems are used.

Photography

Of all forms of cinematography, 16 mm cameras are most frequently chosen because of the cost and the adequacy of the image size. A variety of cameras are available for either the clinical or laboratory setting. Cameras with higher frame rates are necessary for the higher velocity movements used in athletic events, but for clinical and most other purposes frame rates of greater than 64 frames/sec are seldom required. However, many find the disadvantages of time for film processing, cost of the film, and other constraints too limiting for this technique to be frequently used. Similar constraints are associated with panning techniques.

Procedures for reducing data to displacements of joints vary. Location of colored dots at joint centers has been used so that filming from the lateral view can produce sagittal plane motion data that will yield measurements from the screen on which the film is projected. The reader is referred to either Hay (25) or Miller and Nelson (28) for a detailed description of the technique. Location of cameras at multiple angles provides the capability for determination of three-dimensional displacement but simultaneously requires significant methodological attention both in the collection and reduction of the data. Sutherland and Hagy (46) provides the details of this approach. In any case, displacement data can then be used in the velocity and acceleration calculations so that kinetics can be studied.

Other innovative uses of photography have been developed. In 1978 a method using two 35 mm cameras and a system of flashing **light emitting diodes** was detailed (16). These investigators could effectively derive displacement data that could be used, along with kinetic data, in determining hip joint forces. Soderberg and Gabel (43) had previously reported the use of a similar system in describing sagittal plane gait kinematics for both normal and pathological subjects. This methodology essentially produces multi-frame images on a single frame of film. Because the lights flash at a designated frequency, temporal factors can be easily determined. As explained in the above references both linear and angular displacements can be readily determined. Others have used a similar system for both normal and cerebral palsied children, but their data are graphic and not readily quantifiable (3, 4).

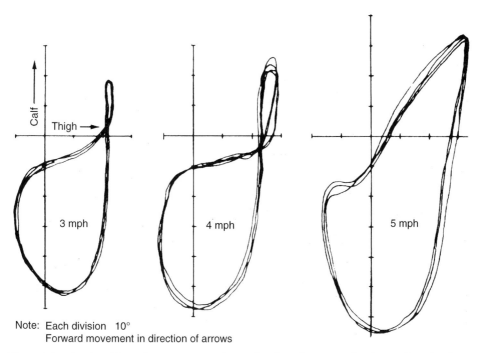

Note: Each division 10°
Forward movement in direction of arrows

Figure 6.4.   Graphs of lower leg versus upper leg angle. This subject completed a number of walking cycles, shown by the multiple lines, at velocities indicated in each plot.

The **strobe** light has also been used in displacement determinations. Richards and Knutsson (37) attached reflective targets to the head or neck and the extremity segments while the subject walked in a strobe-illuminated room in front of an open shutter camera. Figure 6.6 contains the recording of the pattern produced in a normal walking subject. Measurements of angular displacement can be made directly from the film and converted to acceleration and velocity. This system is economical but suffers from limitations associated with planar movements and the requirements for subdued lighting.

Another simple photographic technique is the **sequence camera**. This commercially available low-cost camera takes a series of eight photographs in a temporal sequence that can be preset depending on the velocity of the movement being

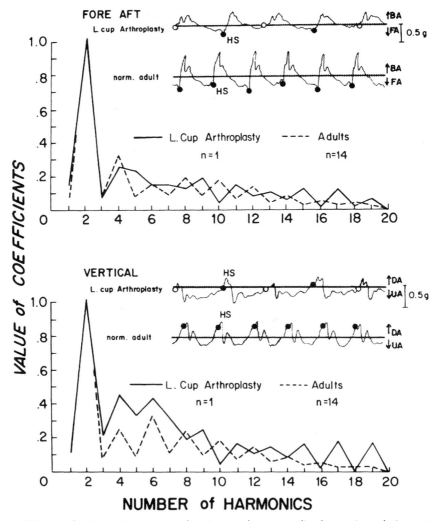

Figure 6.5. Acceleration patterns, in two directions, and corresponding harmonic analysis spectra for normal adults and a subject with arthroplastic surgery of the hip. Accelerations (*A*) are backwards (*B*), forwards (*F*), downwards (*D*), and upwards (*U*). Solid circle is heel strike of normal side and open circle is heel strike of affected side.

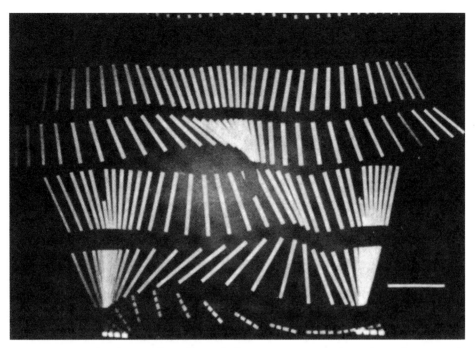

Figure 6.6. Example of a recording of sagittal plane motion using strobographic technique. Strobe frequency was 20 Hz. The horizontal bar represents 30 cm.

photographed. The camera has multiple uses and provides reasonable quality photographs that may be used for descriptive purposes (26).

Video Recorders

Detailed descriptions for use of **video recorders** have been provided in the literature (1, 19, 23, 35, 51). Winter and coworkers (50) have been strong advocates of this form of kinematic analysis, citing a lack of patient encumbrance and the ability to collect multiple trials and analyze them immediately. The technique does require, however, considerable, expensive hardware. Further, specific procedures need to be followed to collect high-quality data.

Now called **photogrammetric reconstruction**, the procedures require the attachment of markers to a subject and then identifying the markers on the videotape. One type of marker is active (maybe small, infrared, light-emitting diodes). The other type is passive (perhaps a light-reflective device). While each system has advantages and disadvantages, in either case the markers will be recorded as "spots" that can be identified for location in space. The appropriate mathematics can then be applied to reconstruct the figure in space, according to data from the multiple camera sources. Computer programming and high-quality display devices are required to avoid tedious data reduction, but again, software is expensive and the desirable engineering support scarce. The product usually constructed is a stick figure, which can then be evaluated in the three planes of motion. Many manipulations are possible, either with software or mathematical techniques (Fig. 6.7).

Video systems can also be linked with other data signals, such as those from load cells used in force plates or from the electromyogram. As a result the kinesiologist,

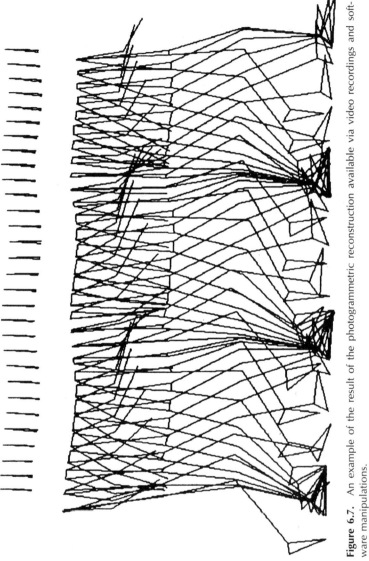

Figure 6.7. An example of the result of the photogrammetric reconstruction available via video recordings and software manipulations.

biomechanician, or clinician can evaluate synchronized data sets that provide a comprehensive set of information. These sets will include kinematic, kinetic, and EMG data, examples of which are shown in this and other chapters. Essential limitations are the time and financial support available for these more complex and sophisticated forms of data collection and analysis; however, many academic and clinical facilities can generate these comprehensive data sets. Referral of patients to these centers by practitioners is well within the scope of practice and should be considered in cases when complete or accurate information is wanted about a movement dysfunction.

Clinical systems using video techniques have also been devised and effectively used. Planar motions have been studied for recording temporal features, walking velocity, stride length, and goniometric angles at the hip, knee, and ankle. Generally, these methods can be used to analyze gait deviations, sitting postures (23), or study outcomes of therapeutic procedures or interventions affecting gait. Equipment required is a reference scale to include in the field of view, a standard video camera, a playback unit, and a standard television monitor. Data can be easily collected and analyzed, but a limitation of the system includes resolution because with the standard camera, film speed is usually limited to 30 Hz, making clear images of the swing phase of gait unlikely. In addition, parallax can be a problem, depending on the set up, the equipment used, and whether or not images are measured in other locations than in the center of the monitor screen. Generally, reliability has been reported as at least good (7, 8, 33, 45, 48). Procedures for this method have been included in the literature and sufficient examples exist as models for a clinician to follow (23, 45). Before investing resources, the clinician must commit to a thorough understanding of the procedure.

Event Markers

Required for analyses of human motion are **event markers** or other devices used as indicators of temporal events. Many kinematic systems, such as the diode and certain cine procedures, have the timing events included on the film and tape. Others need to incorporate a timer into the field of view. Foot switches and other event markers, such as voice or manual controls, are frequently helpful in determining onset and duration of events. Special care must be taken to synchronize the processes if multiple techniques are used simultaneously. Consult Figures 3.13, 6.2, and 6.3 for typical uses of event markers.

Clinical Implications

Each system described in this section has been shown to have adequate reliability for the gathering of kinematic data. Development of the therapist's capability to analyze human motion will be primarily dependent on the purpose of the data gathered. Clinicians would be most interested in the inexpensive methods that provided immediate replay and efficient quantification. Minimal expenditures would be in the hundreds of dollars, depending on whether a videotape system existed in the health care facility in which most professionals are based. Laboratory proven methods require substantial investments, starting with tens of thousands of dollars.

KINETICS

To analyze motion completely, that is, arrive at solutions for joint forces, it is necessary to know how much tension the patient generates and how to calculate the moment.

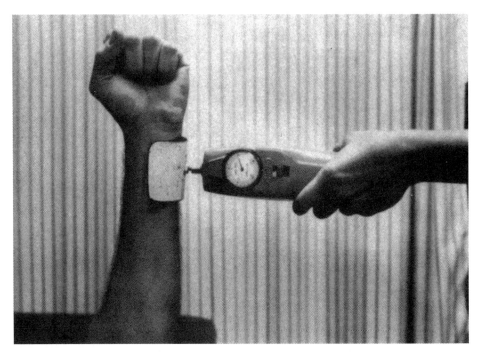

Figure 6.8. An example of a hand held dynamometer. The isometric strength of the extensors of the elbow is being tested here.

To derive kinetic information, a host of force **transducers** are available. Mechanical and electrical strain gauges are all widely used in converting forces to meaningful quantities. Essentially, all work on the principle that strain produces known deformation in materials, which can then be converted to the measure of interest. In kinesiologic applications, force is of most interest; however, many other types of transducers are available for the measurement of forces derived from blood, air, and fluid flow.

Among the most frequently used devices are **cable tensiometers** and **dynamometers**. Hand grip dynamometers are frequently used to evaluate grip strength. Other hand held dynamometers are often used in the clinic. The device measures the compression resulting from an isometric muscle contraction (Fig. 6.8). Output of these devices, in kgf or lbf, is useful because the measure can be used in the calculation of the moment (F × d) being created about the joint axis. A simple measurement of the distance to the joint axis from the perpendicular application of the restraining cable or dynamometer guarantees a measurement unit, torque, that can be used in other comparisons. (See Chapter 1 for further details.)

In this era of miniaturization these hand held units now have great utility in the clinical setting. While more time-consuming to use compared with the more common manual muscle test, the prospect of an objective measure for use in documenting progress and determining outcome is a distinct advantage that should encourage their use. To facilitate the practitioner's treatment goals using these devices, databases for both normal and pathological conditions now need to be created (6, 11, 48).

An example of a force curve generated during isometric knee extension is shown in Figure 6.9. Transducers have also been developed for direct clinical application. One example is an insole that can be inserted into a shoe. By means of electronic circuitry, the clinician can vary the pressure required to produce an output voltage. Many applications exist for the patient with foot dysfunction, such as for the diabetic foot and for today's runner. Example output forms are shown in Figures 6.10 and 6.11 (31).

Transducer output can in turn be processed so that graded degrees or continuous audio tones can be generated, showing the pressure being exerted. A very practical application occurs when the degree of weight bearing needs to be controlled during gait. By adequately calibrating the transducer, the clinician can set the pressure required for feedback to the patient (52).

Forms of **electromechanical dynamometers** are available for clinical use. Many "isokinetic" dynamometers provide output in torque (ft lbs). Because of the wide range of selectable speeds, these devices have applicability to many evaluation and reassessment procedures commonly employed for a variety of patients. Calibrated graphs assist with record interpretation so that data may be interpreted immediately. Because paper readouts, at known speed, are available from the constant velocity exercise, determination of the joint kinematics is easily obtained. Samples of torque curves generated at two different velocities are presented in Figure 6.12 and will be frequently presented in other chapters in this volume. Interpretation of these torque curves are important for treatment and evaluation of patients. Therefore, all clinicians should be prepared to discuss the shape of the torque curve generated for any joint and to compare the normal with the pathological finding.

The other most commonly used transducer for the collection of kinetic information is the **force plate**. Formerly using a system of electromechanical gauges, plates now use piezoresistive or piezoelectric transducers; the plate's response time has been remarkably improved. Output includes the force in the vertical, medial-lateral, and fore-aft directions. Moments about the three principal axes can also be determined, as can the center of pressure. Figure 6.13 shows the three-dimensional forces from a plate for the stance phase of one extremity during gait. Shown in Figure 6.14 are the moment data generated. The ground reaction forces are then used, in concert

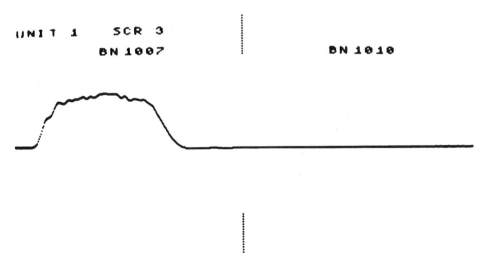

Figure 6.9. Isometric force-time curve for knee extension. This information was obtained by an on-line computer. Peak force was multiplied by distance to obtain torque for a contraction held about three seconds.

with body segment parameter information and kinematic data in calculation of the joint forces acting at the various joints of the lower extremity (21). Innovative use of these plates has led to their installation as part of a treadmill system, allowing the collection of many sequential trials for analysis (18).

Force plates can also be used, as can other similarly manufactured devices, for finding the **center of pressure**. The center of pressure can then be used with time for assessing balance and stability control. As the patient learns control, phase plot diagrams should change (Fig. 6.15). Many patients with injuries of the lower extremity are also subjected to similar test conditions when weight bearing (closed kinetic chains) activities are included in the exercise protocol. Currently only a few devices can monitor the extremity under loading in the clinical environment, but as technology continues to expand other techniques will appear.

Devices have been created to monitor loads of other body parts under a variety of conditions. Force transducers have been fabricated to fit within insoles, allowing the plotting of force magnitudes and distribution patterns during walking and running. These plots (see Fig. 6.11) allow for comparison of abnormal patterns with those considered to be normal. Another application of a similar method is in the monitoring

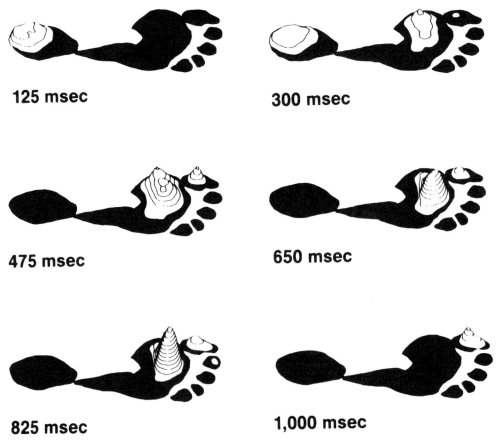

125 msec   **300 msec**

475 msec   **650 msec**

825 msec   **1,000 msec**

Figure 6.10. Time-series plot of plantar pressure during stepping by a patient with diabetes. Contour intervals are 75 kPa.

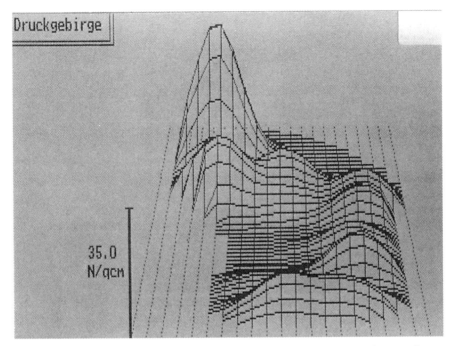

Figure 6.11. Three-dimensional representation of mean maximum pressures during walking.

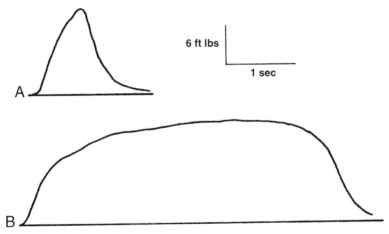

Figure 6.12. Torque curve generated by knee extension at (**A**) 150°/sec and (**B**) 30°/sec. Note that the peak torque is higher at the slower velocity, which is consistent with explanations found in Chapter 2.

of the load under ischial tuberosities during sitting. Here the clinical interest is in monitoring the duration and size of the load so that patients can alter their posture and distribute the load before excessive pressure leads to tissue breakdown (39).

That force patterns are perturbed in pathological gait has been well established. Some have shown the changes in patients with hip disease (Fig. 6.16) (41). Others have used the force plate to collect comprehensive data sets to determine femoral

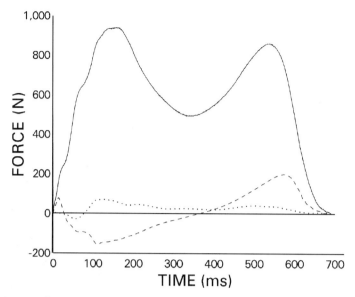

Figure 6.13. Ground reaction forces at the foot during stance phase of walking for a normal subject.

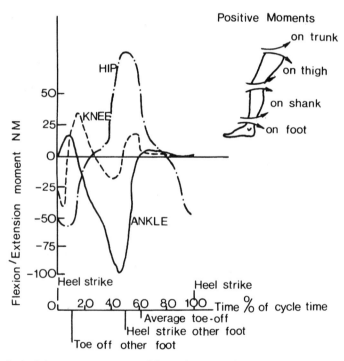

Figure 6.14. Sagittal plane moments generated during the stance phase of walking for a normal individual.

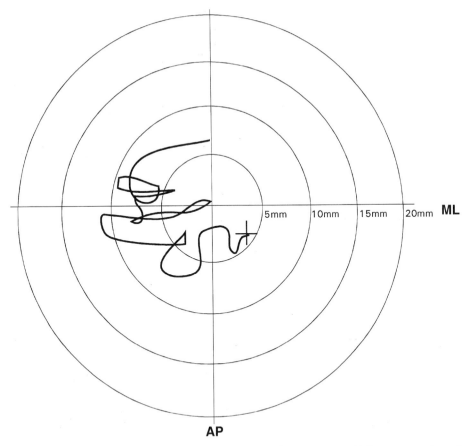

5mm   10mm   15mm   20mm   **ML**

AP

Figure 6.15. Plot showing the center of pressure during standing posture in which sway was voluntarily controlled by the subject.

head forces during activities of daily living (10, 20, 42). By modifying the signal from the force transducer, Cook and Cozzens developed a real time ground reaction force-line visualization technique that uses an optical beamsplitter for superimposition of a scaled vector image as an overlay on the patient image. A sample frame is shown in Figure 6.17. The displayed force vector is directly proportional to the force represented, as is the orientation of the force (15). Other uses include similar determinations for the knee and ankle as well as for studies involving energetics. More details on the work as applied to each joint will be provided in the chapters on the lower extremity.

COMPREHENSIVE ANALYSES OF HUMAN MOTION

The comprehensive study of human motion, particularly dynamic activities, requires the collection and analysis of complete sets of kinematic and kinetic data. For clinical analysis therapists often use manual techniques or functional activities to determine the torque-generating capabilities of their patients. The result of these tests requires that joint forces be generated in and distributed throughout the body. Because clinical methods are limited in their ability to determine generation of the joint forces and

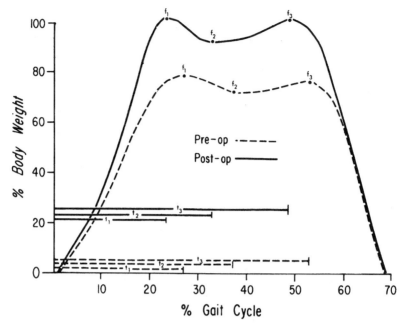

Figure 6.16. Vertical component of the floor reaction force in the hip. The f locates important force points while the t demonstrates how the temporal aspects vary between the normal subject and the patient with hip disease.

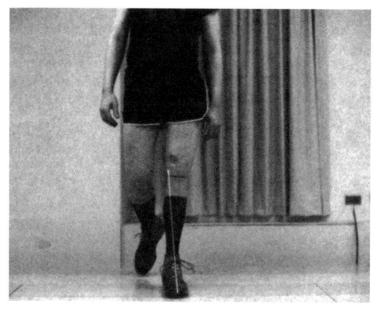

Figure 6.17. Force-line visualization technique for the sagittal plane for a normal subject. Note that the direction and magnitude of the force are both represented.

how they are distributed, comprehensive data sets can be generated and subjected to rigorous analysis. To complete such procedures both theoretical and mathematical analyses are used.

Studies using the more comprehensive methods are becoming available and virtually every joint in the body has been subjected to these analytical techniques. Overall, their purposes are to determine the resultant forces and torques at the joint or joints under study. The problem is complex because the sets of equations that generate the solution are indeterminate; i.e., they cannot be solved because the number of unknowns exceeds the number of equations.

Andrews points out two basic approaches to solving the equations to determine the force and torque resultants at each joint during a given interval. The first method of solution, using **reduction**, makes the equations determinant and places crude upper bound estimates for muscle forces (2). These resultants are then, in effect, distributed to bones, ligaments, and muscles based on certain "limits" set by known physiological information or based on assumptions. For example, kinematic data provide information about muscle length. Subsequently, estimates of available tension can be made. Likewise, knowledge of joint configuration provides data on ligament length that can be related to data from studies of ligament tensile strength. The other process, **optimization**, assumes that the body controls muscle tension to optimize some mechanical or biochemical process. An "objective" function, usually mathematical, is maximized or minimized in this solution process. That is, this technique attempts to model muscle tension by means of a mathematical process. In this latter case validations are frequently done with the electromyographic data derived concurrently with the kinematic and kinetic data. The entry level student of kinesiology and pathomechanics is referred to example studies that have used these techniques (10, 14, 22, 24, 34, 47).

SUMMARY

In summary, all techniques of motion analysis can play a valuable role in the therapist's understanding of normal and pathological function. Therapists should be able to evaluate readily and critically the techniques that appear in the literature and be able to utilize these techniques when applicable in their own clinical setting.

References

1. Allard P, Stokes IAF, Blanchi JP. *Three-Dimensional Analysis of Human Movement*. Champaign, IL: Human Kinetics; 1995.
2. Andrews JG. On the relationship between resultant joint torques and muscular activity. *Med Sci Sports Exerc* 1982;14:361–367.
3. Aptekar RG, Ford F, Bleck EE. Light patterns as a means of assessing and recording gait. I: methods and results in normal children. *Dev Med Child Neurol.* 1976;18:31–36.
4. Aptekar RG, Ford F, Bleck EE. Light patterns as a means of assessing and recording gait. II: results in children with cerebral palsy. *Dev Med Child Neurol.* 1976;18:37–40.
5. Bajd T, Kljajic M, Trnkoczy A, Stanic U. Electrogoniometric measurement of step length. *Scand J Rehabil Med.* 1974;6:78–80.
6. Boenig DD. Evaluation of a clinical method of gait analysis. *Phys Ther.* 1977;57:795–798.
7. Bohannon RW. Test-retest reliability of hand-held dynamometry during a single session of strength assessment. *J Orthop Sports Phys Ther.* 1986;66:206–209.
8. Bohannon RW, Andrews AW. Interrater reliability of hand-held dynamometry. *Phys Ther.* 1987;67:931–933.
9. Boone DC, Azen SP, Lin C, et al. Reliability of goniometric measurements. *Phys Ther.* 1978;58:1355–1360.

10. Brand RA, Crowninshield RD, Johnston RC, et al. Forces on the femoral head during activities of daily living. *Iowa Orthopedic J.* 1982;2:43–49.
11. Brinkman JR. Comparison of a hand-held and fixed dynamometer in measuring strength of patients with neuromuscular disease. *J Orthop Sports Phys Ther.* 1994;19:100–104.
12. Cavanagh PR, Henley JD. The computer era in gait analysis. *Clin Podiatr Med Surg.* 1993;10:71–484.
13. Chao EYS. Justification of triaxial goniometer for the measurement of joint rotation. *J Biomech.* 1980;13:989–1006.
14. Cholewicki J, McGill SM. EMG assisted optimization: a hybrid approach for estimating muscle forces in an indeterminate biomechanical model. *J Biomech.* 1994;27:1287–1290.
15. Cook TM, Cozzens BA. The effects of heel height and ankle-foot-orthosis configuration on weight-line location: a demonstration of principles. *Orthot Prosthet.* 1976;30:43–46.
16. Crowninshield RD, Johnston RC, Andrews JG, et al. A biomechanical investigation of the human hip. *J Biomech.* 1978;11:75–86.
17. Currie G, Rafferty D, Duncan G, et al. Measurement of gait by accelerometer and walkway: a comparison study. *Med Biol Eng Comput.* 1993;30:669–670.
18. Davis BL, Cavanagh PR. Decomposition of superimposed ground reaction forces into left and right force profiles. *J Biomech.* 1993;26:593–597.
19. Foley CD, Quanbury AO, Steinke T. Kinematics of normal child locomotion—a statistical study based on tv data. *J Biomech.* 1979;12:1–6.
20. Givens-Heiss DL, Krebs DE, Riley PO, et al. In vivo acetabular contact pressures during rehabilitation, part II. *Phys Ther.* 1992;700–710.
21. Grieve DW. Electromyography. In: Grieve DW, Miller DI, Mitchelson D, et al. *Techniques for the Analysis of Human Movement.* Princeton: Princeton Book; 1976.
22. Happee R. Inverse dynamic optimization including muscular dynamics, a new simulation method applied to goal directed movements. *J Biomech.* 1994;27:953–960.
23. Harbourne RT, Giuliani C, MacNeela J. A kinematic and electromyographic analysis of the development of sitting posture in infants. *Dev Psychobiol.* 1993;26:51–64.
24. Hardt DE. Determining muscle forces in the leg during normal human walking—an application and evaluation of optimization methods. *J Biomech Eng.* 1978;100:72–78.
25. Hay JG. *Biomechanics of Sport Techniques.* Englewood Cliffs, NJ: Prentice-Hall; 1978.
26. Holt KS, Jones RB, Wilson R. Gait analysis by means of a multiple sequential exposure camera. *Dev Med Child Neurol.* 1974;16:742–745.
27. Johnston RC, Smidt GL. Measurement of hip-joint motion during walking. *J Bone Joint Surg* 1969;51(A):1083–1094.
28. Miller DI, Nelson RC. *Biomechanics of Sport.* Philadelphia: Lea & Febiger; 1973.
29. Morrey BF, Askew LJ, An KN, et al. A biomechanical study of normal functional elbow motion. *J Bone Joint Surg.* 1981;63(A):872–877.
30. Morris JRW. Accelerometry—a technique for the measurement of human body movements. *J Biomech.* 1973;6:729–736.
31. Mueller MJ. Etiology, evaluation, and treatment of the neuropathic foot. *Crit Rev Phys Rehabil Med.* 1992;3:289–309.
32. Muybridge E, Brown LS, eds. *Animals in Motion.* New York: Dover Publications; 1957.
33. Nelson AJ. Functional ambulation profile. *Phys Ther.* 1974;54:1059–1065.
34. Patriarco AG, Mann RW, Simons SR, et al. An evaluation of the approaches of optimization models in the prediction of muscle forces during human gait. *J Biomech.* 1981;14:513–525.
35. Pedersen E, Klemar B. Recording of physiological measurements based on video technique. *Scand J Rehabil Med Suppl.* 1974;3:45–50.
36. Rheault W, Miller M, Nothnagel P, et al. Intertester reliability and concurrent validity of fluid-based and universal goniometers for active knee flexion. *Phys Ther.* 1988;68:1676–1678.
37. Richards C, Knutsson E. Evaluation of abnormal gait patterns by intermittent-light photography and electromyography. *Scand J Rehabil Med Suppl.* 1974;3:61–68.
38. Roebuck JA. Kinesiology in engineering. Presented at the Kinesiology Council, Convention of the American Association for Health, Physical Education and Recreation; March, 1966.
39. Shields RK, Cook TM. Lumbar support thickness: effect on seated buttock pressure in individuals with and without spinal cord injury. *Phys Ther.* 1992;72:218–226.
40. Smidt GL, Arora JS, Johnston RC. Accelerographic analysis of several types of walking. *Am J Phys Med.* 1971;50:285–300.
41. Stauffer RN, Smidt GL, Wadsworth JB. Clinical and biomechanical analysis of gait following Charnley total hip replacement. *Clin Orthop.* 1974;99:70–77.

42. Strickland EM, Fares M, Krebs DE, et al. In vivo acetabular contact pressures during rehabilitation, part I. *Phys Ther.* 1992;72:691–699.

43. Soderberg GL, Gabel R. A light emitting diode system for the analysis of gait: a method and selected clinical examples. *Phys Ther.* 1978;58:426–432.

44. Steindler A. *Kinesiology of the Human Body under Normal and Pathological Conditions.* Springfield, IL: Charles C Thomas; 1935.

45. Stuberg WA, Colerick VL, Blanke DJ, et al. Comparison of a clinical gait analysis method using videography and temporal-distance measures with 16-mm cinematography. *Phys Ther.* 1988; 68:1221–1225.

46. Sutherland DH, Hagy JL. Measurement of gait movements from motion picture film. *J Bone Joint Surg* 1972;54(A):787–797.

47. van den Bogert AJ, Smith GD, Nigg BM. In vivo determination of the anatomical axes of the ankle joint complex: an optimization approach. *J Biomech.* 1994;27:1477–1488.

48. Wadsworth CT, Krishnan R, Sear M, et al. Intrarater reliability of manual muscle testing and hand-held dynametric testing. *Phys Ther.* 1987;67:1342–1347.

49. Wadsworth JB, Smidt GL, Johnston RC. Gait characteristics of subjects with hip disease. *Phys Ther.* 1972;52:829–837.

50. Winter DA. *Biomechanics of Human Movement.* New York: John Wiley & Sons; 1979.

51. Winter DA, Greenlaw RK, Hobson DA. Television—computer analysis of kinematics of human gait. *Comput Biomed Res.* 1972;5:498–504.

52. Wolf SL, Binder-MacLeod SA. Use of the Krusen limb load monitor to quantify temporal and loading measurement of gait. *Phys Ther.* 1982;62:976–982.

7

Shoulder

Both clinicians and investigators have confirmed that function of the human shoulder is complex. The ability to elevate the hand over the head and execute many functional tasks requires great flexibility while maintaining integrity for the multiple joints operative during normal function. At the most proximal series of joints, torque must not be totally sacrificed at the expense of mobility because of frequent need to perform movements that require a great deal of power. This chapter will present the anatomical constraints and functional relationships of the shoulder. Effective function is explained by considering the interaction of the four joints that comprise the shoulder complex. Finally, the altered kinematics and kinetics of selected pathologies will be discussed.

MUSCULATURE

Musculature can be considered to function in isolation or in collective groups. Matsen (54) classifies the musculature as scapulohumeral and claviculohumeral, scapuloradial, scapuloulnar, thoracohumeral, thoracoscapular, and thoracoclavicular. A more functional and less cumbersome classification may be to use the terms scapulohumeral, axioscapular, and axiohumeral. No matter the system selected for classification, the musculature must be thought of in functional terms.

The major muscles of the shoulder complex are the trapezius, serratus anterior, and deltoid. Of these, the **trapezius** has a primary role in support of the upper limb upon the axial skeleton. Bearn (5) has shown the muscle to be electrically quiet during normal postures when no objects are simultaneously held in the hand. Although some activity is produced when weight is supported by the arm, most subjects could cease activity. The passive mechanisms used for support may provide some indication of the postures that lead to difficulties with the vascular and neural tree as each exits the thorax to supply the upper limb. A primary and necessary function of this muscle is to cause and/or maintain upward rotation of the scapula on the thorax.

The **serratus anterior** muscle, by virtue of attachment sites, is dedicated to motion of the scapula on the thorax. A primary responsibility is thought to be the motion of protraction, described to be the anterior gliding of the scapula on the wall of the thorax. The result has been the labeling of the muscle as the boxer's muscle. Another important function is the action of the lower portion of the serratus in effectively assisting with upward rotation of the scapula. Together then, with the trapezius upper and lower fibers, effective scapular upward rotation can be achieved as the arm is elevated over the head (49). Loss of any individual muscle or a collective group of muscles will be specifically discussed in the section on pathokinesiology found later in this chapter.

More important, the trapezius and serratus anterior muscles act as an effective force couple in the accomplishment of scapular upward rotation. To understand this

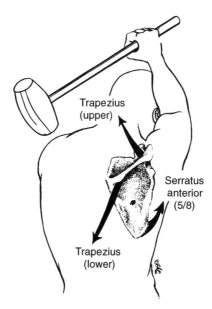

Figure 7.1.   Representation of the action of the serratus anterior and the lower fibers of the trapezius as a force couple.

function, consider the axis of rotation to be in the center of the scapula (Fig. 7.1). As the upper and most lateral fibers of the trapezius pull upwards on the distal aspect of the spine of the scapula, the inferior fibers of the serratus anterior pull the inferior angle of the scapula in a lateral and anterior direction. Thus, the muscles exert torques resulting from effective use of the principle of force couples. Also note that the lower trapezius fibers can act with the serratus anterior, creating another force couple. In relation to this function it is interesting that during man's evolution the trapezius has lost fibers (presumably from lack of use) that run parallel to the spine of the scapula. Further specialization of the serratus anterior is unanticipated since this muscle has already been separated from the levator scapulae muscle by virtue of loss of the intermediate fibers that formerly connected these two muscles (34). The relationship between these two muscles can be shown by their innervation. The levator, supplied by cervical roots 3, 4, and part of 5, and the C 5, 6, and 7 innervation of the serratus anterior, show that these muscles were once continuous with each other (95). Similarly, the rhomboids, teres major, and latissimus dorsi form couples for purposes of lowering the arm to the side. Such action is produced during specific motions such as pull ups or during high velocity activities such as wood chopping.

For the **pectoralis major** muscle, selective activity of the sternal and clavicular heads has long been conceded (79). Superficial and deep layers existed until differentiation took place. In fact, in most animals the pectoralis minor attaches to the humerus instead of the coracoid process (34). However, in human beings, the coracohumeral ligament can be considered a vestige of the former humeral attachment (39). This muscle is unquestionably important for powerful movements of the arm across the trunk. The same may be said about the latissimus dorsi when referring to glenohumeral extension and internal rotation. Together these two muscles account for considerable internal rotation torques that are little used in everyday function.

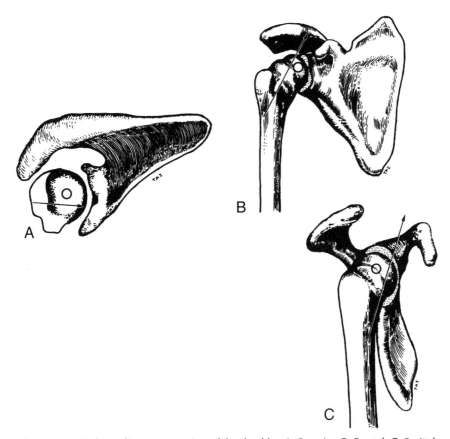

Figure 7.2. Triplanar diagrammatic view of the shoulder. **A.** Superior. **B.** Frontal. **C.** Sagittal.

The increase in the size of the acromion is perhaps indicative of the increase in the deltoid muscle mass. Inman (34) stated in 1944 that the deltoid makes up approximately 41% of the mass of the human abductor group. Today this value would be conservative. The deltoid also formerly contained a lower portion now known as the teres minor, offering a useful tool for remembering the similar axillary (C5–6) innervation of these two muscles (75).

The **deltoid** muscle is of interest because of the relatively large mass and the division of separate fiber groupings into anterior, middle, and posterior. This muscle provides reason to discuss the direction of the muscle's fibers in relation to the axis of rotation for the glenohumeral joint. In Chapter 1 the representation of muscle forces was discussed in relation to their capability to generate tensile loads at some given location with respect to an axis of rotation. The result, depending on the size of the tensile force and the perpendicular distance from which the force is applied determines the resultant torque. If we consider the anterior deltoid fibers while viewing the body in a frontal plane (Fig. 7.2A), the fibers are clearly superior to the axis of rotation. Thus, the muscle's function for this plane is abduction. Considering the same muscle from the superior view (Fig. 7.2B), the muscle essentially passes anterior to the axis of rotation, producing internal rotation. Finally, in the sagittal view (Fig. 7.2C), the anterior location leads to the conclusion that a muscle contraction would cause flexion torque. Similar diagrammatic representations for the middle deltoid would yield functions of abduction but no internal rotation or flexion since for the latter two motions the muscle fibers pass through the instant center of rotation of the joint. Whereas available tension and the muscle "moment arm" are factors involved in producing torques (or lack of torques) about joints, a constant and continual realization of the anatomy of the joint will assist in the conceptualization of the possible and real muscular capabilities as each contributes to joint torques. Conceptualization of the muscle as an effector of three-dimensional motion will be a useful tool in understanding complex interactions as other joint functions are discussed.

In spite of relatively small individual muscle masses, the collective functions of the rotator cuff musculature become important in normal and pathological motion. The **rotator cuff**, composed of the supraspinatus, infraspinatus, teres minor, and subscapularis muscles, is so labeled because of its effect upon the glenohumeral joint. Slips from each muscle are intimately woven into the capsule of the glenohumeral joint, strengthening and reinforcing the capsule. The same may apparently be said about the biceps brachii muscle as it indirectly contributes by increasing the glenohumeral joint's resistance to torsional forces when the joint is in the position of abduction and external rotation (80). Note that the weakest portion of the capsule is inferior, where cuff musculature contributes few reinforcing fibers. Of these muscles the supraspinatus muscle is notable, as it has lost some mass in evolution. More interesting is the teres minor muscle. Because of its attachments, it can depress the head of the humerus in the glenoid during isolated action; however, the teres minor's most important function is probably as a depressor during abduction and/or forward elevation of the arm.

Figure 7.3 shows that the net effect of the contraction of the deltoid and teres minor muscles is rotation by means of a force couple that contributes to effective elevation of the arm away from the body (54, 95). When the arm is still near the body the deltoid elevates the humerus on the glenoid rather than producing the angular rotation required to raise the arm out to the side. This is the case because muscle tension tends to move the humerus vertically. (See the discussion of forces in Chapter 1.) Consequently, in the early part of the range, it is the teres minor (and perhaps the infraspinatus and supraspinatus muscles) that contract to depress the head in the glenoid.

Saha (82) calls the muscles of the rotator cuff "steerers": they are mainly responsible for the head of the humerus rolling in the glenoid in different elevations while the prime mover raises the arm. He uses electromyographic evidence to confirm the role of the subscapularis and infraspinatus as stabilizers in the early range while demonstrating electrical activity in the infraspinatus, almost solely, in the terminal phases of arm elevation.

ARTHROLOGY AND ARTHROKINEMATICS

Anatomical structure and resulting functional capabilities reveal that evolutionary changes associated with the scapula and its movement on the trunk are consistent with the requirements for functional activities. Bechtol (6) has detailed these changes (Fig. 7.4), comparing the scapula of man with other forms of primates. Kent (39) also provides a discussion of the changes in the functional anatomy of the shoulder girdle. She comments that the scapula has increased in length and decreased in width, the primary changes occurring in the infraspinous fossa (Fig. 7.5).

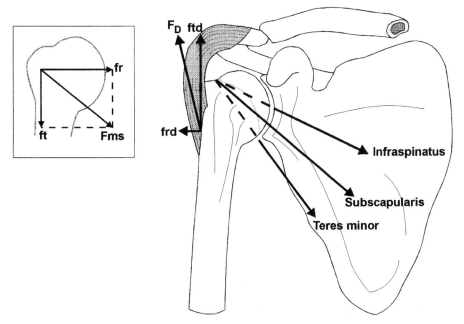

Figure 7.3. Anteroposterior view of the scapula and humerus, showing the force couple of the deltoid (F_D) and the muscles of the rotator cuff. The cuff effect (*Fms*) keeps the head of the humerus in articulation with the glenoid as a result of translational (*ft*) and joint resultant (*fr*) components. F_D results from a translational component (*ftd*) and the rotation component (*frd*). Note that the F_D vector is somewhat parallel to the *Fms* force. If the axis of rotation is placed between these two forces, a couple can be visualized.

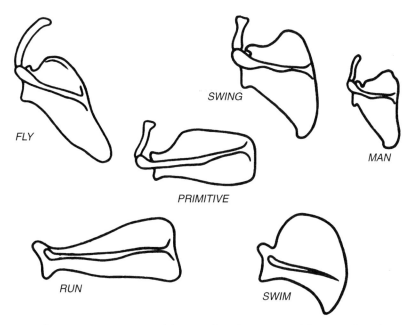

Figure 7.4. Schematic representations of the scapulae of many animal forms. In the adaptations for running and swimming, the scapulae no longer have a clavicular attachment that serves to impede movement of the bone. The scapula is also hinged on the vertical border.

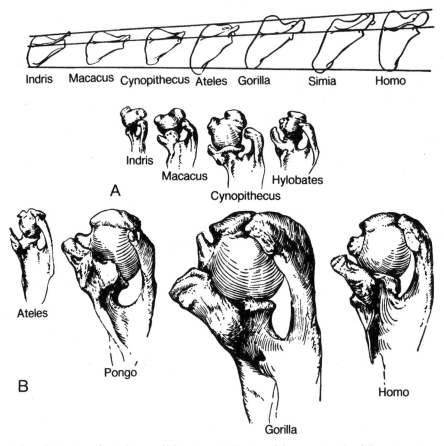

Indris Macacus Cynopithecus Ateles Gorilla Simia Homo

Indris

Macacus   Hylobates

A   Cynopithecus

Ateles

Pongo

B   Homo

Gorilla

Figure 7.5.   Scapular indices and alterations in the size of the acromion for different species.

The clavicle, not present in standing animals, is present in those that use the upper limbs for holding, grasping, and climbing (77). According to Kent's citations (39), several functions have been attributed to the clavicle, including the provision of a bony framework for muscle attachment and for purposes of protecting the peripheral vascular and nervous systems. Further, the clavicle serves as the attachment mechanism for the arm to the body, being at least partially responsible for supporting the weight of the upper limb. Without maintenance of the load with this force in the superior direction the arm would be free to be pulled inferiorly by gravity, potentially resulting in impingement of the vascular and nervous elements that exit the thorax. The clavicle also maintains the position of the scapula and humerus so that the arm can be held away from the body. The effects of congenital absence are seen in Figure 7.6 (84). In addition, the clavicle is said to assist with the transmission of force from the trapezius to the scapula through the coracoclavicular ligament and facilitates a mechanism for increasing the range of motion in the shoulder complex.

Bony changes have also evolved in the humerus. Positioning of the arm in space, as required by man's upright posture, has caused development of torsion in the humeral shaft (Fig. 7.7). That is, as the scapula rotated dorsally the humerus followed, resulting in torsion in the humeral shaft that now amounts to 164°. The deltoid tubercle

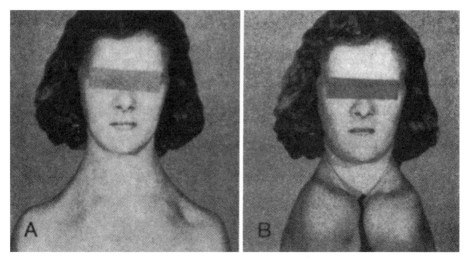

Figure 7.6. **A.** Young girl with cleidocranial dysostosis appears normal when natural posture is assumed. **B.** When the shoulders are brought anteriorly, the absence of the clavicles allows the scapula to move anteriorly so that the glenohumeral joint is now located under the chin.

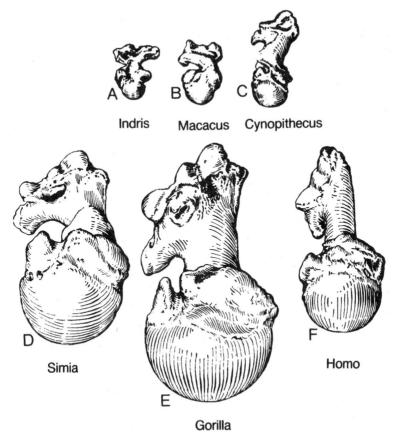

Figure 7.7. Changes in torsion in the humeral shaft relative to the glenoid.

has changed as well; it has migrated distally, thereby increasing the "mechanical advantage" of the deltoid muscle (34).

The scapula, clavicle, and humerus thus make up the bony framework of the shoulder complex. The proximal articulations of each, and the articulations with each other, form four primary joints: the sternoclavicular, acromioclavicular, gleno-humeral, and scapulothoracic joints. An understanding of the motion available at each joint and the interaction among the joints is critical to either normal or pathological motion of the shoulder complex.

The sternoclavicular joint is the only bone to bone attachment of the upper limb to the trunk. Within this synovial joint an intra-articular disc blends intricately with a capsule identified as loose but strong. Additional strength is provided to the joint by the sternocleidomastoid, sternohyoid, and sternothyroid muscles, although the available ranges of motion are accomplished by other muscles of the shoulder complex. Ligaments of significance include the interclavicular, costoclavicular, and the anterior and posterior sternoclavicular.

The acromioclavicular joint is another synovial joint that contains an intra-articular disc. Some disagreement exists as to the overall strength of the capsule, and, with the acromioclavicular joint, ligaments play a primary role in motion that is allowed or achieved as the arm is elevated over the head. The coraco-acromial ligament, blended with the trapezius and deltoid muscle attachments, provides a roof over the humeral head. The coracoclavicular ligament, which runs superiorly and posteriorly from the coracoid process, contains two portions. The conoid or most medial portion is a separate entity from the more laterally directed trapezoid portion. Functionally then, these ligaments provide for more glenohumeral joint abduction while also limiting scapular medial displacement and abduction (95).

The glenohumeral joint is also a synovial joint. The glenoid cavity is pear shaped and is approximately 39 mm in length and 29 mm in width (33). The glenoid is considered approximately 75% as long and 60% as wide as the humeral head. The fibrocartilaginous labrum adds depth to the glenoid, perhaps by as much as 50% (31). The articular radius of curvature of the surface of the glenoid (i.e., the longitudinal distance) is 35–50 mm (54); joint stability is determined not only by its depth but also by its supporting tissue. Evidence for these effects has shown that, with joint compression, the translating force resisted in different directions is variable (Fig. 7.8). Increased compression leads to greater maximum translating force resistance, as expected, while losses in the labrum lead to instabilities (50). Translation also occurs: during elevation an average of 9 mm superior displacement and 4.4 mm anterior displacement has been shown in a study on cadavers. There may be a high likelihood that similar findings would result during in vivo studies (102). Further, the glenoid is, on average, tilted 7° posteriorly (82). In the anatomical position the shaft of the humerus forms an angle of 135° with the glenoid. Retroversion in the humerus causes the humeral head to face posteriorly by 30° (54).

The capsule is attached to the circumference of the glenoid cavity and labrum and the anatomical neck except for the medial aspect attached slightly inferiorly (76). Such an arrangement conveniently adds to the glenohumeral laxity required for arm raising activities. Strength is added by the rotator cuff fibers that are intimately blended with the capsule. Muscles such as the triceps, pectoralis major, and teres major also send slips into the capsule that reinforce its strength. Likewise, the long head of the biceps is continuous with the glenoid labrum and intricately blends with the capsule. Very important are the anterior (or glenohumeral) ligaments. All

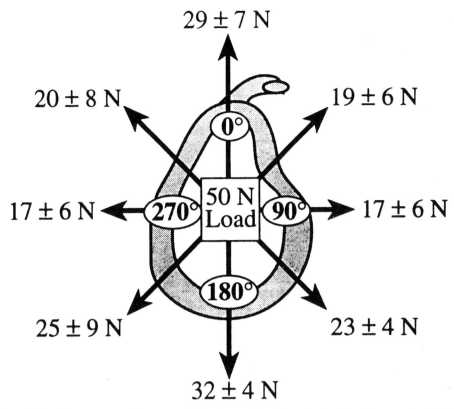

Figure 7.8. The average maximum translating force resisted in each direction (0° = superior, 90° = anterior) by the humeral head compressed into the glenoid concavity with a 50 N load for 10 specimens.

segments, the superior, middle, and inferior, have been credited with strengthening the capsule. Yet, the degree of tightening and subsequent tension for purposes of maintaining the integrity of the joint is dependent on the position of the joint and the structure being considered (35, 69). For example, the middle glenohumeral ligament is "critical" in restraining external rotation when the joint is between 60 and 90° of abduction (22). Similar types of statements can be made about other capsuloligamentous structures as they attempt to control a joint with little inherent stability (8). Also of significance is the anterior superior or coracohumeral ligament from the greater and lesser tuberosities to the coracoid process. Finally, the transverse humeral ligament connects the two primary tubercles on the humerus, forming a tunnel for the passage of the long head of the biceps brachii. In general, the capsule has been identified as loose for motion, primarily anteriorly and inferiorly (95).

Functionally the sternoclavicular joint operates as a ball and socket mechanism. It is generally said to have three degrees of freedom: elevation and depression, protraction and retraction, and rotation (Fig. 7.9). However, translatory motion is also possible at the sternoclavicular joint in both the anterior-posterior and superior-inferior directions. Thus, because of the additional ability to distract and compress the joint, six degrees of freedom can be demonstrated. The acromioclavicular joint is also believed to have three degrees of freedom although the same general principles that apply to the sternoclavicular joint could be advocated for the acromioclavicular

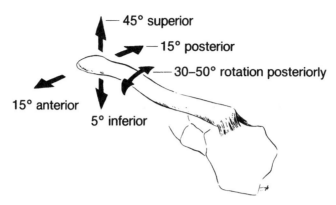

Figure 7.9. Representation of the available ranges of motion in the sternoclavicular joint.

joint. Motion at the acromioclavicular joint exists with upward scapular rotation from 20 to 60° of arm elevation. This motion occurs around an anterior-posterior axis. Another motion often described as winging of the scapula occurs around the vertical axis; 30–50° of winging can ordinarily be produced. Tilting, anterior and posterior, of approximately 30° occurs around the medial-lateral axis (39). The gleno-humeral ("ball and socket") joint allows for large ranges of motion in flexion and extension, adduction and abduction, and in both internal and external rotation. However, constraints are placed on passive movements of all these joints.

Because some motions, such as acromioclavicular, are due to tension in ligaments, active musculature is not required. Further, extremes of ranges of motion require tightening of other ligaments. For example, while glenohumeral abduction and exter-nal rotation are allowed by the relative slack in the inferior capsule, extremes of these motions will produce tightening and eventual achievement of the close packed position (37). Note, however, the influence of the position of the joints of the scapulo-humeral complex on ligamentous tension and the subsequent passive motion. To demonstrate, perform pure abduction to 70° and externally rotate the glenohumeral joint as far as possible. Then abduct an additional 40° and note the increase that has occurred, apparently in the external rotation range of movement. Perhaps the glenohumeral and coracohumeral ligaments have been placed on a relative slack, accounting for the increased motion. In essence, though, the glenohumeral joint demonstrates mobility at the sacrifice of stability.

With an understanding of the structures involved in shoulder motion and the interplay required between the tissues and joints two other aspects are important. The first is the function of the coraco-acromial arch. This area, sometimes labeled as the subdeltoid joint, is important because of the contents of the area and the effect of motion on the contents. To be specific, recall that the coraco-acromial ligament forms a roof over the humeral head. While serving a protective function for the superior elements from direct trauma the unyielding nature of the structure limits the available space for the tendons of the rotator cuff muscles. As a result pathology is focused in this region, in spite of the strategic location of the subdeltoid bursa (81). Discussion of the pathologies related to this functional joint will be presented later in the chapter.

The second feature of import is the relationship of the greater tuberosity to the other structures. In the usually assumed posture with the arm resting at the side, the greater tuberosity is outside the acromion process. However, with 80° of abduction of an internally rotated glenohumeral joint, the tuberosity and the structures superior to the tuberosity are prone to impingement under the acromion process. To avoid the impingement of both the soft and bony structures external rotation of the glenohumeral joint is required. If sufficient range is available in external rotation and if it can take place during abduction, the arm can be elevated completely over the head (85).

SCAPULOHUMERAL RHYTHM

Given an understanding of the joints and their available motions we can now discuss the interaction of the joints that occurs in elevation of the hand over the head. There is general agreement in the literature that during the first 30° of abduction, or the first 60° of forward flexion, the scapula is seeking stability on the thorax. This has been shown in work that has incorporated radiographic analysis (Fig. 7.10) (74). Freedman and Munro (24), on the other hand, have shown total scapular upward

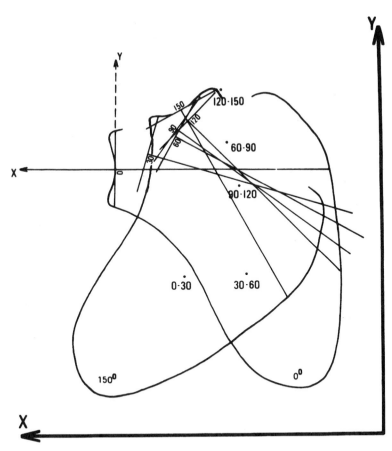

Figure 7.10. Scapular motion, in its own plane, is depicted relative to fixed axes in the body. Dots indicate the center of rotation for each of five positions. The outline of the scapula is also shown for the 0° and 150° positions.

rotation of 65° with total glenohumeral abduction of 103° using radiographic data for five positions of abduction. They concluded that for every two degrees of scapular motion there are three degrees of glenohumeral movement. The discrepancy between the data of Freedman and Munro and that of others may be because motion was allowed to occur in a coronal versus a scapular plane, the latter being 30–45° anterior to the true coronal plane. In another study 1.74° of glenohumeral motion occurred per degree of scapular motion (18). Under loaded conditions the scapular contribution was called for earlier in the range. Overall, the ratio of two degrees of glenohumeral motion to every degree of scapular movement is considered accurate, particularly when the total range of motion was considered (18, 23, 52, 61). Some have shown a 5:4 ratio after 30° of abduction, but a 2:1 ratio for the total range of shoulder motion (74). Overall, most would concede that the range of scapular motion does not exceed 60° while that of the glenohumeral joint does not exceed 120°.

During arm raising the primary motion occurring at the sternoclavicular joint is elevation. Poppen and Walker (74), upon evaluating this motion by means of acromial elevation, reported an approximately 35–45° elevation of the clavicle. Most of this motion occurs during the first 90° of arm elevation. Therefore, 4–5° of elevation occur during each 10° of the first half of the full range of arm elevation. With sternoclavicular elevation, motion also occurs at the acromioclavicular joint. Rotation of the clavicle around its own axis is due to the coracoclavicular ligaments pulling on the inferior aspect of the clavicle. This posterior rotation creates movement of the lateral clavicle on the acromion. Such motion has been detailed in a kinematic model of elevation of the shoulder complex (20). As summarized earlier, during the first 30° and from 135° to maximum elevation, rotation of the acromioclavicular joint occurs around the longitudinal axis of the clavicle (39). The summation of these motions at sternoclavicular, glenohumeral, scapulothoracic, and acromioclavicular joints creates the ability of humans to raise their arms above their heads.

Kapandji (37) states that the range of motion from 0 to 90° is glenohumeral while the motion from 90 to 150° is scapulothoracic. He cites few references, however, making it difficult to know if objective data support his position. Kapandji also states that thoracic extension or contralateral flexion is needed for full flexion or abduction to be achieved to 180°. Observation of patients supports this view, particularly if loads are lifted anteriorly or if unilateral abduction is attempted. Fatigue has also been shown to affect the kinematics of scapulohumeral performance (60).

Each of the four joints involved in motion of the shoulder complex must have the capability for torque generation to participate in elevation of the arm over the head. Whether accomplished in flexion or abduction the serratus anterior and trapezius upwardly rotate the scapula, after the teres minor and deltoid have participated as a **force couple**. The deltoid and supraspinatus are important for glenohumeral joint abduction; apparently, the deltoid is able to compensate for deficiencies in the supraspinatus (101). Also necessary for abduction of the arm is external rotation of the glenohumeral joint. This rotation must occur before 90° so that the greater tuberosity of the humerus not be impinged upon the inferior surface of the acromion process. An example of the activity and the timing of the muscle contractions is shown in Figure 7.11 (43). Other analyses using EMG have also been completed for sports activities to identify the pattern to which an athlete should aspire (10). Simultaneously occurring are passive processes, such as the posterior rotation of the clavicle created by the coracoclavicular ligaments. Alterations of normal kinematics and kinetics result from the pathologies discussed later in this chapter.

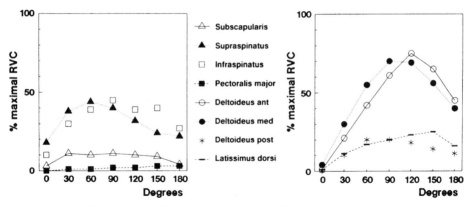

Figure 7.11.   Normalized EMG activity during shoulder abduction for eight muscles.

KINETICS
Torques

Because of the complexity of motions at multiple joints, muscles must create adequate moments to elevate the arm over the head. Recent literature (4, 38, 70, 89, 90) details the muscle geometry and architecture, providing a complete set of data compared with muscle lengths, moment arms, and muscle paths. All this information will assist in the determination of the joint torques, as has been accomplished by many people (12, 25, 46, 55, 56, 57, 71, 88). Table 7.1 summarizes the normal torques for representative studies and provides data clinicians can use to compare with their patients' values. Some caution should be exerted when comparisons are made across devices, as results may not be similar. Variability should also be noted, particularly when it is as large as 29–35%, as has been reported for internal and external rotation (except concentrics) (57).

Others have provided some interesting data based on determinations of moment arms from wire sutures placed directly in muscles. These data, shown in Figure 7.12, are for angles drawn parallel to the face of the glenoid. Evaluation of these graphs shows that the supraspinatus muscle is active throughout the abduction range of motion at a lever arm length of 20 mm. The muscle also maintains an angle with the glenoid of approximately 80°, meaning that the muscle would be effective in producing segment rotation rather than translatory motion. Muscles oriented at relatively small angles to the face of the glenoid would primarily produce shear of the joint rather than rotation. Note also that the anterior and middle deltoids increase their lever arms throughout the range of motion (70, 74). Simultaneously, the subscapularis, latissimus dorsi, and the infraspinatus decrease their moment arms while maintaining a large angle with the face of the glenoid (74).

Forces

At 60° of abduction, forces generated in surrounding musculature have been calculated to be approximately 10 times the weight of the limb. The muscle force required to support the limb at 90° of abduction has been calculated to be 8.2 times the weight of the limb (34). More recently, Walker and Poppen (91) have shown that the joint reaction force can equal approximately 90% of body weight. Others, modeling the shoulder, have calculated the glenohumeral forces to be from 100 to 400 N,

Table 7.1. Shoulder Torques for Subjects Without Pathology

Source Reference	Gender	Age Mean	Age SD	Age Range	n	Activity Level	Movement	Concentric (°/sec)	Eccentric (°/sec)	ROM	Testing Position	Peak Torque Nm	Peak Torque SD	Testing Device
97	m	25	3	18–32	50	normal	abd	180			sitting	80	15*	Biodex
							abd	300				53	19*	
							add	180				89	15*	
							add	300				78	18*	
70	m	26	3	21–35	36	normal	abd	0		0	sit, hip 130	71	3	Cybex II
							abd	0		45		58	2	
							abd	0		90		57	2	
							f	0		0	supine	94	4	
							f	0		45		81	3	
							f	0		90		75	3	
							ir	0		0	sup, sh 90, elb 90	51	2	
							ir	0		45(er)		48	2	
							er	0		0	sup, sh 90, elb 90	43	2	
							er	0		45(er)		35	2	
46	m	24		19–30	21	normal	er	90		60ir–60er	sup, sh abd 45, scaption	39	8	Lido 2.0
							er	210				34	6	
							er	0		0		39	6	
	m	58		50–65	9	normal	er	90		60ir–60er	sup, sh abd 45, scaption	28	6	Lido 2.0
							er	210				24	5	
							er	0		0		30	6	
	f	56		50–65	9	normal	er	90		60ir–60er	sup, sh abd 45, scaption	16	4	Lido 2.0
							er	210				15	3	
							er	0		0		18	4	
	m	24		19–30	21	normal	abd	90		20–120	sit, scaption	70	9	Lido 2.0
							abd	210		20–120		59	11	
							abd	0		90		65	10	
	m	58		50–65	9	normal	abd	90		20–120	sit, scaption	47	10	Lido 2.0
							abd	0		90		52	13	
	f	56		50–65	9	normal	abd	90		20–120	sit, scaption	27	3	Lido 2.0
							abd	0		90		27	6	

Ref	Sex	Age	n		Movement	Speed	Speed 2	Protocol	Position	Mean	SD	Device
92	f	19–25	12		ir	60			sh abd 15, elb 90	30	7	Cybex II
					ir	180				26	7	
					er	60				19	4	
					er	180				16	3	
	f	19–25	12		ir	60			sh abd 90, elb 90	25	5	Cybex II
					ir	180				23	5	
					er	60				19	3	
					er	180				17	4	
	m	34	10		er	60			Cybex II protocol	35	8	Cybex II
					ir	60				57	18	
					er	180				26	8	
					ir	180				43	14	
16	f	26	6		er	60			Cybex II protocol	15	3	Cybex II
					ir	60				23	5	
					er	180				12	3	
					ir	180				19	5	
27	m	21–33	9		ir	60	60	15er–60ir	sh f 45, elb 90	48	11*	Kin-Com
					ir	60				51	11*	
					er	180	180			25	8*	
					er	180				28	7*	
					ir	60	60			43	9*	
					ir	60				49	10*	
					er	180	180			25	7*	
					er	180				30	7*	
	f	21–33	9		ir	60	60	15er–60ir	sh f 45, elb 90	22	5*	Kin-Com
					ir	60				25	7*	
					er	180	180			14	5*	
					er	180				15	4*	
					ir	60	60			22	7*	
					ir	60				28	10*	
					er	180	180			12	3*	
					er	180				18	4*	
	m	21–33	9		ir	60	60	60er–30ir	sh abd 45, elb 90	49	11*	Kin-Com
					ir	60				55	14*	
					er	180	180			31	5*	
					er	180				34	7*	
					ir	60	60			42	8*	
					ir	60				54	13*	
					er	180	180			27	7*	
					er	180				34	7*	

Table 7.1.—*continued*

Source Reference	Gender	Age Mean	Age SD	Age Range	n	Activity Level	Movement	Concentric (°/sec)	Eccentric (°/sec)	ROM	Testing Position	Peak Torque Nm	Peak Torque SD	Testing Device
	f			21–33	9		ir	60		60er–30ir	sh abd 45, elb 90	24	5*	Kin-Com
							ir		60			29	7*	
							er	60				16	3*	
							er		60			18	3*	
							ir	180				22	6*	
							ir		180			29	8*	
							er	180				15	3*	
							er		180			20	4*	
56	f	24	5		19		f	300				24	5	Lido Active
							f	180				25	5	
							f	0				45	13	
							f		60			32	6	
							f		180			40	2	
	f	24	5		19		e	300				32	7	Lido Active
							e	180				32	8	
							e	0				54	12	
							e		60			54	9	
							e		180			57	10	
	f	24	5		19		ir	300				19	3	Lido Active
							ir	180				20	4	
							ir	0				21	7	
							ir		60			25	7	
							ir		180			27	4	
	f	24	5		19		er	300				11	2	Lido Active
							er	180				12	3	
							er	0				15	5	
							er		60			18	4	
							er		180			18	3	
	f	24	5		19		abd	300				18	4	Lido Active
							abd	180				18	4	
							abd	0				28	6	
							abd		60			25	4	
							abd		180			31	5	

Sex	Age			Movement	Speed	Speed	Val1	Val2	Device
f	24	5	19	add	300		23	7	Lido Active
				add	180		22	6	
				add	0		34	9	
				add		60	31	8	
				add		180	39	11	
m	26	4	32	f	300		39	9	Lido Active
				f	180		41	8	
				f	0		68	18	
				f		60	56	13	
				f		180	56	11	
m	26	4	32	e	300		55	15	Lido Active
				e	180		57	12	
				e	0		93	24	
				e		60	78	17	
				e		180	77	10	
m	26	4	32	ir	300		34	8	Lido Active
				ir	180		37	8	
				ir	0		43	12	
				ir		60	46	13	
				ir		180	42	6	
m	26	4	32	er	300		20	6	Lido Active
				er	180		22	5	
				er	0		30	10	
				er		60	30	8	
				er		180	26	4	
m	26	4	32	abd	300		30	8	Lido Active
				abd	180		33	8	
				abd	0		47	12	
				abd		60	41	10	
				abd		180	44	10	
m	26	4	32	add	300		45	18	Lido Active
				add	180		48	13	
				add	0		72	17	
				add		60	55	11	
				add		180	61	14	

Table 7.1.—continued

Source Reference	Gender	Age Mean	Age SD	Age Range	n	Activity Level	Movement	Concentric (°/sec)	Eccentric (°/sec)	ROM	Testing Position	Peak Torque Nm	Peak Torque SD	Testing Device
12	m	29	6	21–38	26		f	60			elb 90	50	12	
							f	300			elb 90	36	11	
							e	60			elb 90	87	18	
							e	300			elb 90	64	15	
	f	29	6	21–40	24		f	60			elb 90	22	5	
							f	300			elb 90	12	5	
							e	60			elb 90	40	7	
							e	300			elb 90	27	6	
	m	29	6	21–38	26		abd	60			scaption, elb 90	39	9	
							abd	300			scaption, elb 90	27	8	
							add	60			scaption, elb 90	80	16	
							add	300			scaption, elb 90	65	14	
	f	29	6	21–40	24		abd	60			scaption, elb 90	20	4	
							abd	300			scaption, elb 90	8	3	
							add	60			scaption, elb 90	39	6	
							add	300			scaption, elb 90	28	8	
	m	29	6	21–38	26		er	60			sh abd 15, elb 90	26	5	
							er	300			sh abd 15, elb 90	14	4	
							ir	60			sh abd 15, elb 90	46	14	
							ir	300			sh abd 15, elb 90	34	13	
	f	29	6	21–40	24		er	60			sh abd 15, elb 90	14	3	
							er	300			sh abd 15, elb 90	4	2	
							ir	60			sh abd 15, elb 90	22	4	
							ir	300			sh abd 15, elb 90	14	4	
63	m	31		26–36	20	untrained	e	0		0	sit, sh abd 0, elb 90	80	4	Force gauge
							f	0		0	sit, sh abd 0, elb 90	104	5	
							f	0		45	sit, sh f 45, elb 90	56	2	
							abd	0		45	sit, sh abd 45, elb 90	55	2	
							add	0		45	sit, sh abd 45, elb 90	103	6	
							ir	0		0	sit, sh abd 0, elb 90	58	3	
							er	0		0	sit, sh abd 0, elb 90	33	1	

Ref	Sex	Age*	n	Range	Subjects	Movement			Position		HHD
	m	62	20	56–66	untrained	e	0	0	sit, sh abd, 0, elb 90	74	3
						f	0	0	sit, sh abd 0, elb 90	84	4
						f	0	45	sit, sh f 45, elb 90	47	2
						abd	0	45	sit, sh abd 45, elb 90	42	2
						add	0	45	sit, sh abd 45, elb 90	82	5
						ir	0	0	sit, sh abd 0, elb 90	44	2
						er	0	0	sit, sh abd 0, elb 90	27	1
	f	29	20	25–35	untrained	e	0	0	sit, sh abd 0, elb 90	53	3
						f	0	0	sit, sh abd 0, elb 90	50	2
						f	0	45	sit, sh f 45, elb 90	33	2
						abd	0	45	sit, sh abd 45, elb 90	27	1
						add	0	45	sit, sh abd 45, elb 90	55	3
						ir	0	0	sit, sh abd 0, elb 90	28	1
						er	0	0	sit, sh abd 0, elb 90	18	1
	f	62	20	60–64	untrained	e	0	0	sit, sh abd 0, elb 90	35	2
						f	0	0	sit, sh abd 0, elb 90	38	3
						f	0	45	sit, sh f 45, elb 90	22	2
						abd	0	45	sit, sh abd 45, elb 90	22	2
						add	0	45	sit, sh abd 45, elb 90	38	2
						ir	0	0	sit, sh abd 0, elb 90	22	1
						er	0	0	sit, sh abd 0, elb 90	15	1
73					non-athlete	e	60	105-0	sup	86	6
						e	180	105-0	sup	70	8
87	m	23	14			er	0	0	sup, sh abd 90	47	
						er	0	0	sup, sh abd 90	49	

Legend: *, mean age; abd, abduction; add, adduction; e, extension; elb, elbow; er, external rotation; f, flexion; ir, internal rotation; scaption, scapular plane; sh, shoulder; sit, sitting; sup, supination.

depending on conditions (89). Maximum shear appears to occur at approximately 60° (89, 91). Figure 7.13 shows that the internal rotation position appears to generate greater joint compression force with some tendency to subluxate the joint. The external rotation position demonstrates greater stability.

Analysis of forces occurring in the shoulder complex is limited for several reasons. First, the motions are composed of complex interactions between multiple joints in multiple planes. Dvir and Berme (20) have addressed these aspects, but because of the complexity of the analytic processes there may be constraints in interpreting these data in light of in vivo considerations. Secondly, interest in forces across the glenohumeral joint has been minimal since the shoulder complex is not subjected to the weight bearing forces produced in the lower limb. Further studies are needed to clarify the interactive relationships among the joints. However, some understanding of the role of the joints and the muscles can be appreciated from the study of injury or paralytic states described in the next section.

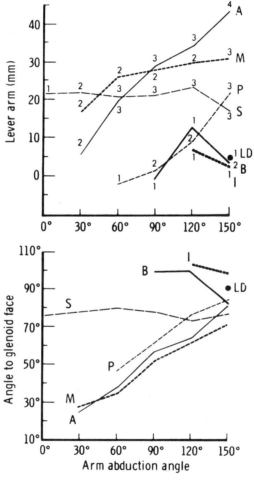

Figure 7.12.   Lever arms and angles to glenoid face plotted against the angle of arm abduction. *Legend*: *A*, anterior deltoid; *M*, middle deltoid; *P*, posterior deltoid; *S*, supraspinatus; *B*, subscapularis; *LD*, latissimus dorsi; *I*, infraspinatus. The numerical values are EMG activity levels on a 0–4 scale.

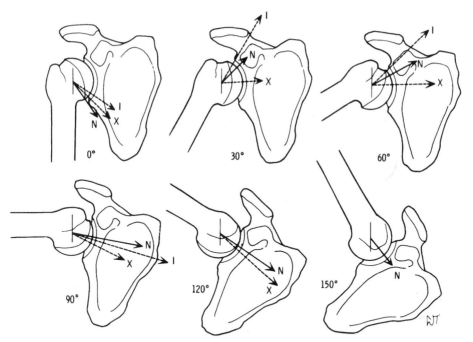

Figure 7.13. Resultant forces at the glenohumeral joint for six positions of the joint. *Legend*: *N*, neutral; *X*, external rotation; *I*, internal rotation.

PATHOKINESIOLOGY

Abnormal motion of the shoulder complex is often a severe and disabling circumstance that can involve acute pain, recurrent minor episodes, or progressive dysfunction. Soft tissue injuries frequently result from work or athletic endeavors. Paralytic lesions can come from pathologies requiring surgery. Further, spinal cord injury produces effects dependent on the level of insult. Each of these areas, and several other more unusual pathologies, will be discussed in this section.

Soft Tissue Injuries

Many **soft tissue injuries** of the shoulder complex have been identified. Common among them are anterior-inferior dislocations of the glenohumeral joint, a requisite of which is laxity but also weakness of this portion of the capsule. Often musculature is also weak. Saha (82) concludes that several factors predispose the glenohumeral joint to instability. Among them are decreased glenoid dimensions, anterior tilt of the glenoid, greater than normal retrotorsion in the humerus, and diminished power of the rotator cuff muscles. The muscular control of the unstable shoulder is an issue of continued debate: some show specific patterns of activity (44, 45, 62, 72), while others suggest that "a balanced muscle envelope" is not required to maintain normal kinematics in the shoulder (32, 94). The import of the rotator cuff has, however, been repeatedly recognized, enough so that the translatory motion at the glenohumeral joint may be diminished by "coordinated activity" of the rotator cuff (102). One study has shown that the subscapularis is the least important anterior stabilizer and that the biceps brachii becomes more important than the rotator cuff when stability in capsuloligamentous structures decreases (36).

Injury also frequently involves the rotator cuff, bursae, the bicipital tendon, and structures involved in "adhesive capsulitis." In these cases, which are relatively common in the elderly (13), no specific injury to tissues should produce long-term effects on function of the shoulder complex. However, as Figure 7.14 shows, a tear of the rotator cuff can produce profound effects on the glenohumeral joint. Figure 7.14B clearly shows the superior movement of the humeral head on the glenoid during maximal abduction effort. Based on what is known about glenohumeral movement there is very ineffective use of the deltoid-teres minor force couple. With such humeral elevation impingement of subacromial structures is likely. There is little doubt that normal kinematics must ultimately be restored in order for normal motion to occur. Where repair has been achieved, recovery is successful when torque testing shows a return to normal values (see Table 7.1 and compare them to those in Table 7.2) (28, 43). Note, however, that pain needs to be controlled (7, 43); in at least one case the instrumented testing did not correlate well with clinical grading of the muscle "power" (78).

Neer has discussed the **impingement lesions** of the shoulder and classified the problem into three stages. According to his observations the problem often occurs against the anterior edge and undersurface of the acromion, the coracoacromial ligaments and the acromioclavicular joint itself. Further, he explains that because of the adjacency of the structures the clinician should consider that two or more structures are involved together (20). In a group of patients with painful arc syndrome the pain was referred to the lateral aspect of the upper arm, occurring between 60 and 120° of abduction. Although the authors point out that the syndrome can be caused by several different lesions, it results from a loss of the normal clearance between the arch formed by the coraco-acromial ligament and the tuberosities below (40). Of some interest is that investigators have determined the forces underneath the coracoacromial vault, peak forces reaching 37.8 N under the acromion, 3.03 N under the coracoacromial ligament, and 6.93 N under the coracoid process. Final stages of arm elevation and "early reverse-elevation" had the most marked increases in forces (100). No matter the location of the specific clinical problem, precise examination techniques are always required to determine effectively which tissues are involved.

For many patients the painful effect of soft tissue injuries is limitation of shoulder use. Subsequently, difficulties arise in putting on a coat, reaching into a high cupboard, or driving a car. Muscle atrophy and weakness is also commonly seen in these patients. Treatment of the specific cause of the lesion should restore normal arthrokinematics and osteokinematics and maintain the usual kinetics required of the muscles. Thus, rehabilitation of shoulder pathology may demand that the specific kinematics of each joint be assessed to determine if any joints are limiting the normal motions described in the scapulohumeral rhythm section of this chapter. Specific examples of treatments and therapeutic exercises that may be necessary in these conditions are documented in the literature (3, 11, 17, 41, 48, 51, 58, 59, 63, 68).

Structural Loss

While the multiple joints in the shoulder complex depend on the bony structure for normal arthrokinematics and osteokinematics, reasonable function can be maintained even when scapulectomy has been required (47). Difficulties are magnified if the glenoid fossa is also lost (93).

Although the glenohumeral joint is subject to relatively small magnitudes of force

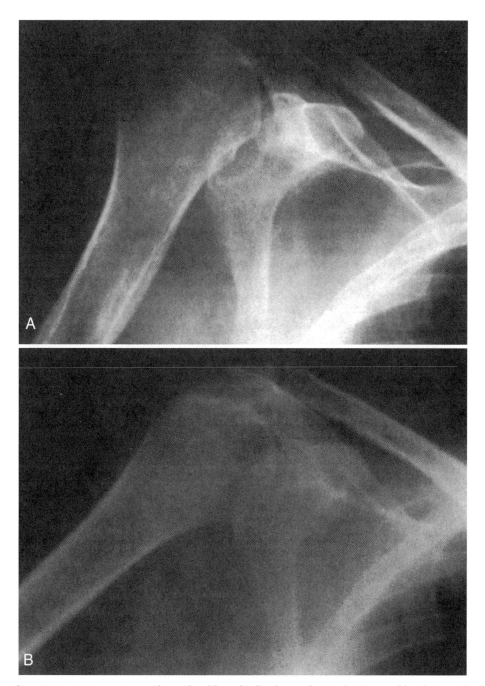

Figure 7.14.   Anteroposterior radiographs of the right glenohumeral joint of a 60-year-old male 6 months post tear. **A.** The joint at rest with elevation of the humerus on the glenoid. **B.** The joint in maximal abduction.

Table 7.2. Shoulder Torque Values for Subjects With Varied Athletic Participation

Source Reference	Gender	Age Mean	Age SD	Age Range	n	Activity Level	Movement	Concentric (°/sec)	Eccentric (°/sec)	ROM	Testing Position	Peak Torque Nm	Peak Torque SD	Testing Device
98	m	25	3	18–32	50	baseball ptchr	abd	180			sitting	75	16*	Biodex
							abd	300				59	19*	
							add	180				94	18*	
							add	300				76	19*	
97	m	23	3	18–32	150	baseball ptchr	er	180			sup, sh abd 45, scaption	48	8	Biodex
							ir	300				73	12	
							er	180				40	7	
							ir	300				66	12	
30	m	16	1	15–18	26	baseball ptchr	ir	90			stand, sh abd 0, elb 90	42	7	Cybex II
							er	90				25	4	
							ir	240				31	8	
							er	240				17	4	
					26		ir	90		90ir–105er	sup, sh abd 90, elb 90	39	7	Cybex II
							er	90				27	6	
							ir	240				26	7	
							er	240				16	4	
99	m			21–30	4	athletic	f	0		0	sh abd 0, elb 90	93		Kin-Com
	f			21–30	4	athletic	f	0		0	sh abd 0, elb 90	29		
53	m	24			26	baseball ptchr	ir	0			prone, sh abd 90, elb 90	48		Lafayette HHD
							er	0			prone, sh abd 90, elb 90	44		
							abd	0			sit, sh abd 90	79		
							mod-abd	0			sit, sh in scaption, ir	58		
	m	25	1		16		ir	0			prone, sh abd 90, elb 90	46		
							er	0			prone, sh abd 90, elb 90	46		
							abd	0			sit, sh abd 90	78		
							mod-abd	0			sit, sh in scaption, ir	60		
73	m	19		18–27	9	baseball ptchr	e	60		105–0	sup	104		Cybex II
							e	180		105–0	sup	83		
	f	19		18–27	15	swimmer	e	60		105–0	sup	102		
							e	180		105–0	sup	89		

1	m	18	14–21	26	baseball ptchr					Cybex II	
						er	90			26	6
						er	120			25	5
						er	210			24	4
						er	300			22	4
						ir	90			39	8
						ir	120			37	7
						ir	210			33	6
						ir	300			32	7
						h-abd	90			50	9
						h-abd	120			48	10
						h-abd	210			43	8
						h-abd	300			38	8
						h-add	90			54	13
						h-add	120			50	12
						h-add	210			44	11
						h-add	300			40	9
						f	90	40e–100f	elb 90	43	10
						f	120	40e–100f	elb 90	41	11
						f	210	40e–100f	elb 90	35	10
						f	300	40e–100f	elb 90	28	9
						e	90	100f–40e	elb 90	83	17
						e	120	100f–40e	elb 90	77	15
						e	210	100f–40e	elb 90	67	14
						e	300	100f–40e	elb 90	58	11
						abd	90	0–100	elb 90	48	12
						abd	120	0–100	elb 90	45	12
						abd	210	0–100	elb 90	38	11
						abd	300	0–100	elb 90	31	9
						add	90	100–0	elb 90	88	16
						add	120	100–0	elb 90	83	15
						add	210	100–0	elb 90	74	14
						add	300	100–0	elb 90	62	14

Legend: *, mean age; abd, abduction; add, adduction; e, extension; elb, elbow; er, external rotation; f, flexion; ir, internal rotation; scaption, scapular plane; sh, shoulder; sit, sitting; sup, supination.

resulting in correspondingly little degeneration, **total joint replacement** is occasionally advised. Criteria for using cemented or uncemented components still seem unclear (15). Neer et al. (66) have reviewed their experience with cemented total shoulder replacements in a consecutive series of 273 shoulders: 60 with old trauma, 56 with rheumatoid arthritis, 55 with osteoarthritis, and 97 with other diagnoses. Glenohumeral stability depended on the height and the version of the prosthetic components. Function depended on reconstruction and the rehabilitation of the rotator cuff and deltoid muscles. In emphasizing the optimum results achieved with the form of unconstrained prostheses used in these patients, the authors specified that the muscles are important to both mobility and stability. Others have specifically indicated the import of the rotator cuff musculature in determining an outcome in a patient series that increased the range of motion by 60° in flexion and 18° in external rotation (29).

One interesting musculoskeletal disorder that affects the shoulder complex is the **snapping scapula syndrome**. Strizak and Cowen (86) reported a case that does not fit the classical etiology of repeated, forceful shoulder action. Thought to produce periosteal microtears along the medial border of the scapula the result is a distinct thump or snapping as the scapula is moved across the thorax. One possible explanation for the syndrome is that the levator scapulae muscle has been weakened by chronic trauma or perhaps has been avulsed.

Neurological Deficit

Paralyses of isolated muscles of the shoulder complex are rare, but when they do occur a profound disruption of scapulohumeral rhythm can occur (83). For example, **trapezius paralysis** may be an unavoidable side effect of surgical procedures in the posterior triangle of the neck (19). In these cases the scapula assumes a position of depression and protraction as the acromion droops. On occasions the sternum can be deviated to the opposite side during full elevation of the arm. The acromion cannot effectively be pulled posteriorly, and weakness in elevation of the arm results (Fig. 7.15).

Although not always the result of isolated or collective paralysis of muscle, poor posture or abnormal positioning can be responsible for dysfunction of the upper limb. This has been well documented for **syndromes of the thoracic outlet**, where impingement of the nerve or vascular bundle will produce definitive symptoms. Often the therapist must make an accurate assessment of the posture and the arthrokinematics and arthrokinetics available to the patient before the problem can be adequately treated.

Serratus anterior paralysis can also be produced in isolation. Such instances have been reported in a young athlete (26) and in cases with an insidious onset (96). Fardin et al. (21) have recently reviewed a series of 10 cases. Nearly all cases were caused by trauma from falls. On occasion the **long thoracic nerve** is sectioned during mastectomy. In these cases of isolated paralysis the scapula becomes winged since virtually no other muscle can hold the inferior angle of the scapula against the thorax. Elevation of the arm overhead may no longer be possible (49). As for isolated paralysis of the trapezius some difficulty can be expected with elevating the arm over the head.

In **combined serratus anterior and trapezius paralysis**, there is distinct difficulty in raising the arm above the head. In these cases all motion must essentially occur at the glenohumeral joint since effective upward rotation of the scapula has been lost. The result is, in effect, static equilibrium: as the arm reaches maximal glenohumeral

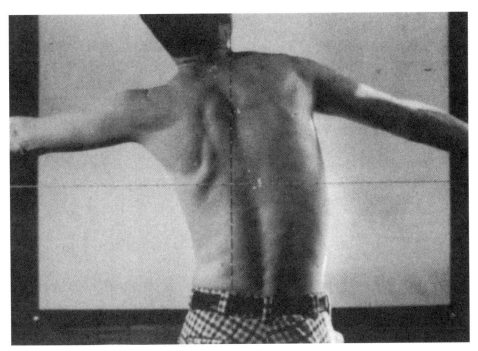

Figure 7.15.   Posterior view of bilateral abduction. Note the normal mechanics of the left side with the abnormal right side. The right glenohumeral joint appears to lack external rotation. To gain more abduction the patient leans to the contralateral side.

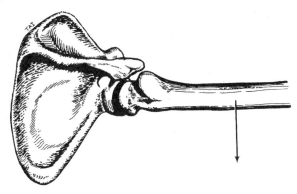

Figure 7.16.   The scapulohumeral complex at the point when full abduction has been reached in the case of paralysis of the shoulder girdle musculature. Note that the scapula assumes a position of downward rotation.

abduction due to the action of the deltoid, the downward moment produced by the weight of the limb balances and prevents further scapular motion (Fig. 7.16). Further abduction of the glenohumeral joint is impossible because the deltoid has been sufficiently shortened so that no further tension is available. As a result the individual can elevate the arm to approximately 60°.

Cases of **facioscapulohumeral muscular dystrophy** also provide useful examples of the effect of scapular stabilization upon the thorax. In these cases the scapula is winged and unable to rotate upwardly (Fig. 7.17). Compare the similarities of the patient photo with the mechanics diagramed in Figure 7.16. To provide for better functional abilities, surgical procedures have been performed with results that have increased abduction by 37% while increasing shoulder strength and endurance (42).

Paralysis or specific involvement of either the **deltoid** or **supraspinatus** produces some weakness at the glenohumeral joint but still allows elevation of the arm over the head. Bechtol (6) has recently suggested that the supraspinatus supplies approximately 20% of the power for arm elevation, and if this muscle is lost the individual has difficulty elevating the arm after 90° (Fig. 7.18). If the deltoid and teres minor are involved because of injury to the axillary nerve, abduction is weak or limited because of the loss of the force-couple at the glenohumeral joint. Etiologies creating this peripheral nerve involvement include subglenoid dislocations, fractures of the humeral head, crutch compression, and/or a severe blow on the shoulder (64).

Spinal cord injury patients provide further examples of disrupted kinetics of the shoulder complex that in turn lead to altered kinematics. The resultant loss will be directly related to the level of the lesion. For purposes of studying the shoulder the C5–6 and C6–7 lesions are of the most interest. Losses above the C5 level leave incompetence of the serratus anterior. The results shown in Figure 7.19 are for attempted arm elevation (67). What results is a scapular downward rotation during a pull forward to the seated position (65). Patients with spinal cord injuries are also noted to have shoulder pain that may be attributed to overuse, impingement, or weakness of the rotator cuff and shoulder girdle musculature. Testing has revealed

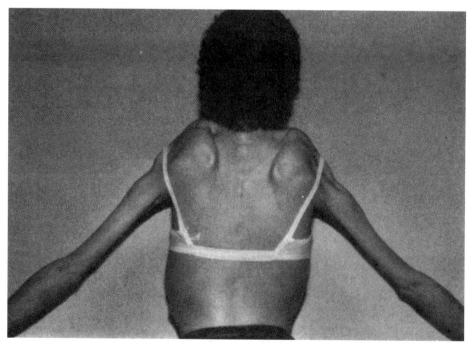

Figure 7.17.   Posterior view of patient with fascioscapulohumeral muscular dystrophy. Note the downwardly rotated position of the scapulae.

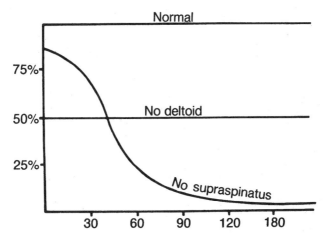

Figure 7.18. Torque, in percent of maximum, is plotted against the range of motion in the normal shoulder. Deltoid loss would still enable abduction of the glenohumeral joint at about 50% of the torque. Loss of the supraspinatus, however, would enable 80% of the torque early in the range, falling rapidly to less than 20% by the midpoint in the range of motion.

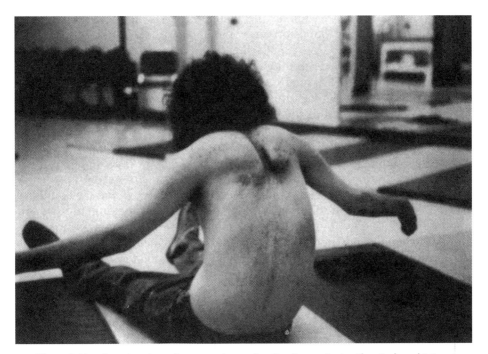

Figure 7.19. Posterior view of attempted arm elevation in a patient with spinal cord injury.

differences in most generated torques, resulting in a greater risk for dysfunction (75). Other lower level cervical injuries that affect the remainder of the arm will be discussed in subsequent chapters.

Other neurological patients are not without movement dysfunction of the shoulder complex. Patients with **hemiplegia** have long been known to exhibit inferior subluxation of the glenohumeral joint secondary to weakness or paralysis, at least in 50% of the cases (9). In postulating that subluxation is caused by brachial plexus lesions Chino (14) suggested that 75% of the supraspinatus and deltoid muscles revealed pathological electromyographic potentials. If in fact the potential incidence is as high as these data suggest, then practitioners must give considerable attention to the glenohumeral joint, including the finding that there is typically decreased range of motion, at least in lateral rotation (2). The suggestion has been made that the shoulder should be in a retracted position or suspended to prevent overstretching (14). Caution should also be exercised against over-aggressive range of motion of the joint. Therapists must be reminded that indiscriminate passive stretching procedures can have deleterious effects on structures that are attempting to provide support. In addition, inert structures can have such great tensile strength that abnormal and/or unwanted arthrokinematics may result from improperly applied therapeutic techniques. That is, motion contrary to the principles applied to joint surfaces, as established in Chapter 4, can result. The therapist must seek a delicate balance to restore or maintain normal arthrokinematics.

SUMMARY

This chapter has discussed anatomical elements in relationship to normal and abnormal motion of the shoulder complex. Fundamental principles of force representation, moments, and couples have been presented as they relate to the shoulder in both normal and pathological circumstances. Finally, various pathologies have been considered with respect to how normal motion is disrupted.

References

1. Alderink GJ, Kuck DJ. Isokinetic shoulder strength of high school and college aged pitchers. *J Orthop Sports Phys Ther.* 1986;7:163–172.
2. Andrews AW, Bohannon RW. Decreased shoulder range of motion on paretic side after stroke. *Phys Ther.* 1989;69:768–772.
3. Ballantyne BT, O'Hare, Paschall JL. Electromyographic activity of selected muscles in commonly used therapeutic exercises. *Phys Ther.* 1993;73:668–677.
4. Bassett RW, Browne AL, Morrey BF, et al. Glenohumeral muscle force and moment mechanics in a position of shoulder instability. *J Biomech.* 1990;23:405–415.
5. Bearn JG. An electromyographic study of the trapezius, deltoid, pectoralis major, biceps and triceps muscles, during static loading of the upper limb. *Anat Rec.* 1961;140:103–108.
6. Bechtol CO. Biomechanics of the shoulder. *Clin Orthop.* 1980;146:37–41.
7. Ben-Yishay A, Zuckerman JD, Gallagher M, et al. Pain inhibition of shoulder strength in patients with impingement syndrome. *Orthopedics.* 1994;17:685–688.
8. Bowen MK, Warren RF. Ligamentous control of shoulder stability based on selective cutting and static translation experiments. *Clin Sports Med.* 1991;10:757–782.
9. Boyd EA, Goudreau L, O'Riain MD, et al. A radiological measure of shoulder subluxation in hemiplegia: its reliability and validity. *Arch Phys Med Rehabil.* 1993;74:188–193.
10. Bradley JP, Tibone JE. Electromyographic analysis of muscle action about the shoulder. *Clin Sports Med.* 1991;10:789–805.
11. Brewster C, Moynes D, Schwab DR. Rehabilitation of the shoulder following rotator cuff injury or surgery. *J Orthop Sports Phys Ther.* 1993;18:422–426.
12. Cahalan TD, Johnson ME, Chao EYS. Shoulder strength analysis using the Cybex II isokinetic dynamometer. *Clin Orthop.* 1991;271:249–257.
13. Chakravarty K, Webley M. Shoulder joint movement and its relationship to disability in the elderly. *J Rheumatol.* 1993;20:1359–1361.
14. Chino N. Electrophysiological investigation on shoulder subluxation in hemiplegics. *Scand J Rehabil Med.* 1981;13:17–21.
15. Cofield RH. Uncemented total shoulder arthroplasty. *Clin Orthop.* 1994;307:86–93.

16. Connelly-Maddux RE, Kibler WB, et al. Isokinetic peak torque and work values for the shoulder. *J Orthop Sports Phys Ther.* 1989;10:264–269.

17. Davies GJ, Dickoff-Hoffman S. Neuromuscular testing and rehabilitation of the shoulder complex. *J Orthop Sports Phys Ther.* 1993;18:449–458.

18. Doody SG, Freedman L, Waterland JC. Shoulder movement during abduction in the scapular plane. *Arch Phys Med Rehabil.* 1970;51:595–604.

19. Dunn AW. Trapezius paralysis after minor surgical procedures in the posterior cervical triangle. *South Med J.* 1974;67:312–315.

20. Dvir Z, Berme N. The shoulder complex in elevation of the arm: a mechanism approach. *J Biomech.* 1978;11:219–225.

21. Fardin P, Negrin P, Dainese R. The isolated paralysis of the serratus anterior muscle: clinical and electromyographical follow-up of 10 cases. *Electromyogr Clin Neurophysiol.* 1978;18:379–386.

22. Ferrari DA. Capsular ligaments of the shoulder-anatomical and functional study of the anterior superior capsule. *Am J Sports Med.* 1990;18:20–24.

23. Frankel VH, Nordin M. *Basic Biomechanics of the Skeletal System.* Philadelphia: Lea & Febiger; 1980.

24. Freedman L, Munro RR. Abduction of the arm in the scapular plane: scapular and glenohumeral movements. *J Bone Joint Surg.* 1966;48(A):1503–1510.

25. Frisiello S, Gazaille A, O'Halloran J, et al. Test-retest reliability of eccentric peak torque values for shoulder medial and lateral rotation using the Biodex isokinetic dynamometer. *J Orthop Sports Phys Ther.* 1994;19:341–344.

26. Gregg JR, Labosky D, Harty M, et al. Serratus anterior paralysis in the young athlete. *J Bone Joint Surg.* 1979;61(A):825–832.

27. Hageman PA, Mason DK, Rylund KN, et al. Effects of positions and speed on eccentric and concentric isokinetic testing of the shoulder rotators. *J Orthop Sports Phys Ther.* 1989;11:64–69.

28. Hartsell HD. Postsurgical shoulder strength in the older patient. *J Orthop Sports Phys Ther.* 1993;18:667–672.

29. Hawkins RJ, Bell RH, Jalley B. Total shoulder arthroplasty. *Clin Orthop.* 1989;242:188–194.

30. Hinton RY. Isokinetic evaluation of shoulder rotational strength in high school baseball pitchers. *Am J Sports Med.* 1988;16:274–279.

31. Howell SM, Galinat BJ. The glenoid-labral socket—a constrained articular surface. *Clin Orthop.* 1989;243:122–125.

32. Howell SM, Kraft TA. The role of the supraspinatus and infraspinatus muscles in glenohumeral kinematics of anterior shoulder instability. *Clin Orthop.* 1991;263:128–134.

33. Iannotti JP, Babriel JP, Schneck SL, et al. The normal glenohumeral relationships—an anatomical study of one hundred and forty shoulders. *J Bone Joint Surg.* 1992;74(A):491–500.

34. Inman V, Saunders M, Abbott LC. Observations on the function of the shoulder joint. *J Bone Joint Surg.* 1944; 26(A):1–30.

35. Itoi E, Grabowski JJ, Morrey BF, et al. Capsular properties of the shoulder. *Tohoku J Exp Med.* 1993;171:203–210.

36. Itoi E, Newman SR, Kuechle DK, et al. Dynamic anterior stabilisers of the shoulder with the arm in abduction. *J Bone Joint Surg.* 1994;76(B):834–836.

37. Kapandji IA. *The Physiology of the Joints.* 5th ed. Edinburgh: Churchill Livingstone; 1982;1.

38. Karlson D, Peterson B. Towards a model for force predictions in the human shoulder. *J Biomech.* 1991;25:189–199.

39. Kent BE. Functional anatomy of the shoulder complex: a review. *J Am Phys Ther Assoc.* 1971;51:867–888.

40. Kessel L, Watson M. The painful arc syndrome: clinical classification as a guide to management. *J Bone Joint Surg.* 1977;59(B):166–172.

41. Kessler RK, Hertling D. *Management of Common Musculoskeletal Disorders.* Philadelphia: Harper & Row; 1983.

42. Ketenjian AY. Scapulocostal stabilization for scapular winging in facio-scapulohumeral muscular dystrophy. *J Bone Joint Surg.* 1978;60(A):476–480.

43. Kirschenbaum D, Coyle MP, Leddy JP. Shoulder strength with rotator cuff tears—pre and postoperative analysis. *Clin Orthop.* 1993;288:174–178.

44. Kronberg M, Németh G, Broström L-Å. Muscle activity and coordination in the normal shoulder. *Clin Orthop.* 1990;257:76–85.

45. Kronberg M, Németh G, Broström L-Å. Differences in shoulder muscle activity between patients with generalized joint laxity and normal controls. *Clin Orthop.* 1991;269:181–192.

46. Kuhlman JR, Iannotti JP, Kelly MJ, et al. Isokinetic and isometric measurement of strength of external rotation and abduction of the shoulder. *J Bone Joint Surg.* 1992;74:1320–1333.
47. Kumar VP, Satku SK, Mitra AK, et al. Function following limb salvage for primary tumors of the shoulder girdle: 10 patients followed 4 years. *Acta Orthop Scand.* 1994;65:55–61.
48. LaStayo P, Jaffe R. Assessment and management of shoulder stiffness: a biomechanical approach. *J Hand Ther.* 1994;7:122–130.
49. Lehmkuhl LD, Smith LK. *Brunnstrom's Clinical Kinesiology.* 5th ed. Philadelphia: FA Davis; 1996.
50. Lippitt S, Matsen F. Mechanisms of glenohumeral joint stability. *Clin Orthop.* 1993;291:20–28.
51. Litchfield R, Hawkins R, Dillman CJ, et al. Rehabilitation for the overhead athlete. *J Orthop Sports Phys Ther.* 1993;18:433–441.
52. MacConaill MA, Basmajian JV. *Muscles and Movements: A Basis for Human Kinesiology.* Baltimore: Williams & Wilkins; 1969.
53. Magnussen SP, Bleim BW, Nicholas JA. Shoulder weakness in professional baseball pitchers. *Med Sci Sports Exerc.* 1994;26:5–9.
54. Matsen FA. Biomechanics of the shoulder. In: Frankel VM, Nordin M, eds. *Basic Biomechanics of the Skeletal System.* Philadelphia: Lea & Febiger; 1980:221–242.
55. Malerba JL, Adams ML, Harris BA, et al. Reliability of dynamic and isometric testing of shoulder external and internal rotators. *J Orthop Sports Phys Ther.* 1993;18:543–552.
56. Mayer F, Horstmann T, Röcker K, et al. Normal values of isokinetic maximum strength, the strength/velocity curve, and the angle at peak torque of all degrees of freedom in the shoulder. *Int J Sports Med.* 1994;15:S19–S25.
57. Mayer F, Horstmann T, Kranenberg U, et al. Reproducibility of isokinetic peak torque and angle at peak torque in the shoulder joint. *Int J Sports Med.* 1994;15 (S1):S26–31.
58. McCann PD, Wootten ME, Kadaba MP, et al. A kinematic and electromyographic study of shoulder rehabilitation exercises. *Clin Orthop.* 1993;288:179–188.
59. McClure PW, Flowers KR. Treatment of limited shoulder motion: a case study based on biomechanical considerations. *Phys Ther.* 1992;72:929–936.
60. McQuade KJ, Wei SH, Smidt GL. Effects of local muscle fatigue on three-dimensional scapulohumeral rhythm. *Clin Biomech.* 1995;10:144–148.
61. Michiels I, Grevenstein J. Kinematics of shoulder abduction in the scapular plane—on the influence of abduction velocity and external load. *Clin Biomech.* 1995;10:137–143.
62. Moseley JB, Jobe FW, Pink M, et al. EMG analysis of the scapular muscles during a shoulder rehabilitation program. *Am J Sports Med.* 1992;20:128–134.
63. Murray MP, Gore Dr, Gardner GM, et al. Shoulder motion and muscle strength of normal men and women in two age groups. *Clin Orthop.* 1985;192:268–273.
64. Narakas AO. Paralytic disorders of the shoulder girdle. *Hand Clin.* 1988;4:619–632.
65. Neer CS. Impingement lesions. *Clin Orthop.* 1983;173:70–77.
66. Neer CS, Watson KC, Stanton FJ. Recent experience in total shoulder replacement. *J Bone Joint Surg.* 1982;64(A):319–337.
67. Neumann D. Iowa City, Iowa, personal communication; 1983.
68. Nicholson GG. Rehabilitation of common shoulder injuries. *Clin Sports Med.* 1989;8:633–655.
69. O'Connell PW, Nuber GW, Mileski RA, et al. The contribution of the glenohumeral ligaments to anterior stability of the shoulder joint. *Am J Sports Med.* 1990;18:579–584.
70. Otis JC, Jiang C-C, Wickiewicz TL, et al. Changes in the moment arms of the rotator cuff and deltoid muscles with abduction and rotation. *J Bone Joint Surg.* 1994;76(A):667–676.
71. Otis JC, Warren RF, Backus SI, et al. Torque production in the shoulder of the normal young adult male—the interaction of function, dominance, joint angle, and angular velocity. *Am J Sports Med.* 1990;18:119–123.
72. Peat M, Grahame RE. Electromyographic analysis of soft tissue lesions affecting shoulder function. *Am J Phys Med.* 1977;56:223–240.
73. Perrin DH, Robertson RJ, Ray KL. Bilateral isokinetic peak torque, torque acceleration energy, power and work relationship in athletes and non-athletes. *J Orthop Sports Phys Ther.* 1987;9:184–189.
74. Poppen NK, Walker PS. Normal and abnormal motion of the shoulder. *J Bone Joint Surg.* 1976;58(A):195–201.
75. Powers CM, Newsam CJ, Gronley JK, et al. Isometric shoulder torque in subjects with spinal cord injury. *Arch Phys Med Rehabil.* 1994;75:761–765.
76. Pratt NE. Anatomy and biomechanics of the shoulder. *J Hand Ther.* 1994;7:65–76.
77. Quiring DP, Boroush EL. Functional anatomy of the shoulder girdle. *Arch Phys Med.* 1946;27:90–96.

78. Rabin SI, Post M. A comparative study of clinical muscle testing and Cybex evaluation after shoulder operations. *Clin Orthop*. 1990;147–156.

79. Rasch PJ, Burke RK. *Kinesiology and Applied Anatomy: The Science of Human Movement*. 6th ed. Philadelphia: Lea & Febiger; 1978.

80. Rodosky MW, Harner CD, Fu FH. The role of the long head of the biceps muscle and superior glenoid labrum in anterior stability of the shoulder. *Am J Sports Med*. 1994;22:121–130.

81. Rothman RH, Marvel JP, Heppenstall RB. Anatomic considerations in the glenohumeral joint. *Orthop Clin of North Am*. 1975;6:341–352.

82. Saha AK. Dynamic stability of the glenohumeral joint. *Acta Orthop Scand*. 1971;42:491–505.

83. Saha AK. Mechanics of elevation of glenohumeral joint: its application in rehabilitation of flail shoulder in upper brachial plexus injuries and poliomyelitis and in replacement of the upper humerus by prosthesis. *Acta Orthop Scand*. 1973;44:668–678.

84. Shands AR. *Handbook of Orthopedic Surgery*. 5th ed. St. Louis: CV Mosby; 1971.

85. Sohier R. *Kinesitherapy of the Shoulder*. Bristol, England: John Wright and Sons; 1967.

86. Strizak AM, Cowen MH. The snapping scapula syndrome. *J Bone Joint Surg*. 1982;64(A):941–942.

87. Sullivan SJ, Chesley A, Hebert G, et al. The validity and reliability of hand held dynamometry in assessing isometric external rotator performance. *J Orthop Sports Phys Ther*. 1988;10:213–217.

88. Tata GE, Ng L, Kramer JF. Shoulder antagonistic strength ratios during concentric and eccentric muscle actions in the scapular plane. *J Orthop Sports Phys Ther*. 1993;18:654–660.

89. Van der Helm FCT. Analysis of the kinematic and dynamic behavior of the shoulder mechanism. *J Biomech*. 1994;27:527–550.

90. Van der Helm FCT, Veeger HEJ, Pronk GM, et al. Geometry parameters for musculoskeletal modelling of the shoulder system. *J Biomech*. 1991;25:129–144.

91. Walker PS, Poppen NK. Biomechanics of the shoulder joint during abduction in the plane of the scapula. *Bull Hosp Jt Dis*. 1977;38:107–111.

92. Walmsley RP, Szybbo C. A comparative study of the torque generated by the shoulder internal and external rotator muscles in different positions at varying speeds. *J Orthop Sports Phys Ther*. 1987;9:217–222.

93. Ward B, McGarvey C, Lotze MT. Excellent shoulder function is attainable after partial or total scapulectomy. *Arch Surg*. 1990;125:537–542.

94. Warner JJP, Micheli LH, Aarslanian LE, et al. Scapulothoracic motion in normal shoulders and shoulders with glenohumeral instability and impingement syndrome. *Clin Orthop*. 1992;285:191–199.

95. Warwick R, Williams PL, eds. *Gray's Anatomy*. 37th British ed. Philadelphia: WB Saunders; 1989.

96. Watson CH, Schenkman M. Physical therapy management of isolated serratus anterior muscle paralysis. *Phys Ther*. 1995;75:194–202.

97. Wilk KE, Andrews JR, Arrigo CA, et al. The strength characteristics of internal and external rotator muscles in professional baseball pitchers. *Am J Sports Med*. 1993;21:61–66.

98. Wilk KE, Arrigo CA, Andrews JR. Isokinetic testing of the shoulder abductors and adductors: windowed versus nonwindowed data collection. *J Orthop Sports Phys Ther*. 1992;15:107–112.

99. Winters JM, Kleweno DG. Effect of initial upper-limb alignment on muscle contributions to isometric strength curves. *J Biomech*. 1993;26:143–153.

100. Wuelker N, Plitz W, Roetman B. Biomechanical data concerning the shoulder impingement syndrome. *Clin Orthop*. 1994;303:242–249.

101. Wuelker N, Plitz W, Roetman B, et al. Function of the supraspinatus muscle-abduction of the humerus studied in cadavers. *Acta Orthop Scand*. 1994;65:442–446.

102. Wuelker N, Schmotzer H, Thren K, et al. Translation of glenohumeral joint with simulated active elevation. *Clin Orthop*. 1994;309:193–200.

8

Elbow

The joints that make up the elbow are in an important functional relationship to the use of the upper limb. The elbow is made up of at least three joints, each having a specific function in positioning the hand in space. In this chapter each joint will be discussed and their interaction described. Sections dealing with the kinematics and kinetics are included. The chapter concludes with a presentation of various pathologies that affect the elbow.

MUSCULAR FUNCTION
Anatomical Organization

The musculature affecting the elbow is frequently described topographically: an above elbow group, i.e., the flexors and extensors, and a below elbow group consisting of three subgroups. The below elbow group consists of a radial group (the brachioradialis, extensor carpi radialis longus, and the extensor carpi radialis brevis muscles), a dorso-ulnar group (wrist extensor-supinator muscles), and a volar medial group (the muscles originating from the medial epicondyle) (41). Functionally the muscles may be thought of as flexors and extensors, supinators, and pronators. For example, some authors and clinicians keep the flexor and extensor designation and divide the below elbow mass into a flexor-pronator and an extensor-supinator group (60). If this latter system is used, one must include the muscles of the hand and wrist that originate above the elbow and subsequently have a potential elbow or radio-ulnar joint function.

Flexor Function

There is some disagreement, and perhaps less than adequate data, regarding the function of the elbow and radio-ulnar joint musculature. Based on known anatomical locations, however, certain muscles have single joint functions while other muscles have multiple ones. A variety of studies, most of which have employed electromyography, have attempted to clarify the situation. Among the earliest was a study that evaluated the functions of the chief flexors of the elbow (8). From the resulting data the **biceps** was demonstrated to be an effective flexor of the forearm only if it had been prepositioned in supine or if it were under significant load. However, the muscle played little or no role in flexion of the elbow even when a load of 2 pounds was lifted. Furthermore, they discovered that the biceps brachii is not a supinator of the extended arm unless supination is firmly resisted. During slow supination of the radio-ulnar joint almost no activity is required of the biceps. The lap test demonstrates this phenomenon. With the forearm completely supported in the lap of the seated subject, the fingers of the opposite hand are used to palpate the prominent tendon of the biceps brachii muscle. Very slow supination from the initial position of pronation elicits no contraction of the biceps, but if resistance is supplied or the velocity

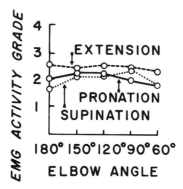

Figure 8.1.   Graph of EMG activity from anconeus during supination, pronation, and extension of the elbow.

of forearm supination increased, the biceps contracts. Some have used this motion to "test" the supinator after a peripheral nerve injury. Without the supinator, no matter how slow the forearm is supinated, the biceps tenses. Generally the biceps can generate most power for either supination or flexion when the elbow is flexed at 90°. Mechanical features identified in Chapter 1, specifically the angle of insertion, may be primarily responsible.

The **brachialis** muscle is located ideally to complete elbow flexion. The brachialis was found to be active during flexion "under all conditions" and generally active during most movements and postures (8). Because of this study, the muscle was labeled the **workhorse** of the elbow joint. Note also that the length-tension relationship in this muscle does not change with pronation/supination due to the insertion on the ulna. The function of the **brachioradialis** muscle is less clear. Identified by early anatomists as the supinator longus, there is little doubt that this muscle is a flexor. Fick, as cited by Lehmkuhl and Smith, also stated that the muscle could perform some pronation from the fully supinated position and somewhat less supination from the fully pronated position (41). Electromyographic data contradict these theoretical functions unless the movements are strongly resisted (8). Under these circumstances the muscle may be serving a stabilization function.

Extensor Function

Extensor muscle function is less difficult to analyze since there are only the **triceps** and **anconeus** muscles to consider. Further, there is no effect on the radio-ulnar joint to consider because of the ulnar attachments of musculature. As for the triceps, Kapandji (33) has stated that the medial triceps is most active, making it the workhorse of the extensors. The lateral triceps is considered the strongest while the long head is the quietest. There appear to be no data to confirm or deny these statements. On the other hand more extensive studies have been completed on the function of the anconeus muscle. Some have found this muscle to be electrically active in the early phases of elbow extension. The muscle also appeared to have a stabilizing function during other upper limb motions such as pronation and supination (53). The anconeus has also been shown to be active at levels comparable to those achieved during extension (Fig. 8.1). Activity levels of the anconeus and the triceps were judged by the same investigators to be comparable (7) (Fig. 8.2). The suggestion by Duchenne

(19) that the anconeus causes ulnar abduction during pronation is more likely a demonstration of a stabilization effect.

It is also interesting that the pectoralis major and anterior deltoid muscles can be effective extensors of the elbow. Such a motion occurs when the hand is fixed or when heavy objects are pushed away from the body. Using the former case as the example, visualize the front leaning rest position assumed in the pushup. As one pushes the body up from the ground, forward flexion of the humerus onto the trunk and elbow extension occur simultaneously. However, because the hand is fixed the pectoralis major and anterior deltoid may, at least, facilitate elbow extension. This example demonstrates the concept of reversal of the origin and insertion so that muscles may perform functionally. Another way to consider this effect is that the kinetic chain is closed when the hand becomes fixed, thus invoking the reversal of actions, by which the trunk moves on the humerus.

Supination-Pronation Function

Relatively little information is available about the function of the **supinator** and **pronator** musculature. Lehmkuhl and Smith (41) compare the pronators quadratus and teres concerning cross section and available shortening. They state, with assumptions, that the pronator quadratus pronates unaided by other muscles if performed slowly without resistance and active elbow flexion. The influence of elbow position upon the effective action of the pronator teres must be taken into account, since the moment arm of the muscle is significantly decreased in full elbow extension. Supination by the supinator muscle is not dependent on the degree of elbow flexion because of its origination site on the ulna and lateral humeral epicondyle. Fick, according to Lehmkuhl and Smith, says that at 90° elbow flexion, the biceps is four times as effective a supinator as the supinator muscle (41). At full elbow extension the difference diminishes to a factor of two. Repeating the lap test confirms the ability of the supinator to act alone under conditions of low load and low velocity. These findings from palpation have been electromyographically confirmed (8).

Anatomical Influences

An interesting study (3) of the muscles crossing the elbow joint suggested that most muscles with "rather discrete origins and insertions" assumed the **parallelepipedon** form. In this configuration the muscle fibers are of uniform length and the tendons

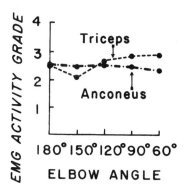

Figure 8.2.   Comparison of medial head of the triceps and anconeus during elbow extension.

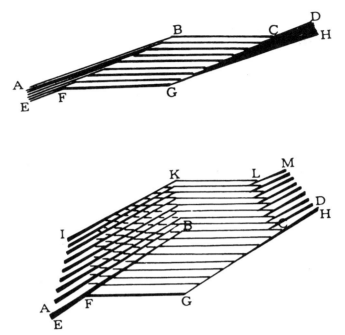

Figure 8.3.   Demonstration of the parallelepipedon shape of muscle fibers. Various letters are used in the description of fiber shape and location.

became progressively thicker as they assumed more fibers (Fig. 8.3). Other muscles, such as the brachialis, supinator, and medial and lateral heads of the triceps, do not readily conform to the parallelepipedon shape. Furthermore, some muscles that remained more muscular than tendinous had muscle fiber variations where longer fibers were situated farther from the joint. The import of these factors will be discussed in the section on kinetics found later in this chapter.

Integrated Action

Muscular actions across the elbow also should be considered from a collective viewpoint. For example, the biceps and triceps have a reciprocal relationship not only at the elbow but also at the glenohumeral joint. Recall that the biceps flexes the elbow and supinates the radio-ulnar joint. In addition, the muscle is anterior to the glenohumeral joint and therefore able to create flexion. Assume that a subject wishes to bring closer an object in front of the body. This functional activity requires flexion at the elbow and extension at the glenohumeral joint. Because the former motion shortens the muscle at the elbow and the latter motion lengthens the muscle at the shoulder, the biceps can maintain an appropriate length so that sufficient tension can be generated throughout the range of motion. The triceps performs similarly yet conversely in pushing objects away from the body. The concept of links and chains as discussed in Chapter 4 is another interpretation. If the length of the biceps and triceps is truly not changing then these muscles are adding stability to the kinetic chain but not producing the motion. Rather, single joint muscles such as the latissimus dorsi and teres major must be extending, the infraspinatus and teres minor controlling rotation, and the coracobrachialis flexing the glenohumeral joint.

Other muscles are most probably involved in controlling these motions. If necessary, the importance of these features should be reviewed in the length-tension section of Chapter 2 and the links and chains section in Chapter 4.

Elbow musculature also demonstrates excellent examples of **synergy.** Consider the case of turning doorknobs. In this activity supination of the forearm by the biceps brachii would also tend to flex the elbow, moving the hand away from the knob. To prevent the biceps from carrying out all its actions, the triceps muscle is activated to neutralize the flexion tendency so that effective supination can be completed. Driving a wood screw yields similar results, particularly when resistance is met. Even under light manual resistance to supination triceps muscle activity can be palpated.

Also recall the differences in contraction type discussed in Chapter 1. Consider bringing a fork to the mouth, a task of simple elbow flexion combined with slight radio-ulnar supination. These motions can be completed by concentric action of the biceps brachii muscle. On return to the starting position elbow extension and radio-ulnar pronation follow. However, performance of these motions is not accomplished by action of the triceps brachii muscle and pronators. Instead, the same muscles that did the concentric work now do eccentric work. That is, the muscles "let" the weight of the arm lower the segment to the table by means of a slow, controlled lengthening of the biceps brachii and/or the supinator. If, in fact, the extensors and pronators contracted, the result would be a rapid extension of the elbow that could meet with disastrous results. This principle of controlled eccentric contraction is an important concept that must be ingrained in the therapist's motion analysis technique. Otherwise, incorrect interpretations can be applied. Virtually any time that gravity assists motion eccentric contraction will be called into play. Primary examples include the descent to the seated position from standing, lowering the foot to the floor before beginning the stance phase in gait, and the control of one's body weight during the descent of stairs. Other examples will be provided in other chapters.

The motions of flexion-extension and supination-pronation have also been studied in a context in which movements are combined and/or used in control strategies. Most of these works lend clarification about how truly integrated the movements of multiple joints are performed. In at least some situations, there is co-contraction (24, 30, 58), while in other situations the cooperation is called coordination (56) or synergy (9, 12, 32). The therapist should realize that many tasks, although appearing to be simple, are carried out by a complex interaction of multiple muscles. This interaction may be called **dynamic synergism,** although the degrees of freedom of movement at the joint may be limited.

ARTHROLOGY AND ARTHROKINEMATICS

The bony structure of the elbow and radio-ulnar joints comprise an interesting framework around which motions occur (23). The spherical end of the proximal radius is unique in provision for the rotary requirements of the forearm. The ulna seems to have a cradling effect on the distal end of the humerus, perhaps for purposes of stability. Figure 8.4 shows that the joint has been likened to a ball and spool on the same axis. Note that the distal end of the humerus acts as a male surface projecting anteriorly at an angle of 45°. A similar arrangement occurs at the proximal portion of the ulna in that the olecranon and coronoid processes are also 45° offset in an anterior direction. Kapandji (33) has likened the distal humerus to fork prongs sticking anteriorly from the axis of the humerus and the ulna. Such a structure, along with

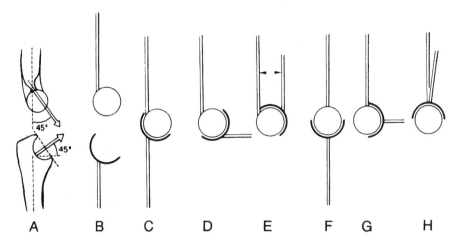

Figure 8.4.   The articulation of the humerus and ulna. **A—E.** The normal configuration of the bony structures. **F.** In this position flexion is limited to 90° (**G**). **H.** This position leaves no room for muscle mass.

the depth of the coronoid and olecranon fossae, provides an increased range of motion for elbow flexion without creating impingement of the ulna upon the humerus. Figure 8.4F–H demonstrates the results if the bony offsets at 45° did not exist. Asymmetry of the trochlea may also play a role in laterally angulating the ulna on the humerus. The purpose of this angulation, known as the **carrying angle,** is considered a means of keeping the arm away from the side while carrying objects. Considerable doubt as to this purpose must be expressed on the basis that objects, particularly heavy objects, are virtually always carried with the forearm in the middle of the supination-pronation range. Such a maneuver tends to negate any potential effect of the carrying angle. The angle has been found to be 10–15° in males and 20–25° in females. Steindler (59), in his classic treatise on kinesiology, maintained that in part due to the osteology, a gap opened on the medial side of the olecranon during extension of the elbow. Conversely, on extreme flexion the gap opened at the lateral olecranon border.

All of the joints at the elbow, ulnohumeral, radiohumeral, and radio-ulnar, are synovial joints. Reinforcement and medial-lateral constraint is provided by the medial and lateral ligaments. The medial, or ulnar, collateral ligament has anterior, intermediate, and posterior sets of fibers, of which the anterior fibers help reinforce the annular ligament of the radio-ulnar joint (62). Studies have revealed that the range of motion determines which part of what ligament is taut or slack at any particular time. For example, the anterior medial collateral ligament and the radial collateral ligament were taut throughout most of flexion while the posterior medial collateral ligament was taut only when the elbow was in a flexed position (55). The lateral, or radial, ligament is intimately associated with the annular ligament that surrounds the head of the radius and maintains the proximal radius in articulation with the ulna (28). Furthermore, some significance has been assigned to the attachment of this ligament to the tubercle of the supinator muscle (crista supinatoris) (45). The posterior portion of the ulnar collateral ligament is taut in maximal flexion. Conversely, of the three anterior bundles, one is taut in extension, another in intermediate positions between mid and full flexion, and the third is always taut. Because this bundle guides joint movement, it is known as a **guiding bundle.** Even the tightness of ligament component fibers changes during joint range of motion (25), demonstrating the remarkable influence exerted on bony congruity maintenance while allowing appropriate arthrokinematics.

Understanding the specifics of ligament action and control can improve the therapist's outcome, because specific therapeutic procedures may need to be altered based on which ligament is taut at any given joint configuration. Tightness in the ligaments is also relevant to surgeons with considerations associated with total joint replacements and other repairs, assuring that stability will be provided without the sacrifice of range of motion (45). Without such considerations the therapeutic outcome and the patient's function will not be maximized because of tissue constraints inherent in mechanical properties (see Chapter 5).

BIOMECHANICS

Only recently have comprehensive studies adequately addressed the kinesiology and biomechanics of the joints that make up the elbow complex. Most have considered the elbow a pure hinge joint in spite of a known mechanical influence of the radio-ulnar joints.

Studies of the three-dimensional rotation of the elbow (14) and analyses of forearm pronation-supination and elbow flexion-extension (64) have been completed. Performed on cadaver specimens, both studies used different methodologies and provided useful information about elbow and radio-ulnar motion. Both studies evaluated the kinematics of the elbow and found the long axis of the elbow to rotate about 5° internally during early elbow flexion and about 5° externally during the later phases. In finding that the carrying angle varied linearly as a function of flexion, some authors have noted that the elbow proceeded from valgus in extension toward varus in flexion (14). Youm and colleagues (64) differ in that four of six specimens showed a sinusoidal relationship (Fig. 8.5) rather than the linear form demonstrated in two elbows. At least part of the explanation may be that the latter study showed no medial-lateral movement of the proximal ulna on the humerus during the flexion-extension motion. Both studies determined that the locus of the axis of rotation was through the trochlea, confirming work done at the turn of the century by Fischer as cited by Chao and Morrey (14). Figure 8.6 shows the displacement of the axis during elbow flexion. Youm (64) further identified the radio-ulnar axis, specifying the location as ranging from the center of the capitulum to the distal end of the ulna.

The kinematics of elbow motion have also been studied using a radiographic technique on humans. Results showed the instant centers of rotation to be tightly clustered in the center of the trochlea except during the extremes of the range of motion. For the last 5–10° of flexion the axis was displaced toward the coronoid fossa while during the same extreme of extension the displacement was toward the olecranon fossa. London (43) also studied the axis of the radiohumeral joint and found similar anterior and posterior displacements of the axes in the terminal ranges of flexion and extension. Location of the instant centers is of practical import because the osteokinematics can be described based on this information. For example, with the elbow, motion of the ulnohumeral and radiohumeral joint is gliding, except at the extremes of flexion and extension. During these ranges the axis moves, indicating that gliding motion changes to rolling. The specific therapeutic import can be seen in patients with limited range. Because rolling will be important to restoration of

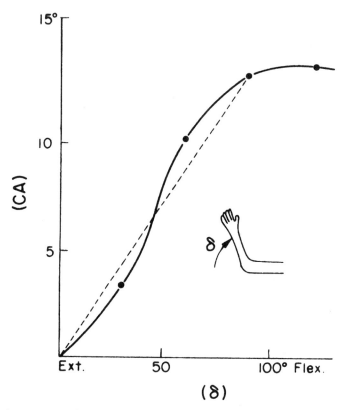

Figure 8.5. The carrying angle (*CA*) plotted versus the elbow angle (*δ*). Two specimens showed a linear change while four others demonstrated a flat sinusoidal curve up to 90°. All of the elbows behaved similarly after this point in the range of motion.

normal kinematics required for a full range of motion, therapeutic efforts to maintain these ranges are likely to assist with positive treatment results. For specific techniques aimed at achieving these motions the reader is referred to Kessler and Hertling (34) and similar works.

Therapeutic consideration must also be given to maintenance or restoration of the ranges of motion required for normal function. Usually, the total range of elbow flexion is 140°. In reporting that most activities of daily living can be accomplished with 30–130° of flexion and from 50° of pronation to 50° of supination, they have defined limits for clinical use. Figures 8.7 and 8.8 represent the arcs of motion required during the activities studied (47).

KINETICS

Muscular Forces

In 1911, Fick (22) published his well-known work on anatomy. According to his measurements the total cross-sectional area of the elbow flexors is 26.5 cm², which exceeded the 20.3 cm² area of the extensors. He was the first to claim that the biceps area exceeded the cross section of the brachialis muscle by only a slight margin; however, some published results differ (3, 31). Hui et al. (31) state that the brachialis,

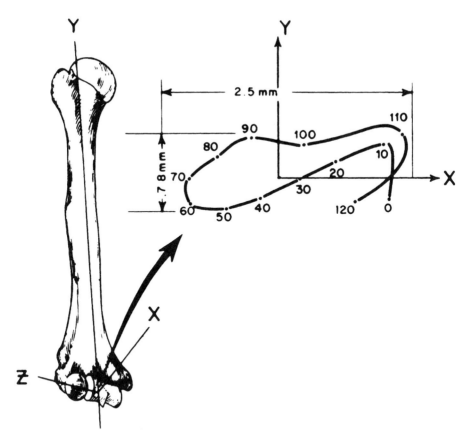

Figure 8.6. Instantaneous center of rotation for the sagittal plane for the elbow joint.

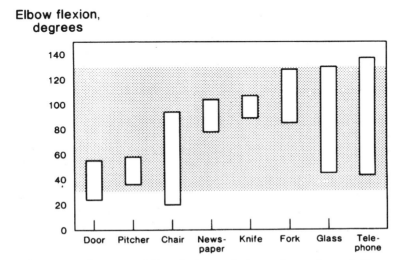

Figure 8.7. The ranges of elbow flexion required to perform various activities.

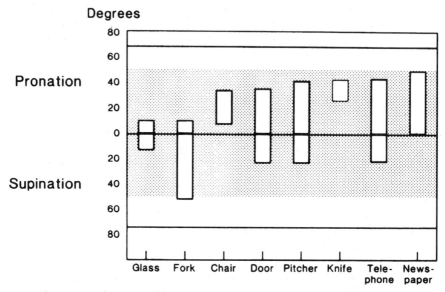

Figure 8.8.   The ranges of forearm rotation required to perform various activities.

in terms of cross sectional area, is consistently the strongest flexor although no specific data are cited. The 1981 work of An et al. (3) includes a specific analysis of all muscles that affect the elbow. The cross section for both heads of the biceps muscle totaled 4.5 cm² while the brachialis was 7.0 cm². Total area for the triceps was cited as 18.8 cm². Probably because the fibers of the biceps and brachioradialis muscles are relatively long, the cross-sectional area is relatively small.

Others have attempted to measure elbow flexor and extensor force. In 1966 Little and Lehmkuhl (42) measured elbow extension force in three positions. Cable tensiometer values, with the restraining cuff positioned just proximal to the wrist, were between 18.0 and 25.2 pounds. In another study (17), extensor force was measured with the elbow in 60°, 90°, and 120° of flexion. Cable tensiometer values showed that the greatest values (48.8 lbf) were reached at the 90° position. Although the 120° angle produced values only 4 lbf less, the 60° angle involved values of 35.8 lbf. That the two studies used both men and women accounts for their different results. Larson (40) also used similar techniques in evaluating the effect of forearm positioning on flexor force. With the cuff at approximately mid-forearm, results showed supination force at 95 pounds, mid-position at 97 pounds, and pronation at 88 pounds. These results are difficult to interpret because the values were not converted to torque measurements, which would have allowed for comparison within and between subjects as well as across studies.

Anatomical Considerations

As is well known, considering the factors determining torque includes (a) the physiological characteristics that contribute to force and (b) the moment arm length. The study by An et al. (3) included a complete set of moment arm data for all musculature affecting the elbow and the radio-ulnar joints. Among other comments, and although various positions of supination-pronation and flexion-extension were studied, these investigators concluded that the brachioradialis, biceps, brachialis, and extensor carpi radialis muscles were the major flexors. They provided an interesting array of diagrams that show the potential moment contribution of each muscle. One such representation is shown in Figure 8.9. Hui et al. (31) say that the brachioradialis, based on moment arm, is consistently the most "efficient" muscle. In discussing the influence of mechanical factors, the gain in moment production, allowed by an increasing moment arm upon elbow flexion, is not completely negated by the tension loss that ordinarily accompanies a "slackened" muscle. The net result is that a flexed elbow can resist more load than an extended elbow. Winters and Kleweno (63) have also strongly suggested that this moment production may be due to a greater contribution by force-length features than changes in moment arms, which is consistent with an apparently small role played by the passive element in these muscles (4).

In an interesting sidelight, Andersson and Schultz (5) calculated rough estimates of the **maximum voluntary contractile strength** per cross-sectional area. Using estimates of shapes and area, they determined stress to be 100 N/cm^2. Although not of particular significance to the kinesiology or pathokinesiology of the elbow, the data offer some explanation as to the potential for muscle rupture. The mechanisms that pertain to the biceps brachii muscle will be discussed in the section on pathokinesiology.

Torques

Many data have been published regarding the torque generated about the elbow. Some of these, judged upon review to have used appropriate methodology, are shown in Table 8.1. Other works have produced agreeable results but are not reported

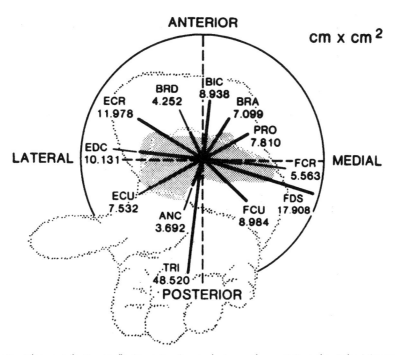

Figure 8.9. The contribution to flexion-extension and varus-valgus rotation about the joint center for the extended-supinated position of the elbow. The moment contribution of each muscle was estimated by multiplying the moment arm (cm) by its physiological cross-sectional area (cm^2).

Table 8.1. Compilation of Torque Values for the Joints at the Elbow

Source Reference	Gender	Age Mean	Age SD	Age Range	n	Movement	Concentric (°/sec)	Eccentric (°/sec)	ROM	Testing Position	Peak Torque Nm	Peak Torque SD	Testing Device
6	m	41	12	23–75	50	f	0		90	sh abd 0, elb 90, fa 0	71	15	custom HHD
						e	0		90		41	11	
						pro	0		0		7	2	
						sup	0		0		9	2	
	f	45	16	21–79	50	f	0		90	sh abd 0, elb 90, fa 0	33	8	
						e	0		90		21	6	
						pro	0		0		4	1	
						sup	0		0		4	1	
37	m	24	6		352	e	0		90		54	12	Cybex II
						f	0		90		67	15	
						e	30				43	10	
						e	90				38	10	
						e	180				30	7	
						f	30				50	12	
						f	90				33	8	
						f	180				26	6	
57	f	20		20–25	20	f	0		80	elb 80, fa sup	82		custom load cell
						e	0		80	elb 80, fa sup	53		
						f	0		100	elb 100, fa sup	87		
						e	0		100	elb 100, fa sup	51		
38	f	25	4		15	e	0		70	elb 70, fa 0	42		Cybex II
						f	0		90	elb 70, fa 0	40		
						e	36				33		
						e	108				28		
						e	180				25		
						f	36				28		
						f	108				25		
						f	180				20		
	m	26	4		16	e	0		70	elb 70, fa 0	73		Cybex II
						f	0		90	elb 70, fa 0	79		

Ref	Sex	n	Age	Age range	n₂	Movement	°/s or angle	°/s	Elbow (°)	Position	Mean	SD	Equipment
63	m	40	12	21–30	4	e	36				60		
						e	108				50		
						e	180				43		
						f	36				58		
						f	108				49		
						f	180				40		
	f	41	12	21–30	4	f	0		90	sh abd 0, elb 90, fa sup	74		KinCom
						f	0		90	sh abd 0, elb 90, fa pro	74		
						f	0		90	sh abd 0, elb 90, fa sup	34		
						f	0		90	sh abd 0, elb 90, fa pro	33		
28	m	30	7		40	f	30	30			68	12	KinCom
						f	120	120			67	10	
						f	30				53	9	
						f	120				45	8	
	f	28	6		50	f	30	30			35	7	KinCom
						f	120	120			35	7	
						f	30				25	6	
						f	120				21	5	
39	m				21	pro	0			sh abd 10, elb 90, fa sup 10	12	4	BTE
						sup	0			sh abd 10, elb 90, fa sup 10	11	3	Cybex II
						pro	0			sh abd 10, elb 90, fa sup 10	13	3	BTE
						sup	0			sh abd 10, elb 90, fa sup 10	11	3	Cybex II
	f				22	pro	0			sh abd 10, elb 90, fa sup 10	6	2	
						sup	0			sh abd 10, elb 90, fa sup 10	6	1	
						pro	0			sh abd 10, elb 90, fa sup 10	7	2	
						sup	0			sh abd 10, elb 90, fa sup 10	6	1	
15	m			21–60	22	e	0		90	elb 90, fa sup	34	7	strain gauge
						f	0		90	elb 90, fa sup	64	11	
	m			60–102	10	e	0		90	elb 90, fa sup	35	10	
						f	0		90	elb 90, fa sup	61	15	
	f			18–60	17	e	0		90	elb 90, fa sup	20	4	
						f	0		90	elb 90, fa sup	36	6	
	f			60–85	7	e	0		90	elb 90, fa sup	17	5	
						f	0		90	elb 90, fa sup	32	11	

Legend: BTE, Baltimore Therapeutic Equipment; *e,* extension; *elb,* elbow; *f,* flexion; *fa,* forearm; *HHD,* hand held dynamometer; *pro,* pronation; *sh,* shoulder; *sup,* supination.

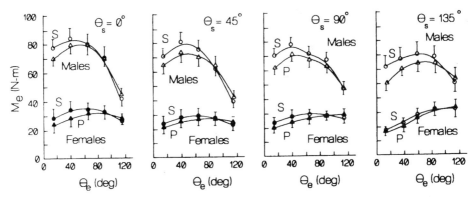

Figure 8.10. Averaged male and female elbow strength curves. Each plot includes both male (open symbols) and female (filled symbols) data, both with the wrist supinated (circles or S) and pronated (triangles or P). From left to right, the shoulder flexion angles are 0°, 45°, 90°, and 135°. Standard deviation bars only in one direction.

in the table because of some lack of clarity in their methodology (5, 6, 9, 13, 27, 39, 48). Generally, in most works the radio-ulnar joint position was altered as both flexion and extension were studied. A family of data is shown in Figure 8.10. Although not shown in this figure note that elbow flexion torque is from 25 to 50% greater than the extension torque in all positions (21, 54) (see Table 8.1).

In summarizing the collective results, the mid-position of pronation-supination produced the greatest torque for flexors and extensors. A similar finding for extension, when compared with flexion, is interesting in that there should be no hypothetical differences because of the anatomical arrangements for the extensors. The results are perhaps explainable on the basis of moment arm and muscle length. Analyses of the length and "mechanical advantage" of the elbow flexors (Fig. 8.11) have been completed (61). Thus, as to function, therapists should readily recognize that because of mechanics, the length-tension relationship, and anatomical factors, muscles may have varying roles as the joint proceeds through a dynamic range of motion.

Functional Capacity

Kapandji's first volume on the physiology of joints (33) includes a discussion of function in man as it relates to "efficiency" of the flexor and extensor muscles. In discussing how the "power" of the muscle groups varies with shoulder position, he maintains that once the arm is stretched vertically above the shoulder, an additional 43 kg(f) can be exerted in extension of the arm overhead. However, with the arm stretched above the shoulder and attempting to pull oneself upward, the force is equivalent to 83 kg(f). Further, flexion forces, i.e., in rowing, are almost twice as great as forces available for pushing heavy loads forward. Thus, at least in the upper limb, man is well adapted for climbing.

Joint Forces

Many clinicians and basic scientists have discounted the importance of resultant joint forces at the elbow because the upper limb is non-weight-bearing. Some have discounted this argument, stating that maximal isometric flexion in the extended position yields joint contact forces equivalent to twice body weight. Shear forces in the specimens studied, although somewhat difficult to interpret from the data, also seemed considerable (31). In a very comprehensive analysis of elbow joint forces, forearm abduction and adduction as well as elbow flexion and extension were analyzed. How these forces produced at the humero-ulnar and humeroradial joints are distributed across the joint (Fig. 8.12) is an important factor in most circumstances where prostheses have been implanted (2). That the greatest forces through the radial head have been found with the joint pronated may also have implication for reparative procedures and the resultant rehabilitative process (46).

During more **functional activities,** Nicol, as cited by Matsen (44), found that dressing and eating create joint reaction forces of 300 newtons. Activities requiring pulling of heavy objects or assisting standing from sitting produce peak forces up to 1700 newtons. Using a different reporting mechanism, the maximum axial force at the elbow was between 40 and 50% of body weight during the pushup exercise, no matter how the hands were positioned on the floor (18).

PATHOKINESIOLOGY

Injuries affecting the joints of the elbow are usually not as disabling as those that affect either the shoulder or the wrist and hand. In cases with neurological origin, the result is frequently satisfactory kinesiologically because of the differing innervations of the muscles serving the elbow and radio-ulnar joints. However, other pathologies can be acute, chronic, or require extensive surgery or immobilization. In this section the more common pathologies will be discussed.

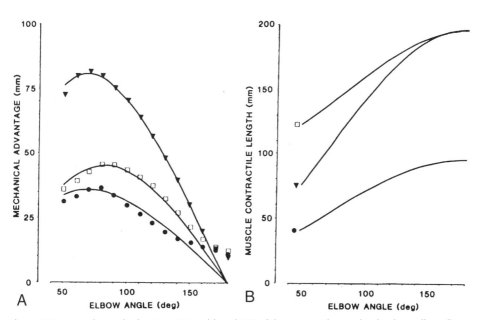

Figure 8.11. Mechanical advantage (**A**) and length (**B**) of the contractile part for the three elbow flexor muscles: brachialis (*circles*), biceps (*squares*), and brachioradialis (*triangles*) as a function of elbow angle. Solid lines give the model results. Points in **A** indicate the data of Braune and Fischer (11). Symbols in **B** indicate that the given model results apply to the corresponding muscles in **A**.

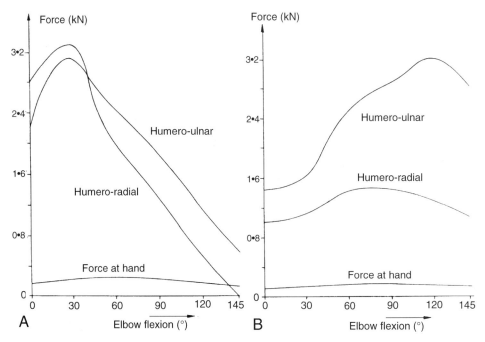

Figure 8.12. Forces at the humerocoronoid, humeroradial, and humero-ulnar joints during isometric contractions. **A.** Flexion with triceps antagonism. **B.** Extension with biceps brachii antagonism.

Neurological Injuries

Unless a patient suffers massive injury to the brachial plexus, the functional abilities associated with elbow and radio-ulnar joint motions from **peripheral nerve injury** are usually preserved. However, in blast injuries, as occasionally occur due to gunshot wounds or high pressure air hose explosions, limitations of the entire distal limb can be extremely debilitating. Fortunately, the biceps and brachialis are innervated by the musculocutaneous nerve, since in rare injuries of this well-protected nerve, the brachioradialis (radial nerve) and pronator teres (median nerve) muscles are spared. Rarely, such as with post poliomyelitis patients, are all elbow flexors lost. In such cases, patients have been known to flex the elbow with the extensor carpi radialis longus and the extensor carpi radialis brevis muscles. The point is that if an adequate moment arm and tension are available, a movement can be accomplished, even by a substitution.

The supination function can be carried out reasonably well by the supinator alone. However, heavy load manipulation can be difficult for patients with these injuries. Elbow flexion will be obviously weak. Injury to the radial nerve causes loss of the extensors and supinator, severely limiting the ability to extend the elbow. Du Toit and Levy (20) have suggested the transposition of the latissimus dorsi to substitute for such a loss. Because the musculocutaneous nerve and the biceps muscle are still intact, the supination function is within normal limits. Finally, loss of the median nerve affects only pronation in the forearm, though its loss is disastrous to the thumb. However, because both pronator muscles are eliminated, effective pronation is lost.

Spinal cord injured patients also show demonstrable examples of altered muscle function. For example, consider the C6 patient with no triceps available for elbow extension. However, if the hand is fixed on a surface, such as in pushups from the seated position, the clavicular portion of the pectoralis major can serve to assist elbow extension by pulling the upper arm across the chest. Often, the torque producing capability of this arrangement is enough to allow successful completion of the maneuver.

Central nervous system disorders also affect the muscles' ability to generate tension. For example, elbow flexion forces after stroke have been found to be about 50% of the nonparetic extremity when using a break test and about 35% when using a make test (10). Other evidence shows that the elbow flexors are relatively more weakened than the extensors on the hemiparetic side, a finding contrary to a commonly held belief (15). Specific testing by the therapist should result in the application of the most appropriate therapeutic procedures.

Soft Tissue Injuries

Soft tissue injuries are a common occurrence at the elbow. The capsule, ligaments, or tendons can be involved in inflammatory processes, sprains, or acute ruptures. **Lateral epicondylitis** has been related to involvement of many tissues, among them bursa, ligaments, and tears of the originations of the extensor musculature. Produced by overuse and often related to tennis playing the syndrome is felt by some to be a microscopic rupture and poor resulting natural repair of the origin of the extensor carpi radialis brevis (49, 50). On the other side of the elbow **medial epicondylitis**, sometimes known as "Little League elbow," has been biomechanically analyzed. Some have hypothesized that throwing breaking pitches generates higher medial loading (29). Gainor et al. (26) determined torques and kinetic energy in the arm and also cited overloading as predisposing the humeral condylar to changes that produce the symptoms frequently seen in the clinic. Several interesting cases, including a spiral fracture of the humerus, are included in their paper.

Inability of the soft tissues to constrain motion adequately occasionally results in the "**pulled radial head**" encountered in children. In these and other soft tissue injuries, treatment is directed toward care of the symptoms, but some attention must be paid to the osteokinematics described in earlier sections.

A key factor in effective treatment appears to be temporal elements associated with periods of **immobilization.** Frequently the long-term results of elbow dislocations are unsatisfactory because of the inability of the patient to achieve a complete range of motion in either flexion or extension. Some effects of immobilization discussed in Chapter 2 may explain the difficulty in achieving treatment goals. Although sufficient time for healing must be allowed, ultimate mobility cannot be sacrificed. That immobilization is common is well known and well founded in certain clinical elbow conditions such as post fractures and burns (1). That strategies change because of immobilization or simulate arthrodesis has also been documented (16, 52). However, more direct evidence for the advantages of early mobilization of tendons and joints is needed. More specific discussion of this topic is included in Chapters 9 and 11.

One injury of reasonable frequency that affects the elbow is **rupture** of the biceps brachii muscle. Occurring more frequently in the long head of the muscle in middle aged persons, the result is immediate and permanent unless surgery is performed. Many causes have been postulated. Weakness in the tissue can be produced by degenerative changes so that relatively inconsequential movements result in tensions that exceed the rupture strength of the musculotendinous unit. Also recall that the biceps brachii is a multiple joint muscle in that joints affected are the radio-ulnar,

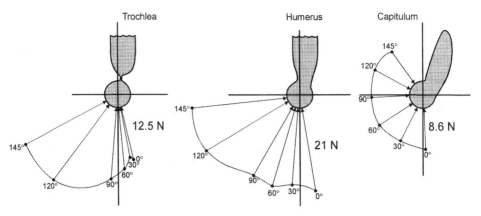

Figure 8.13.   Location and magnitude of the forces at the articular surface of the humerus during extension. Forces are per unit of force at the hand.

elbow, and glenohumeral. As An et al. have shown, the fibers are relatively long (3). So, in sum and substance, the pronated elbow, accompanied by elbow and glenohumeral extension, could put considerable stretch on the biceps brachii muscle. Then, if additional force is added to the muscle by means of either contraction or quick stretch, the rupture point may be reached, resulting in avulsion of the long head of the muscle from the glenoid labrum. Thus, as the muscle cannot produce any effective tension across the joint as intended, weakness results. Discomfort obviously results in the more acute stages, but muscles not repaired function quite adequately in the long term.

Joint Replacement

Much of the motivation for the study of the kinematics and kinetics of the elbow has been due to the more recent interest in total elbow prostheses. Based on the data of several investigative groups (14, 43, 64), a uniaxial hinged prosthesis has been recommended. However, caution must be exercised because either the ulnar rotation or the change in joint motion from sliding to rolling at the terminal phases of the range may be cause for loosening of the prosthetic components. London (43) has also postulated that the axis of the device may not be aligned with the true axis, thus producing another potential cause of loosening. A review of the prosthetic problem has been presented (2), showing the forces on various components at different angles of elbow extension (Fig. 8.13). These authors suggest that designers consider the inclusion of a flange on the lateral aspect of the olecranon to distribute shear forces. More recently, studies have been conducted on a variety of total elbow prostheses, defining the amount of varus and valgus angulation and laxity that can occur under a variety of conditions (35, 36). That each of these prostheses is essentially unconstrained (35, 36) and that soft tissues resist some forces and moments that would have been transferred to the prosthesis-bone interface (51) can effectively decrease the incidence of loosening. Concern for this issue lends credence to the joints at the elbow being multiple, thus requiring the accommodation for six degrees of freedom.

Finally, that those treated with total elbow joint arthroplasty improve significantly in torque has been demonstrated in a group of 27 patients (48). Although the location of the prosthetic axis proximal or anterior to the normal axis was responsible for decreases, patients still improved by 69% in supination, 63% in pronation, and 92% in flexion. Extension measures were equivocal, showing great differences between the subjects with rheumatoid arthritis and those with hemophilia/traumatic arthritis. The therapeutic implication is that clinicians need to attend to specific measures of assessment that will lead to the adoption of the most meaningful approach in any given situation.

SUMMARY

This chapter has presented a discussion of the muscular contributions to the motions available in the multijoint elbow. Kinematics and kinetics were described in relation to their contribution to normal motion and possible role in pathological circumstances. Although considered a pure hinge joint, new information is confirming that this approach is an oversimplification of the real conditions required for normal motion.

References

1. Ader PB, Nadel E, Wingate L. A survey of postoperative elbow immobilization approaches. *J Burn Care Rehabil.* 1992;13:365–370.
2. Amis AA, Dowson D, Wright V. Elbow joint force predictions for some strenuous isometric actions. *J Biomech.* 1980;13:765–775.
3. An KN, Hui FC, Morrey BF, Linscheid RL, Chao EY. Muscles across the elbow joint: a biomechanical analysis. *J Biomech.* 1981;14:659–669.
4. An K-N, Kaufman KR, Chao EYS. Physiological considerations of muscle force through the elbow joint. *J Biomech.* 1989;22:1249–1256.
5. Andersson GBJ, Schultz AB. Transmission of moments across the elbow joint and the lumbar spine. *J Biomech.* 1979;12:747–756.
6. Askew LJ, AN K-N, Morrey BF, Chao EYS. Isometric elbow strength in normal individuals. *Clin Orthop.* 1987;222:261–266.
7. Basmajian JV, Griffin WR. Function of anconeus muscle: an electromyographic study. *J Bone Joint Surg.* 1972;54(A):1712–1714.
8. Basmajian JV, Latif A. Integrated actions and functions of the chief flexors of the elbow: a detailed electromyographic analysis. *J Bone Joint Surg.* 1957;39(A):1106–1118.
9. Bechtel R, Caldwell GE. The influence of task and angle on torque production and muscle activity at the elbow. *J Electromyogr Kinesiol.* 1994;4:195–204.
10. Bohannon RW. Make versus break tests for measuring elbow flexor muscle force with a hand-held dynamometer in patients with stroke. *Physiother Can.* 1990;42:247–251.
11. Braune W, Fischer FO. *Die Rotationsmomente der Beugemuskeln am Ellebogengelenk des Menshshen.* Abh sächs Akad. Wiss 15 Nr. III. Leipzig; 1889.
12. Buchanan TS, Rovai GP, Rymer WZ. Strategies for muscle activation during isometric torque generation at the human elbow. *J Neurophysiol.* 1989;62:1201–1212.
13. Caldwell GE, Van Leemputte M. Elbow torques and EMG patterns of flexor muscles during different isometric tasks. *Electromyogr Clin Neurophysiol.* 1991;31:433–445.
14. Chao EY, Morrey BF. Three dimensional rotation of the elbow. *J Biomech.* 1978;11:57–73.
15. Colebatch JG, Ganderia SC, Spira PJ. Voluntary muscle strength in hemiparesis: distribution of weakness at the elbow. *J Neurol Neurosurg Psychiatry.* 1986;49:1019–1024.
16. Cooper JE, Shwedyk E, Quanbury AO, et al. Elbow joint restriction: effect on functional upper limb motion during performance of three feeding activities. *Arch Phys Med Rehabil.* 1993;74:805–809.
17. Currier DP. Maximal isometric tension of the elbow extensors at varied positions. *Phys Ther.* 1972;52:1043–1049.
18. Donkers MJ, An K-N, Chao EYS, Morrey BF. Hand position affects elbow joint load during push-up exercise. *J Biomech.* 1993;26:625–632.
19. Duchenne GBA; Kaplan EB, trans-ed. *Physiology of Motion Demonstrated by Means of Electrical Stimulation and Clinical Observation and Applied to the Study of Paralysis and Deformities.* Philadelphia: JB Lippincott; 1949:98–105.

20. Du Toit GT, Levy SJ. Transposition of latissimus dorsi for paralysis of triceps brachii. *J Bone Joint Surg.* 1967;49(B):135–137.

21. Elkins EC, Leden UM, Wakim KG. Objective recording of the strength of normal muscles. *Arch Phys Med.* 1951;32:639–647.

22. Fick R. *Anatomie und Mechanik der Gelenke. Teil III, Spezielle Gelenk und Muskel Mechanik.* Fisher: Jena; 1911.

23. Fischer O. Zur kinematik der gelenke vom typus des humeroradial gelenkes. *Abh Math-Phys Cl Sk K Sachs Ges*; 1909;32:3–77.

24. Funk DA, An K-N, Morrey BF, Daube JR. Electromyographic analysis of muscle across the elbow joint. *J Orthop Res.* 1987;5:529–538.

25. Fuss FK. The ulnar collateral ligament of the human elbow joint. Anatomy, function and biomechanics. *J Anat.* 1991;175:203–212.

26. Gainor BJ, Piotrowski G, Puhl J, et al. The throw: biomechanics and acute injury. *Am J Sports Med.* 1980;8:114–118.

27. Griffin JW. Differences in elbow flexion torque measured concentrically, eccentrically, and isometrically. *Phys Ther.* 1987;67:1205–1208.

28. Griffin JW, Tooms RE, VanderZwaag, Bertorini TE, O'Toole ML. Eccentric muscle performance of elbow and knee muscle groups in untrained men and women. *Med Sci Sports Exerc.* 1993;25:936–944.

29. Hang YS, Lippert FG, Spolek GA, Frankel VH, Harrington RM. Biomechanical study of the pitching elbow. *Int Orthop.* 1979;3:217–223.

30. Hébert LJ, DeSerres SJ, Arsenault AB. Cocontraction of the elbow muscles during combined tasks of pronation-flexion and supination-flexion. *Electromyogr Clin Neurophysiol.* 1991;31:483–488.

31. Hui FC, Chao EY, An KN. Muscle and joint forces at the elbow during isometric lifting. Paper presented at the 24th annual meeting of the Orthopedic Research Society; February, 1978; Dallas, Texas.

32. Jamison C, Caldwell GE. Muscle synergies and isometric torque production: influence of supination and pronation level on elbow flexion. *J Neurophysiol.* 1993;70:947–960.

33. Kapandji AI. *The Physiology of the Joints.* 5th ed. New York: Churchill Livingstone; 1982.

34. Kessler R, Hertling D. *Management of Common Musculoskeletal Disorders.* Philadelphia: Harper & Row; 1983.

35. King GJW, Itoi E, Niebur BL, Morrey BF, An K-N. Motion and laxity of the capitellocondylar total elbow prosthesis. *J Bone Joint Surg.* 1994;76(A):1000–1008.

36. King GJW, Itoi E, Risung F, Niebur BL, et al. Kinematics and stability of the Norway elbow: a cadaveric study. *Acta Orthop Scand.* 1993;64:657–663.

37. Knapik JJ, Ramos MV. Isokinetic and isometric torque relationships in the human body. *Arch Phys Med Rehabil.* 1980;61:64–67.

38. Knapik JJ, Wright JE, Mawdsley RH, Braun J. Isometric, isotonic and isokinetic torque variations in four muscle groups through a range of joint motion. *Phys Ther.* 1983;63:938–947.

39. Kramer JF, Nusca D, Bisbee L, et al. Forearm pronation and supination: reliability of absolute torques and nondominant/dominant ratios. *J Hand Ther.* 1994;7:15–20.

40. Larson RF. Forearm positioning on maximal elbow-flexor force. *J Am Phys Ther Assoc.* 1969;49:748–756.

41. Lehmkuhl LD, Smith LK. *Brunnstrom's Clinical Kinesiology.* 4th ed. Philadelphia: FA Davis; 1983.

42. Little AD, Lehmkuhl D. Elbow extension force measured in three positions. *J Am Phys Ther Assoc.* 1966;46:7–17.

43. London JT. Kinematics of the elbow. *J Bone Joint Surg.* 1981;63(A):529–535.

44. Matsen FA. Biomechanics of the elbow. In: Frankel VM, Nordin M, eds. *Basic Biomechanics of the Skeletal System.* Philadelphia: Lea & Febiger; 1980.

45. Morrey BF, An K-N. Functional anatomy of the ligaments of the elbow. *Clin Orthop.* 1985;201:84–90.

46. Morrey BF, An K-N, Stormont TJ. Force transmission through the radial head. *J Bone Joint Surg.* 1988;70(A):250–256.

47. Morrey BF, Askew LJ, An K-N, et al. A biomechanical study of normal functional elbow motion. *J Bone Joint Surg.* 1981;63(A):872–877.

48. Morrey BF, Askew LJ, An K-N. Strength function after elbow arthroplasty. *Clin Orthop.* 1988;234:43–50.

49. Nirschl RP, Pettrone FA. Tennis elbow: the surgical treatment of lateral epicondylitis. *J Bone Joint Surg.* 1979;61(A):832–839.

50. Noteboom T, Cruver R, Keller J, et. al. Tennis elbow: a review. *J Orthop Sports Phys Ther.* 1994;19:357–366.

51. O'Driscoll SW, An K-N, Korinek S, Morrey BF. Kinematics of semi-constrained total elbow arthroplasty. *J Bone Joint Surg.* 1992;74(B):297–299.

52. O'Neill OR, Morrey BF, Tanaka S, An K-N. Compensatory motion in the upper extremity after elbow arthrodesis. *Clin Orthop.* 1992;281:89–96.

53. Pauly JE, Rushing JL, Scheving LE. An electromyographic study of some muscles crossing the elbow joint. *Anat Rec.* 1967;159:47–53.

54. Provins KA, Salter N. Maximum torque exerted about the elbow joint. *J Appl Physiol.* 1955;7:393–398.

55. Regan WD, Korinek SL, Morrey BF, An K-N. Biomechanical study of ligaments around the elbow joint. *Clin Orthop.* 1991;170–179.

56. Sergio LE, Ostry DJ. Coordination of mono- and bi-articular muscle in multi-degree of freedom elbow movements. *Exp Brain Res.* 1994;97:551–555.

57. Singh M, Karpovich PV. Isotonic and isometric forces of forearm flexors and extensors. *J Appl Physiol.* 1966;21:1435–1437.

58. Solomonow M, Baratta R, Zhou BH, D'Ambrosia R. Electromyogram coactivation patterns of the elbow-antagonist muscles during slow isokinetic movement. *Exp Neurol.* 1988;100:470–477.

59. Steindler A. *Kinesiology of the Human Body under Normal and Pathological Conditions.* Springfield, IL: Charles C Thomas; 1955.

60. Stroyan M, Wilk KE. The functional anatomy of the elbow complex. *J Orthop Sports Phys Ther.* 1993;17:279–288.

61. vanZuylen EJ, van Velzen A, van der Gon JJD. A biomechanical model for flexion torques of human arm muscles as a function of elbow angle. *J Biomech.* 1988;21:183–190.

62. Warwick R, Williams PL, eds. *Gray's Anatomy.* 36th British ed. Philadelphia: WB Saunders; 1980.

63. Winters JM, Kleweno DG. Effect of initial upper-limb alignment on muscle contributions to isometric strength curves. *J Biomech.* 1993;26:143–153.

64. Youm Y, Dryer RF, Thambyrajah K, et al. Biomechanical analyses of forearm pronation-supination and elbow flexion-extension. *J Biomech.* 1979;12:245–255.

9

Wrist and Hand

The wrist and hand are a group of joints that dictate functional capabilities unique to man. The importance of the hand is manifested by the large area of the central nervous system devoted to its control. Capable of extremely fine movements such as threading a needle, the wrist and hand must also regularly perform gross tasks requiring considerable force. This chapter presents the arthrology and arthrokinematics, biomechanics, and kinetics associated with both normal and pathological motion of the wrist and hand.

MUSCULAR ACTIONS
Wrist

The musculature at the wrist may be conveniently categorized by function: flexion, extension, and radial deviation, and ulnar deviation. Of these motions the most important are extension and flexion. The three primary extensors, carpi radialis longus, carpi radialis brevis, and carpi ulnaris, are dedicated to wrist control. The other tendons pass to distal insertions and assist with control of wrist extension. Included within this assistive group are extensors digitorum, digiti minimi, pollicis longus, and indicis proprius. All the extensor muscles are innervated by the radial nerve, which is of practical significance because effective hand function is ultimately dependent upon positioning of the wrist in extension.

Flexion is the responsibility of two muscles: flexors carpi radialis and ulnaris. Another muscle, the palmaris longus, may play a role in wrist flexion, but its importance is probably minimal since it is often absent unilaterally or bilaterally. Its presence may provide a "spare" tendon for potential surgical transfer, however. The flexors digitorum superficialis and profundus provide strong assistive function, but only if the muscles are not being used simultaneously for flexion of the digits. Finally, the flexor pollicis longus may assist wrist flexion.

Radial and ulnar deviation at the wrist are the result of synergistic contraction of muscles whose primary actions are either extension or flexion of the wrist. For example, radial deviation is carried out by the simultaneous action of the flexor and extensor carpi radialis muscles. Assistance during powerful movements may be obtained from the musculature arising from the forearm and passing to the thumb. Conversely, ulnar deviation is accomplished by contraction of the flexor and extensor carpi ulnaris muscles. Furthermore, all muscles can be cyclically contracted to perform circumduction (circling) of the wrist. Because of the location of the wrist extensors and flexors, many examples of antagonistic and synergistic contraction may be cited. Study of a cross section taken through the wrist confirms the actions of these muscles (Fig. 9.1). Note that the moment arms vary considerably and that many combinations of tension (synergistic action) could produce the desired result.

The radial and ulnar carpi muscles function synergistically in certain wrist positions

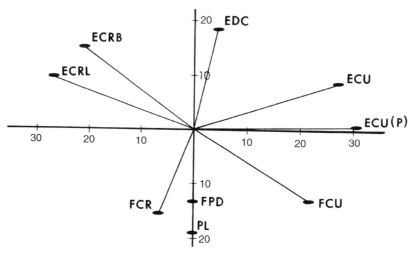

Figure 9.1.   The location of the muscles that cross the wrist is shown in terms of location from the axis of motion. All distances are in millimeters. *Legend*: *ECRL*, extensor carpi radialis longus; *ECRB*, extensor carpi radialis brevis; *EDC*, extensor digitorum; *ECU(S)* and *ECU(P)*, extensor carpi ulnaris with forearm supinated and pronated, respectively; *FCU*, flexor carpi ulnaris; *FPD*, flexor digitorum profundus; *PL*, palmaris longus; *FCR*, flexor carpi radialis.

but act antagonistically in radial and ulnar deviation. To determine the role of musculature in wrist stability, EMG activity has been recorded in several wrist muscles during flexion-extension and radio-ulnar deviation with the forearm in pronated and supinated positions. Results showed that the extensor carpi ulnaris, the abductor pollicis longus, and the extensor pollicis brevis were active during both flexion and extension. Differences in activity were recorded when the supinated position was compared with the pronated position. Because minimal displacements of the tendons were noted during wrist flexion, the conclusion was drawn that these three muscles could be considered an adjustable collateral system that provides support at the wrist (28).

In another study, wrist muscle activity was evaluated during grasping motions of the normal hand (43). Extensor activity was observed primarily in the extensor carpi radialis brevis. Increased gripping efforts resulted in increased activity seen first in the extensor carpi ulnaris and then in the extensor carpi radialis longus. Other cases of synergistic action are included in later sections of this chapter.

Hand

Musculature of the hand is complex. A comprehensive discussion of hand anatomy is contained in such classic works as Landsmeer (31). Anatomical relationships are confounded by the presence of two special digits, the thumb and index finger, and because the muscles controlling the digits arise from the forearm. That these muscles also cross the wrist means that wrist position and dynamic function will influence muscular control of these digits.

The thumb has a complex arrangement of muscles, with four intrinsic to the hand and four extrinsic from the forearm (67). The four muscles arising from the forearm include only one brevis (the extensor pollicis) and three pollicis longi: the flexor, abductor, and extensor. Those intrinsic to the hand include two pollicis brevi (the flexor and abductor) along with the opponens and adductor pollicis. This arrangement allows one to draw the thumb across the hand and to oppose the pad of the thumb with the medial aspect of the hand or little finger. Without such capability, the function of the hand would be severely compromised.

The index, long, and ring fingers have a common muscular arrangement. Extension of all phalangeal joints is directly produced or influenced by the extensor digitorum (34). Some consider the extensor digitorum to extend only the metacarpophalangeal (MP) joints, with full extension of the proximal and distal joints (PIP and DIP) by the intrinsics via the dorsal hood. Warwick and Williams (69) state that the intrinsics place tension on the dorsal hood, allowing the extensor digitorum to extend the interphalangeal (IP) joints. In addition, both the interossei and lumbricals flex the MP joints of their respective fingers while the interossei can abduct or adduct the digit to which they are attached (Fig. 9.2). The lumbricals are unique in that they can relax their own antagonist via their proximal attachment to the flexor digitorum profundus tendons. As they contract, the distal portions of the profundus tendons are slackened, allowing greater IP extension while the lumbricals also tighten the extensor expansion.

Extensive study of the extensor expansion has been undertaken because this apparatus is important for normal hand function. As discussed earlier, fiber expansions of

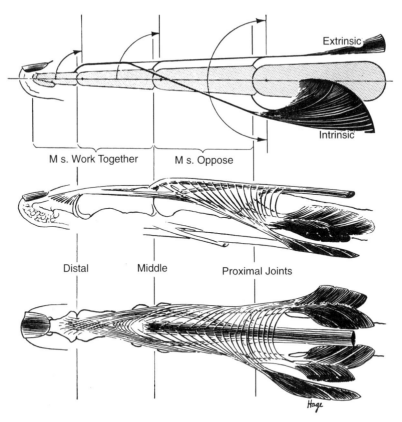

Figure 9.2.   Three views of the musculature of the fingers, exclusive of the thumb. The top two are lateral views, the lowest a view of the dorsal surface.

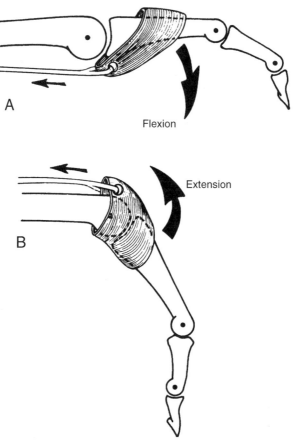

Figure 9.3.   The transverse and sagittal bands of the MP joint. **A.** The transverse fibers of the interosseus facilitate MP joint flexion. **B.** The sagittal bands of the extensor tendon insert into the volar plate, acting as an extensor.

the interossei and extensor digitorum essentially serve to assist both IP extension and MP flexion. This is accomplished via insertion of the interosseus tendons into the transverse fibers of the expansion, producing MP flexion. In addition, the remainder of the insertion goes to the extensor expansion for IP extension. In addition, the sagittal bands are used for effective MP joint extension (Fig. 9.3) (56). Other detailed accounts of the anatomy of the expansion are found in the literature (29, 67, 69).

Comprehensive accounts of the anatomy of the intrinsic musculature are contained in other works (19). Flexion of the MP joint is produced by both the flexors digitorum superficialis and profundus. As these muscles project distally, however, the superficialis divides and send slips to the base of the middle phalanx, allowing the profundus to pass to the base of the distal phalanx.

The little finger has anatomical features common to fingers index, long, and ring, but also has special features related to functional requirements. Abduction is produced by the abductor digiti minimi muscle, similar to the first dorsal interosseous muscle and in contrast to those of the third and fourth digits. Hollowing of the palm, an action used to hold water in the palm of the hand or to grasp a cylinder, is facilitated by the opponens digiti minimi. Finally, the MP joint has an additional flexor: the digiti minimi brevis. Table 9.1 provides a summary of the motions and the responsible musculature.

Combined Motions

The result of these anatomical arrangements is a meaningful and coordinated pattern of movement. Effective function comes from the power of the extrinsic musculature while fine control is left to the intrinsic musculature of the hand. Effective motion is created by interaction of the various segments as a particular task is accomplished. For example, extension of the IP joints is accomplished by the intrinsic muscles when the MP joint is concurrently being extended by the extensor digitorum muscle. Conversely, flexion of the MP joint is completed by the intrinsics as the extensor digitorum extends the IP joints. Furthermore, the long finger flexors can affect motion of the proximal finger and wrist joints if the more distal joints are stabilized. Or, if the proximal joints are stabilized, the long flexors can effectively function through their attachments at the distal joints. The interaction of these muscles allows motions such as simultaneous IP joint flexion and MP joint extension by respective action of the long finger flexors and the extensor digitorum. Or, all joints of the fingers may simultaneously extend or flex, with the former by action of both the extensor digitorum and the intrinsics. Other combinations are possible but these are the most important combinations required for functional activities (69).

To perform these functions effectively the wrist must be held in a position that

Table 9.1. Wrist and Hand Muscle Actions

	WRIST				MP				PIP 1st		DIP 2nd		CMC				
	Flexion	Extension	Abduction	Adduction	Flexion	Extension	Abduction	Adduction	Flexion	Extension	Flexion	Extension	Flexion	Extension	Abduction	Adduction	Opposition
Flexor carpi radialis	P		S														
Flexor carpi ulnaris	P			S													
Palmaris longus	P																
Extensor carpi radialis longus		P	S														
Extensor carpi radialis brevis		P	S														
Extensor carpi ulnaris		P		S													
Flexor digitorum profundus	S				S						P						
Flexor digitorum superficialis	S				S				P								
Extensor digitorum		S				P				P		P					
Extensor indicis		S				P				P		P					
Extensor digiti minimi		S				P	S			P		P					
Lumbricals					P					P		P					
Dorsal interossei					P		P			P		P					
2nd, 3rd, and 4th palmar interossei					P			P		P		P					
Abductor digiti minimi							P										
Flexor digiti minimi brevis					P												
Opponens digiti minimi					P												
Extensor pollicis longus		S	S							P						S	
Extensor pollicis brevis			S			P									S		
Abductor pollicis longus	S		S											S	P		
Abductor pollicis brevis													S		P		
Flexor pollicis longus	S				S				P				S				S
Flexor pollicis brevis													P			P	
Opponens pollicis													P				P
Adductor pollicis																P	

Abduction-adduction at MP joints is relative to line located along long axis of long finger. For thumb muscles PIP is equivalent to IP joint. *Legend: MP*, metacarpophalangeal joint; *PIP*, proximal interphalangeal joint; *DIP*, distal interphalangeal joint; *CMC*, carpometacarpal joint of thumb; *P*, primary function; *S*, secondary function.

will allow the musculature to develop or maintain the required tension. Chapter 2 discussed the length-tension relationship for human muscle. Because many muscles that affect finger motion originate in the forearm and pass across the wrist, the *length* of these muscles can be significantly influenced by altering the position of the wrist. Consider the case where the wrist is placed in full flexion. In this configuration, as happens in radial nerve injuries, the long finger flexor musculature has simultaneously been shortened. Because significantly less tension is available when the muscle is extremely shortened, only limited tension is available in the flexor digitorum superficialis and profundus. As a result, little grip strength can be achieved with the wrist in full flexion. Full and forceful wrist flexion may even cause an assailant to lose an effective grip on an intended weapon. Consequently, the optimal position for hand function is at 20–30° of wrist extension. Similar effects on finger extension can be seen if the wrist is completely extended. In this case the extensor digitorum muscle is slackened, preventing sufficient extension torques to be generated at the MP and IP joints.

Mechanical implications arise from these anatomical features. The arrangement of the flexor digitorum profundus and superficialis muscles provides an example. Because the profundus tendon passes deep to the superficialis at a point near the proximal IP joint, the profundus can act to elevate the superficialis tendon and increase its angle of insertion into the base of the middle phalanx. Another example comes from the lumbrical and interosseous muscles. Although the interossei have twice the cross-sectional area, the lumbrical muscles have a longer possible excursion. However, the lumbricals have a better mechanical advantage because their line of action is farther from the joint axis. Therefore, they are considered to have an overall advantage for creating joint torque during grasping.

Synergistic actions can also be readily displayed in the wrist and hand. Warwick and Williams (69), among others, cite one interesting case. When the abductor digiti minimi muscle contracts to abduct the fifth finger at the MP joint, the flexor carpi ulnaris can be palpated to contract, exerting a countertraction on the pisiform bone from which the abductor originates. To prevent the flexor carpi ulnaris from producing ulnar deviation and wrist flexion, the abductor pollicis longus contracts to neutralize both motions. Many other complex events such as typing, piano playing, and object manipulation require serial synergistic events. This remarkable coordination can leave us in awe of our own abilities.

Much of the functional capacity of the hand comes from the thumb's special abilities, in particular its opposition to the other digits. Opposition is usually thought of as pulp-to-pulp (pad-to-pad) contact of the thumb with any of the other digits. In addition, the thumb can assume other relationships with the fingers, accounting for many other hand postures. Many classifications of hand function have been developed. Kapandji (27) mentions six modes of prehension, of which four require the thumb. **Terminal opposition,** in which a fine object is held between the thumb and index finger, is the most precise mode of prehension. Another mode is **prehension by subterminal opposition,** probably the most commonly used manipulative technique. An example of this mode is the grasp of a pencil or a piece of paper between the thumb and index finger.

Some other modes specified by Kapandji are similar to a more commonly accepted classification described by Flatt (19): tip, palmar, and lateral. **Tip grip** uses PIP joint flexion as the very tips of the digits oppose each other. The **palmar grip** uses more of a pad-to-pad opposition. The third type, **lateral or key grip,** uses the thumb against the side of the finger, usually the radial side of the first PIP of the index finger. Palmar grip is the most frequently used mechanism, especially for holding or picking up objects.

ARTHROLOGY AND ARTHROKINEMATICS

As for other joints in the body, the bony framework and configuration is responsible for the resulting kinematics. The close interrelationship between the wrist and hand must be kept in mind although they will be considered separately in this section.

Wrist

Because of the many bones comprising the wrist, the analysis of motion is complex. Some specific joints have undergone thorough biomechanical analysis (24, 74). Most sources distinguish a proximal and a distal row of carpals (32, 47, 52). Some disagree on how the two rows of carpals operate as nearly separate segments yet with an integrated relationship (32, 47, 52, 65). That the distal row bones remain relatively tightly bound likely depends on the ligamentous structures (47). In fact, movements of the distal carpal row have been noted to closely resemble the movements of the hand (50). Conversely, the proximal row is more unstable (32). From a cineradiographic analysis, simultaneous movement is observed in the radiocarpal joint and the midcarpal joints (28). The literature frequently notes the action of the scaphoid compared with other bones: it serves as a mechanical link between the carpal rows by articulation with capitate, lunate, radius, trapezium, and trapezoid bones and via ligamentous structures (28, 32, 52). The effect is to provide synchronous angulation of both carpal rows that encourages radio-ulnar deviation (32). In all these motions the ligaments play an important role, the tension dependent on the position of joints (1, 51, 70). Generally, however, the function of the ligaments is still an unsolved problem (52).

MacConaill (35) states that in complete extension (the close-packed position), the carpus rotates toward supination. This rotary movement occurs at the junction of the scaphoid and the radius because the other articulations have already achieved their respective **close-packed positions.** Others state that upon flexion-extension, the scaphoid moves more with respect to the forearm than do the lunate and triquetrum. This asymmetrical motion produces tension in the joint capsules and ligaments during extension, resulting in the close-packed position. Other rotations occur during radial and ulnar deviation, with the former producing the close-packed position of the midcarpal (intercarpal) joint (29). Another analysis of wrist kinematics modeled the normal wrist after a tight, universal joint in that little or no longitudinal rotation is allowed between one segment (hand) and the other (forearm) (3). Such constraints as these may make work of this nature invalid.

Specific components of wrist movement have been studied by a number of investigators. In 1977, one group studied flexion and extension in a roentgenographic analysis of 55 normal wrists. Average measurements showed that 40%, or 26°, of flexion occurred at the radiocarpal joint. The remaining 60% occurred during the 40° of motion at the midcarpal joint. Conversely, the radiocarpal joint involved two thirds of the extension in comparison with one third at the midcarpal joint. A summary of these findings is shown in Figure 9.4. The functional significance of this study was the conclusion that the scaphoid belongs to the second row of carpals during extension and to the first row during flexion (48).

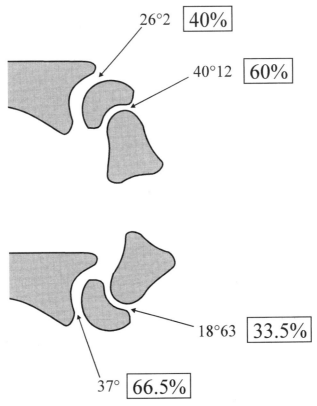

Figure 9.4. Motion in the wrist. Flexion is shown in the upper view and extension in the lower. Both actual motion in degrees and percentages are shown for the radiocarpal and midcarpal motions.

The **center of rotation** of the wrist during flexion, extension, radial deviation, and ulnar deviation has been identified. During these motions, the center is found at the base of the capitate bone, being slightly more proximal during flexion-extension than radial-ulnar deviation (Fig. 9.5) (72). These same investigators also found that for passive radial deviation from neutral to 20°, motion was minimal in the proximal row. However, for passive ulnar deviation up to 37° of motion occurred at both the radiocarpal and midcarpal joints.

The articulation of the metacarpals with the carpals varies from the radial to the ulnar side of the hand. The joints are limited in range for the index and long, but for the ring and little fingers there is increased motion. This can be observed by viewing the dorsal surface of the hand while going from a light to a strong grip. The increased motion apparently allows for more effective grip and cupping of the hand.

Hand

The MP and IP joints have also been examined from an arthrokinematic viewpoint. Flatt (19) noted that the narrow metacarpal head allows for lateral movement at the MP joint in full extension. However, upon full flexion, the collateral ligaments tighten from the shape of the head of the metacarpals. Youm et al. (73), in a companion work to their efforts on the wrist, studied the kinematic behavior of the MP joint and quantified radial-ulnar deviation at the joint during various positions of MP flexion and extension. They measured 40° of radial-ulnar deviation in neutral, only 10° in full flexion, and 25° at a position 30° past full extension. They found the center of rotation of the MP joint to be fixed on the midline of the metacarpal, at a point proximal to the joint line by one-tenth the metacarpal length.

The DIP and PIP joints lack a collateral ligament tightening mechanism. In fact, some state that the collateral ligaments are tight in all positions of the IP joints (19). Study of the distal IP joints displays some unique features associated with joint surfaces. Asymmetries of the metacarpal head are the rule, causing an incomplete fit and resulting accessory motions. Furthermore, because the condyles of the phalanges do not extend distally the same amount, the long axes of the ring and middle finger can deviate (23). The effect is that, on flexion, the fingers rotate toward the thumb, helping to maximize the function of the hand.

Special consideration should be given to the thumb because of its importance to effective hand function. In fact, some consider the thumb to be 40% or greater of the hand's functional value (67). Techniques of wire fixation, goniometry, and cineradiography have been used to study the function of the carpometacarpal (CMC) joint. Others, however, have presented quantitatively derived, in vivo data. With respect to a reference system associated with the third metacarpal, the CMC joint had 53° of flexion-extension, 42° of adduction-abduction, and 17° of rotation. A key finding was that the 17° occur with the four primary movements of flexion, extension, abduction, and adduction. The motions of the CMC and the MP joint of the thumb, which together are responsible for opposition, are a result of joint surface geometry, muscle action, and limitations imposed by ligamentous structures (15).

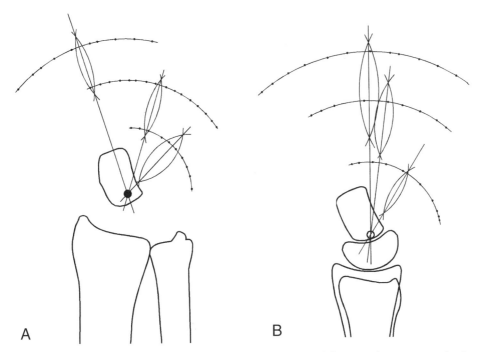

Figure 9.5.   Centers of rotation during radial-ulnar deviation (**A**) and flexion and extension (**B**) for the wrist, indicated by the circle in the proximal capitate.

BIOMECHANICS

Published information relating to the biomechanics of the wrist and hand has usually been specific to either kinematics or kinetics. More comprehensive studies are difficult or impossible because of the complexity of the articulations, which creates many variables that cannot be controlled. In spite of these problems, the anatomy and applied mechanics of the hand provide an opportunity to further knowledge of the significance of altering mechanics by injury or surgical repair. For example, the results of tendon transfer are directly related to altering the "mechanical advantage" (moment arm) and/or the excursion capability of the transferred muscle. Because the clinician and the patient assess effectiveness of tendon transfers in terms of function and because the long finger muscles are frequently used in transfers, most of the current information concerns these muscles (12).

As can be anticipated from knowledge of the extensor mechanism, the **moment arm** of the extensor tendons remains virtually constant throughout the range of flexion and extension. Conversely, as the MP joint moves from extension to full flexion, the moment arm of the flexors increases about 50% (73). An et al. (2) studied the influence of excursions of the index finger joints and confirmed previous work. Figure 9.6 shows relatively constant moment arms for the extensors and minor changes produced in the radial and ulnar interossei muscles during MP joint flexion. Note, however, the increase for the long flexors produced by MP joint flexion, but little effect produced by MP abduction-adduction.

Other methods have been used to evaluate muscles of the forearm and hand. Extensive dissection and calculations were completed to determine mean fiber length and "physiological" cross section of various muscles. Based on data for all forearm muscles, a **tension fraction** was calculated for each muscle, yielding a determination of its "tension" compared with all other muscles in the forearm and hand. These data are valuable because excursion values, one determinant of function, are also included in the analysis (10). Others have also studied tendon excursion in the hand. One group determined that tendon excursions of the long flexors generally exceeded 20 millimeters when the MP joint was moved from 30° of extension to 90° of flexion. Little change in tendon excursion occurred in the interossei during MP flexion-extension, and only slightly more was noted on finger abduction-adduction. These investigators also pointed out that MP joint stability is dependent on the action of the intrinsic muscles in the neutral position (73).

An et al. (2) displaced all joints of the index finger in evaluating tendon excursion. A representative result is shown in Figure 9.7. Negative values suggest shortening while positive values show elongation. Note the essentially linear changes in the long flexors and extensors and the tendency for the intrinsic muscles to reach their peak change at mid range. Excursions for the IP joints and the MP joint in adduction-abduction were relatively small when considered in relationship to the changes produced by MP flexion.

KINETICS

Forces delivered to the various joints of the thumb, hand, and wrist are critical to the function of the hand. The **balance of forces** is carefully regulated within the normal hand by many phenomena, some of which are unknown and others precisely known (9). When an imbalance is created by injury or disease, restoration of function is contingent on generating sufficient tension in the correct temporal sequence.

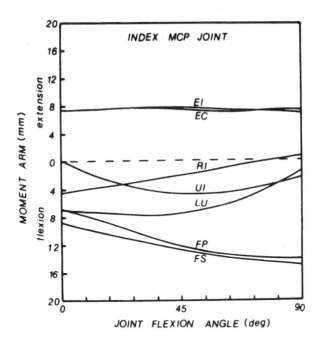

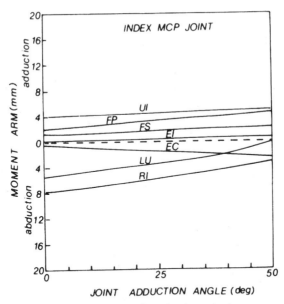

Figure 9.6. Moment arms of the index finger muscles. The determinations were made at the MP joint for flexion and extension (*top*) and abduction and adduction (*bottom*). *Legend*: *FS*, flexor digitorum superficialis; *FP*, flexor digitorum profundus; *EC*, extensor digitorum communis; *EI*, extensor indicis; *RI*, radial interosseous; *LU*, lumbrical; *UI*, ulnar interosseous.

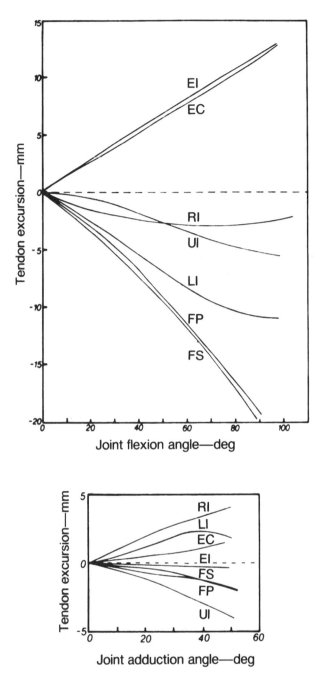

Figure 9.7.   Tendon excursion plotted versus joint angle at the MP joint for flexion (*top*) and adduction (*bottom*). Positive values are elongations (distal) displacements, negative are shortening (retraction) movements of the tendons. *Legend*: *FS*, flexor digitorum superficialis; *FP*, flexor digitorum profundus; *EC*, extensor digitorum communis; *EI*, extensor indicis; *RU*, radial interosseous; *LI*, lumbrical; *UI*, ulnar interosseous.

However, little is known about the true forces exerted by the musculature in the forearm and hand.

Tension generated in muscles can be estimated from the cross-sectional area of the individual muscles. Cross-sectional areas must be taken perpendicular to the fiber direction to determine precisely the available tension. Studies specifying the cross section have been completed, but the work of Brand and coworkers (10) is the first to calculate tension fractions based on the individual muscle's contribution to the total mass of the forearm and hand (see earlier discussion of tension fraction).

Theoretical work has also been completed on the static forces in the thumb. Results showed tendon forces that varied from 0.9 to 3.52 kg for the tip grip and from 1.29 to 5.61 kg for the lateral grip. During grasp, tendon forces reached over 50 kg in the abductor pollicis longus muscle (14). Studies with a more practical focus have also been completed. One has recorded the following "strength" values for men and women, respectively: wrist extension, 13 and 7 kg; MP extension, 6 and 4 kg; thumb MP extension, 3 and 2 kg. The absence of information on the location of the force measurement, however, limits the usefulness of this study (46). Therefore, no calculation of torques can be completed for purposes of measurements with either previously recorded or prospective measurements. A summary table of some known torques at the wrist and fingers is shown in Table 9.2.

Of most significance is the force within any given tendon, as therapists often mobilize tendons actively or passively after injury or surgery. Most of the effort in this area has been accomplished either in animals or post immobilization. Thus, the primary discussion of this issue will be in the following section on pathokinesiology. Implications also exist for the positions of the wrist and fingers during splinting procedures and when active mobilization may be used (49). Related to this is the moment arms of the tendons as they attempt to create forces across the wrist. That the six major muscles uniquely contribute to wrist forces and that none of four common prosthetic implants duplicated normal wrist kinetics may prove surprising to many (62).

Joint forces have not been studied frequently in the upper limb because of its non- weight-bearing role and the few pathological changes created by its relatively low compression forces. In one study, shear, rotation, bending, and compression forces were determined for all of the joints in the thumb. Generally, the magnitudes of these joint forces were 2 kg or less at all joints for 1 kg of tip or key grip force. Joint compressive force, however, reached as much as 120 kg at the CMC joint during strong grasp (14). Volz et al. (65) showed that small compressive loads are transmitted through the scaphoid, lunate, and distal radius. As the load is increased, compressive load is also transmitted through the distal radio-ulnar fibrocartilage surfaces. Perhaps the load is quite equally divided between the scaphoid-trapezium-trapezoid, scaphoid-capitate, lunate-capitate, and triquetrum-hamate joints in the midcarpal joint (64). The key point to remember with upper extremity kinetics, however, is that the size of forces is usually quite low.

While significant forces do occur in the tissues of the wrist and hand it is unlikely that they will lead to the same degree of degenerative joint disease that occurs in lower extremity joints. The requirements during functional activities have had limited assessment and more information is needed (13). Disruption of kinetics resulting from pathologies such as arthritis or trauma or from surgical procedures may lead to deformity and dysfunction. How such disruptions in kinematics and kinetics are manifested is discussed in the next section.

Table 9.2. Normative Wrist and Finger Torque Values

Source Reference	Gender	Age Mean	Age SD	Age Range	n	Movement	Concentric (°/sec)	Eccentric (°/sec)	ROM	Testing Position	Peak Torque Nm	Peak Torque SD	Testing Device
63	f	22	2		24	wr f	0		0	sit, sh f 15, elb 90, wr sup	22		Cybex II
						wr f	60			sit, sh f 15, elb 90, wr pro	20		
						wr f	60			sit, sh f 15, elb 90, wr sup	19		
						wr e	0		0	sit, sh f 15, elb 90, wr pro	8		
						wr e	60			sit, sh f 15, elb 90, wr pro	4		
						wr e	60			sit, sh f 15, elb 90, wr sup	5		
						rd	0		0	sit, sh f 15, elb 90, wr 0	9		
						rd	60			sit, sh f 15, elb 90, wr pro	8		
						ud	0		0	sit, sh f 15, elb 90, wr 0	8		
						ud	60			sit, sh f 15, elb 90, wr pro	7		
	m	22	2		6	wr f	0		0	sit, sh f 15, elb 90, wr sup	13		Cybex II
						wr f	60			sit, sh f 15, elb 90, wr pro	11		
						wr f	60			sit, sh f 15, elb 90, wr sup	18		
						wr e	0		0	sit, sh f 15, elb 90, wr pro	12		
						wr e	60			sit, sh f 15, elb 90, wr pro	7		
						wr e	60			sit, sh f 15, elb 90, wr sup	12		
						rd	0		0	sit, sh f 15, elb 90, wr 0	18		
						rd	60			sit, sh f 15, elb 90, wr pro	16		
						ud	0		0	sit, sh f 15, elb 90, wr 0	15		
						ud	60			sit, sh f 15, elb 90, wr pro	12		
4	m			50–60	5	wr e	0		0	elb 120	13		Cybex II
	f			50–65	5	wr e	0		0	elb 120	7		
71	m			21–30	4	pro	0		0	sh abd 0, elb 90	9		Kin-Com
						sup	0		0	sh abd 0, elb 90	9		
	f			21–30	4	pro	0		0	sh abd 0, elb 90	4		
						sup	0		0	sh abd 0, elb 90	4		
36	m			20–24	29	grip	0			sh abd 0, elb 90	121	21	Jamar HHD
				35–39	25	grip	0			sh abd 0, elb 90	120	24	
				55–59	21	grip	0			sh abd 0, elb 90	101	27	
				75+	25	grip	0			sh abd 0, elb 90	66	21	

Ref	Sex	n	Age	n	Test		Velocity	ROM	Position	Mean	SD	Device
	m		20–24	29	tip pinch	0			sh abd 0, elb 90	18	3	Jamar HHD
			35–39	25	tip pinch	0			sh abd 0, elb 90	18	4	
			55–59	21	tip pinch	0			sh abd 0, elb 90	17	3	
			75+	25	tip pinch	0			sh abd 0, elb 90	14	3	
	m		20–24	29	key pinch	0			sh abd 0, elb 90	26	4	Jamar HHD
			35–39	25	key pinch	0			sh abd 0, elb 90	26	3	
			55–59	25	key pinch	0			sh abd 0, elb 90	24	4	
			75+	25	key pinch	0			sh abd 0, elb 90	20	5	
	m		20–24	29	palmar pinch	0			sh abd 0, elb 90	27	6	Jamar HHD
			35–39	25	palmar pinch	0			sh abd 0, elb 90	26	4	
			55–59	21	palmar pinch	0			sh abd 0, elb 90	24	5	
			75+	25	palmar pinch	0			sh abd 0, elb 90	19	4	
	f		20–24	26	grip	0			sh abd 0, elb 90	70	15	Jamar HHD
			35–39	24	grip	0			sh abd 0, elb 90	74	11	
			55–59	21	grip	0			sh abd 0, elb 90	57	13	
			75+	25	grip	0			sh abd 0, elb 90	43	11	
	f		20–24	26	tip pinch	0			sh abd 0, elb 90	11	2	Jamar HHD
			35–39	24	tip pinch	0			sh abd 0, elb 90	12	3	
			55–59	21	tip pinch	0			sh abd 0, elb 90	12	2	
			75+	25	tip pinch	0			sh abd 0, elb 90	10	3	
	f		20–24	26	key pinch	0			sh abd 0, elb 90	18	2	Jamar HHD
			35–39	24	key pinch	0			sh abd 0, elb 90	17	3	
			55–59	21	key pinch	0			sh abd 0, elb 90	16	3	
			75+	25	key pinch	0			sh abd 0, elb 90	13	2	
	f		20–24	26	palmar pinch	0			sh abd 0, elb 90	17	2	Jamar HHD
			35–39	24	palmar pinch	0			sh abd 0, elb 90	18	4	
			55–59	21	palmar pinch	0			sh abd 0, elb 90	16	3	
			75+	25	palmar pinch	0			sh abd 0, elb 90	12	3	
5	m	41 12	23–75	50	grip	0	0.36*	0	sh abd 0, elb 90, wr 0	5	1	custom HHD
	f	45 16	21–79	50	grip	0	0.93*	0	sh abd 0, elb 90, wr 0	3	1	custom HHD
68	f	22	19–24	12	wr e	0	1.64*	30e–30f	wr pro	9		custom load cell
					wr e			30e–30f	wr pro	10		
					wr e			30e–30f	wr pro	10		
					wr e			30e–30f	wr pro	11		

Legend: *, cm/sec shortening of muscle; *abd*, abduction; *e*, extension; *elb*, elbow; *f*, flexion; *HHD*, hand held dynamometer; *pro*, pronation; *rd*, radial deviation; *sh*, shoulder; *sup*, supination; *ud*, ulnar deviation; *wr*, wrist.

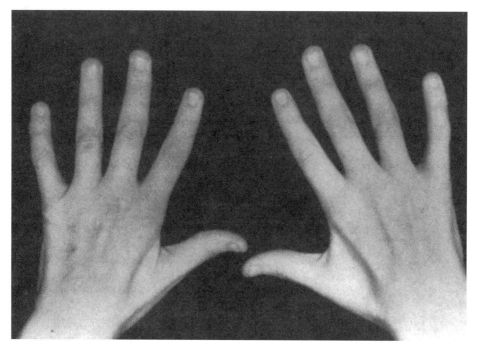

Figure 9.8.   Dorsal view of the hands, resulting from lesions of the ulnar nerves.

PATHOKINESIOLOGY

As the distal portion of the upper limb was freed by the assumption of the upright posture, the wrist and hand became essential to human function. Gross positioning of the limb in space is essentially ineffective if objects cannot be manipulated or functions cannot be carried out by a dexterous hand. Simple experiences with hands that have become extremely cold are demonstration enough of the loss of abilities upon which humans so depend. Subsequently, any loss created by neurological or musculoskeletal injury has the potential to be devastating. The remainder of this chapter will discuss how commonly encountered pathologies affect function of the wrist and hand.

Nerve Injuries

The effects of peripheral nerve injury are well established. Individual or collective loss of the radial, median, and ulnar nerves have differing effects, the size of which depends on the degree and site of injury.

Ulnar nerve injuries that are proximal, i.e., above the innervation site for the flexor digitorum profundus muscle, will cause loss of abduction and adduction of all the fingers. Flexion power will also be decreased, particularly in the ring and little fingers. Typically, the hand assumes a clawlike posture. More distal injury to the ulnar nerve leaves the flexor profundus and flexor superficialis muscles intact. Thus, the effect on gripping is not as pronounced. Loss of the lumbricals for the ring and little finger, in combination with the loss of the interossei and thumb adduction, produces significant changes (Fig. 9.8). The ring and little fingers are unable to flex at the MP joints or extend at the IP joints, resulting in the ulnar "claw hand" (Fig. 9.9). A further implication is that the long finger flexors cause IP flexion, preventing opposition to the thumb. Sensory changes are apparent over the ulnar two fingers and the ulnar surface of the hand. The ulnar half of the long finger may also show loss in some patients.

Median nerve injury affects the thumb, in severe cases so much so that the thumb remains extended. The thenar eminence is markedly flattened (Fig. 9.10). Because of the effect on the index and long fingers (superficialis and profundus muscles), the hand assumes the posture of a brachiating ape. Sensory changes predominate over the palmar surface of the hand on the radial side, including the thenar eminence.

Combined high median and ulnar nerve losses will paralyze all interossei, lumbricals, superficialis, and profundus muscles, thus causing total loss of all finger flexing ability. Combined paralysis of distal (forearm) ulnar and median nerves produces a hand in which no intrinsic (lumbricals and interossei) muscles are functional. The result is the intrinsic minus hand in which the MP joint is hyperextended and the IP joints are flexed (Figs. 9.11–9.13). To study the effects, movement patterns of the MP and IP joints in 141 fingers were evaluated. The conclusion was that the long flexors and extensors produced simultaneous rather than successive MP flexion and PIP extension. Although equal range of motion was achieved at MP and PIP joints, the latter was achieved without excessive motion at the PIP joint. In extension PIP movement lagged behind MP extension so much that full extension was not achieved even when the MP joint was maximally extended (59).

Radial nerve palsies may result from humeral fractures, shoulder dislocations, and other causes. The resulting loss of wrist extension, called "wrist drop," prevents

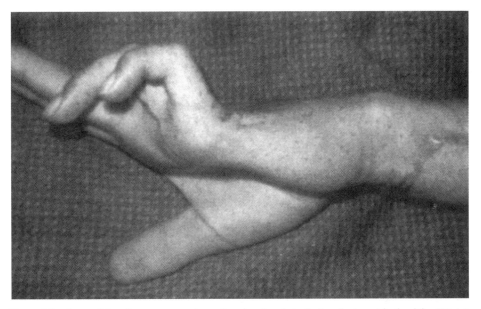

Figure 9.9. Loss of the ulnar nerve produces the claw hand, including flexion at both of the IP joints of the ring and little fingers.

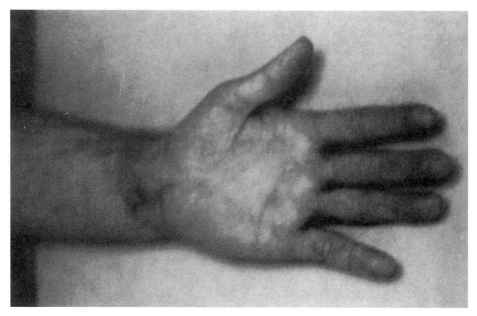

Figure 9.10. Typical appearance of the hand following long-term injury to the median nerve. Note specifically the flattening of the thenar eminence.

effective grip because the long finger flexors do not have a stabilized wrist across which finger flexion can occur. This is because as the flexors attempt to close the fingers they also act to flex the wrist. Due to the simultaneous flexion at the MP, IP, and wrist, effective tension is unavailable because the muscles have undergone significant shortening. Additional losses resulting from radial nerve injury include extension of the MP joints by the extensor digitorum and extension of the thumb

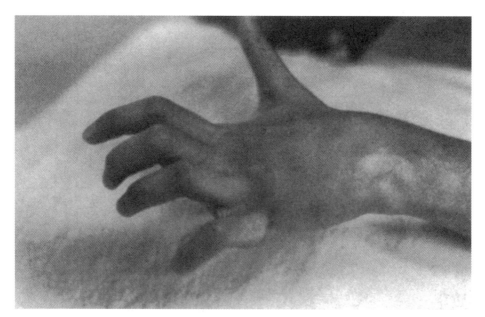

Figure 9.11. Combined loss of the distal portion of the median and ulnar nerves produces loss of both the lumbricals and the interossei and results in this hand posture.

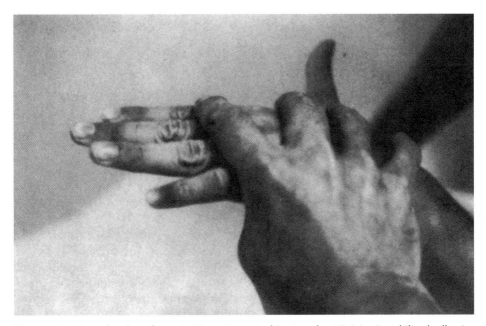

Figure 9.12. Same hand as shown in Figure 9.11. In this view the MP joint is stabilized, allowing extension of the IP joints by the extensor digitorum.

(56). At least sometimes, although muscle mass was recovered after radial nerve injury, the force generating capability is significantly altered (8).

Some **spinal cord injured patients** may benefit from a flexor tenodesis, a procedure that removes a length of the flexor tendon(s). As a result, passive tension is created in the flexors because stretch can be applied when maximal wrist extension is achieved. Subsequently, more effective hand function, i.e., finger closure, can be accomplished because some finger grip is restored.

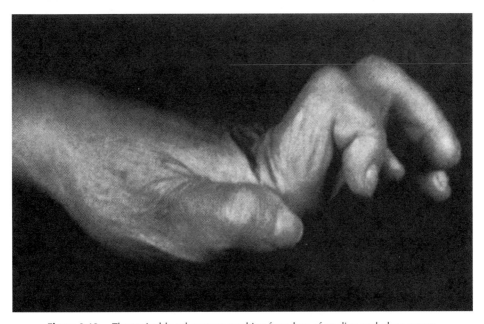

Figure 9.13. The typical hand posture resulting from loss of median and ulnar nerves.

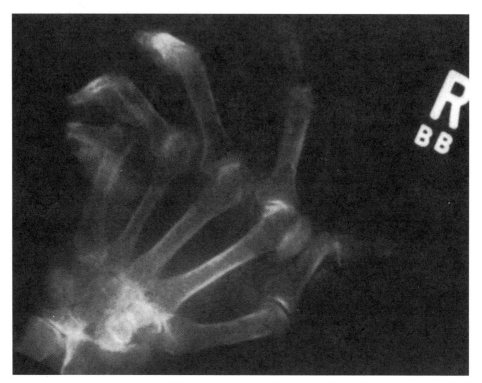

Figure 9.14.   Radiograph of the hand and wrist of a rheumatoid arthritic. Note the deformity, particularly at the MP joints where ulnar drift is obvious. The wrist is also deviated in all but the radial direction.

Rheumatoid Arthritis

The hand of the patient with **rheumatoid arthritis** provides an interesting clinical example of hand pathology. Because of the nature of the pathology, anatomical factors, and existing forces, several reasons for the resulting deformity and disability have been advanced. Among the reasons for ulnar drift at the MP joints are the smaller ulnar condyles of the intercarpals, the larger ulnar collateral ligaments, and the larger muscle mass associated with the little finger. Other forces known to facilitate ulnar drift include gravity, thumb pressure in the ulnar direction, and ulnar deviation associated with the power grip. These anatomical and force elements are coupled with factors associated with rheumatoid changes, such as decreased stability of the proximal phalanx. In addition, flexor and extensor tendons are displaced in the ulnar direction, facilitating ulnar deviation of the MP joint concurrently with radial deviation of the wrist (Fig. 9.14).

Hand postures are also frequently altered because of pathological changes. One example is a condition known as "swan-neck" deformity: flexion of the MP and distal IP joints and hyperextension of the proximal IP joint (Figs. 9.15 and 9.16). This "intrinsic plus" condition significantly disturbs kinetic balance. Although multiple causes for the deformity have been proposed, some authors agree that tightness of the intrinsics produces the flexion deformity of the MP joint. Laxity of the proximal IP joint secondary to the disease facilitates hyperextension of this joint, again by tightness of the intrinsics. The net result of MP flexion and IP hyperextension is

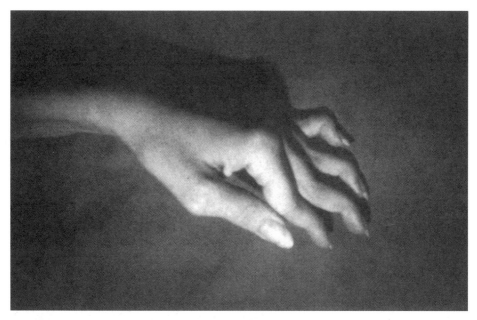

Figure 9.15. Swan neck deformity in the rheumatoid arthritic. Note the MP and IP positions described in the text.

tension in the flexor profundus tendon, resulting in a flexion deformity at the distal IP joint and completing the clinical "swan-neck" picture (61).

Observing the gross deformities that can occur in rheumatoid hands demands considerable attention to the loss of functional abilities. The coming of joint replacement procedures has greatly assisted the rehabilitation process associated with advanced stages of the pathology (17, 57) (Fig. 9.17).

Total finger joint replacements, such as the Flatt, Niebauer, Swanson, and Steffee,

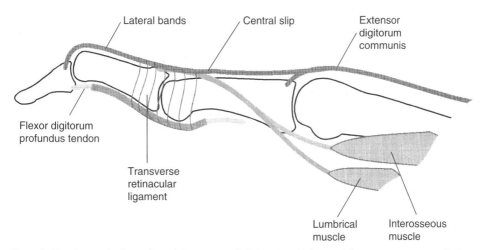

Figure 9.16. Anatomical correlate of the swan-neck deformity with laxity of the transverse retinacular ligament.

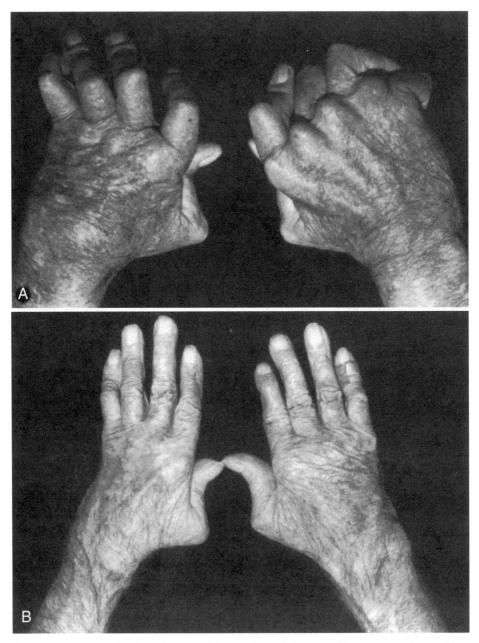

Figure 9.17. Preoperative (**A**) and postoperative (**B**) views of rheumatoid hands undergoing total joint replacement of the MP finger joints, exclusive of the thumb.

have been used frequently but with varied success. What success they have enjoyed is probably because the MP and IP joints are essentially non-weight-bearing and operate almost as hinges. Prostheses are, however, subject to breakage, loosening, and difficulty in achieving sufficient joint movement. A sample of these results is provided in studies that evaluated patients with MP replacements required by rheumatoid arthritis (33, 42). Performance of tip prehension and grasp were improved while power grip, pinch force, and lateral prehension remained unchanged. The effects shown in the latter group were explained by prosthetic looseness.

Comprehensive results of MP joint arthroplasties have also been presented. In separate studies, silastic and metallic hinge prostheses were evaluated in long-term follow-up on many patients. Despite some ulnar deviation recurrence and some failures, functional ranges of motion were retained. This latter finding, coupled with high patient satisfaction, apparently establishes the worth of the procedure (6, 7). Unfortunately, 20% of the replacements eventually fractured (42). Other work has evaluated the effect of MP reconstruction, showing that motion varies depending on the procedure performed and the time elapsed from the surgery (16). Results for total wrist replacement show that muscle imbalance, loosening, and prosthesis dislocation are potential problems (37). In other work, results have been judged to be 72% good or excellent (38). There is, however, evidence that arthritics have a loss of volitional wrist extensor control during closing motions of the hand. If the mechanism is one of inhibition due to pain, reeducation procedures for the wrist extensors may be necessary (66).

Soft Tissue and Trauma

The hand is subject to a number of soft tissue pathologies due to traumatic events. Many conditions could be discussed in this section, but only a few relatively common problems produce pathological motion.

One soft tissue anomaly related to rheumatoid arthritis is the **boutonnière or buttonhole deformity**. In this case, the central slip of the extensor tendon is avulsed, or sufficiently stretched, from the base of the middle phalanx to allow the lateral bands of the extensor hood to pass to the volar surface of the proximal IP joint. Subsequently, the PIP joint projects through the lateral bands as a button would pop through a hole (61) (Fig. 9.18).

Trigger finger is a condition that can affect any of the long finger flexors. An increase in connective tissue of the tendon may cause thickening or even a nodule. As the tendon attempts to pass through the flexor sheath near the MP joint, the thickening or nodule catches on the small-diameter opening and hinders smooth passage. Increased tension, however, may cause the thickening to squeeze through the opening, resulting in a fast flexion of the finger and in a snapping movement (44). Similar findings occur when passive tension is created during finger extension.

Another pathological condition indirectly affecting the tendons is **Dupuytren's contracture**. Proliferation of fibrous tissue of the palm, usually more pronounced on the medial aspect, causes the ring and little fingers to be drawn toward the palm of the hand (Fig. 9.19). This progressive degenerative disease ultimately prevents the fingers from extending (44).

Because tendons are subject to trauma, high tensile loads, and degenerative processes, **repairs** are often necessary. After surgery, care must be taken with mobilization of tendons because high tensile loads can lead to rupture at the repair site. Therapists should note that the tensile strength of individual flexor tendons may be reduced by as much as 66% compared with losses of only 26% in hand grip strength (16). This reinforces the need to respect even small deficits in grip strength as possibly suggesting quite remarkable weakness in the individual tendons.

The literature shows an overall increased trend, since the first report in the 1970s (30), toward early controlled **mobilization** of finger segments postsurgery and immo-

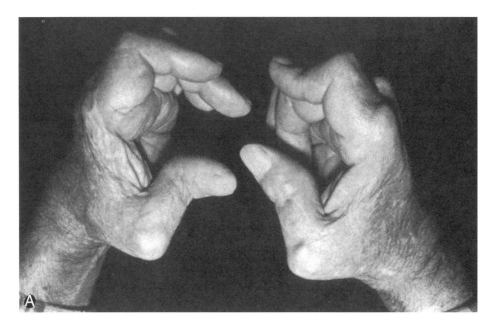

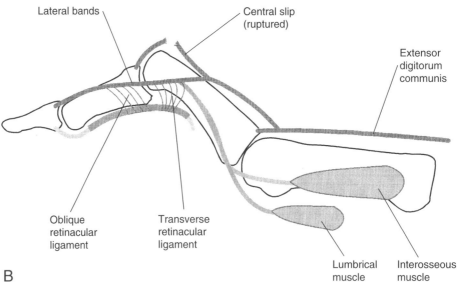

Figure 9.18.   Clinical appearance (**A**) and anatomical view (**B**) of the Boutonnière deformity in the index finger of the right hand.

bilization. Controlled motion usually starts at day three, with progressive increases in range. Such a therapeutic program has been shown to positively affect range of motion and adhesion formation (26, 53, 54, 55). Mechanical changes have also been noted, specifically via increases in strain, stiffness, rupture load, energy absorbed, and stress (20). Type of procedure may have an effect (22, 25); however, as can be noted in a study that showed that the increase in the passive range of motion was proportional to how much time the finger joint was held at its end range (21). These data were in support of the **total end range time theory** as applied to motion of the finger joints. Little information is available about the force that can be applied (18). Nordin and Frankel (40) note that human tendon does not regain normal strength until 40–50 weeks post surgery. Several surgical repair procedures are compared in their text. Although some disagreement exists as to the proper duration of immobilization and aggressiveness of treatment, 5–6 weeks is a general minimum time necessary for repair strength to develop. Allowing too much time before encouraging motion can lead to adhesions between the tendon and its surrounding tissues.

A confounding issue in the assessment of hand function is that many techniques are available as a measure of hand function. Therapists need to be familiar with the methods to know how to interpret the literature since the results vary from one technique to another (58, 60).

The influence of immobilization on tissues has been noted elsewhere in this book. Because immobilization is often a treatment of choice, therapists need to be familiar with its effects and with therapeutic regimens most effective in reversing changes in tissues. While significant muscle degeneration has not been shown, the deficits in "strength" at the wrist approximate 30% (39). Specific studies on the effect of mobilization are conflicting, but may be due to differences in the administration of the treatment (41, 45). More study in this area is needed to be of more direct assistance to the clinician.

Other effects on finger function occur from changes within the flexor sheaths. Trauma, complications of surgery, or arthritis can create **bowstringing** of the flexor tendons across the volar surface of the MP joint (Fig. 9.20). Although bowstringing creates a better moment arm for flexion of the MP joint, it has been known to seriously weaken the IP joint flexors due to muscle shortening. In fact, this loss in

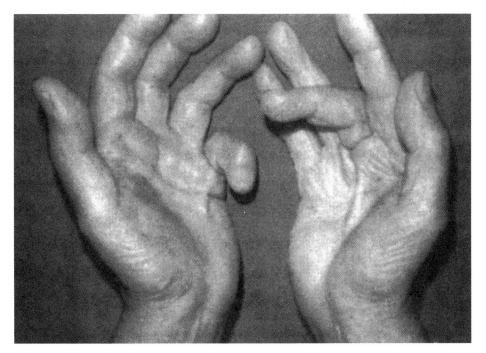

Figure 9.19. Dupuytren's contracture.

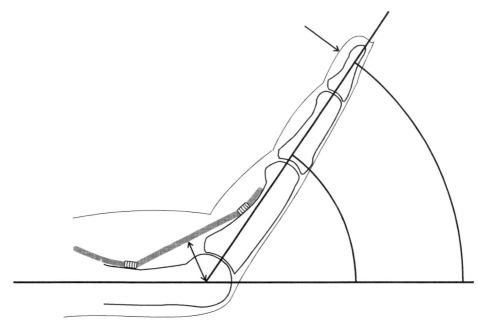

Figure 9.20. The mechanical effects of "bowstringing" of the flexor tendons across the MP joint are apparent. The moment arm is obviously increased, but the shortening of the muscle significantly affects the patient's ability to generate effective moments at the distal joints.

grip strength is equivalent to that created by 40° of wrist flexion. Brand and coworkers (11) also point out that the surgical procedure known as pulley advance is advocated for intrinsic paralysis although it does not increase the mechanical advantage when the MP joint is in full extension or hyperextension. This case points out the necessity of appropriate mechanical evaluation before beginning surgical procedures. Thus, to restore finger function, kinetic balance must be evaluated and monitored. These elements have been aptly pointed out. Key points include the ability of the muscle to adapt (modification of the number of sarcomeres) by about 1 mm per day, the importance of constant versus intermittent stress (which tends to make tissue thicker and stronger), and the recommendation to assure between one and two hours of activity per day to keep joints mobile (9, 13). Compliance with these principles should provide more effective results for the therapist dealing with patients who have disorders of the hand and wrist.

SUMMARY

The anatomy and functional biomechanics of the hand are complex, complicating the ability of clinical kinesiologists to understand both normal and pathological motion. As more sophisticated repair techniques become available, therapists will continue to be called upon not only to evaluate pathological motion comprehensively but also to apply biomechanical principles to treatment regimens. Patients depend on our understanding of hand function; ultimately, the critical role played by the hand in human development challenges us to reach a greater understanding.

References

1. Acosta R, Hnat W, Scheker LR. Distal radio-ulnar ligament motion during supination and pronation. *J Hand Surg (Br)*. 1993;18:502–505.
2. An KN, Ueba Y, Chao EY, Cooney WP, Linscheid RL. Tendon excursion and moment arm of index finger muscles. *J Biomech*. 1983;16:419–426.
3. Andrews JG, Youm Y. A biomechanical investigation of wrist kinematics. *J Biomech*. 1979;12:83–93.
4. Arner M, Hagberg L. Wrist flexion strength after excision at the pisiform bone. *Scand J Plastic Reconstr Surg*. 1984;18:241–245.
5. Askew LJ, An K-N, Morrey BF, Chao EYS. Isometric elbow strength in normal individuals. *Clin Orthop*. 1987;222:261–266.
6. Blair WF, Shurr DG, Buckwalter JA. Metacarpophalangeal joint implant arthroplasty with a silastic spacer. *J Bone Joint Surg*. 1984;66(A):365–370.
7. Blair WF, Shurr DG, Buckwalter JA. Metacarpophalangeal joint arthroplasty with a metallic hinged prosthesis. *Clin Orthop*. 1984;184:156–163.
8. Bosnjak RF, Dolenc VV, Sepe A, Demsar F. Force, fatigue, and the cross-sectional area of wrist extensor muscles after radial nerve grafting. *Neurosurg*. 1992;31:1035–1041.
9. Brand PW. Biomechanics of balance in the hand. *J Hand Ther*. 1993;6:247–251.
10. Brand PW, Beach RB, Thompson DE. Relative tension and potential excursion of muscles in the forearm and hand. *J Hand Surg*. 1981;6:209–219.
11. Brand PW, Cranor KC, Ellis JC. Tendon and pulleys at the metacarpophalangeal joint of a finger. *J Bone Joint Surg*. 1975;57(A):779–784.
12. Brand PW, Hollister A. *Clinical Mechanics of the Hand*. St. Louis: Mosby Year Book; 1993.
13. Brumfield RH, Champoux JA. A biomechanical study of normal functional wrist motion. *Clin Orthop*. 1984;187:23–25.
14. Cooney WP, Chao EYS. Biomechanical analysis of static forces in the thumb during hand function. *J Bone Joint Surg*. 1977;59(A):27–36.
15. Cooney WP, Lucca MJ, Chao EYS, Linscheid RL. The kinesiology of the thumb trapeziometacarpal joint. *J Bone Joint Surg*. 1981;63(A):1371–1381.
16. Ejeskar A. Finger flexion force and hand grip strength after tendon repair. *J Hand Surg*. 1982;7:61–65.
17. El-Gammal T, Blair W. Motion after metacarpophalangeal joint reconstruction in rheumatoid disease. *J Hand Surg*. 1993;18A:504–511.
18. Evans RB, Thompson DE. The application of force to the healing tendon. *J Hand Ther*. 1993;6:266–284.
19. Flatt AE. *Kinesiology of the Hand. American Academy of Orthopaedic Surgeons: Instructional Course Lectures XVIII*. St. Louis: CV Mosby; 1961.
20. Feehan LM, Beauchene JG. Early tensile properties of healing chicken flexor tendons: early controlled passive motion versus postoperative immobilization. *J Hand Surg*. 1990;15A:63–68.
21. Flowers KR, LaStayo P. Effect of total end range time on improving passive range of motion. *J Hand Ther*. 1994;7:150–157.
22. Gelberman RH, Woo SL-Y, Amiel D, et al. Influences of flexor sheath continuity and early motion on tendon healing in dogs. *J Hand Surg*. 1990;15A:69–77.
23. Gigis PI, Kuczynski K. The distal interphalangeal joints of human fingers. *J Hand Surg*. 1982;7:176–182.
24. Hollister A, Buford WL, Myers LM, et al. The axes of rotation of the thumb carpometacarpal joint. *J Orthop Res*. 1992;10:454–460.
25. Hume EL, Hutchinson DT, Jaeger SA, Hunter JM. Biomechanics of pulley reconstruction. *J Hand Surg*. 1991;16A:722–730.
26. Hung LK, Chan A, Chang J, et al. Early controlled active mobilization with dynamic splintage for treatment of extensor tendon injuries. *J Hand Surg*. 1990;15A:251–257.
27. Kapandji AI. *The Physiology of Joints*. 5th ed. New York: Churchill Livingstone; 1982.
28. Kauer JMG. Functional anatomy of the wrist. *Clin Orthop*. 1980;149:9–20.
29. Kessler R, Hertling D. *Management of Common Musculoskeletal Disorders*. New York: Harper & Row; 1983.
30. Kleinert HE, Spokevicius S, Papas NH. History of flexor tendon repair. *J Hand Surg*. 1995;20A: S46–S52.
31. Landsmeer JMF. Anatomical and functional investigations on the articulation of the human fingers. *Acta Anat*. 1955:25:Supplementum 24.
32. Linscheid RL. Kinematic considerations of the wrist. *Clin Orthop*. 1986;202:27–39.

33. Linscheid RL, Dobyns JH. Total joint arthroplasty: the hand. *Mayo Clin Proc.* 1979;54:516–526.
34. MacConaill MA, Basmajian JV. *Muscles and Movements: A Basis for Human Kinesiology.* Baltimore: Williams & Wilkins; 1969.
35. MacConaill MA. Mechanical anatomy of the carpus and its bearing on surgical problems. *J Anat.* 1941;75:166–175.
36. Mathiowetz V, Kashman N, Volland G, et al. Grip and pinch strength: normative data for adults. *Arch Phys Med Rehabil.* 1985;66:69–74.
37. Menon J. Total wrist replacement using the modified Volz prosthesis. *J Bone Joint Surg.* 1987;69A:998–1006.
38. Meuli HC, Fernandez DL. Uncemented total wrist arthroplasty. *J Hand Surg.* 1995;20A:115–122.
39. Miles MP, Clarkson PM, Bean M, et al. Muscle function at the wrist following 9 days of immobilization and suspension. *Med Sci Sports Exerc.* 1994;26:615–623.
40. Nordin M, Frankel VH. Biomechanics of collagenous tissue. In: Frankel VH, Nordin M, eds. *Basic Biomechanics of the Skeletal System.* Philadelphia: Lea & Febiger; 1980.
41. Nørregaard O, Jakobsen J, Nielsen KK. Hyperextension injuries of the PIP finger joint. *Acta Orthop Scand.* 1987;239–240.
42. Opitz JL, Linscheid RL. Hand function after metacarpo-phalangeal joint replacement in rheumatoid arthritis. *Arch Phys Med Rehabil.* 1978;59:160–165.
43. Radonjic D, Long CL. II: Kinesiology of the wrist. *Am J Phys Med.* 1971;50:57–71.
44. Ramamurti CP. *Orthopaedics in Primary Care.* Baltimore: Williams & Wilkins; 1979.
45. Randall T, Portney L, Harris BA. Effects of joint mobilization on joint stiffness and active motion of the metacarpal-phalangeal joint. *J Orthop Sports Phys Ther.* 1992;16:30–36.
46. Richards RR, Gordon R, Beaton D. Measurement of wrist, metacarpophalangeal joint, and thumb extension strength in a normal population. *J Hand Surg.* 1993;18A:253–261.
47. Ruby LK, Cooney WP, An K-N, Chao EYS. Relative motion of selected carpal bones: a kinematic analysis of the normal wrist. *J Hand Surg.* 1988;13A:1–10.
48. Sarrafian SK, Melamed JL, Goshgarian GM. Study of wrist motion in flexion and extension. *Clin Orthop.* 1977;126:153–159.
49. Savage R. The influence of wrist position on the minimum force required for active movement of the interphalangeal joints. *J Hand Surg.* 1988;13B:262–268.
50. Savelberg HHCM, Otten JDM, Kooloos JGM, et al. Carpal bone kinematics and ligament lengthening studied for the full range of joint movement. *J Biomech.* 1993;26:1389–1402.
51. Schuind F, An K-N, Berglund L, et al. The distal radioulnar ligaments: a biomechanical study. *J Hand Surg.* 1991;16A:1106–1113.
52. Seenwald GR, Zdravkovic V, Kern H-P, et al. Kinematics of the wrist and its ligaments. *J Hand Surg.* 1993;18A:805–814.
53. Silfverskiöld KL, May EJ, Oden A. Factors affecting results after flexor tendon repair in zone II: a multivariate prospective analysis. *J Hand Surg.* 1992;18A:654–662.
54. Silfverskiöld KL, May EJ, Törnvall AH. Tendon excursions after flexor tendon repair in zone II: results with a new controlled-motion program. *J Hand Surg.* 1993;18A:403–410.
55. Singer M, Maloon S. Flexor tendon injuries: the results of primary repair. *J Hand Surg.* 1988;13B:269–272.
56. Smith RJ. Balance and kinetics of the fingers under normal and pathological conditions. *Clin Orthop.* 1974;104:92–111.
57. Smith RJ, Kaplan EB. Rheumatoid deformities at the metacarpophalangeal joints of the fingers. *J Bone Joint Surg.* 1967;49(A):31–47.
58. So YC, Chow SP, Run WK, et al. Evaluation of results in flexor tendon repair: a critical analysis of five methods in ninety-five digits. *J Hand Surg.* 1990;15A:258–264.
59. Srinivasan H. Patterns of movement of totally intrinsic-minus fingers. *J Bone Joint Surg.* 1976;58(A):777–785.
60. Stegink-Jansen CW, Watson MG. Measurement of range of motion of the finger after flexor tendon repair in zone II of the hand. *J Hand Surg.* 1993;18A:411–417.
61. Swezey RL. Dynamic factors in deformity of the rheumatoid arthritic hand. *Bull Rheum Dis.* 1971–72;22:649–656.
62. Tolbert JR, Blair WF, Andrews JG, Crowninshield RD. The kinetics of normal and prosthetic wrists. *J Biomech.* 1985;18:887–897.
63. Vanswearingen JM. Measuring wrist muscle strength. *J Orthop Sports Phys Ther.* 1983;4:217–228.
64. Viegas ST, Patterson RM, Todd PD, McCarty P. Load mechanics of the midcarpal joint. *J Hand Surg.* 1993;18:14–18.

65. Volz RG, Lieb M, Benjamin J. Biomechanics of the wrist. *Clin Orthop.* 1980;149:112–117.
66. Volz RG. Total wrist arthroplasty. *Clin Orthop.* 1984;187:112–120.
67. Wadsworth CT. Clinical anatomy and mechanics of the wrist and hand. *J Orthop Sports Phys Ther.* 1983;4:206–216.
68. Walmsley RP, Pearson N, Stymiest P. Eccentric wrist extensor contractions and the force velocity relationship in muscle. *J Orthop Sports Phys Ther.* 1986;8:288–293.
69. Warwick R, Williams PL, eds. *Gray's Anatomy.* 35th British ed. Philadelphia: WB Saunders; 1973.
70. Weaver L, Tencer AF, Trumble TE. Tension in the palmar ligaments of the wrist. I. The normal wrist. *J Hand Surg.* 1994;19:464–474.
71. Winters JM, Kleweno DG. Effect of initial upper limb alignment on muscle contributions to isometric strength curves. *J Biomech.* 1993;26:143–153.
72. Youm Y, McMurtry RY, Flatt AE, Gillespie TE. Kinematics of the wrist: I. An experimental study of radial-ulnar deviation and flexion-extension. *J Bone Joint Surg.* 1978;60(A):423–431.
73. Youm Y, Gillespie TE, Flatt AE, Sprague BL. Kinematic investigation of normal MCP joint. *J Biomech.* 1978;11:109–118.
74. Zancolli EA, Ziadenberg C, Zancolli E. Biomechanics of the trapeziometacarpal joint. *Clin Orthop.* 1987;220:14–26.

10

Hip

The mechanics and control of the hip joint present an interesting set of circumstances for the student of kinesiology and biomechanics. As the most proximal joint of the lower limb, the hip provides stability and gross control in space for the rest of the leg. Activities such as stair climbing and lifting require that hip muscles exert large forces for generating appropriate moments; overall, anatomical structure reflects functional requirements for effective performance. Joint pathology is rather common, mostly because of large and/or repetitive loading that occurs in the joints of the lower limb. This chapter will present kinesiology and biomechanics as related to the hip and then discuss some pathologies that disrupt the normal kinematics and kinetics.

MUSCULAR ACTIONS
Extensors-Flexors

The extensor group, mostly contributed to by the gluteus maximus and the hamstrings, is supplemented in action by muscles such as the gemelli, the obturator internus, and the adductor magnus, all of which have other primary functions. When considered as a whole the extensors comprise a powerful group with a physiological cross section of more than 150 cm^2 (32). If "accessory" muscles of the hip are excluded, a cross-sectional area of over 113 cm^2 remains. Specific functions in which these accessory muscles are particularly useful include rising from a chair, stair climbing, powering the prosthesis of the above-knee amputee, and propulsive activities such as running.

Fischer and Houtz (17) analyzed individual hip extensors with the use of electromyography. Several activities requiring hip extension were performed in different positions to assess contraction of the gluteus maximus. Analysis revealed that the greatest activity occurred during isometric muscle setting, and during maximal contractions in a position of hyperextension, external rotation, and abduction. The authors commented that extension of the flexed thigh was accomplished by the hamstrings muscles. Some caution should be exercised in deriving conclusions from these data, however, because recorder response characteristics were limited to less than the optimal suggested for EMG signals.

Musculature responsible for flexion includes two primary muscles, the psoas major and the iliacus. By virtue of attachment to the lumbar spine, the psoas has potentially profound effects on the hip and spine, the latter to be discussed thoroughly in Chapter 13. In any case, the combined contraction of the psoas major and the iliacus can participate in powerful although infrequently needed hip flexion movements. Secondary hip flexors include the tensor fasciae latae, rectus femoris, sartorius, and the adductors. Other muscles, such as the gracilis and quadratus femoris, assist with flexion in only a tertiary fashion (16).

Abductors-Adductors

In general, the hip adductor group has been believed to be of minor importance. Because the large cross-sectional areas are inconsistent with any need for adduction torque, perhaps secondary functions are of greater importance. For example, the adductors regularly contract early in the swing phase of the gait cycle. The participation of these muscles in hip rotation and extension (depending upon the position of the thigh) is further evidence of their role as accessory muscles.

The abductor group serves an important function, particularly during weight bearing. A specific discussion of this mechanism is discussed later in the section on biomechanics. Besides the gluteus medius and minimus, the tensor fasciae latae and piriformis appear to play some role in abduction. Years ago, theoretical calculations were made that showed the ratio of the average muscle masses relative to each other: medius, 4; minimus, 2; tensor fascia latae, 1 (24). Since the advent of computed tomography, data are available that confirm the mass and line of actions of the abductors of the hip. Calculations show that with a cross-sectional area of 25.3 cm² the gluteus medius muscle accounts for 59% of the total area, the gluteus minimus 20%, the tensor fasciae latae 11%, and the piriformis 10% of all the muscles studied (10). Creation of such ratios essentially establishes the relative import of each muscle.

Merchant (36) also completed a study that analyzed the abductor muscle force required as the superincumbent body weight varied from 20 to 60 pounds. By altering the position of the femur and pelvis, this investigator noted that the tension in the abductors varied considerably. For example, with the femur externally rotated 30° while the pelvis was maintained in neutral, the tensor fasciae latae muscle accounted for more than 50% of the tension required to keep the model in equilibrium. Conversely, with the femur rotated internally and the pelvis neutral, no tension existed in the tensor; therefore, a large dependence of position on function is obviated.

Rotation

The rotator musculature of the hip has been relegated to a much less important position than the rotators of the glenohumeral joint. Although internal rotation may be accomplished by as many as nine muscles, Favill (16) considers the anterior fibers of the gluteus medius and gluteus minimus to be the primary movers. External rotation may be a dedicated function of the obturator externus and quadratus femoris, but portions of the adductor magnus, gluteus minimus, and long head of the biceps femoris also contribute. The gemelli, obturator internus, and piriformis externally rotate when the hip is in extension. The mass of the rotators and other muscles is considerable. Kapandji (28) states that the power of the medial rotators is only about one-third that of the lateral rotators. Certainly the relatively low amount of force the medial rotators are required to generate bears witness to their seeming unimportance.

Geometry and Function

The multiple actions of the hip musculature have been addressed earlier in this chapter. These actions result from the known geometric relationships that the muscles have with the hip joint. Still to be considered, however, is the relationship of the muscles to the hip as the joint is moved through its range of motion. Extensive work in modeling the hip has provided a complete set of data for 27 of the muscles. The hip was moved through ranges of motion while the effect on the moment arm vector component was determined. An exemplary result is provided in Figure 10.1 for the fibers representing the anterior portion of the gluteus medius muscle. From these

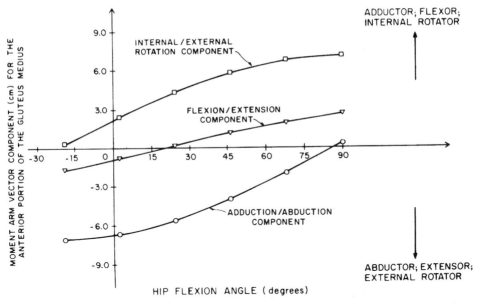

Figure 10.1. Changes in the moment arm vector component of the anterior portion of the gluteus medius for the motion of hip flexion. Motions in the respective planes are given at the far right. See text and Table 10.1 for further description.

data it is possible to determine the effect of any hip position upon the potential action of any of the muscles included in the analysis. The effects of the ranges of motions studied are shown in Table 10.1 (14, 15). Therapists may find such a description of the changes in muscle function with joint position useful in assessing and treating patients. Such changes occur at all joints, and once objectively measured, they will offer the same application to patient care.

Other information available about the function of the hip musculature indicates that the gluteus medius can be divided into at least three segments. In this work, fine-wire EMG was used to simultaneously record from anterior, middle, and posterior segments of the muscle during a variety of functional activities. Results definitively showed that subjects selectively activated different segments of the muscle during some of these activities. For example, during forward leaning from the standing position the anterior portion of muscle becomes relatively quiet while the posterior segment increases in activity as the lean increases (54). Another study has also demonstrated that the anteromedial and posterolateral fibers of the tensor fasciae latae muscle also produce different EMG output during gait and other selected activities (46). Considering that the tensor can act at the knee joint via the iliotibial band, these findings may have implications for control of the knee deficient of ligaments, particularly the anterior cruciate. Specific functional roles of different muscle segments make possible fine control over the size and direction of joint torque. Consequently, therapists must be aware that certain training procedures may be needed to ensure that specific segments of muscle are active instead of a gross contraction of the whole muscle.

Some **biarticular muscles** about the hip affect several joints. Included in this category are the muscles psoas major, rectus femoris, tensor fasciae latae, gracilis,

Table 10.1. Classification of Muscles According to Action at 0, 40, and 90 Degrees of Hip Flexion

Degrees	Action					
	Extension	Flexion	Adduction	Abduction	Internal Rotation	External Rotation
All	BF ST SM AP AMG	RF SR IP TFL[c]	ADB ADL AMN AMG[a,b] GR PC[c]	TFL[a,b] PR[c]		QF[b,c]
0 and 40 only		PC[a]	OE	GMDA[a] GMDM GMDP GMNA[a] GMNM GMNP		GS OI GI
0 and 90 only			AP[b,c]	SR[b,c] RF[b,c]		
40 and 90 only	QF[a]			GS[a]	GMDA GMNA GMDM[a] GMNM[a]	OE[a]
0 only	GM[d]	ADL[b]	QF			PR
40 only						GMDP[c]
90 only	GR[b] AMN[b] ADB[b] ADL[b]			OI	GMDP GMNP PR[b]	

Legend: ADB, adductor brevis; *ADL*, adductor longus; *AP*, adductor magnus (posterior); *AMG*, adductor magnus (middle); *AMN*, adductor minimus; *BF*, biceps femoris; *GM*, gluteus maximus; *GMDA*, gluteus medius (anterior); *GMDM*, gluteus medius (middle); *GMDP*, gluteus medius (posterior); *GMNA*, gluteus minimus (anterior); *GMNM*, gluteus minimus (middle); *GMNP*, gluteus minimus (posterior); *GR*, gracilis; *GI*, gemelli inferior; *GS*, gemelli superior; *IP*, iliopsoas; *OE*, obturator externus; *OI*, obturator internus; *PC*, pectineus; *PR*, piriformis; *QF*, quadratus femoris; *RF*, rectus femoris; *SR*, sartorius; *ST*, semitendinosus; *SM*, semimembranosus; *TFL*, tensor fascia lata.

[a] Secondary action at 40°.

[b] Secondary action at 90°.

[c] Secondary action at 0°.

[d] Model not valid for flexed configurations.

sartorius, biceps femoris, semitendinosus, and semimembranosus. Motion at one joint alters muscle length, which then affects the muscle's function at adjacent joints. Length-tension relationships again become important if we are to consider function effectively. A discussion of the interactive effects of hip and knee joint musculature is included in the next chapter.

ARTHROLOGY AND ARTHROKINEMATICS

Anatomical characteristics of the hip joint are different from upper limb joints. The primary reason for the differences is the necessity for the joints of the lower limb to bear the superincumbent body weight. Another reason is that the lower limb contains more massive musculature necessary to meet larger torque requirements. This section of the chapter presents a summary of the relevant anatomy and discusses the influence of these anatomical features on function.

The hip is generally considered a "ball-and-socket" joint whose center is approximately 1 cm inferior to the mid-position of the inguinal ligament (61). According to Radin and Paul (49), both the acetabular and femoral components are mainly trabecular bone. The acetabulum faces anteriorly, laterally, and inferiorly and is encircled by a labrum that serves to deepen the socket (30). The functional articular surface is the portion known as the lunate surface (Fig. 10.2). This ring is covered by articular cartilage that is thickest superiorly and absent inferiorly (61).

The femoral head, forming about two-thirds of a sphere, is regarded by most to be symmetrical (30). Rydell (53), however, indicates this is not true, because the head is slightly compressed in the anterior-posterior direction. Hoaglund and Low (22) provide a summary that corroborates this position based on radii and intersubject variability. The head is completely covered with articular cartilage except in the location of the fovea, tapering to a "neck" that joins the femoral head and shaft. In turn the neck joins the femoral shaft at an angle of approximately 135° (61). Study of the architecture of the femoral neck is important, because this section of the femur is frequently involved in pathologies. Studies have shown that the cross section of the neck is virtually symmetric near the femoral head and elliptical near the trochanters. This fact may account for some pathology due to trauma and provide clues why some surgical repairs fail (1). Furthermore, the axis of the elliptical segment is not aligned with the long axis of the femoral shaft, thus producing further potential difficulties in load bearing (53). These issues will be discussed in the section on pathokinesiology.

Another anatomical feature that can influence hip mechanics is torsion in the femoral shaft. Antetorsion (anteversion) means that the shaft of the femur has been rotated such that the femoral neck forms a larger than usual angle with the transverse

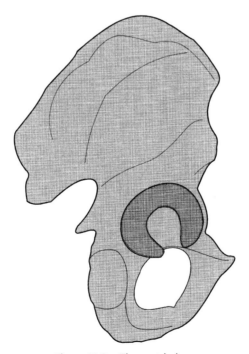

Figure 10.2. The acetabulum.

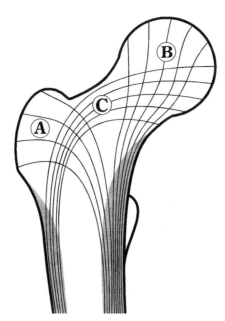

Figure 10.3.   The three main networks of trabeculae: lateral (*A*), medial (*B*), and the arcuate (*C*).

axis of the femoral condyles, as measured in a horizontal plane. **Retrotorsion** is the converse: a smaller than usual angle. Thought to begin in fetal life, **antetorsion** amounts to about 35° in the "average" newborn. During growth, however, the angle diminishes to only 14° in the typical adult (53). The significance of this factor will be discussed in the section on biomechanics.

Trabecular patterns in the proximal femur and pelvis have also been considered important. Virtually any article on the biomechanics of the hip will discuss this issue in detail (28, 30, 53). Although stating that trabeculae have been overemphasized from a mechanical point of view, Rydell describes medial, lateral, and arcuate **trabecular systems** (Fig. 10.3) (53). The lateral portion has been given credit for resisting tensile forces applied by the abductor mechanism, while the medial group resists compressive forces through the head of the femur. The arcuate portion of the trabeculae is responsible for resisting the bending moment through the femoral neck. Note also that areas of pattern intersection have greater strength than those areas where none exists (30).

Ligaments and the extensive joint capsule also are integral aspects of the functional biomechanics of the hip joint. Three strong ligaments are of special significance. The **iliofemoral,** or ligament of Bigelow, simulates an inverted Y as the fibers originating from the pelvis spiral anteriorly and inferiorly to insert along the anterior intertrochanteric line (Fig. 10.4). Note how the fibers attach along the entire length of the line. Two important ligaments arise posteriorly. The **pubofemoral** ligament, in a more inferior location, is stretched most significantly on abduction. The **ischiofemoral ligament,** which also lies posteriorly, resists hip extension and internal rotation as does the anteriorly located iliofemoral ligament (30). These major ligaments blend with and strengthen the expansive capsule. Other ligaments are of little functional importance. The capsule is strongest anteriorly and superiorly, because substantial resistance to hip extension is required for commonly assumed postures. That the fibers of the capsule adopt both a circular and longitudinal orientation has no apparent mechanical significance (61). The bursae found around the joint also have no remarkable features although involvement is not uncommon in various pathologies.

As for any joint, the anatomical structures influence arthrokinematics. A deep acetabulum, receiving much of the femoral head, provides for maximal stability. Further support is provided by ligamentous and capsular structures. Surface joint movement occurs according to the principles of motion as described in Chapter 4. In the lower limb, however, compression due to body weight and consequent muscle contraction increases the shear forces between the joint surfaces. In practice, smaller degrees of arthrokinematic motions are likely to exist because of the nature of the joint structure. Thus, clinicians may regard these joint motions to be of lesser importance.

BIOMECHANICS
Joint Congruence

The hip joint is interesting because of the arthrology and myology associated with its requirements for stability while bearing relatively large loads. However, large ranges of motion exist in the three primary movements. Joint congruence, an important aspect of hip arthrology, has been detailed by Kapandji (28). Simple observation of the human skeleton confirms that, in the upright posture, the femoral head is not covered by the anterior-superior rim of the acetabulum. This finding results from a different planar orientation of the acetabulum relative to the head of the femur. Full congruence can be achieved by either moving the pelvis on the femur or moving the femur on the pelvis. In either case, maximal congruence can be achieved at about 90° of flexion and small amounts of abduction and lateral rotation.

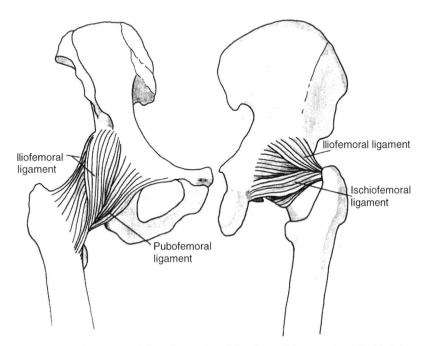

Figure 10.4.   The anterior (*left*) and posterior (*right*) views of the capsule of the hip joint.

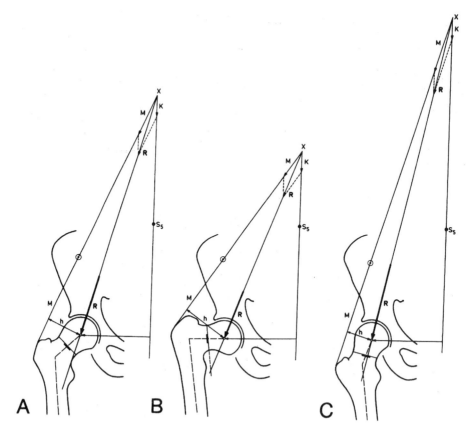

Figure 10.5. Mechanical effects of the position of the hip. **A.** The normal hip. **B.** The varus hip. **C.** The valgus hip. *Legend*: *M,* abductor muscle force; *h,* the moment arm relative to the center of the hip; *R,* the resultant force at the joint; *X,* the intersection of the muscle line of insertion with the line of action of the partial body weight *K.*

Achieving this hip position while weight bearing through the limbs requires the assumption of the quadruped position. (The upright posture requires decreased articular congruence at the hip.)

Confusion may arise as to the difference between congruence achieved in the quadruped position and the close-packed position involving hip extension, abduction, and internal rotation. Recall that a requirement for achieving the close-packed position is tension in the ligaments and joint capsule, a condition only satisfied when the hip is in extension. Paraplegics and amputees usually assume standing postures that cause the line of gravity to fall posterior to the hip joint. In this circumstance, the resistive force that limits hip hyperextension and allows a relaxed standing posture is supplied by the anterior ligaments.

Bony Configuration

Anatomical features decidedly influence hip biomechanics. One is the **angle of inclination,** or the angle in a frontal plane made by the neck and shaft of the femur. Considerable variation in this angle across the human population has been well documented. Figure 10.5 shows an average angle and two structural deviations of the hip known as **coxa vara and valga**. In the varus hip, the angle between the shaft and neck is less than that of the normal 135° configuration. Such a position markedly increases the bending moment in the proximal femur, because the force transmitted along the long axis of the femur has a larger moment arm in respect to the hip joint. Pauwels (47) has demonstrated that the size of tensile and compressive forces produced by the bending moment vary depending on the angle of inclination of the hip. These mechanical considerations affect the design of hip prostheses, in particular the selection of prosthetic materials that can bear anticipated bending moments without fracture. Examples of these problems will be presented in the pathokinesiology section in this chapter. Conversely, the position of valgus (Fig. 10.5C) minimizes the bending moment because the load along the shaft of the femur can be transmitted more directly into the joint.

Other influences stem from the angle of inclination, the position and mass of the greater trochanter, and the antetorsion in the femur. Radin (49) has commented that a decreased angle of inclination (i.e., greater varus) results in greater mechanical advantage of the gluteus medius muscle for controlling the pelvis (described in the following section). Compared with the lever arm of body weight, considered relative to rotation at the center of the hip joint, the lever arm of the abductors is quite small (perhaps 2 to 1). Thus, any advantage that can be provided to the abductor musculature is probably beneficial. Also, remember that considerable hip joint compression is due to contraction of the muscles spanning the joint. Therefore, a beneficial therapeutic approach would be to decrease the muscular forces required to generate or control the moments at the hip. This may be the mechanism for surgical procedures performed with the intent of decreasing pain or alleviating hip joint dysfunction. Radin also suggests that increased antetorsion leads to an increased moment arm for the gluteus maximus, and consequently lengthening of the muscle, together increasing the advantage for this muscle (49). Should this hypothesis be proven true, then two factors may account for increased gluteus maximus mechanical advantage with femoral antetorsion: the increased moment arm and increased muscular tension available due to the length-tension relationship.

Abductor Mechanism

Virtually any analysis of hip mechanics requires discussion of the role of the abductor mechanism. To best understand the function of this muscle, consider the origin and the insertion of the gluteus medius and minimus muscles to be reversed from the classical anatomical description. That is, the origin of the abductors should be considered to be on the greater trochanter of the femur. Then, when standing on one leg, the gluteus medius and minimus can pull the rim of the pelvis toward the greater trochanter of the femur. An understanding of this function is important for several reasons. As one walks, swinging a leg forward requires that balance be momentarily maintained over the leg remaining in contact with the ground. To maintain balance and allow the foot of the swinging leg to clear the ground, the abductors of the stance leg must contract to prevent the pelvis from dropping on the opposite side. This potential drop is caused by the weight of the trunk and swinging leg. Figure 10.6 shows the free body diagram with body weight acting to create a moment about the center of the hip. The force and moment arm of the gluteus medius and minimus have also been added to demonstrate that the system is in equilibrium. Without this balance of moments, the system would not be in equilibrium, resulting in rotation in the direction of the greatest moment. The equation representing this free body

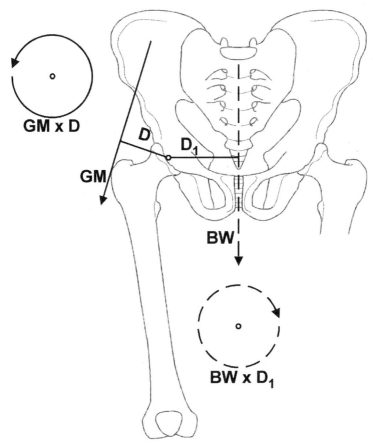

Figure 10.6. Mechanical representation of the hip describing the function of the abductor mechanism. Moments are taken about the center of the hip. To maintain balance and equilibrium, the product of body weight *BW* and D_1 must equal the product of the tension in the gluteus medius (*GM*) and *D*.

diagram would be BW × D_1 = GM × D. Should the mechanics be altered the situation may favor instability, for example, a decrease in abductor force or moment arm. Instability would also be more likely to occur with either an increase in body weight or an increase in the moment arm through which the weight acts relative to the center of the hip joint. Thus, mechanics dictate why patients with hip joint disease or pain may be advised to lose weight, i.e., to reduce the abductor muscle force required to maintain equilibrium while concurrently diminishing compressive load across the hip (26). How patients compensate for pathology will be discussed in the section on pathokinesiology.

The importance of the abductor mechanism has led to a series of studies on tension generating capabilities under a variety of conditions. One study assessed the influences of muscle length changes, called "stretch weakness" by some, on the production of abductor torques in right and left hips. Results showed that between hip differences existed at the −10 and 0 degree test angles. The right hip abductors produced greater torques (Fig. 10.7) (44). The effect of changes in muscle length on tension generation in humans subjected to long-term postures is important so that

clinicians understand the true or potential effect on results of clinical testing procedures. Also remember the issues attendant to immobilization of tissues discussed in
Chapter 2: the assumption of postures can be considered a form of immobilization
and potentially influence tension generation or create "imbalances" that may
need intervention.

As noted earlier, the size of the load across the hip is a result of the intensity of the
contraction of the hip abductor musculature. Carrying loads, however, is frequently
required during daily activities. The greatest electrical activity in the abductors is
produced when loads are carried contralateral to the hip being evaluated (41).
Further, there is some evidence that loads should be carried bilaterally to reduce the
force across the hip joint (42). Finally, because of a higher incidence of osteoarthritis in
the right hip there may be a causal relationship to the size of the activity in the right
hip abductors of right-handed people. Higher levels of EMG have been measured,
although not significantly different, on the side of the subject's handedness (43).

KINETICS

Large muscles are required to generate the torques necessary to function, particularly
under conditions involving large loads. In producing these large torques, however,
muscles also create compression of the joints they span. The compression produced
by a muscle is dependent not only on the tension generated but also on the direction
of the muscle pull relative to the joint surface. Specifically, the greatest compression

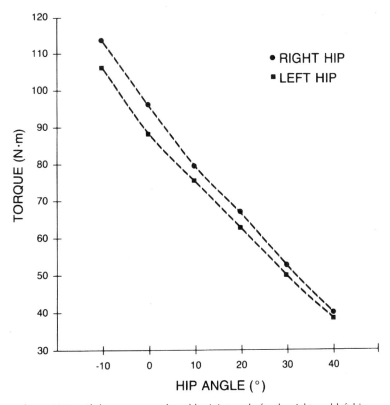

Figure 10.7.   Abductor torque plotted by joint angle for the right and left hips.

of the joint surface will occur on a plane perpendicular to the muscle's direction of pull no matter the curvature in the convex and concave surfaces. Conversely, note that muscles that are parallel with the joint surface produce greater shear at the joint in that they will tend to drag the joint surfaces across each other. To better understand these factors as related to the hip joint this section will discuss torques and joint forces.

Torques

Many studies have been completed on the tension generated in the hip musculature. For example, Jarvis (25) evaluated "strength" of the hip rotators while apparently imposing a force gauge between the leg tested and the manual resistance applied by the examiner. She included a left-to-right comparison of the subjects' legs in various test positions. She noted that the internal rotators generated greater tension than external rotators when the hip was in flexion. However, upon placing the hip in extension, the external rotators were found to exert greater tension than the internal. This reversal was not because they gained mechanical advantage in extension, but because the internal rotators lost mechanical advantage while that of the external rotators remained unchanged. Haley (20) subsequently completed a similar study that addressed the issue of rotator muscle length. Although finding no correlation between joint range and joint torque, the study noted differences in torques in the sitting versus the supine testing position. For example, sitting position torques were 23% and 5% greater than supine for internal and external rotation, respectively. A more recent study, which fails to cite either of the other two studies, also assessed the effect of position on the torque of hip rotators (34). Their results showed that torques were largely dependent on test position, with highest torques being produced in the sitting position. Average peak torques were 64 ft-lbs for internal rotation and 39 ft-lbs for external rotation for the female subjects. Data from the males were 103 and 62 ft-lbs, respectfully. Internal rotation torques exceeded the external rotation torques with one exception, making their data different from that of others. When the literature is considered across all studies, the ratios for internal/external rotation torques approximate 1.0 (6).

   The findings of these and other studies (Table 10.2) point to the importance of standardizing the method and the position across trials and therapists. Chapter 1 pointed out that the correct method for equating "strength" data across subjects and therapists is to use torque directly or calculate torque from the measured force. Because many hip functions are influenced by altering the position of at least one joint crossed by a two-joint muscle, Nemeth et al. (39) studied the effect of knee position on isometric hip extension moment. These investigators determined that knee angle did not influence maximal hip extension torque. The moment values produced, however, decreased as the hip angle progressed from 90° of flexion to full extension. Torques combined across all male and female subjects were at a maximum of 245 Nm at 90° and diminished to 55% of this value at full hip extension. The loss of torque results from the shortening of the muscles. Always, when the hip extensor moment was tested at knee angles of 0, 30, 60, and 90°, the hip extensor torque decreased by approximately equal magnitudes (Fig. 10.8). Few reports appear in the literature about hip flexor torques, presumably because of our need to generate high torques only rarely. In one case flexion torques generated at 30°/sec ranged from 270 Nm for 18-year-olds to less than 120 Nm for subjects in their 60s and 70s. Measurements of flexion torques are, however, of probably more esoteric than clinical

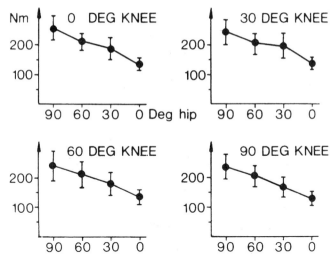

Figure 10.8.   Mean maximum hip extensor muscular moments (n = 10, confidence intervals = .05) at four different angles of the knee.

interest (7). It also now appears likely that passive components contribute usually less than 10% of the total moment generated at the hip in flexion or extension (60).

Torques produced by the abductor musculature have been of longstanding interest because of their role in controlling lateral motion of the trunk during gait. As early as 1947, Inman (24) calculated theoretical abductor torques and then measured peak values of between 1000 and 1100 kg-cm in the standing position. Almost 20 years later, Murray and Sepic (38) studied both abductor and adductor torques at neutral and at 25° of abduction. Although values for both positions tested ranged from 749 to 1390 kg-cm for middle-aged females and young males, respectively, their grand mean value of 1067 agreed quite closely with the Inman data. When the test was completed at 25° of abduction, the abductor torque fell to around 60% of the value produced at the neutral position. More recent data have further demonstrated the influence of joint position (44) (see Fig. 10.7). Considering the antagonist muscle group, the adductor torques, as expected, increased from 1140 kg-cm in neutral to 1287 kg-cm at 25° of abduction (38). These changes further document the influence of muscle length on the ability of muscle to generate torque.

Because torques will vary significantly due to gender, the clinician should consider this factor when measurements are made in the clinical setting. Variances in torques between genders are generally between 30 and 50%, depending on the conditions of testing, age of subjects, and other factors. We also know that the differences are due to multiple factors, but in particular the force that can be generated and the moment arm associated with the force are the two factors (f × d) that account for the torque value. An example of how the moment arms vary is available in the literature. The values are 65 mm for men and 54 mm for women for the gluteus medius muscle. That the moment arms for the gluteus minimus and the tensor fasciae latae muscles are 48 and 42 mm for women and 57 and 46 mm for men show some differences between muscles (40).

Torque values generated for hip abduction while in the supine position were

Table 10.2. Normative Hip Torque Values

Source Reference	Gender	Age Mean	Age SD	Age Range	n	Movement	Concentric (°/sec)	Eccentric (°/sec)	ROM	Testing Position	Peak Torque Nm	Peak Torque SD	Testing Device
31	f	24			20	abd	0		10	sup, hip abd 10	49	22	Spark HHD
		68			20	abd	0		10	sup, hip abd 10	77	17	
6	m	28		20–39	18	f				standing	152	50	Cybex II
						f				standing	126	50	
						f				standing	102	47	
						e				standing	91	50	
						e				standing	177	42	
						e				standing	163	49	
						e				standing	142	49	
						abd				standing	125	52	
						abd				standing	103	26	
						abd				standing	79	20	
						abd				standing	57	20	
						add				standing	45	20	
						add				standing	121	26	
						add				standing	103	32	
						add				standing	85	32	
						add				standing	66	39	
						er				sit, hip 60, kn 90	65	24	
						er				sit, hip 60, kn 90	49	24	
						er				sit, hip 60, kn 90	43	20	
						er				sit, hip 60, kn 90	36	18	
						ir				sit, hip 60, kn 90	72	17	
						ir				sit, hip 60, kn 90	53	19	
						ir				sit, hip 60, kn 90	42	15	
						ir				sit, hip 60, kn 90	34	14	
						f	0		10	standing	167	30	
						f	0		45	standing	108	23	
						e	0		45	standing	160	42	
						e	0		90	standing	204	50	
						abd	0		10	standing	120	23	
						abd	0		0	standing	108	19	
						abd			10	standing	89	18	

	Cybex II

Sex	Age	Range	n
m	54	40–81	17

Movement	0	Angle	Position		
add	0	0	standing	83	27
add	0	10	standing	111	26
add	0	20	standing	129	29
er	0	10ir	sit, hip 60, kn 90	67	21
er	0	0	sit, hip 60, kn 90	62	21
ir	0	10er	sit, hip 60, kn 90	68	22
ir			sit, hip 60, kn 90	85	25
f			standing	113	21
f			standing	84	21
f			standing	68	17
e			standing	57	20
e			standing	157	22
e			standing	132	32
abd			standing	122	34
abd			standing	111	44
abd			standing	75	18
add			standing	63	19
add			standing	46	15
add			standing	32	23
er			standing	99	18
er			standing	83	28
er			standing	55	25
ir			standing	33	26
ir			sit, hip 60, kn 90	50	15
ir			sit, hip 60, kn 90	38	12
f			sit, hip 60, kn 90	30	9
f			sit, hip 60, kn 90	23	10
e			sit, hip 60, kn 90	61	21
e			sit, hip 60, kn 90	41	16
abd			sit, hip 60, kn 90	32	14
abd			sit, hip 60, kn 90	27	14
f	0	10	standing	166	37
f	0	45	standing	89	23
e	0	45	standing	156	65
e	0	90	standing	203	70
abd	0	10	standing	108	26
abd	0	0	standing	90	19
abd	0	10	standing	73	22

Table 10.2.—*continued*

Source Reference	Gender	Age Mean	Age SD	Age Range	n	Movement	Concentric (°/sec)	Eccentric (°/sec)	ROM	Testing Position	Peak Torque Nm	Peak Torque SD	Testing Device
						add	0		0	standing	77	26	
						add	0		10	standing	104	29	
						add	0		20	standing	107	33	
						er	0		10ir	sit, hip 60, kn 90	65	20	
						er	0		0	sit, hip 60, kn 90	54	14	
						ir	0		0	sit, hip 60, kn 90	62	18	
	f	27		20–39	21	ir	0		10er	sit, hip 60, kn 90	75	24	Cybex II
						f				standing	91	24	
						f				standing	70	26	
						f				standing	57	29	
						f				standing	46	16	
						e				standing	110	37	
						e				standing	97	41	
						e				standing	85	34	
						e				standing	77	34	
						abd				standing	66	19	
						abd				standing	54	20	
						abd				standing	43	21	
						abd				standing	32	19	
						add				standing	82	26	
						add				standing	62	32	
						add				standing	50	25	
						add				standing	39	22	
						er				sit, hip 60, kn 90	43	13	
						er				sit, hip 60, kn 90	31	12	
						er				sit, hip 60, kn 90	25	9	
						er				sit, hip 60, kn 90	20	7	
						ir				sit, hip 60, kn 90	47	13	
						ir				sit, hip 60, kn 90	36	14	
						ir				sit, hip 60, kn 90	25	9	
						ir				sit, hip 60, kn 90	22	9	
						f	0		10	standing	105	26	
						f	0		45	standing	66	16	
						e	0		45	standing	95	35	
						e	0		90	standing	126	45	

Cybex II

					abd/add/etc	angle		position	value	SD
f	53	40–64	16		abd	0	10	standing	81	19
					abd	0	0	standing	72	17
					abd	0	10	standing	55	15
					add	0	0	standing	58	19
					add	0	10	standing	70	26
					add	0	20	standing	79	30
					er	0	10ir	sit, hip 60, kn 90	47	13
					er	0	0	sit, hip 60, kn 90	38	9
					ir	0	0	sit, hip 60, kn 90	46	13
					ir	0	10er	sit, hip 60, kn 90	58	13
					f	30		standing	67	21
					f	90		standing	46	17
					f	150		standing	37	13
					f	210		standing	27	12
					e	30		standing	101	27
					e	90		standing	70	26
					e	150		standing	60	22
					e	210		standing	45	21
					abd	30		standing	48	14
					abd	90		standing	38	13
					abd	150		standing	23	9
					abd	210		standing	11	9
					add	30		standing	63	17
					add	90		standing	44	19
					add	150		standing	25	14
					add	210		standing	17	15
					er	30		sit, hip 60, kn 90	32	11
					er	90		sit, hip 60, kn 90	21	8
					er	150		sit, hip 60, kn 90	15	5
					er	210		sit, hip 60, kn 90	12	5
					ir	30		sit, hip 60, kn 90	34	9
					ir	90		sit, hip 60, kn 90	22	7
					ir	150		sit, hip 60, kn 90	15	6
					ir	210		sit, hip 60, kn 90	12	5
					f	0	10	standing	86	24
					f	0	45	standing	51	18
					e	0	45	standing	82	27
					e	0	90	standing	110	34

Table 10.2.—*continued*

Source Reference	Gender	Age Mean	Age SD	Age Range	n	Movement	Concentric (°/sec)	Eccentric (°/sec)	ROM	Testing Position	Peak Torque Nm	Peak Torque SD	Testing Device
						abd	0		10	standing	69	20	
						abd	0		0	standing	55	20	
						abd	0		10	standing	46	22	
						add	0		0	standing	49	17	
						add	0		10	standing	59	17	
						add	0		20	standing	62	19	
						er	0		10ir	sit, hip 60, kn 90	36	8	
						er	0		0	sit, hip 60, kn 90	31	7	
						ir	0		0	sit, hip 60, kn 90	34	11	
						ir	0		10er	sit, hip 60, kn 90	45	12	
34	m	26	3		30	ir	60			sup, hip 0, kn 0	37	8	Cybex 340
						er	60			sup, hip 0, kn 0	33	7	
						ir	60			sup, hip 0, kn 90	90	17	
						er	60			sup, hip 0, kn 90	72	13	
						ir	60			sit, hip 90, kn 90	140	27	
						er	60			sit, hip 90, kn 90	85	21	
	f	24	3		30	ir	60			sup, hip 0, kn 0	26	6	Cybex 340
						er	60			sup, hip 0, kn 0	21	5	
						ir	60			sup, hip 0, kn 90	58	12	
						er	60			sup, hip 0, kn 90	47	11	
						ir	60			sit, hip 90, kn 90	87	20	
						er	60			sit, hip 90, kn 90	53	12	

Legend: *abd*, abduction; *add*, adduction; *e*, extension; *er*, external rotation; *f*, flexion; *HHD*, hand held dynamometer; *ir*, internal rotation; *kn*, knee; *sup*, supine.

slightly less than 1000 kg-cm. These data further confirm aspects of functional muscle mechanics (Fig. 10.9). Concentric contractions at a constant velocity of approximately 13°/sec produced lower torques than isometric trials. Conversely, eccentric contractions performed under similar conditions and compared at similar points in the range of motion produced higher values than did isometric trials (45). All data are in strong agreement with the force-velocity relationship for shortening and lengthening contractions, except the terminal phase of the eccentric range of motion.

Joint Forces

Forces in the hip joint potentially alter the condition of the joint surfaces or alter the bone because of the stress and strain produced through **loading**. The area of contact in the hip is about 25–30 cm^2. However, much of the load through the hip joint is transmitted superiorly and somewhat medially into the acetabulum. Concentration of the load in these areas explains the pattern of wear commonly seen in degenerative joint disease. Radin (49) remarks that the spongy composition of the head of the femur and the acetabulum provides a degree of elasticity. Such elastic compliance serves to decrease the force per unit area since spreading occurs. That joint congruity is less than maximal in the unloaded condition but increased under loading is further evidence of the structure's ability to adjust for increased joint forces. Thus, flattening of the subchondral bone increases surface area, thereby keeping the loads within tolerable limits.

Indirect techniques can be used in arriving at the hip joint forces. Brand et al. (4) have presented an example of indirect measurement of forces on the femoral head

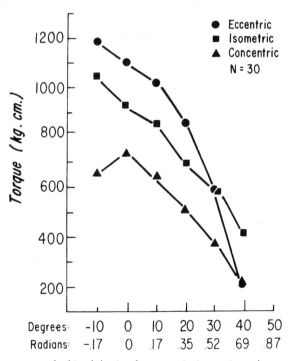

Figure 10.9. Torques curves for hip abduction for eccentric, isometric, and concentric contractions.

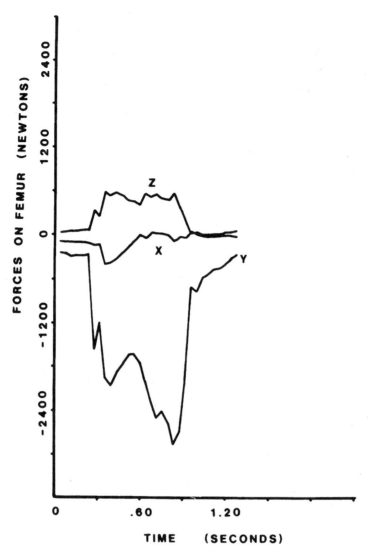

Figure 10.10.   Forces on the femoral head in the three orthogonal directions. The component of greatest magnitude is in the vertical direction (Y).

in three orthogonal directions. Notice in Figure 10.10 that the force on the femoral head exceeds 2400 newtons. Stair climbing caused forces exceeding 3500 newtons, equivalent to approximately six times body weight. Body weight itself contributes only a small portion of this total force; most of this relatively high value is from muscle contraction that creates force across the joint. Rydell (53) has found that straight leg raising from the supine position creates a hip joint force of 1.5 times body weight—further evidence that muscle contraction plays a significant role in creating joint compression. Even tightening of the capsule can lead to increased joint force. Such tightening may occur during less than full extension in the stance phase of the gait cycle if the capsule is shortened due to hip pathology.

As discussed earlier in this chapter, joint forces at the hip are primarily the result of two factors: body weight and muscular contraction. Considering only the effect of body weight, hip joint force in erect posture would be one-half of body weight minus the weight of the legs. However, the typical force across the joint occurring during the single limb support phase of gait ranges from 2.5 to 4 times body weight (26).

Years ago Rydell (53) implanted a prosthesis instrumented with strain gauges, allowing direct measurement of joint forces. Single limb standing produced forces of about 2.5 times body weight. Although stance phase forces were not as large as expected, the swing phase forces were larger than expected. Forces of 4.5–5 times body weight occurred during running. In the late 1980s reports of patient performances with instrumented prostheses became available in the literature. One such study reported, up to 31 days postoperatively, joint contact forces of up to 2.8 times body weight during the stance phase of gait. Stair climbing forces were 2.6 times body weight and the force was always on the anterosuperior portion of the femoral head. Straight leg raising and functional activities such as getting in and out of bed produced forces of less than 1.8 times body weight (12). At the same time, reports were published about the implantation of a similar prosthesis in a 73-year-old healthy woman (19, 23, 33, 57). Early in the recovery process some patient activities were over 80% of the value of 3.4 MPa achieved during parallel bar ambulation. Rising from a chair produced values as high as 18 MPa at 12 months postoperatively, but these decreased to 7.5 MPa by 24 months postoperatively. High **pressures** occurred, particularly in the superior and posterior aspects of the acetabulum (23, 57). The work was then extended up to 5 years postoperatively, during which the effects of some exercises were evaluated. Resisted isometric hip abduction exercise was the most variable over time. The clinical investigative group concluded that hip pressures may be limited by controlling muscle force and movement velocity (19).

Since many therapeutic interventions for hip pathologies ultimately are designed to decrease joint forces, therapists and others treating these patients need to be aware of the mechanics of the surgical and supportive therapy. Complete information about the patient will be helpful in determining the most effective intervention likely to succeed in the shortest period. Some examples of the considerations that should be given are discussed in the next section.

PATHOKINESIOLOGY

Many pathological conditions are manifested in the hip joint. The reasons for these pathologies are the frequency, size, and mechanism for transmission of hip loads (50). The presentation of the pathologies in this section will emphasize principles of mechanics related to the condition and to principles of potentially effective treatment.

Painful Hip

No matter the etiology, pain is a symptom common to most hip pathologies, and is sufficient to affect hip mechanics. In such cases, patients assume postures that diminish the force through the hip joint. During normal standing the magnitudes of the forces are low and are usually tolerable. However, single limb stance during gait significantly increases the joint force due to the abductor muscle force required to keep the pelvis from dropping on the opposite side. To avoid these joint forces the patient has several alternatives available. The section on biomechanics explained that these alternatives are limited, since major changes in body weight are difficult

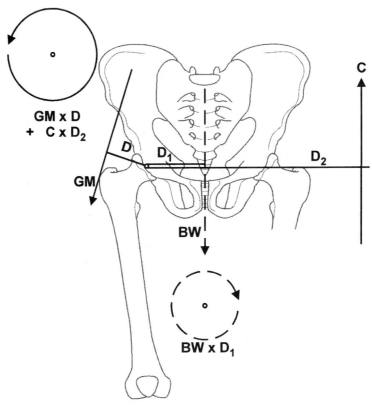

Figure 10.11.   A mechanical representation of the hip similar to Figure 7.6, except, in this instance, the product of the cane force (C) and the distance D_2 is added to the moment for the gluteus medius. To balance the moments, gluteus medius (GM) force can be reduced, which will lower the force at the hip.

to achieve. Therefore, the patient must resort to mechanical means. Often, the method selected is an alteration in the line of gravity associated with body weight. This is accomplished by a lateral lean of the body weight toward the side of the stance limb, effectively diminishing the moment arm of the body weight relative to the center of rotation at the hip. This can be seen in Figure 10.6 by finding the line of force through the body weight closer to the center of rotation of the hip about which moments are being considered. This clinical picture is described as an **abductor** or **gluteus medius lurch.** Similar mechanics occur with weakness in the abductor mechanism, because balance of the trunk over the hip is less difficult to accomplish with a decreased moment arm.

Another alternative is to instruct the patient in the use of an assistive device. Two crutches, for example, allow the patient to bear minimal weight on the involved limb, thereby decreasing the resultant joint force. A cane, held in the opposite hand, also significantly reduces the force necessary in the abductor musculature and diminishes the resultant hip joint force. This reduction is possible due to a large moment arm through which the force on the cane is applied (Fig. 10.11), requiring only a moderate force on the cane. Using the cane on the ipsilateral side of the pathology is not as effective in decreasing joint force and generally is not recommended due to mechanical reasons. In addition, use of the cane in the same hand as the diseased hip narrows the patient's base of support and alters the gait pattern by not allowing for contralateral arm swing.

Congenital Dislocation

Analogous circumstances arise in congenital dislocation of the hip. In this situation the hip does not form a fixed fulcrum or center of rotation about which moments may be generated. In addition, because of the lack of a specific location for joint forces, the acetabulum develops incompletely and the femoral head loses its spherical shape. A further complication is that the head of the femur is superior and posterior to the usual location within the acetabulum, markedly affecting the length of the abductor musculature and diminishing its tension-generating abilities. Diminished tension on the greater trochanter results in lower vertical compressive forces that in turn lead to the tendency for a diminished angle of inclination (valgus deformity) of the femoral neck. Treatment is virtually always directed toward correcting the altered mechanics (Fig. 10.12).

Closed reduction is frequently elected because treatment goals can be accomplished by nonsurgical means such as casting or splinting. These procedures can place the hip in abduction so that adductor and abductor forces are redirected into the acetabulum, increasing their compressive and shear components. Thus, the acetabulum and head of the femur are stimulated to mold to each other, decreasing the tendency toward subluxation. In cases of inadequate bony development, surgical

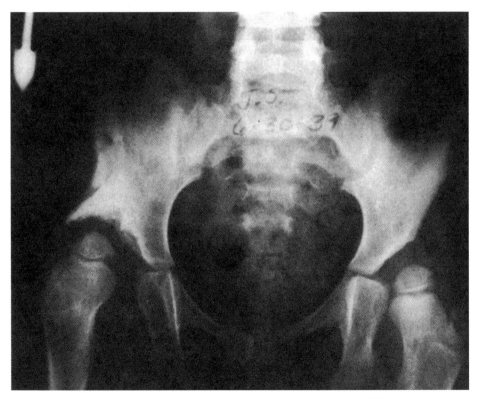

Figure 10.12. Bilateral congenital dislocation of the hips. In the right hip stability is provided by a surgically constructed bony shelf.

creation of a bony shelf may be necessary to provide a stable hip. In other situations varus or valgus osteotomies may be necessary (51). Hip dysplasia models are being developed and elaborated so that the best position for the hip can be achieved to maximize the effect of treatment (55). These procedures will be discussed more thoroughly under the category of degenerative joint disease.

The origin of congenital hip dislocation may be traced to faulty hip development in utero. Studies of neonates permit extrapolation to the developing fetus, demonstrating that hip positions at the extremes of the range of motion create more articular cartilage deformation than do more moderate positions. Frequency and mechanism of loading have been the focus of considerable attention in both the painful and dislocated hip (21). Special note should be made, however, that the time factor of loading is also important. Often one can readily observe the patient avoiding sudden (impulsive) loading in favor of a long interval to avoid pain in the joint.

Muscular Losses

Muscular control of the hip is provided by many massive muscles that can effect large torques. Examples of these torques were cited earlier in this chapter. Much less is known about hip torques under pathological situations. Often, clinicians can only estimate the torque production of their patients from knowledge of normal function. Only recently has work been done that adds to the kinesiologist's and clinician's understanding of hip function. The data reported by Markhede and Stener (35) are valuable, because the 46 patients studied had undergone excision of various hip and thigh musculature because of tumor development. In their series the hip was tested both isometrically and isokinetically so that derived torques could be compared with the opposite limb. The loss of the gluteus maximus created only a slight decrease in extension torque, but the loss of all hamstrings produced significant reductions. For flexion, iliopsoas loss in two patients was apparently responsible for weakness only at the extreme of flexion. Rectus femoris loss in six subjects accounted for a 37% loss in flexion torque and a 17% loss in isokinetic torque. Interesting findings also were produced by the series of eight patients who lost most of the abductor musculature. Even with those suffering extensive loss, the available torque ranged from just under 50% to 80% of the opposite limb. Functional losses were also evaluated, and although some changes such as a positive Trendelenburg sign were noted, the general pattern showed little impairment. Thus, remaining musculature must undergo hypertrophy to offset the losses created by the surgical procedures. The torques required might result from forces generated in other muscles that are less mechanically advantaged to perform the functional activity.

Muscular power also plays a substantial role in treatment of the pathological hip. The **Mustard procedure,** using the iliopsoas, and the **Thomas method,** using the external oblique, are examples of tendon transfer techniques that often provide positive results in stabilizing the hips of young patients. In these procedures, the respective muscles are removed from their attachment and relocated onto the greater trochanter of the femur, usually by passing the muscle through an opening created in the wing of the ilium. Cabaud et al. (5), in a retrospective study, provide evidence that these transfer procedures were effective for 23 of 38 patients in improving stability and pain. Success was thought to be primarily due to the redirection of forces. Specifically, an iliopsoas transfer converts a flexion and adduction force to an abduction force. That 37 brace-dependent patients could function without braces establishes the value of primary muscular support of the hip.

Degenerative Joint Disease

A complication to the normal function of the hip joint is degenerative joint disease, or osteoarthritis. As the most common disease of axial and peripheral joints, the condition is characterized by deterioration and diminution of articular cartilage (48). The problem is found most frequently in the hip, knee, and hand but other joints are often involved. Much work has been done on the pathogenesis of the disease; the primary effects are manifest at the articular cartilage. Earlier in this chapter, the mechanisms available for articular cartilage to absorb loads were presented. Since deformation of the cartilage is possible because of the viscoelastic properties of the tissue and its contents, loss of the cartilage severely impedes normal joint kinematics and kinetics. Radin (47), in discussing joint degeneration, states that cracking and tearing begin in the surface layer due to tensile stress. Stresses continue to be propagated into the remaining tissues although they are specifically designed to dissipate load to adjacent structures. Following these degenerative changes the joint's smooth articular surface is lost, sometimes lost completely. Because the joint no longer possesses low friction surfaces, movement frequently becomes painful.

A practical method of dealing with degenerative joint disease is to diminish the loading through the hip. Some mechanisms have been presented earlier, but others, such as the tenotomy, are also used. This muscle lengthening technique is often applied to several muscles crossing the joint. By performing this procedure, the muscles heal with noncontractile elements that cannot contribute to the tension-generating capacity of the surgically incised muscle. Because the muscles are now weaker, the joint resultant force will be decreased, allowing time for healing in the joint to occur.

Another mechanical alternative in management of the degenerated hip joint is a femoral osteotomy. Two choices exist: the varus or the valgus procedure. A varus osteotomy may indeed increase the area of the load-bearing surface of the joint (Fig. 10.13) and the moment arm for the abductor muscles. For reasons previously discussed, these increases are highly desirable by-products of the technique. Also note that this method will cause the operated leg to be shorter than the contralateral limb. A short leg causes the pelvis to drop on the involved side, and results in greater contact area of the articular surfaces (51). Although a valgus osteotomy may also increase the total joint contact area, its decrease of the abductor moment arm may require a tenotomy to offset this disadvantage (Fig. 10.14) (51).

Total Joint Replacement

Degenerative and rheumatoid arthritis of the hip have led to the development and refinement of procedures for **joint surface and total joint replacement.** Extensive analyses of both anatomical and mechanical factors provide data that improve clinical outcomes. Total joint replacement is, in fact, an excellent example of mechanics applied to the biological specimen. The procedure cannot totally compromise anatomy. Freeman (18) pointed out the importance of adequate blood supply to the head of the femur. Elaborations earlier in this chapter explained the need for caution against indiscriminate sectioning of muscles or translocation of bony prominences to which muscles attach. Some surgeons use techniques that remove and reattach the greater trochanter of the femur. The reattachment site is usually more distal and lateral than the original, therefore providing a larger abductor moment arm (Fig. 10.15). Some data exist, however, that caution against a direct lateral approach for

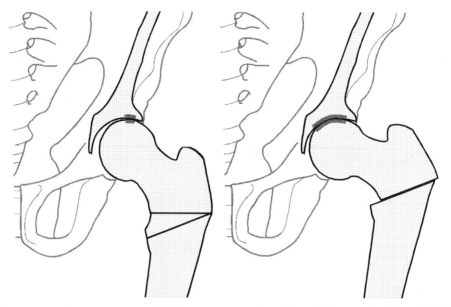

Figure 10.13.   A varus osteotomy of the hip removes a wedge of bone (*left*). Note the change in load-bearing surface and the moment arm for the abductor muscles.

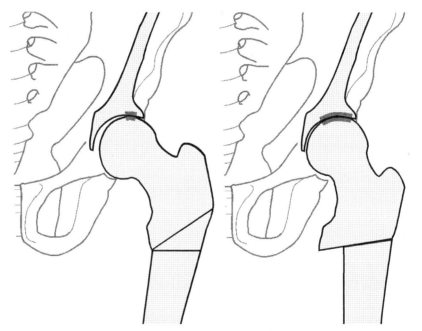

Figure 10.14.   A valgus osteotomy removes a wedge-shaped piece of bone (*left*). The wedge shape differs from Figure 10.13. Note that the moment arm of the abductor muscles has been shortened.

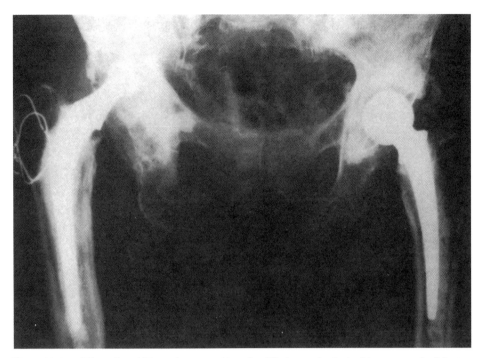

Figure 10.15.   Bilateral total hip replacement. Note the differing angles in the hips as a result of the two procedures. A wire used to reattach the greater trochanter resembles thread around the right hip.

a total hip replacement based on denervation and subsequent muscle weaknesses that result from potential section of the inferior branch of the superior gluteal nerve (2).

Another important matter is **prosthesis design.** Certain alloys of lesser strength may have the advantage of being lighter in weight when compared with other materials. In view of the incidence of fracture in the components used in total hip arthroplasty, strength of the materials used is important to the patient. For example, the femoral neck may have a small range of tolerance for a bending moment. Usually, the success or failure of total joint replacement depends on the stresses imposed by loading. Stresses exist not only in the prosthetic components themselves but also at the interfaces between the components' cement and bone. Stress caused by bending of the femoral component could be alleviated by increasing the valgus in the femoral component or by decreasing the length of the neck of the prosthesis. Strength could also be increased by increasing the cross section of the prosthetic component, but the weight also will be commensurately increased (51). Debate continues as to the mechanisms responsible for prosthesis loosening. Experimental work is continuing in an attempt to determine the nature and magnitude of the forces responsible (9).

Shear forces probably are responsible for the stress occurring at the interfaces. One mechanism used to offset this problem is to decrease the size of the femoral head, which serves to reduce shear forces in the joint commensurately. Clarke (11) speculates on other reasons, including socket impingement by the femoral neck at extremes of motion and contact forces generated by joint forces.

Stauffer (56), in a 10-year follow-up study of total hip replacements, states that

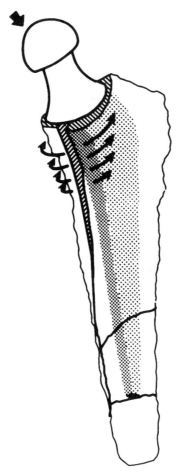

Figure 10.16.   Loosening at the cement-prosthesis interface.

the most common type of **loosening** resulted from prosthesis-cement interface failure due to splitting of the cement mantle (Fig. 10.16). Circumferential stresses are generated due to the axial loading of the tapered and wedge-shaped component inserted into the femur. The incidence of loosening at 10 years was 11.3% for the acetabular component and 29.9% for the femoral component. Johnston and Crowninshield (27) reported another 10-year follow-up of total hip arthroplasty patients, stating that component loosening is the major long-term problem. Their assessment of bone resorption and radiolucency as related to prosthesis loosening showed that 9% of the patients had femoral component loosening at 10 years post replacement, but they observed no correlation between femoral loosening and calcar resorption. Although the incidence of acetabular loosening was only 10.9%, the data indicated that the association of calcar resorption and acetabular loosening was important. Each of these studies points out that both the loading of the hip and the components used in the replacement procedures are significant. The actual mechanisms causing the changes and the resulting loosening are not yet precisely clear. Radin has indicated that components not adequately supported or fixed on the femur also may loosen (48). As further understanding of the conditions that produce component loosening is made possible through clinical, experimental, and theoretical testing, higher success rates will be achieved.

Alternative forms of reconstruction are being offered as means of overcoming the biomechanical faults of the earlier techniques (8). **Cementless total hip arthroplasty** involves different designs and fixation by threads, pegs, screws, self-locking mechanisms or a pore coated prosthesis-bone interface. These models essentially use the principle of increased surface area for facilitating fixation by bony ingrowth. Also, the trend is to use less rigid, elastic implants that overcome stress propagation of more rigid implants. Others prefer to use cementless arthroplasty for the patient age 40 or under who requires an arthroplasty: newer materials undergo less wear, and the absence of cement allows bony ingrowth directly into the prosthesis, resulting in less loosening (37). Principles associated with the treatment of the joint all remain similar, focusing on reducing the likelihood of component loosening. However, a cementless prosthesis requires a much longer non-weight-bearing period, to allow component fixation to occur. The physical therapist is thus challenged to gain or maintain motion without disturbing alignment and while avoiding extreme losses of muscle strength due to disuse.

A comment about **wear:** many laboratory and clinical retrieval studies show the importance of wear in the performance of total joint arthroplasties. Principles of friction must also be applied because the mechanical systems implanted cannot match the low friction of natural human joints. Wear, craters, and the role of debris all have been associated with changes in articular surfaces, and lead to potentially undesirable results. In addressing some aspects associated with polyethylene wear, Rose and Radin remark that relatively high wear may occur even without acrylic debris (52). Materials are being refined with an aim to reduce friction and resulting wear significantly.

For the present, knowledge of the role of these factors in disrupting normal joint kinematics is essential for effective clinical results. Furthermore, little is known about how these factors influence the therapist's treatment. One can only speculate that the extremes of the range of motion, particularly those with forceful movements, should be avoided. The same may be said for impact loading. That is, the extremity that contains the prostheses should not have high loads placed on it in short periods.

Little data exist about whether range of motion is best gained with active exercise or passive stretch. We do know, however, that no significant improvement was made in hip flexion and abduction one year after total replacement. Adduction and both rotation motions were improved at the last follow-up visit, which was an average of 7.5 years later (62). We also do not know whether the patient's ability to generate torque will be best accomplished with isometric or dynamic exercise. Selection of surgical procedure has been clearly shown to affect the moment generating capability (58); however, others have shown no difference in abductor torque generating capability no matter whether **trochanteric osteotomy** was part of the total hip replacement procedure (3). Another work shows that treated patients significantly improve abductor torques between the postoperative measurement intervals of 1, 6, 12, and 24 weeks (59). Only after more data are generated and communicated will the therapist have a sufficient pool of knowledge on which to judge the clinical procedures necessary for the most effective patient care.

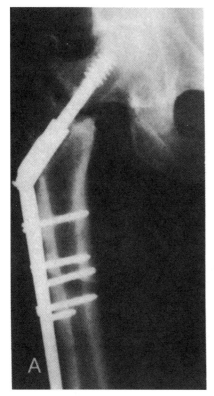
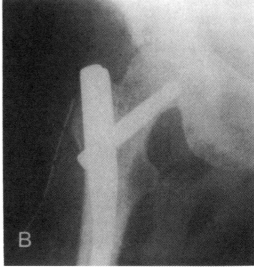

Figure 10.17. Compression screw-plate for fractured femur (**A**) and a Zickel nail in a patient with metastasis in the femur secondary to breast cancer (**B**). The nailing was performed to prevent fracture and prolong function.

Fractures and Repairs

Biomechanics and material properties also play a role in the treatment of fractures. Extensive analyses of materials, insertion site, failure, and other biomechanical features have been aggressively evaluated by surgeons and manufacturers. In failures of adequate treatment of the intertrochanteric fracture, the clinician is often reminded of the large force that must be transmitted across the fracture site. Many of these fractures have been treated by closed techniques that require prolonged inactivity before healing allows weight bearing through the fracture site. Thus, treatment by **internal fixation** (open reduction) is often the treatment of choice, because improved mobility avoids unsatisfactory results. The fixation device and method must be able to tolerate loading by body weight and that created by frequent and high muscle forces. In discussing the treatment of hip fractures, Kaufer (29) states that of five possible variables, only bone quality and fragment geometry cannot be modified. The other factors—reduction, the implant, and implant placement—are all controllable. The ideal is always to achieve a stable reduction. Usually this requires sufficient medial and posterior cortical contact between the proximal and distal segments to oppose the tendency toward varus and posterior displacement that occurs in intertrochanteric fractures.

Figure 10.17 presents two devices used as **implants:** the compression plate and intramedullary devices. Note that both are inserted into the trabecular bone of the proximal segment. The distal fragment is reattached to the external femoral cortex by the angulated nail plate, and the intramedullary device contacts the internal cortical surface. These devices offer either a fixed or adjustable angle of inclination between 130 and 150°. Provision of an option that would allow greater varus in the hip would only invite complications caused by large bending moments during lower limb loading. So, the choice of a device that gives the fracture patient a stable hip is determined by the consideration given to material properties and their ability to tolerate loading. Upon thorough evaluation of all aspects of mechanics, treatment will more likely yield a positive result.

The evaluation of surgical repairs will continue and will be simplified by the extensive use of modeling. Valid results will likely be produced by these procedures. Subsequent treatments will then in turn need clinical evaluation. One example is the work on the Chiari pelvic osteotomy. Here the surgical parameters evaluated

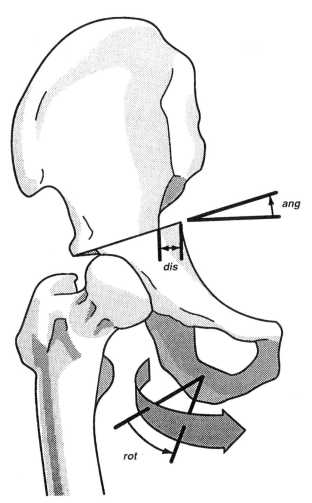

Figure 10.18. Surgical parameters used in the evaluation of the Chiari osteotomy procedure. Labels indicate angulation of the osteotomy (*ang*), distance of medial displacement (*dis*), and the internal rotation angle (*rot*).

were the angulation of the osteotomy, the distance of the medial displacement, and the internal rotation angle (Fig. 10.18). Having a set of abductor torque data, the variables could be entered into a biomechanical model to simulate various surgical procedures. Results showed that a high angulation and a large medial displacement reduced gluteus medius abductor torque up to 65%. This combination of parameters may account for some instances of the postoperative limp seen in some of these patients (13). If enough patients undergo these procedures, then therapists can be actively engaged in determining the functional outcome.

SUMMARY

The hip joint, by virtue of its location in the body, has the unenviable task of providing both large ranges of motion and large torques in attempting to meet the requirements imposed by human motion. Loads that must be tolerated by the joint create special degenerative pathologies that provide applications of biomechanics. As further information becomes available on load-bearing joints and their clinical management, the application of biomechanical principles will become even more important in assuring that patients are left with minimal dysfunction.

References

1. Backman S. The proximal end of the femur. *Acta Radiol Suppl.* 1957;146:1–166.
2. Baker AS, Bitounis VC. Abductor function after total hip replacement. *J Bone Joint Surg.* 1989;71B:47–50.
3. Borja F, Latta LL, Stinchfield FE, et al. Abductor muscle performance in total hip arthroplasty with and without trochanteric osteotomy. *Clin Orthop.* 1985;197:181–190.
4. Brand RA, Crowninshield RD, Johnston RC, et al. Forces on the femoral head during activities of daily living. *Iowa Orthop J.* 1982;2:43–49.
5. Cabaud HE, Westin GW, Connelly S. Tendon transfers in the paralytic hip. *J Bone Joint Surg.* 1979;61(A):1035–1041.
6. Cahalan TD, Johnson ME, Liu S, et al. Quantitative measurement of hip strength in different age groups. *Clin Orthop.* 1989;246:136–145.
7. Cahalan TD, Liu SH, Chao EY. Isokinetic and isometric strength analysis of hip musculature. Presented at the 33rd Annual Meeting of the Orthopedic Research Society; February, 1987; San Francisco.
8. Capello WN. Surface replacement. *Iowa Orthop J.* 1983;3:50–54.
9. Cheal EJ, Spector M, Hayes WC. Role of loads and prosthesis material properties on the mechanics of the proximal femur after total hip arthroplasty. *J Orthop Res.* 1992;10:405–422.
10. Clark JM, Haynor DR. Anatomy of the abductor muscles of the hip as studied by computed tomography. *J Bone Joint Surg.* 1987;69(A):1021–1031.
11. Clarke IC. Biomechanics. *Orthop Clin North Am.* 1982;13:681–707.
12. Davy DT, Kotzar GM, Brown RH, et al. Telemetric force measurements across the hip after total arthroplasty. *J Bone Joint Surg.* 1988;70(A):45–50.
13. Delp WL, Bleck EE, Zajac FE, et al. Biomechanical analysis of the chiari pelvic osteotomy—preserving hip abductor strength. *Clin Orthop.* 1990;254:189–198.
14. Dostal WF. *The Prediction of Coordinates of Bony Landmark and Hip Muscle Attachment Points.* Iowa City, IA: Graduate College, University of Iowa; 1979. Ph.D. thesis.
15. Dostal WF, Andrews JG. A three dimensional biomechanical model of hip musculature. *J Biomech.* 1981;14:803–812.
16. Favill J. *Outline of the Spinal Nerves.* Springfield, IL: Charles C Thomas; 1946.
17. Fischer FJ, Houtz SJ. Evaluation and function of the gluteus maximus muscle. *Am J Phys Med.* 1968;47:182–191.
18. Freeman MAR. Some anatomical and mechanical considerations relevant to the surface replacement of the femoral head. *Clin Orthop.* 1978;134:19–24.
19. Givens-Heiss, Krebs DA, O'Riley PO, et al. In vivo acetabular contact pressures during rehabilitation, Part II: postacute phase. *Phys Ther.* 1992;72:700–705.
20. Haley ET. Range of hip rotation and torque of hip rotator muscle groups. *Am J Phys Med.* 1953;32:261–270.

21. Hjelmstedt A, Asplund S. Congenital dislocation of the hip: a biomechanical study in autopsy specimens. *J Ped Orthop*. 1983;3:491–497.

22. Hoaglund FT, Low WD. Anatomy of the femoral neck and head, with comparative data from caucasians and Hong Kong Chinese. *Clin Orthop*. 1980;152:10–16.

23. Hodge WA, Carlson SM, Fijan RS, et al. Contact pressures from an instrumented hip endoprosthesis. *J Bone Joint Surg*. 1989;71(A):1378–1386.

24. Inman VT. Functional aspects of the abductor muscles of the hip. *J Bone Joint Surg*. 1947;29(A):607–619.

25. Jarvis DK. Relative strength of the hip rotator muscle groups. *J Am Phys Ther Assoc*. 1952;32:500–503.

26. Johnston RC. Mechanical considerations of the hip joint. *Arch Surg*. 1973;107:411–417.

27. Johnston RC, Crowninshield RD. Roentgenologic results of total hip arthroplasty. *Clin Orthop*. 1983;181:92–98.

28. Kapandji IA. *The Physiology of the Joints: Volume Two—Lower Limb*. Edinburgh: Churchill Livingstone; 1970.

29. Kaufer H. Mechanics of the treatment of hip injuries. *Clin Orthop*. 1980;146:53–61.

30. Kessler R, Hertling D. *Management of Common Musculoskeletal Disorders*. Philadelphia: Harper & Row; 1983.

31. Kramer JF, Vaz MD, Vandervoot AA. Reliability of isometric hip abductor torques during examiner and belt-resisted tests. *J Gerontol*. 1991;46:M47–51.

32. Lehmkuhl LD, Smith L. *Brunnstrom's Clinical Kinesiology*. Philadelphia: FA Davis; 1983.

33. Levin R. Pressures measured in live hip joint. *Science*. 1986;232:1192–1193.

34. Lindsay DM, Maitland ME, Lowe RC, et al. Comparison of isokinetic internal and external hip rotation torques using different testing positions. *J Orthop Sports Phys Ther*. 1992;16:43–50.

35. Markhede G, Stener B. Function after removal of various hip and thigh muscles for extirpation of tumors. *Acta Orthop Scand*. 1981;52:373–395.

36. Merchant AC. Hip abductor muscle force. *J Bone Joint Surg*. 1965;47(A):462–476.

37. Morscher EW. Cementless total hip arthroplasty. *Clin Orthop*. 1983;181:76–91.

38. Murray MP, Sepic SB. Maximum isometric torque of hip abductor and adductor muscles. *Phys Ther*. 1968;48:1327–1335.

39. Nemeth G, Ekholm J, Arborelius UP, et al. Influence of knee flexion on isometric hip extensor strength. *Scand J Rehabil Med*. 1983;15:97–101.

40. Nemeth G, Ohlsen H. Moment arms of hip abductor and adductor muscles measured in vivo by computed tomography. *Clin Biomech*. 1989;4:133–136.

41. Neumann DA, Cook TM. Effect of load and carrying position on the electromyographic activity of the gluteus medius muscle during walking. *Phys Ther*. 1985;65:305–311.

42. Neumann DA, Cook TM, Sholty RL, et al. An electromyographic analysis of hip abductor muscle activity when subjects are carrying loads in one or both hands. *Phys Ther*. 1992;72:207–217.

43. Neumann DC, Sobush DC, Paschke S, et al. An electromyographic analysis of the hip abductor muscles during a standing work task. *Arthritis Care Res*. 1990;3:116–126.

44. Neumann DA, Soderberg GL, Cook TM. Comparison of maximal isometric hip abductor muscle torques between hip sides. *Phys Ther*. 1988;68:496–502.

45. Olson VL, Smidt GL, Johnston RC. The maximum torque generated by the eccentric, isometric, and concentric contractions of the hip abductor muscles. *Phys Ther*. 1972;52:149–157.

46. Pare EB, Stern JT, Schwartz JM. Functional differentiation within the tensor fasciae latae. *J Bone Joint Surg*. 1981;63A:1457–1471.

47. Pauwels F. *Biomechanics of the Normal and Diseased Hip*. Berlin: Springer-Verlag; 1976.

48. Radin EL. Biomechanics of the human hip. *Clin Orthop*. 1980;152:28–34.

49. Radin EL, Paul IL. The biomechanics of congenital dislocated hips and their treatment. *Clin Orthop*. 1974;98:32–38.

50. Radin EL, Simon SR, Rose RM, et al. *Practical Biomechanics for the Orthopedic Surgeon*. New York: John Wiley & Sons; 1979.

51. Rodnan GP, Schumacher HR, eds. *Primer on the Rheumatic Diseases*. Atlanta, GA: Arthritis Foundation; 1983.

52. Rose RM, Radin EL. Wear of polyethylene in the total hip prosthesis. *Clin Orthop*. 1982;170:107–115.

53. Rydell N. Biomechanics of the hip joint. *Clin Orthop*. 1973;92:6–15.

54. Soderberg GL, Dostal WF. Electromyographic study of three parts of the gluteus medius muscle during functional activities. *Phys Ther*. 1978;58:691–696.

55. Spoor CW, vanLeeuwen JL, deWindt FHJ, et al. A model study of muscle forces and joint-force direction in normal and dysplastic neonatal hips. *J Biomech*. 1989;22:873–884.

56. Stauffer RN. Ten-year follow-up study of total hip replacement. *J Bone Joint Surg.* 1982;64(A): 983–990.
57. Strickland EM, Fares M, Krebs DE, et al. In vivo acetabular contact pressure during rehabilitation, part I: acute phase. *Phys Ther.* 1992;72:691–699.
58. Vasavada AN, Delp SL, Mahoney WJ, et al. Compensating for changes in muscle length in total hip arthroplasty—effects on the moment generating capacity of the muscles. *Clin Orthop.* 1994;302: 121–133.
59. Vaz MD, Kramer JF, Rorabeck CH, et al. Isometric hip abductor strength following total hip replacement and its relationship to functional assessments. *J Orthop Sports Phys Ther.* 1993;18:526–531.
60. Vrahas MS, Brand RA, Brown TD, et al. Contribution of passive tissues to the intersegmental moments at the hip. *J Biomech.* 1990;23:357–362.
61. Williams PL, Warwick R, eds. *Gray's Anatomy.* 37th British ed. Philadelphia: WB Saunders; 1989.
62. Woolson ST, Maloney WJ, Schurman DJ. Time-related improvement in the range of motion of the hip after total replacement. *J Bone Joint Surg.* 1985;67(A):1251–1254.

11

Knee

The knee has been subjected to more clinical and investigative attention than any other joint for at least three good reasons. This joint, by virtue of its bony and soft tissue structure, epitomizes arthrokinematics that demand motion beyond the typical one degree of freedom. It also makes for an interesting study of load transmission given its cartilaginous pads between joint surfaces. Finally, the knee's location between the body's longest bony segments predisposes the joint to traumatic injury and other pathologies that bear further study. This chapter will discuss these and other aspects of the kinesiology and pathokinesiology of the knee.

MUSCULAR ACTIONS

The quadriceps muscle group has been well studied because of its importance in controlling the joint. Little information is available on the flexor musculature because it plays a comparatively less significant role in knee control. Considered as a whole, the extensors are composed of a cross-sectional area of approximately 148 cm², approximately three times that of the hamstring musculature (81). The flexor group is supported functionally by the sartorius, gracilis, popliteus, and gastrocnemius muscles. Each of these has at least one additional function and therefore cannot be considered as a primary knee flexor.

The musculature responsible for controlling knee motion is important to understand because most of the key components also serve at either the hip or the ankle. For example, of all the flexor musculature, only the popliteus can claim a single joint action (101); on the extensor side, the rectus femoris can play an important role in hip motion. Thus, in any considerations of knee motion the therapist must be aware of both the proximal and distal joint positions to test or interpret patient performance accurately. Considering all possible combinations patients may use in generating joint torques will assist the therapist's understanding of the interactions that produce effective function in the lower limb.

The most frequently used functional combinations are knee extension–hip extension and hip flexion–knee flexion. The extension "synergy" is commonly found in activities such as rising from a chair or in ascending stairs. Gait is also a useful example: if appropriate moments were not simultaneously generated during stance phase at the hip and knee, flexor moments would result in the tendency for the upper body to rotate around the most distally fixed segment. Control of the extended position of these joints is by the hamstrings at the hip and the quadriceps at the knee, respectively. However, these muscles also have antagonistic actions, i.e., knee flexion for the hamstrings and hip flexion for the rectus femoris. So, if both muscle groups generate tension, it prevents motion and results in isometric contractions. This situation demonstrates an important lesson in mechanics. The explanation for our ability to complete the simultaneous knee and hip extension movement appears to rest in the findings of Elftman (35), who in 1939 published the lengths of moment arms for the muscle groups in a representative individual. He stated that the 4.4 cm rectus femoris moment arm at the knee exceeds the moment arm of 3.9 cm at the hip. Conversely, the 6.7 cm moment arm of the hamstrings at the hip exceeded the moment arm of 3.4 cm at the knee. Because the moment arms favor knee extension for the rectus femoris and hip extension for the hamstrings, simultaneous motions can occur. This has another beneficial effect. As the knee is extended, the hamstring musculature is lengthened at the knee. Thus, because the muscle is lengthened at the knee while tension is needed at the hip, the motions maintain the muscle at an appropriate length for tension generation. The lengthening of the rectus femoris at the hip functions similarly. More information about knee function and the production of moments from changes in moment arms is available in the literature (65, 147).

One further extension of the multiple joint phenomenon is the effect on the gastrocnemius muscle. We have already seen that hip extension essentially facilitates knee extension. It should also be clear that knee extension lengthens the gastrocnemius muscle, which is then able to exert effective tension for plantar flexion of the ankle. The result is an interdependency among the joints responsible for propulsion and maintenance of the upright posture. These relationships also hold true during eccentric phases of muscle activity: for an easy demonstration, palpate the muscles during the transition from sitting to standing.

The combination of hip flexion and knee flexion occurs in ascending stairs, albeit with passive knee flexion. Active control of both motions is, however, most frequently achieved by eccentric contractions of the hip and knee extensors. Here, the rectus femoris is simultaneously shortening at the hip and elongating at the knee.

The quadriceps can complete knee extension–hip flexion. This straight-leg-raising maneuver is limited, however, for two reasons. First, the musculature comprising the quadriceps is shortening at both the hip and the knee, thereby limiting the muscle's tension-generating ability. This limitation has been called **active insufficiency** (91). Second, the antagonistic hamstrings are being stretched to the point of limiting the range of motion. Thus, **passive insufficiency** can also be demonstrated. The hamstrings also work in reciprocity during knee flexion–hip extension. In fact, active insufficiency can be easily shown: when standing on one leg, a person cannot touch the heel to the buttock by actively contracting the knee flexors of the free leg.

Of the many analyses of quadriceps component function, most have used electromyographic techniques. Brunnstrom (91), however, used descriptive anatomy and palpation to conclude that the rectus femoris is activated after the early part of the knee extension range of motion and particularly when overcoming considerable resistance. Other more extensive and objective studies have since been completed, particularily on the influence of hip position on the rectus femoris. An early study evaluated the EMG activity of the rectus femoris during knee extension in the supine and sitting positions. Rectus femoris and vasti activity occurred simultaneously during supine knee extension, but sitting knee extension produced rectus femoris activity only at terminal extension (28). This tendency would likely be confirmed by visual analysis of other supine and sitting data, at least for the trials completed from the supine position. The sitting trials (116) do not corroborate the earlier data (28). However, a 1980 study showed that the rectus femoris contracted only near the limit of knee extension. In analyzing the quadriceps during other activities these investigators also found high levels of activity in the rectus femoris during the initial range of the straight leg raise and throughout hip flexion with the knee flexed

(43). Thus, making specific conclusions about the functions of these quadriceps components during various positions is difficult.

Because the function of the quadriceps is regarded as an important measure of rehabilitation, some work has been done to assess the actions of the quadriceps muscles during therapeutic exercises. The primary purpose of these works has been to learn whether the musculature plays a different role in various portions of the range of motion. Pocock (124) investigated the temporal phase of action of the three superficial quadriceps femoris muscle components during various clinically useful quadriceps exercises. EMG activity was measured during active knee extension under several resistive loading conditions. The most important conclusion was that temporal sequence varied little among the three quadriceps components and that the EMG patterns were similar throughout the range of knee extension. These findings have since been verified by other investigators who have evaluated the potential specificity of activity of the vastus medialis muscle in the terminal portion of knee extension (16, 34, 72, 131).

Other studies have evaluated levels of muscle activity during rehabilitation exercises. The straight leg raise and the isometric quadriceps setting exercise frequently have been compared. One study showed that the greatest quadriceps activity occurred during isometric contraction for 25 subjects; greatest quadriceps activity occurred for only 6 subjects during the straight leg raise (60). Another work concluded that none of the three superficial quadriceps muscles are as active during straight leg raising as during knee extension at the same relative workload (85). In yet another study, Soderberg and Cook (141) reported results that compared the quad setting and straight leg raising exercises during EMG recording from the vastus medialis and the rectus femoris muscles. Forty normal subjects completed maximal effort trials, showing highly significant differences between the activity levels of the two muscles. In the straight leg raise, the mean normalized level of rectus activity was 93% of the maximum while that of the vastus medialis was only 63% of its maximum. Conversely, for the quadriceps setting exercise the rectus activity was only 52% as compared to 103% for the vastus medialis. Because of differences displayed by the quadriceps and in the biceps femoris and gluteus medius muscles the exercise selected should be based on therapeutic purposes. Similar findings have also been reported in a group of patients with knee pathologies (142).

The distal and most oblique portion of the **vastus medialis** has also been of interest to researchers. Because of the position of its fibers, this portion is better located to provide a medial force on the patella rather than assist the quadriceps muscle with knee extension. Some speculation has been offered about the importance of this function in resisting lateral displacements, or even dislocations, of the patella.

To better define the role of the oblique fibers of the vastus medialis, EMG data were derived simultaneously from the three other components of the quadriceps and from the long and oblique portions of the vastus medialis. Results showed that the EMG signal amplitude from the oblique portion was twice that of the other components with no other significant differences among the other components. These authors also found no consistent variation in EMG pattern to suggest that any one muscle studied had a "predominant" responsibility for knee extension in any part of the range of motion (94). Offering an opposite view, Reynolds et al. (127) confirmed no specific role for the oblique in their study of muscle function during terminal knee extension. Comparison of EMG data derived from the medialis oblique and the lateralis showed low and insignificant differences between the activity of the two muscles.

Lieb and Perry (95), in a frequently cited classic study of knee mechanics, undertook an analysis of the role of muscular forces in creating knee extension. Among the parameters assessed were the fascial coverings and fiber alignments of the quadriceps muscles. The vastus medialis was divided into a longus section and an oblique section because of differences in the angle of pull: 15–18° for the longus from the long axis of the femur compared with 50–55° for the oblique segment. To study mechanical effects they inserted cables into the tendons of each of the five muscular components. Results showed that almost twice as much quadriceps force was required to produce full extension than to extend the knee 15° short of the full range of motion. To assess the capability of the vastus medialis oblique in performing the terminal phase of extension, isolated loads were applied to this muscle. Because this isolated loading did not produce extension and other testing demonstrated medial alignment effects, the authors concluded that the only selective function of the vastus medialis is patellar alignment. Although there is early and clinically recognizable atrophy of the vastus medialis, the prominence of the muscle and the thinness of the fascial covering often lead the therapist into a misimpression of specific rather than general quadriceps atrophy.

Other muscles that affect the knee have also been studied. Because the flexors are attached either medially or laterally to the tibia, they tend to rotate the knee. The effectiveness of the hamstrings has also been analyzed by establishing the line of action and the moment arms associated with various knee angles (65). In essence, this study showed that the moment arms can increase more than three times when the joint goes from full extension to 130° of flexion. These results have bearing if the muscles are in fact generating tensions during these ranges of motion. If they do so while contracting, there may be an increased contraction at larger knee angles and at higher velocities (140). Lateral rotators include the biceps femoris and the tensor fascia latae. Kapandji states that the tensor muscle loses the ability to flex and rotate when the knee is extended, in effect becoming only a knee extensor (81). Of all the muscles posterior to the knee that may have a role in rotation, only the short head of the biceps femoris (lateral rotation) and the popliteus (medial rotation) are monarticular muscles.

Specifically, the popliteus is potentially important because of the role it may serve in "unlocking" the knee. Other functions of this muscle have been purported to be posterior displacement of the lateral meniscus and the control of forward motion of the femur on the tibia. EMG studies have shown the popliteus to be most active on medial rotation of the shank segment. Action during flexion was small. Prevention of forward displacement of the femur and posterior motion of the meniscus, although not unequivocally established, were supported by this study (8). The popliteus has also been studied during planned exercises and gait, which confirmed the medial rotation function of the muscle, partly via the phasic activity associated with internal tibial rotation required during the gait cycle. The internally rotated position of the tibia on the femur throughout most of the stance phase was also apparently maintained by the popliteus (100).

Little information is available about the function of the gastrocnemius at the knee. Because of the bilateral composition of the muscular insertion into the femur, little rotary component could be mustered. The ability of the muscle to create knee flexion is well recognized, however, and may be demonstrated in the control of knee hyperextension.

ARTHROLOGY AND ARTHROKINEMATICS

The knee joint is essential for carrying out many normal functional activities. Joint surfaces and structures must successfully tolerate loads about as great as those cited for the hip joint. However, inherent hip stability is not present at the knee joint. Furthermore, the joint is found between the two longest levers in the body, therefore subjecting the joint to or requiring great torques. Because the joint has a large range of motion in only one plane, the bony and soft tissue structures must withstand considerable loads and/or externally applied torques. A thorough understanding of the arthrology and arthrokinematics is required, therefore, to comprehend the affect of structure on normal and abnormal function.

Arthrology

Osteology

The bony makeup of the tibiofemoral joint appears superficially simple. However, the **femoral condyles** should be considered as individual convex surfaces because of marked differences in the shape of both the femoral and tibial condyles. Gross examination of the femur shows that the medial condyle projects extensively, both longitudinally and medially, to offset the lateral-medial angulation of the femur as the shaft progresses distally. The femoral condyles differ in anterior-posterior dimension and configuration, a factor that is important to joint movement. For example, the medial and lateral condyles both decrease their radii from anterior to posterior. That is, the distance from the center of rotation in the condyles is greatest towards the anterior bony surface, progressively decreasing as one moves along the distal edge of the bone to the posterior surface. Other differences exist, however, in that the medial condyle is longer anteroposteriorly while the lateral condyle is flatter (81). The lateral condyle is more prominent anteriorly, probably to control the tendency for lateral displacement of the patella via the pull of the quadriceps muscles.

The medial and lateral compartments of the **tibial plateau** also have demonstrable bony differences. Some texts state that the tibial plateaus are convex in both the mediolateral and the anteroposterior directions, although the latter direction is not uniform (162). Kapandji (81) states that anteroposteriorly the medial tibial condyle is concave superiorly, while the lateral condyle is convex superiorly. Further, because the radii of curvature of these bony segments are not equal, the articular surfaces are not congruent. That the medial tibial surface is longer than the lateral anteroposteriorly, and slightly concave to the lateral side, may have implications for knee kinematics (162). Neither can the intercondylar eminence be ignored because of the mechanical resistance that may be offered to the femoral condyles during rotatory motions of the knee.

The **patella** must also be considered because of the significant role it plays in knee mechanics and pathologies. Imbedded in the patellar tendon, the posterior aspect of the bone is well endowed with articular cartilage. Respective facets articulate with the femoral condyles, while some show special locations during specific points between motion of flexion and extension (12, 162). Figure 11.1 provides one example of the articular surfaces in contact with the femur during the range of motion of the knee.

Finally, osteological considerations at the knee would be incomplete without a brief discussion of the **proximal tibiofibular joint.** Although not a part of the knee joint proper, this joint has distinct soft tissue connections that bear on the arthrokinematics of the knee. Little information is available on the specific impact of the

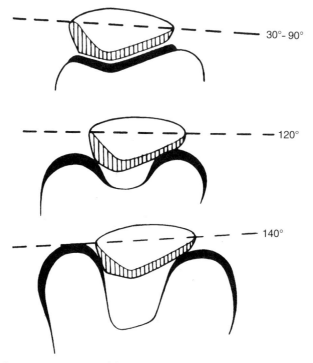

$30°- 90°$

$120°$

$140°$

Figure 11.1. Position of the patella at different angles of knee flexion.

anatomy and kinematics of this joint. One study, however, supplied both radiographic and anatomical data that classified the joint geometry into either horizontal or oblique configurations. The horizontal had greater surface area and rotary mobility than the oblique. Based on the results of this study the author concluded that the primary functions of the proximal tibiofibular joint are to dissipate lateral tibial bending moments and torsional stresses applied at the ankle. The role of the joint in tensile versus compressive loading is probably not clear or of any particular significance (115).

Ligaments

Anatomical locations of soft tissue structures are relevant because of their effect on the joint motion. Ligaments of primary interest are the **tibial and fibular collateral** and the **anterior and posterior cruciate ligaments** (ACL, PCL). The tibial or medial collateral ligament extends from a posterior-superior position on the femur to the medial aspect of the medial tibial plateau. It is generally agreed that the tibial collateral and its posterior oblique fibers blend with the capsule of the joint. The ligament is attached to the medial meniscus (81, 162). The lateral collateral ligament is much smaller than the medial as it traverses the joint from the posterior and superior lateral femoral condyle to the fibular head. In general, the shape of this ligament is much rounder and thinner than the medial collateral ligament (162).

The anterior and posterior cruciate ligaments are believed to at least control anterior and posterior translatory movement of the two bony segments on each other. As implied by its name, the anterior cruciate runs from the anterior middle portion of the tibia in a superior and posterior direction to an attachment on the medial aspect of the lateral femoral condyle. Conversely, the posterior cruciate has attachments between the middle of the posterior tibial plateau and the anterolateral aspect of the medial femoral condyle. The importance of these attachment sites will become clear when the kinematics of the joint are presented.

The **ligamentum patellae,** which forms the central portion of the common tendon of the quadriceps, is approximately 8 cm long from the patella to the tibial tuberosity (162). Considerable tensile strength can be managed by this structure and has been shown to be very high.

Both anterior and posterior portions of the **meniscofemoral ligaments** emanate from the lateral meniscus, ultimately running in close association with the posterior cruciate ligament. Their effects will also be explained later in this chapter.

Capsule

The complicated and very large **capsule** of the knee receives extensive reinforcement, particularly from the collateral and patellar ligaments. The posterolateral aspect is frequently damaged in traumatic injuries. Reinforcement of the capsule is provided by the arcuate or fabellofibular ligaments alone or collectively. In over two-thirds of knees studied, the fabellofibular ligaments were responsible for the reinforcement (133). Few detailed studies of this region have been undertaken. One such study, including 35 dissections, has shown that the lateral structures of the knee can be divided into three layers. The deepest part of the lateral aspect of the capsule divides into two laminae just posterior to the overlying iliotibial tract. These laminae encompass the arcuate, fabellofibular, and lateral collateral ligaments. Also recall that the posterior capsule is specifically reinforced by the deep and posterior oblique portions of the medial collateral ligament (83). Further reinforcement posteriorly is provided by the oblique popliteal ligament, derived from the semimembranosus muscle (162). Further strength is gained via muscular tendons: the patellar and quadriceps tendons anteriorly, the iliotibial band laterally, and the tendons of the pes anserine medially. The most important additional posterior support comes from the tendons of the biceps femoris, the gastrocnemius, and the popliteus muscles. For further descriptions of the intricacies of the knee joint the reader should refer to an anatomy text.

Menisci

When considering the knee joint, the **menisci** must also be included. Both the medial and lateral menisci are semilunar in shape, although the lateral forms a greater part of a circle than does the medial. These wedge-shaped structures have been credited with protecting the capsule while deepening the articulation and providing a buffer for pressure (144). The peripheral tibial and ligamentous attachments, and lack of central attachments, are critical to an understanding of the joint arthrokinematics; that is, the unattached internal edge of a meniscus allows for considerable freedom of movement. On the other hand, because of the attachment of the medial meniscus to the semimembranosus and the medial collateral ligament, mobility of the peripheral portion is limited. This potentially affects the type of internal derangement that may result from traumatic injury of the knee. Generally, the lateral meniscus is considered more mobile than the medial, in spite of the attachment to the popliteus muscle.

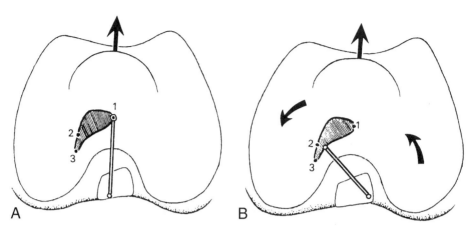

Figure 11.2. View of the distal end of the femur, just prior to maximal extension; the arrow pointing up shows the extension direction of the femoral shaft. **A.** Position of the hypothetical "sagittal" posterior cruciate ligament guiding bundle. **B.** Position of the real posterior cruciate ligament guiding bundle. The curved arrows show the direction of rotation.

Arthrokinematics

Rotation

Movement of the knee, whether active or passive, demands interaction among the structures described earlier in this chapter. Although the largest movement is in the sagittal plane, i.e., flexion-extension, rotational movements are crucial to normal function. During extension of the non-weight-bearing knee, external rotation of the tibia occurs during the last 30° of extension. Circumstances are different for weight bearing, however, because the tibia is now the fixed segment. As a result, the 5–7° of rotation that occur under the latter condition most probably result from combined tibial external rotation and femoral internal rotation. The final result of this motion is the close-packed position of the knee joint, indicative of maximum congruity of the surfaces.

Many explanations have been offered concerning this rotational movement. The unequal curvature of the femoral condyles has been suggested, because different degrees of rotation would be required by the different bony geometry. A similar rationale can be applied to the different anteroposterior femoral condyle dimensions as a reason for the rotation. Soft tissue influences have also been cited. Included in this category are tightening of either or both the anterior and posterior cruciate ligaments. Perhaps the ligaments wind on themselves during the terminal phases of knee extension. Even a tightening of the collateral ligaments has been postulated (161). Perhaps the most likely explanation is that change in position or length of these and other structures combine to produce the close-packed position. This conclusion is supported by the detailed work of Fuss (50), who has thoroughly examined the effect of the ACL, PCL and curvature of the medial femoral condyle in relationship to the rotation of the knee during terminal extension. Specifically, a section of the PCL called the guiding bundle is constantly taut, producing a torque between the two bone segments (Fig. 11.2). Further, the ACL becomes too short during the end phase of extension, a result of the shape of the articular surfaces. Finally, during knee terminal knee extension the medial femoral condyle is deflected by the medial tubercle of the intercondylar eminence, causing the subsequent rotation. Thus, this may be the first work that has identified simultaneous occurrences that all produce the same effect.

Menisci and their motion also are a factor in knee arthrokinematics. Because they are deformable and mobile, reconfiguration of the joint moves the horns of the menisci. Also recall that various muscles send slips to the menisci, producing a direct effect on the motion that occurs. Steindler has stated that in knee extension the menisci are forced forward and stretched, increasing the pressure on these cartilaginous discs (144). Although essentially in agreement, Kapandji (81) specifies that during active knee extension the menisci are pulled forward by the meniscopatellar fibers. Even the posterior horn of the lateral meniscus is pulled anteriorly, during extension, by tension developed in the meniscofemoral ligament as the PCL becomes taut. Active knee flexion also causes posterior menisci movement, the medial via tension in the semimembranosus and the lateral by tension in the popliteus expansion. In rotational movements and during passive knee motion the menisci follow the femoral condyles.

Surface Motions

The femoral, or convex surface, in articulation with the tibial or concave surface, provides an excellent example of joint movements. As discussed in Chapter 4, the surfaces act in a prescribed manner. As the tibia is extended on the femur, rolling and sliding occur in the same direction (Fig. 11.3). Now consider the movement in which the femoral condyles move. Unless the femur slides anteriorly on the tibia during the joint flexion the femur would literally roll off the posterior margin of the

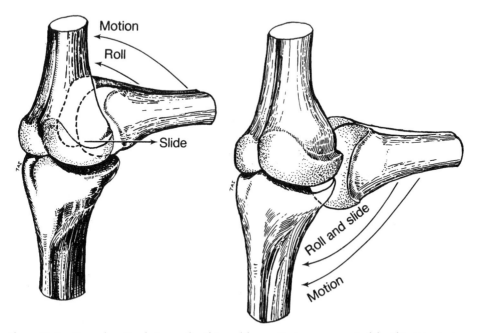

Figure 11.3.   Normal motion between the tibia and femur. During movement of the tibia (concave) on the femur (convex), the rolling and sliding are in the same direction. If the femur moves on the tibia, roll and slide must be in opposite directions for normal movement.

tibia (Fig. 11.4). Accomplishing this sliding motion allows the femur to use the total surface of the femoral condyle. Thus, as the convex moves on the concave, the roll and slide occur in opposite directions. In moving these surfaces on each other congruity has been maintained. Without the existence of such a mechanism, joint integrity would be sacrificed so much that little stability would remain.

The patellofemoral joint cannot be ignored, primarily because of the mechanical effect in both normal and pathological motion. During flexion and extension of the knee the patella moves vertically as much as 8 cm in the intercondylar groove. While flexion is accomplished, the patella and patellar tendon are also displaced posteriorly: when viewed from a lateral projection, the angle of attachment of the tendon to the tibial tuberosity is progressively diminished (Fig. 11.5). Finally, during rotation of the knee the patella is displaced laterally during internal rotation of the tibia and medially during lateral rotation of the tibia (81). Without these motions, considered accessory by some, the normal arthrokinematics cannot be demonstrated in the knee.

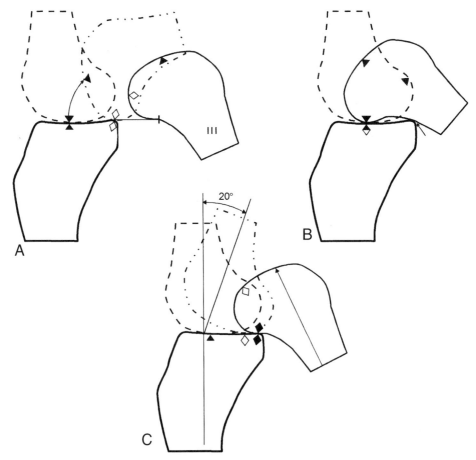

Figure 11.4.   Abnormal motion between the tibia and femur. **A.** The femur would fall off the posterior aspect of the tibia if slide did not occur in the opposite direction. **B.** The effect of too much slide. **C.** The normal condition. The diamonds are contact points for each portion of the range of motion.

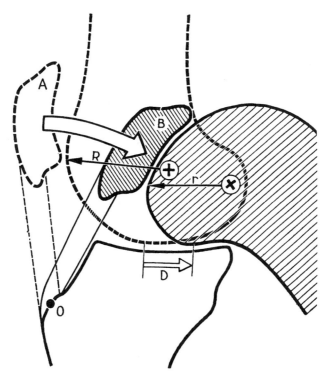

Figure 11.5. Two superimposed lateral views of the knee. The position of the patella in extension (*A*) and in flexion (*B*) is shown. The decreased distance (*R* and *r*) of the patella from the axis of rotation (+) is also shown. The displacement of the contact point between the two bones (*D*) and the attachment of the patellar ligament (*O*) are also shown.

BIOMECHANICS
Kinematics

The kinematics of the knee have been well described by many clinicians and investigators. The sagittal plane range of motion consists of approximately 10° of hyperextension to 145° of flexion. Achievement of the fully extended or close-packed position negates rotation and adduction and abduction (valgus and varus). However, up to 45° each of internal and external rotation are available when the knee is at 60 or more degrees of flexion (88). Electrogoniometry has allowed for quantification of the knee motion necessary to perform activities of daily living: 83° was the mean value recorded for stair climbing, 93° for sitting, and 106° for shoe tying (90). During normal gait, 65–70° of knee flexion is required.

Instant Center of Rotation

Several attempts have been made to identify the location of the instant center of rotation for the **sagittal plane** motion of the knee. The technique and the results have been thoroughly described by Frankel and Burstein (45) and others. These studies have established the semicircular pathway shown in Figure 11.6. The centers fall within a circle with a diameter of 2.3 cm. All points were on axes that penetrated the lateral femoral condyle (139), similar to the work of Hollister and coworkers

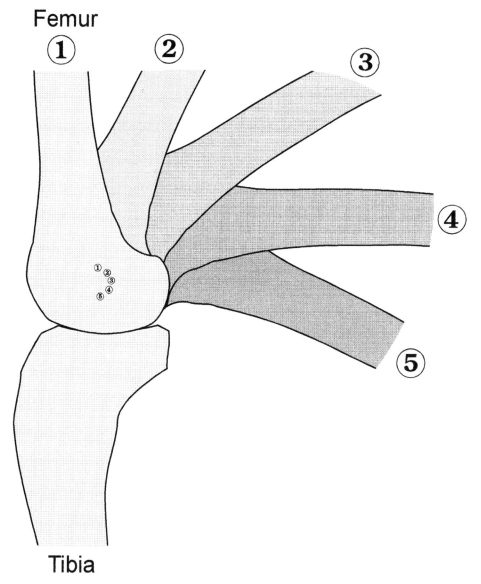

Figure 11.6. The instant center of rotation plotted for the femur and tibia.

who say that the axis is "constant" (67). Little information is available as to the axis for **transverse plane** knee rotation. According to Steindler the **vertical axis** of the knee passes through the medial condyle (144), but according to Hollister it is anterior and not perpendicular to the axis for flexion-extension axis (67). However, with the knee being used as an example, the difficulties associated with instant center analysis have been addressed (143). Whatever the precise location for the instant center, the knee cannot be considered a true hinge joint. Furthermore, and perhaps more important, bony and soft tissues produce changes in the arthrokinematics during a range of motion because the location of the center of rotation moves.

Effects of Motion on Ligaments

Consider the position of the medial collateral ligament in knee extension (Fig. 11.7). Then, study the ligament configuration with the knee in the flexed position and note that several events have occurred. First, the contact point of the femur on the tibia has moved posteriorly. In addition, the menisci have also been required to assume a new position. The mechanisms available for these movements were discussed previously in this chapter. The patellar ligament can be seen to have decreased its angle of insertion in relationship to the tibia. Finally, the joint motion has required changes in the length of the anterior and posterior segments of the long fibers of the medial collateral ligament. These changes, though relatively small, create **elongation** of the anterior portion of the ligament and concurrent slack in the posterior segment. Realize also that length changes concurrently take place in the lateral collateral and cruciate ligaments of the knee. Changes also occur in the capsule, the most important of which is the slack produced in the posterior portion.

Because of the **stress** in the ligaments and the capsule, many workers have evaluated the role of ligaments in restraining motion in the knee. In vitro and in vivo studies have been performed during anteroposterior, valgus, and varus motion, and during induced torques. Results from some of these studies improve our understanding of knee function and have implications for treatment indications and contraindications.

Regarding the cruciate ligaments, Cabaud has provided a summary of the function of the ACL. It has been strongly documented that this ligament resists anterior displacement of the tibia on the femur (51, 165). Other works have documented that

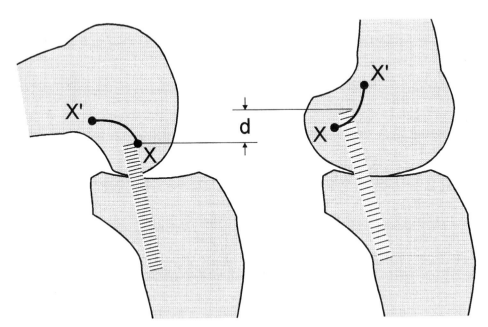

Figure 11.7. Lateral view of the knee in flexion and extension, showing the effects on the medial collateral ligament. Due to the location of the center of rotation the anterior portion of the ligament may become taut during flexion while the posterior is placed on a slack. The length of the ligament is shown as *d*, the centers of curvature of the condyles as *x* and *x'*.

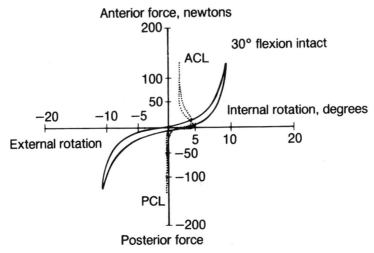

Figure 11.8. Tibial rotation resulting from application of anteroposterior force with the knee at 30° of flexion. The dotted line shows the result after either isolated section of the anterior or posterior cruciate ligament (ACL, PCL).

various portions of the ACL and PCL become taut in certain parts of the range of knee flexion and extension (51, 87). Probably less recognized is the anterior cruciate's primary role in resisting internal rotation (21). This function has been reinforced by findings that, in 7 of 17 cadaver knees, rotation significantly increased with sectioning of this ligament (97). Cabaud further summarizes, while ignoring any twist within the ligament, that the posterior fibers of this ligament are longest in the position of knee extension while the anterior fibers are most tense in flexion (21). The posterior cruciate is given primary credit for resisting posterior displacement of the tibia on the femur (51). Less is known about the rotation function of this ligament although data have shown a marked loss of rotation with insufficiency of the cruciate ligaments; that is, intact ligaments produced concurrent rotation. As a result they concluded that the cruciates also constitute a primary mechanism in the production and control of rotation during anterior and posterior knee motion (49). An example of their results is shown in Figure 11.8.

Because in many patients the cruciate ligaments are deficient, some researchers are also interested in determining which structures provide secondary restraint to motion. This issue has been specifically addressed by performing the anteroposterior drawer sign in human knees. With the loss of the anterior cruciate, the iliotibial tract and band, the middle third of the medial and lateral capsules, and the medial and lateral collateral ligaments all serve to restrain this motion. Secondary restraints for posterior motion were provided by the posterior lateral capsule and popliteus complex combined and also by the medial collateral ligament. The authors noted, however, that if the cruciates are torn, only minimal support exists from these secondary structures (20). Finally, Kapandji (81) describes the mechanical role of the cruciates and makes a case that during flexion the anterior cruciate is responsible for the anterior sliding movement of the femur as the condyles roll posteriorly. This is achieved via induced ligamentous tension as the femoral attachment of the ligament attempts to move farther away from the tibial attachment. Because the ligament will not significantly elongate, the resulting motion is the anterior movement of the femur. Similar mechanics explain how the posterior cruciate ligament produces posterior slide of the femur during knee extension.

Additional work has been completed on the effects of rotary testing of the knee, partly for discovering the role of the capsule in restraining motion. The posterolateral complex has been sectioned, finding increased internal rotation in specimens with concurrently destroyed anterior cruciate ligaments. Their work also revealed that section of the anterolateral capsule produced no increase in either internal or external rotation. However, when the posterolateral capsule was divided, external rotation was significantly increased (97). This result confirmed earlier work that also demonstrated large increases in anteroposterior laxity when the medial collateral ligament and posterior capsule were sectioned in combination (104). Similar results, i.e., large increases in anterior posterior motion, have also been found when the medial meniscus is sacrificed after the isolated section of the anterior cruciate ligament (92). The position of the knee has also been varied for the different tests. As expected, the posterior capsule is less prone to injury when the knee is in the flexed position because the structure is relatively slack (56). As also may be anticipated, axial load and intact menisci reduce rotary laxity (160).

Researchers have used both bench tests and clinical tests to study anterolateral and anterior **laxity** in cadaver knees before and after cutting the anterior cruciate ligament. Results from the translatory tests showed more than twice as much movement when the anterior cruciate ligament was sectioned alone. Relatively minor effects were seen when the iliotibial band and lateral capsule were sectioned. Rotation tests showed similar results. In general, data suggest that the primary laxity, whether in translatory or rotary motion, results from an approximately 100% increase in anteroposterior translatory and only a 15% increase in rotation laxity (112). Resistance to anterior translation has also been shown to increase markedly with internal prerotation (1). An example of the results for the pivot shift maneuver is shown in Figure 11.9.

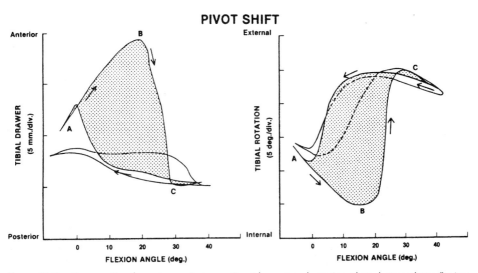

Figure 11.9.   Knee motion for anteroposterior motion (drawer) and rotation plotted versus knee flexion prior to (open circle) and after (dotted circle) ligament sectioning. *A*, starting position; *B*, maximum subluxated position; *C*, reduced position.

In summary, the different results of in vivo and in vitro knee ligament testing can be difficult to interpret; however, the following is a general consensus:

medial collateral	tight in extension and external rotation
lateral collateral	tight in extension and probably external rotation
anterior cruciate	tight in extension, controls anterior glide of tibia on femur
posterior cruciate	tight in flexion, selected fibers tight on extension, controls posterior glide of tibia on femur

Patellofemoral Joint

Two key biomechanical features of the patellofemoral joint should be understood. The first is that the patella increases the moment arm of the quadriceps tendon so that adequate extensor torques can be generated. That the moment arm varies over the range of motion has been shown by Smidt (139). From 90° of flexion to 45° short of complete extension, the moment arm increases from 3.8 to 4.9 cm and then decreases to 4.4 cm at full extension. This may be why the greatest quadriceps torques can be generated at 45° of flexion. A decreased moment arm and shortened muscle length would account for the smaller torques that can be generated at the end of the range of movement.

A second feature is the generation of **patellofemoral joint forces.** The patella is not pulled strictly vertical in the patellar groove on the femur, although primarily guided by soft tissue action (62) through most of the range of motion. Near complete extension the retinaculi has been reported to be "more noticeable" at full extension (62) and "small in all knee positions" (63). All these tissues contribute to the resulting contact force between these two bones. Therefore, assuming the same quadriceps tension, patellofemoral contact (reaction) force decreases as the knee is extended (Fig. 11.10). Conversely, with greater knee flexion, such as during stair climbing and the squat exercise, patellofemoral contact forces will rise markedly due to both the mechanics and increased quadriceps tension (46). Apparently, however, the tension in the quadriceps tendon and patellar ligament cannot be considered equal. Investigators have found that a ratio of the tensions in the two structures changes little in the first 15° of flexion but that patellar ligament tension was reduced to 50% of that in the quadriceps tendon when the knee was flexed from 80 to 100° (36). These results have implications for analyses that calculate patellofemoral joint reaction force.

KINETICS

The tibiofemoral and patellofemoral joints can both tolerate considerable load. Weight bearing requires the tibiofemoral joint to bear considerable load during activities of daily living. Shear forces are also a factor, both at the patellofemoral joint and between the tibial and femoral surfaces during joint movement. This section will cover joint torque, forces incurred during compression and shear, and the role of the joint structures in distributing pressure.

Torque

Many studies have evaluated torque of the knee extensors and flexors (5, 19, 86, 95, 98, 137, 148, 157, 158) under a variety of circumstances (19, 54, 64, 80, 119, 120, 122, 154, 155). Recorded values have varied due to differences in techniques used to record data. With the arrival of sophisticated dynamometers, isokinetic testing data are continually being gathered. Because the testing of both normal and pathological subjects has been done under isometric, concentric, and eccentric conditions, torque differences resulting from the different contractions can be studied. Application of data resulting from these contractions is relevant, however, because all contraction forms are used in completion of activities required for effective human function.

Comparison of **isometric torques** is complicated by variance in the angle of the knee joint. For example, for knee extensors the highest maximum values have usually

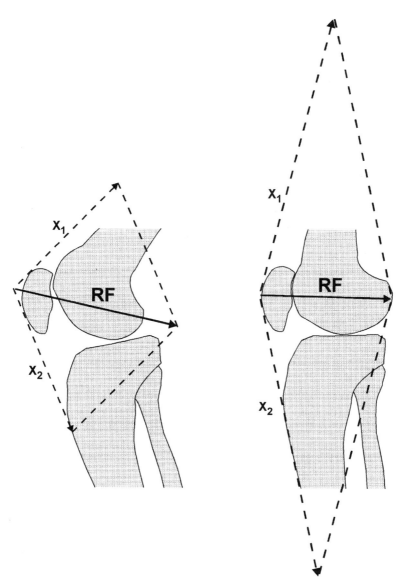

Figure 11.10. Lateral view of the knee showing the alteration in the patellofemoral joint reaction force (*RF*) with knee angle. Quadriceps tendon (x_1) and patellar ligament (x_2) tensions are also indicated.

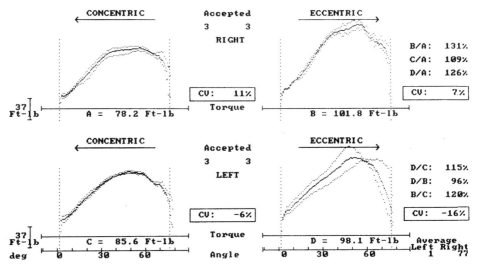

Figure 11.11. Knee extensor torque curves generated at 60°/sec for right (*top*) and left (*bottom*) knees. Ratios are provided for comparison. Heavy line is mean of contractions, the dotted lines the variation.

been recorded at 45° of flexion. With normal subjects in the side lying position, Smidt recorded values close to 1200 kg cms (120Nm) (139). Another group of workers calculated the maximal extending moment to be 226 Nm, a value not usually attained in experimental studies (96). Still another group assessed the moment during the vigorous knee extension required during kicking and found 260 Nm to be the highest torque achieved by any subject. The mean value for all the kicks was 151 Nm (158). Considering that kicking is a dynamic activity that requires concentric contraction, the determination of a value that exceeds the isometric value could be considered unusual.

An analysis of the representative results shown in Table 11.1 reveals several points of which the clinician should be aware when testing or interpreting knee joint torque data. As should be expected, concentric torque values are less when comparable tests are completed at higher **velocities**. Change is primarily dependent on the size of the velocity change, although data suggest that velocity has less effect on flexion torques (132). **Contraction type** also has a demonstrable effect, increasing with the eccentric contractions that cause the lengthening of muscle (Fig. 11.11). Data from the torque curves readily show that there are differences at each joint angle (Figs. 11.11, 11.12) due to the optimal quadriceps force production and moment arm at a position of 60° from complete extension during a quadriceps muscle contraction. Furthermore, **other joints crossed** by muscles that contribute to the knee joint torques have a bearing on the results (42). For example, Lunnen et al. varied the hip position while the subject remained seated; they recorded 39 Nm at 0° of hip flexion, 49 Nm at 45°, 57 Nm at 90°, and 65 Nm at 135° (99). Thus, it is clearly shown that hip angle influences knee flexion torque. Sitting upright distinctly stretches the hamstrings across the posterior aspect of the hip, allowing for greater torque generation. The implication is that therapists must be consistent in their procedures since not only knee position, but also hip position, exerts a powerful influence on the recorded torque. Finally, **age** and **gender** are both significant factors in torque production (109).

Torque measurements have also been used to evaluate the **quadriceps/hamstrings ratio** (78). This parameter is of some interest because reconditioning of athletes and others is occasionally based on returning torques to a normal ratio. Although data are more commonly available for males, studies now exist on female athletes (71) and mixed samples (68). Some have attempted to use isokinetic dynamometry of the knee to establish normative data for use in the clinical setting. Maximal extension/ flexion torque ratios were 2.19/1 for males and 2.32/1 for females. These authors also use their data to develop norms so that at 30°/sec the ratio of 2.25/1 is normal, 3.25/1 is abnormally high, and 1.25/1 is abnormally low. Further, they (arbitrarily) contend that rehabilitation is not complete unless the extensor/flexor ratio is approximately 2/1 with the weaker extensors not less than 60° as strong as the extensors of the opposite limb (53). Use of a higher percentage may clinically be more justifiable. Another assessment of this ratio reports values for both males and females. Ratios, reported in percentages, were virtually the same in each of the two samples of 50 men and 50 women. For all testing, the hamstring values were less. Hamstring/ quadriceps ratios at tests of 60°/sec were 71–72% at 60°/sec, increasing to 83–85% at the highest test speed of 300°/sec. These investigators comment that their results show higher values than the ratio of 63% at 60°/sec as had been previously reported. As the test velocity was increased, the differences in torque values decreased (166). As evidenced by the data, the population from which the information is collected is obviously a primary factor in determining the appropriate ratio to use clinically. In general, the ratio is likely to be highly variable (79), of potential use in evaluating patients (82), and likely dependent on velocity (68). Its utility is also limited by inherent difficulties associated with the formation of ratios and the potentially false assumption that the opposite extremity yields valid data.

Because rotation of the knee is often involved in the production of pathology, **rotary torque** data may assist the therapist in making a determination of the criterion level to be used in treatment of the unstable knee. To establish such norms, 28 young adult subjects were tested to determine both internal and external rotary torques. Testing was completed at both 45° and 90° of knee flexion. Mean torques, greater

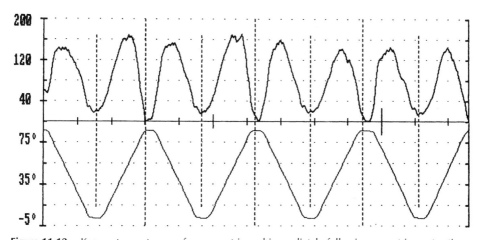

Figure 11.12.   Knee extensor torques for concentric and immediately following eccentric contractions. Torque in foot pounds is plotted on the upper portion and the joint angle on the bottom. Velocity was 60°/sec.

Table 11.1. Knee Normative Torque Values

Source Reference	Gender	Age Mean	Age SD	Age Range	n	Activity Level	Movement	Concentric (°/sec)	Eccentric (°/sec)	ROM	Testing Position	Peak Torque Nm	Peak Torque SD	Testing Device
52	m			18–25	100		e	60			sit, hip f 110	260		Biodex B-2000
							e	120				219		
							e	300				149		
							f	60				142		
							f	120				126		
							f	300				88		
							e		60			257		
							e		120			260		
							f		60			166		
							f		120			168		
58	m			10–20	4		e	60			hip 90, knee 90	117		Cybex II
							f	80				84		
							e	60				84		
							f	80				74		
	f			10–20	6		e	60				80		
							f	80				50		
							e	60				37		
							f	80				32		
	m			20–40	12		e	60				137		
							f	80				98		
							e	60				93		
							f	80				79		
	f			20–40	14		e	60				80		
							f	80				63		
							e	60				52		
							f	80				55		
	m			40–60	6		e	60				118		
							f	80				80		
							e	60				72		
							f	80				65		
	f			40–60	10		e	60				73		
							f	80				49		
							e	60				41		
							f	80				37		
	m			60–80	8		e	60				73		
							f	80				53		

No.	Sex	n	n (sub)	Age range	Age	Activity	Action	Speed (°/s)	ROM	Position	Value	SD	Device
134	f			60–80	16		e	60	90–0		38	33	Kin-Com
							f	80	0–90		39	51	
							e	60	90–0		49	26	
							f	80	0–90		42	52	
							e	60			32	19	
							f	80			36	27	
156	m	26		19–37	15		e	60	90–0		65	16	Kin-Com
	f	25		19–37	15		e	60	0–90		65	27	
	f	25	3	20–29	26		e	45	90–10	hip 80	61	17	
	f	73	6	68–89	26		e	90	90–10		57	23	
	f	25	3	20–29	26		e	45			137	14	
	f	73	6	68–89	26		e	90			151	24	
							e	45			131	8	
							e	90			152	20	
							e	45		hip 80	72	10	
							e	90			94	20	
							e	45			61		
							e	90			100		
							f	45	10–90		68		
							f	90	10–90		85		
							f	45			64		
							f	90			85		
							f	45			37		
							f	90	10–90		60		
							f	45			36		
							f	90			64		
41	f	19	1		25	soccer player	e	60			63	12	Cybex II
							f	60			118	22	
							e	240			34	14	
							f	240			62	12	
14	f	28	6		14		e	60		sit, hip 95	124	26	Cybex II
							e	60		sit, hip 150	90	18	
							f	60		sit, hip 95	77	13	
							f	60		sit, hip 150	52	8	
15	m	20			27	mod active	(R)e	90	90–0	hip 90, knee 90	231	32	Cybex II
		20			26		(R)e	150			180	24	
		30					(R)e	90			207	38	
		30			21		(R)e	150			158	34	
		50					(R)e	90			186	36	
		50					(R)e	150			145	27	
		70			21		(R)e	90			143	24	
		70					(R)e	150			113	22	

Table 11.1—*continued*

Source Reference	Gender	Age Mean	Age SD	Age Range	n	Activity Level	Movement	Concentric (°/sec)	Eccentric (°/sec)	ROM	Testing Position	Peak Torque Nm	Peak Torque SD	Testing Device
	f	20			26	mod active	(R)e	90			hip 90, knee 90	143	25	Cybex II
		20					(R)e	150				110	18	
		30			30		(R)e	90				138	22	
		30					(R)e	150				108	19	
		50			17		(R)e	90				122	18	
		50					(R)e	150				94	16	
		70			21		(R)e	90				98	17	
		70					(R)e	150				74	12	
	m	20			27	mod active	(R)e	0		90	hip 90, knee 90	301	56	Cybex II
		30			26		(R)e	0				255	47	
		50			21		(R)e	0				229	51	
		70			21		(R)e	0				187	38	
	f	20			26	mod active	(R)e	0		90	hip 90, knee 90	169	34	Cybex II
		30			30		(R)e	0				147	34	
		50			17		(R)e	0				123	23	
		70			21		(R)e	0				116	23	
	m	20			27	mod active	(L)e	90		90–0	hip 90, knee 90	217	27	Cybex II
		20					(L)e	150				179	22	
		30			26		(L)e	90				196	35	
		30					(L)e	150				160	28	
		50			21		(L)e	90				177	32	
		50					(L)e	150				143	30	
		70			21		(L)e	90				145	30	
		70					(L)e	150				113	21	
	f	20			26	mod active	(L)e	90		90–0	hip 90, knee 90	137	24	Cybex II
		20					(L)e	150				106	19	
		30			30		(L)e	90				134	20	
		30					(L)e	150				107	15	
		50			17		(L)e	90				114	17	
		50					(L)e	150				92	14	
		70			21		(L)e	90				93	15	
		70					(L)e	150				70	11	
	m	20			27	mod active	(L)e	0		90	hip 90, knee 90	280	59	Cybex II
		30			26		(L)e	0				240	44	
		50			21		(L)e	0				224	50	
		70			21		(L)e	0				179	40	

Sex	Age	Activity	Action	Velocity (°/s)	Angle (°)	ROM	Position	Torque	SD	Dynamometer
f	26	mod active	(L)e	0	20	90	hip 90, knee 90	156	32	Cybex II
	30		(L)e	0	30			139	28	
	17		(L)e	0	50			116	18	
	21		(L)e	0	70			105	22	
m	27	mod active	(R)f	90	20	0–90	hip 90, knee 90	122	21	Cybex II
	26		(R)f	150	20			96	19	
	21		(R)f	90	30			113	23	
	21		(R)f	150	30			91	26	
	26		(R)f	90	50			98	24	
	30		(R)f	150	50			82	23	
	17		(R)f	90	70			78	26	
	21		(R)f	150	70			61	23	
f	26	mod active	(R)f	90	20	0–90	hip 90, knee 90	68	21	Cybex II
	30		(R)f	150	20			49	19	
	17		(R)f	90	30			61	15	
	21		(R)f	150	30			46	14	
	27		(R)f	90	50			52	13	
	26		(R)f	150	50			36	13	
	21		(R)f	90	70			39	13	
	21		(R)f	150	70			28	8	
m	27	mod active	(L)e	90	20	0–90	hip 90, knee 90	113	21	Cybex II
	26		(L)e	150	20			91	19	
	21		(L)e	90	30			108	29	
	21		(L)e	150	30			87	25	
	26		(L)e	90	50			91	25	
	30		(L)e	150	50			76	25	
	17		(L)e	90	70			77	23	
	21		(L)e	150	70			60	26	
f	27	mod active	(L)e	90	20	0–90	hip 90, knee 90	66	17	Cybex II
	26		(L)e	150	20			46	16	
	21		(L)e	90	30			58	13	
	21		(L)e	150	30			42	12	
	26		(L)e	90	50			51	13	
	30		(L)e	150	50			38	11	
	17		(L)e	90	70			38	13	
	21		(L)e	150	70			25	9	
m (59), n 3	12		e	60			hip 90, knee 90	152	57	Cybex II
n 6	20		e	60				240	49	
n 6	17		e	60				203	37	
f, n 5	15		e	60			hip 90, knee 90	140	28	Cybex II
n 3	12		e	60				117	35	
n 6	20		e	60				146	32	

Table 11.1—*continued*

Source Reference	Gender	Age Mean	Age SD	Age Range	n	Activity Level	Movement	Concentric (°/sec)	Eccentric (°/sec)	ROM	Testing Position	Peak Torque Nm	Peak Torque SD	Testing Device
	m	50	6		21		e	60			hip 90, knee 90	113	24	Cybex II
		69	6		17		e	60				91	17	
		15	3		12		e	180				98	38	
		30	6		20		e	180				172	31	
		49	6		17		e	180				135	29	
	f	70	5		15		e	180			hip 90, knee 90	79	19	Cybex II
		15	3		12		e	180				75	29	
		30	6		20		e	180				89	22	
		50	6		21		e	180				62	20	
		69	6		17		e	180				46	13	
	m	15	3		12		f	60			hip 90, knee 90	108	37	Cybex II
		30	6		20		f	60				153	36	
		49	6		17		f	60				140	27	
		70	5		15		f	60				111	22	
	f	15	3		12		f	60			hip 90, knee 90	83	23	Cybex II
		30	6		20		f	60				93	17	
		50	6		21		f	60				80	14	
		69	6		17		f	60				72	15	
	m	15	3		12		f	180			hip 90, knee 90	95	35	Cybex II
		30	6		20		f	180				132	36	
		49	6		17		f	180				118	31	
		70	5		15		f	180				89	19	
	f	15	3		12		f	180			hip 90, knee 90	74	24	Cybex II
		30	6		20		f	180				70	17	
		50	6		21		f	180				66	18	
		69	6		17		f	180				60	16	
166	m	29			50		e	60			sit, hip 75–80	186	30	Cybex II
							f	60				133	18	
							e	180				133	18	
							f	180				104	18	
							e	300				91	16	
							f	300				75	15	
	f	28			50		e	60			sit, hip 75–80	108	19	Cybex II
							f	60				77	16	
							e	180				79	14	
							f	180				62	14	
							e	300				52	11	
							f	300				42	11	

n	sex	age			age range		°/s	angle	position	value	SD	apparatus
44	m	35	7	10		e	60		sit, hip 75–80	205	33	Cybex II
						f	60			112	20	
						e	120			174	22	
						f	120			106	17	
						e	240			132	24	
						f	240			76	14	
	f	24	2	11		e	60		sit, hip 75–80	131	23	Cybex II
						f	60			172	16	
						e	120			107	18	
						f	120			65	16	
						e	240			78	12	
						f	240			50	10	
163	m	28		10	21–45	e	0	30	sit	171	14	Cybex II special transducer
42	m			36	20–29	e	0	90	hip 90, knee 90	200	10	
				21	30–39	e	0	90		197	5	
				18	40–49	e	0	90		195	5	
				16	50–59	e	0	90		170		
				16	60–69	e	0	90		150		
				9	70–79	e	0	90		112		
	f			29	20–29	e	0	90		113	5	
				20	30–39	e	0	90		109	5	
				20	40–49	e	0	90		105		
				21	50–59	e	0	90		97		
				38	60–69	e	0	90		76		
				25	70–79	e	0	90		65		
66	m	22		24	19–28	e	120			195	18	
						f	120			118	9	
						e	240			179	18	
						f	240			102	8	
32	f	21		241	18–28	e	60		sit, hip 110	131	28	Cybex II
						f	60			70	16	
61	f	21	2	14		e	60		sit, hip 105	135	25	Kin-Com
						f	60			57	11	

Table 11.1—*continued*

Source Reference	Gender	Age Mean	SD	Range	n	Activity Level	Movement	Concentric (°/sec)	Eccentric (°/sec)	ROM	Testing Position	Peak Torque Nm	SD	Testing Device
55	m	40	12		40		e	30				183	29	Kin-Com
							e	120				158	23	
							e		30			229	39	
							e		120			232	39	
	f	41	12		50		e	30				116	26	
							e	120				95	20	
							e		30			157	35	
							e		120			154	34	
	m	40	12		40		f	30				93	15	
							f	120				82	14	
							f		30			110	19	
							f		120			109	19	
	f	41	12		50		f	30				55	13	
							f	120				48	11	
							f		30			67	15	
							f		120			67	15	
110	f			20–30	16		e	60				76	12	Cybex II
							e	180				49	19	
							f	60				42	9	
							f	180				24	11	
	m			20–30	9		e	60				90	23	
							e	180				58	8	
							f	60				62	25	
							f	180				41	15	

Legend: e, extension; f, flexion; L, left; R, right.

at the 90° position, ranged from 121 to 151 Nm, with little difference between knees or between direction of rotation (118). Rotary torques have also been measured at 20° and 90° of flexion. At the neutral position of rotation values ranged from 25 to 31 Nm, again with little difference between direction of rotation (135). The large differences between the results of these studies may be partly accounted for by differing methodologies. This discrepancy makes it extremely difficult for therapists to apply these data to their own clinical situations, probably requiring that normative data be developed according to individual testing protocols.

Joint Loading

As has been implied already, **load transmission** by the knee is important because of the repetitive loading cycles required during locomotion. In the frequently cited work of Morrison (107), mean peak compression force of just more than three times body weight was measured for the early and late phases of stance. When ramps or stairs were ascended, the peak values increased to 4–4.25 times body weight. The values reported for the knee are somewhat less than those for the hip, probably because of the decreased need for muscular forces.

It is well known, however, that muscular contraction of the extensors and flexors affect **compression** and **shear** at the knee. Force magnitudes are dependent on loading conditions such as weight-bearing or non-weight-bearing, point of load application, and intensity of muscular contraction. For example, extension during quadriceps contraction while non-weight-bearing was responsible for 132 kgf of compression. The hamstrings produced 268 kgf compression at the position of knee extension but less than 10 kg compression when the knee was positioned at 90° of flexion. In a flexed position the quadriceps contributed 274 kgf of compression effect. Taking into account muscle length change and angle of insertion, the relative changes could have been predicted. Shear production, so important in rehabilitation exercises, was at a maximum of 34.7 kgf for the quadriceps with a distally applied load when the non-weight-bearing knee was 15° short of full extension. The ability of the hamstrings to exert a maximum posterior shear of 151 kgf at 90° of flexion is of considerably less importance unless the posterior cruciate ligament is injured or unless this force is considered a potential restraint to the anterior motion of the tibia on the femur because of quadriceps contraction (139). Another study has reported maximum values of 1780 N for anterior shear at 90° of knee flexion and 285 N for posterior shear at 30° of knee flexion (100). Anterior shear, however, may be limited to the range for 40° to full extension, while posterior occurs at angles from full flexion to 40° short of full extension (82). Further, a direct comparison of open versus closed chain exercises has shown that the closed chain increases the compression, increases the amount of muscular cocontraction, and reduces the magnitudes of the anterior and posterior shear forces (100).

How loads are transmitted through the joint is another factor to consider. Because the contact area determines the **pressure** per unit area, the fully extended position that offers maximal contact area would be the position of choice. Furthermore, one study has noted that the area of the medial plateau is about 60% larger than that of the lateral plateau (84). Considering that the cartilage of the medial plateau is approximately three times thicker than the lateral the combined effect is that the medial aspect can more easily tolerate higher imposed forces (46).

Although debated before more sophisticated analytical techniques became available, evidence now exists that the menisci participate in load bearing. It may be that

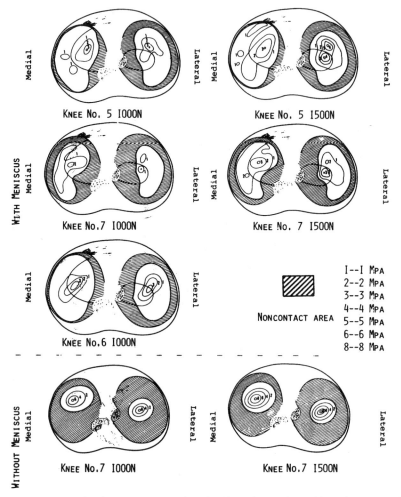

Figure 11.13. Pressure distribution patterns with and without the meniscus. Note changes, particularly on the lateral side.

distribution of the load is more effective and that pressure is reduced when the menisci are intact. Fukubayashi and Kurosawa (48) have provided specific data on this problem; the peak pressures were three MPa with the menisci and six MPa without them at compressing loads of 1000 N. Their work also showed that the contact area decreased to less than one-half of that of the intact knee. Figure 11.13 shows an example from their data. Note both the shape and size of the pressure pattern. The tibial fixation, meniscal structure, and femoral condyle geometry all seem to suggest that the menisci bear load throughout the knee range of motion, perhaps as much as 45% of the total in the human knee joint (136).

Stability of the knee during loading is of practical concern because the joint is usually loaded to some extent in situations that create pathologies. In fact, in clinical circles, the effect of loading has been well accepted. In examination of the knee, for example, apparent ligamentous laxity created by destruction of the articular cartilage requires that traction (distraction) loads be exerted to rule out the possibility of pseudo-laxity. Conversely, the knee loaded in compression assumes a more close-packed position; thus, a greater degree of stability is noted upon examination. For example, Markolf et al. (103) found that while a tibiofemoral compressive force was applied, stiffness was increased. Laxities decreased in anteroposterior, mediolateral, torsional, and varus-valgus testing. Apparently no matter whether the joint load is produced by gravitational, dynamic, or muscular force, the effect is to protect the ligaments from strain. Because of meniscal removal the authors also noted that the knee is looser in the unloaded, but not in the loaded, knee.

Patellofemoral Joint

The kinetics of the patellofemoral joint are also a factor in consideration of knee motion because often the levels of the forces exceed tolerable limits and/or produce pathology. A frequently cited work on the patellofemoral joint is that of Reilly and Martens (126), who in 1972 studied the joint reaction forces and the quadriceps forces during straight leg raising and other activities. The lowest value for patellofemoral joint reaction force (PFJR) was during walking, amounting to .5 times body weight. Stair climbing required PFJR of 3.3 times body weight while the largest force of 7.6 times body weight was produced during the squat activity. These values appear to have been confirmed via radiographic and mathematical analysis of 15 normal knees (105). Figure 11.10 showed the mechanical effects of different joint positions on the patellofemoral joint reaction force. Although subjected to degenerative and other disease processes, the patello-femoral joint can withstand high loads while assuring that friction is minimal as the tendon and inferior surface of the patella move over the femur. The size of these forces has been reported to be as high as 600 N with certain patellar lengths and patellar ligament lengths (138).

Other consideration needs to be given to conditions of weight bearing versus knee extension of the free distal portion of the extremity. Specifically, in standing with full knee extension, the quadriceps force is minimal, but increases with greater knee flexion (i.e., the squat). If extending against resistance while in the sitting position with the knee at 90° of flexion, the quadriceps force requirement is zero, increasing as extension follows (70). These factors, coupled with changes in contact area of the patella on the femur offer potential explanation for understanding that some exercises can produce significant forces at this joint. Further discussion of these features is in the next section on pathokinesiology.

Because these forces are distributed over a potentially limited area, i.e., the inferior surface of the patella, the **contact stresses** per unit area can be very large. Investigators have determined that between 13 and 38% of the patellar surface bears joint load, and have calculated patellofemoral contact stresses to vary between 1.3 and 12.6 newtons per square mm (105). Methods of reducing these forces resort to altering the mechanical conditions producing the high loads. One technique used is to reduce the load supported, for example by decreasing the weight of the patient or avoiding maneuvers such as the squat. Another technique used is the advancement of the tibial tuberosity. This surgical procedure has been shown to reduce the PFJR force by about 50%, thereby potentially resulting in diminished pain in patients suffering from osteoarthritis of this joint (102).

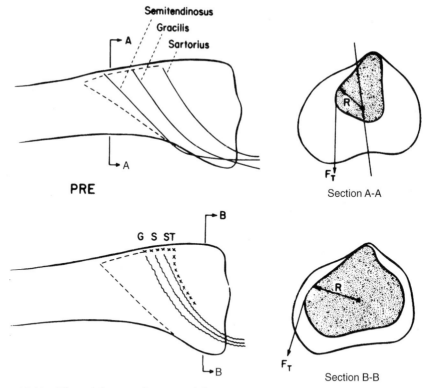

Figure 11.14. Effect of the transplantation of the pes anserine to a more proximal location on the tibia. Cross sections are shown for two locations. Note the change in the moment arm R. Force (F_T) is also represented.

PATHOKINESIOLOGY

Knee injuries cause many conditions that demonstrate pathological motion. This section of the chapter will be primarily devoted to the effects induced by damage or repair of soft tissue. Joint replacement procedures will also be discussed, as will the mechanical implications resulting from changes in the patellofemoral joint.

Pes Anserine Transfer

One surgical procedure, although now used less commonly, is the proximal transfer of the pes anserine insertion at the tibia. The pes is made up of tendinous insertions of the sartorius, gracilis, and semitendinosus muscles, and its location on the proximal tibia makes for accessibility for surgical relocation. The mechanical effects are shown in Figure 11.14. The basic premise of the transfer is to provide additional stability during terminal knee extension (screw-home mechanism). As predicted by the result shown in Figure 11.14, proximal transposition of the pes causes an increased moment arm for rotation. If the muscle lengths have not been significantly shortened, causing reduced tension generation, the effective moment for rotation should be increased. To test such a hypothesis both flexion and rotation forces were measured in cadaver specimens. As was anticipated when all test positions were considered, the flexion force was decreased by as much as 36%. This loss of flexion force is due to the decrease of the moment arm for flexion from the proximal relocation of the pes insertion. However, rotation forces were significantly increased at 90, 60, and 30° of flexion, but not in the fully extended position. This "wind up" effect was considered advantageous in the control of rotation in the knee (113).

Several laboratory and clinically based studies have evaluated the effectiveness of the procedure. DiStefano and coworkers (33) evaluated 15 postsurgical subjects for changes in torque generated in internal rotation. Although the 60° knee angle produced the greatest torque of 28.5 Nm in the postsurgical knee, the only test position in which torque increased preoperatively to postoperatively was the 30° test position (+9.2%). Osternig and colleagues (117) also evaluated 15 postsurgical subjects and found no significant differences between postsurgical and nonsurgical contralateral limbs for any of the positions tested. Internal rotation torque for nonsurgical limbs tested at 90° of flexion while in 5° of tibial rotation, were about 37 Nm. Others have performed clinical evaluations of the results of the transfer. Retrospective analyses provided mixed results. D'Arcy (26) found improvement of stability during activity in 42 of 51 knees while Chick et al. (30) stated that 89% of patients followed after 6.1 years had a combined rotary instability of the knee. Freeman et al. (47) reported more positive results; symptomatic improvements occurred in many patients. However, the results were not felt to be adequate for the patients used in the population in which the procedure was completed. In spite of these results function of the pes in providing stability has been demonstrated. Electromyographic comparison of normals with those in which the pes had been transferred showed that increased levels of activity occurred in those with transfers. Thus the conclusion was that these muscles were being used to control any potential instability in the knee (123).

In summary, attempts have been made to control anteromedial knee instability with transfers of the pes anserine. Although the procedure is based on known mechanical effects, the results have generally been discouraging. Because elongation of transposed muscle-tendon can occur with time, the long-term effect of this procedure is perhaps not optimal.

Anterolateral Instability and Ligament Insufficiencies

Although anterolateral instability has been recognized since 1972, progressively more attention has been given to this relatively common problem. The instability, also known as the **pivot shift,** is considered either the subluxation or reduction (or both in rapid succession) of the loaded joint. The pathology is manifested (as subluxation) as the femur twists externally or the tibia rotates internally. Occurring mainly in the lateral compartment of the knee, the anterior cruciate ligament (ACL) and the lateral and posterolateral segments of the capsule are considered deficient. Because the joint is in the close-packed position in full extension and because the iliotibial band may control the subluxation after 40 or 50° of flexion, the shift should be evaluated within this range of motion (98). Noyes et al. suggest that the mechanics are significantly influenced via the position of the iliotibial band. They point out that this band, as an extension of the tensor fascia latae muscle, is an extensor until 30° of flexion and a flexor beyond 40° (112). Anterior drawer movement of the lateral tibial component followed by sudden reduction of the tibiofemoral joint at 30–40° produces abnormal rotation (108). Although some suggest that under low stress, translational motion dominates angular motion (2), evidence is also available that changes can be seen during the pivot shift in the movement pattern of the instant axis of rotation within the sagittal condylar silhouette. The findings suggest that in the late stages of extension rolling predominated, followed by a marked change to a gliding motion. Data reduced from the radiographs also indicated that excessive friction and compressive forces existed in patients with anterolateral instability (148).

Ligamentous function and passive restraints that may produce certain joint motion can be related to the pivot shift by way of analyzing which structures are deficient in the knee demonstrating abnormal motion. As already discussed in this chapter, the anterior cruciate ligament is the most commonly disrupted structure in the knee. There is also evidence that the posterolateral capsule is stretched to allow room for the lateral femoral condyle during subluxation. Changes may occur in the fabello-fibular and arcuate ligaments, but consistent findings in this area have not been shown (98) except in the series of 12 surgically repaired cases (31).

Among the surgical procedures attempted to control abnormal rotation are surgical advancement of the biceps femoris insertion toward Gerdy's tubercle and the Ellison and the Losee methods, both of which involve transferring the iliotibial band. The latter procedure involves transposition of the tendon of the iliotibial band by passing the attachment and bone fragment under the fibular collateral ligament to an insertion on the anterolateral aspect of the tibia (37).

The effectiveness of these transfers has differed depending on the patient population and the precise procedure used. For example, one study reported on a group of 60 patients in which the distal iliotibial band was transferred to the fibular collateral ligaments. Although early scores that rated such factors as instability and pain were improved, the results at the end of a 40-month period indicated that the transfer did not function satisfactorily (114). On the other hand, Benum (10) used a segment of the patellar ligament and adjoining patella on six patients, five of which had increased stability and good function. Perhaps if the patients in the latter study had been followed for more than 17 months the results for his patient group would have shown similar deterioration. As with many transfers the primary deterrent to a continuing good result is tissue elongation from stretch, whether this is applied incidentally or intentionally. Knowing the surgical procedure and the motion required, indications and contraindications may assist with yielding better long-term results from transfer procedures.

Passive restraint normally controls the pivot shift, but, in the abnormal case, dynamic muscular control may achieve functional goals. Similar comments may also be made about the patient with deficiency of the ACL. In fact, some have detailed the anterior translation of the tibia on the femur during quadriceps muscle contraction, noting that undesirable and excessive motions may occur (69). For example, one investigator said that for knee extension performed with a long leg cast or knee brace as much as 12.3 kgf would be applied in the direction of anterior shear (74). If in fact the anterior cruciate had been injured or if surgical reconstructions had been completed, there is a clear danger that muscle contraction can induce unwanted or too great a stress in the tissues (6). This is apparently true particularly for the last 30° of knee extension (57).

To counteract the **anterior translation of the tibia** considerable attention has been focused on the role of the hamstring musculature. Studies have focused on the contraction of these muscles during simple exercises and during more complex activities. Some have suggested that the hamstring muscles at least contribute to the "protective reflex" so that translation is limited (7, 9). Evidence is also available concerning differences in the temporal onsets and durations of muscle activity during activities such as walking (77, 89). Such information is important for the return of these patients to normal activities, since without normal durations and magnitudes of muscle contractions, normal function is unlikely. Thus, the implication is that hamstrings activation may be critical to normal function (76, 106, 152, 159).

Therefore, some seriously question the efficacy of quadriceps exercises without cocontraction of the hamstrings during the rehabilitative phases, although it has been shown that the maximal quadriceps contraction results in less anterior displacement than manual or instrumented "drawer" readings (62). Because ligamentous strength may take more than a year to return to reasonable levels, the use of quadriceps exercises must at least be cautiously approached. In recognition of this problem many therapists will limit the range of motion to only 60° of flexion or use exercise programs that require cocontraction of the hamstrings. These exercises are thought to resist or restrain the tendency for anterior shear of the tibia. One such exercise suggested is the step-up exercise. A purported advantage of this exercise is that contractions of both the quadriceps and hamstrings are required, reducing the tendency for joint shear. Because little evidence existed as to the magnitude of tension required in these muscles to perform the step-up and down, Brask and coworkers (18) performed an electromyographic study on these muscles during the exercise. Their results revealed that the average values for muscular activity, depending on the height and the direction of the step, ranged from 24 to 60% of maximum EMG for the vastus medialis and 8 to 23% for the rectus femoris. Activity in the biceps femoris was only 3–9% and in the semimembranosus/semitendinosus muscles of the order of 4–9% of the maximum value. Thus, in spite of the attempt to control for shear, the hamstrings may not be generating sufficient tension to be able to do so. Other exercise techniques have also been studied in search of a better exercise technique; however, forward and backward bicycle riding, use of a stair stepper, and rotations on a balance board have all proved ineffective in creating optimal timing and levels of hamstring muscle contractions.

Instead, weight bearing may be the critical factor in controlling shear, since the joint is more congruous under these conditions. This statement is supported by studies (153, 167) that show translation to decrease by as much as 71% in ACL sectioned knees (153). Functional testing of these patients, which may be more applicable in the weight bearing position, has shown that most patients with ACL deficiency reduce the net quadriceps moment when the knee is near full extension (3). Reductions in the intensity of quadriceps effort have also been shown during walking, the result of which may be to decrease the effect of an anterior pull on the tibia (11, 17).

In summary, there will continue to be special focus on the ACL (38). In general, there is gathering support for the importance of controlling anterior shear in the knee, particularly for injuries of the ACL. Many support the notion that hamstrings are an important component of this control; however, considering the mechanics and current analyses, at least some skepticism must be offered that adequate control can be exerted by the hamstrings or any other posterior structures in and around the knee. Closed kinetic chain exercises may offer an effective approach but should still be monitored closely for the effects on the osteokinematics and arthrokinematics in the knee. Biomechanical analyses of the knee extension exercise may also lend additional information that will be useful to the therapist in making clinical judgments (24).

Ligamentous Reconstructions

Ligament reconstructions are designed to increase stability and improve joint function following injury. Ligamentous, capsular, and musculotendinous units have all been used. Always, surgical repairs should be designed such that joint kinematics and the resulting kinetics will not be altered, particularly in structures used in the repair procedure (23). Mechanics, those either required by functional activities or invoked by well-meaning therapeutic exercises, can produce abnormal forces that will lead to potential failure of the procedure. Translocation may also lead to abnormal shear forces at locations where ligaments or structures are required to pass through or over bone or over new soft tissue structures (73). Knowledge of the procedure used is helpful to the therapist's understanding of necessary postoperative therapeutic procedures.

Although simple ligament relocations are done, such as the anterior and distal advancement of the medial collateral ligament for medial instability, most of this section will deal with reconstructions associated with anterior cruciate ligament insufficiencies. The type of reconstruction can be direct or by extra-articular substitution and intra-articular augmentation. Fascia latae allografts and temporary supportive prostheses are also available, but less frequently used (129). In any case, Butler (Butler DL, personal communication, 1983) has developed criteria for replacement of the anterior cruciate ligament. The tissue should have (a) adequate mechanical properties (strength and stiffness), (b) vascular viability, (c) availability, and (d) access to bone at both ends of the graft. In addition, the procedure should be (e) technically feasible, and (f) have a low mobility. Whether the procedures have developed the criteria or vice versa, the patellar ligament, iliotibial band, and semitendinosus tendon have all been used in the surgical procedures (27, 130, 168, 169). Judging function based on functional activities, and in some cases on the return to competitive sports, results could be considered encouraging at the least. One example is a follow-up which used patellar tendon reconstruction. Many patients (69%) had good to excellent results. Arthrosis and parapatellar pain were the most frequent factors that contributed to failure (75). Unsuccessful reconstructions result from inattention to the classic criteria or for reasons cited in the section on anterolateral instabilities. Because of the debilitating nature of the injury and the subsequent surgical procedure, rehabilitative techniques should be instituted. However, consideration must be given to both the extra-articular and intra-articular mechanics associated with any therapeutic procedure.

Patellar Mechanics

As discussed earlier in this chapter, the patella is responsible for mechanical effects that are facilitative to knee extension. Losses, such as in **patellectomy** (Fig. 11.15), have an influence on the ability of the patient to perform knee extension, resulting in the common condition known as **extensor lag** (Fig. 11.16). Although some contend that such a lag should not be seen with proper surgical technique, postoperative immobilization in extension, and rehabilitation procedures, the losses are difficult to overcome. Both theoretical and clinical studies have revealed that extension capability is reduced from 15 to 49% (121, 146). The primary reason for this loss appears to be due to the decreased moment arm through which the quadriceps mechanism can now act. Thus, a significant loss in moment arm means that higher tensions must be generated in the extensors to offset the loss. Because these patients

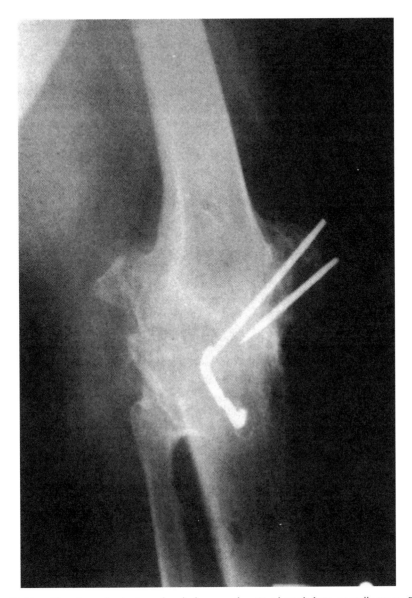

Figure 11.15. AP radiograph of a knee fused after poor functional result from a patellectomy. Due to excessive bone formation, it is difficult to discern the absence of the patella.

are likely to suffer from quadriceps weakness due to factors that precipitated the patellectomy, the therapist is forced to deal with a doubly difficult problem: loss of tension and loss of the adequate moment arm.

In contrast to the patellectomy is elevation or displacement of the tibial tubercle. This technique relieves abnormally high patellofemoral joint forces and the pain that may result. Figure 11.17 shows a free body diagram of the preoperative and postoperative conditions. With the tibial tubercle elevated, and maintained by the assistance of a bone block, two significant mechanical changes have occurred. First, note that the distance d, from F_p to the instant center of rotation has increased,

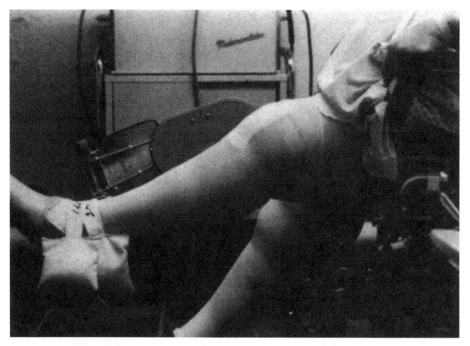

Figure 11.16. Post-patellectomy patient attempting to extend the knee with three pounds suspended at the distal shank. Although the center of the hip is difficult to find, significant extensor lag exists due to insufficient extensor moment.

resulting in the improved ability for the generation of an extension moment. Secondly, note that the angle between F_p and F_q has increased, the result of which is a decrease in patellofemoral contact force as shown by a reduction in vector F_c. Thus, the procedure achieves two changes that should facilitate extension moments in the knee (Fig. 11.18). Although slow return to full function and poor cosmesis are two disadvantages, the results seem to justify the continued use of the procedure, particularly with as much as 50% of the joint reaction force (under certain conditions) (25). That a half inch elevation may be optimal is at least of some help in controlling the unsightly tibial prominence (39, 40).

Patellofemoral joint reaction forces are a factor to consider in exercise techniques, not only because some patients' pathologies are associated with the patella (149, 150, 151). Often patients cannot tolerate a dynamic knee extension movement due to pain/discomfort from the reaction forces. Because the area of the patella in contact with the femur increases with knee flexion, the area over which forces are distributed also increases. The effect is to distribute the load over a broader area. Conversely, during extension the opposite occurs. The result is that at some point in the range the compression will exceed the physiological loading occurring during weight bearing. This is at 52° short of complete knee extension. A practical example can be produced from a plot of the patellofemoral joint reaction forces during knee extension with a resistance of a 9 kg weight boot added to the foot of the subject (Fig. 11.19). The peak force would occur approximately 40° from complete knee extension, a point in the range of motion that may be difficult for a patient with patellofemoral joint pathology. Also note that after this point in the range of motion the force decreases rapidly because tension in the quadriceps and patellar tendon produce mostly joint shear at this position rather than compressive force (70). Thus, therapists need to consider pressure rather than force to make a conclusion. Although contact force decreases with extension, if contact area decreases at a faster rate, an increase in pressure results. These mechanics offer the reason why many patellofemoral patients have no symptoms at 52° or greater, and severe pain at angles of less than 52°.

Other pathologies of the extensor mechanism also occur with regularity. **Patellar malalignment** problems can be so great that the patella can dislocate laterally. In these cases, transposition tightening or "reefing" of medial structures may best solve a problem that tends to recur. In less severe malalignments, functional training of the quadriceps with setting and straight leg raising exercises may arrest the persistent symptoms. Another useful exercise is the manual displacement of the patella slightly laterally, having the patient return it to neutral via quadriceps muscle contraction.

Ruptures of the extensor mechanisms, both in the quadriceps tendon and in the patellar ligament, have been reported. In either case, it is difficult for the therapist to return the patient to normal extensor torque because of the delay required to allow sufficient healing before resistive exercise can begin. The therapist must carefully minimize dynamic loading that increases the tension in the tendon or ligament to a point where the high tensile stress would lead to rupture (Fig. 11.20).

Therapists should also be aware that joint position and state of **effusion** can

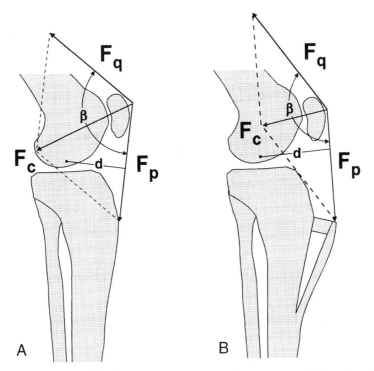

Figure 11.17. Lateral view of the knee, preoperative (**A**) and postoperative (**B**) elevation of the tibial tubercle. Compared to the preoperative knee, the contact force (F_c) decreases due to change in angle of β and the increase in the patellar moment arm d. Force in the quadriceps and patellar ligament is shown with F_p and F_q, respectively.

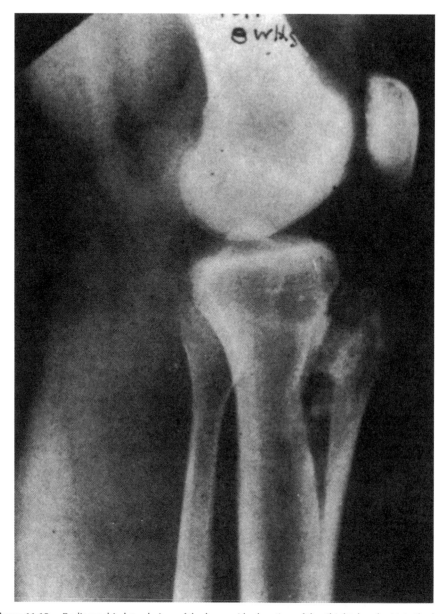

Figure 11.18. Radiographic lateral view of the knee with elevation of the tibial tubercle. Note the bone block used to maintain the position of the tubercle.

influence the level of contraction that can be produced (164). This is significant because many knee patients display effusions from either trauma or surgery or both. In one study, decreased EMG activity was shown at the fully extended position when compared to the position of 30° of flexion (145). Another study established that when comparing operated and nonoperated limbs, types of exercise and joint position caused differences in the resulting EMG values (86). However, the fully extended position, being close-packed, provides a decreased area of volume available for joint fluid. Therefore, the effused knee often adopts a degree of flexion and is inhibited from full extension by increased fluid pressure that distends the capsule. These results point to the importance of taking into account information about neural control mechanisms when applying therapeutic interventions.

Total Joint Replacements

The knee has been a popular joint for replacement because of its high incidence of degenerative disease and problems of malalignment. These **arthroplasties** are completed primarily to reduce pain and improve range of motion. Stability, however, must be maintained. Multiple prosthetic designs are available to the surgeon. One may classify these replacements into three major types (125). Unconstrained implants are intended for those patients with ligamentous integrity because these passive structures will, of necessity, be responsible for maintaining the stability of the joint. At the other extreme is the constrained device, which is not dependent upon ligaments for alignment. These components, however, may be more likely to loosen because other joint structures may not be able to manage the forces. A compromise is the semi-constrained replacement (Fig. 11.21). This device tries to select the positive features of each of the other two devices. No matter the procedure, failure rates, for a variety of reasons, have continued to be a concern. Many studies summarize some of these mechanisms and discuss tibial loosening as related to tilt and sink, compression, torsion, and other mechanical groupings. Further confounding problems include infection, loss of bone, and patellar subluxation (13, 22). In general, therapists can expect that additional designs will be marketed, tested, and implanted

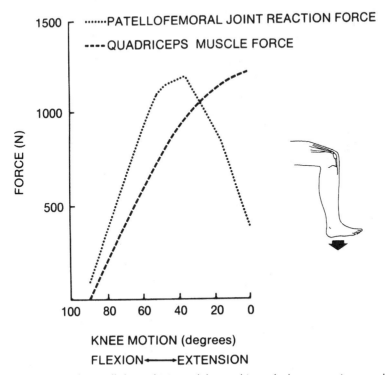

Figure 11.19. Force in the patellofemoral joint and the quadriceps for knee extension completed with a boot weighing 9 kg, the subject seated, and the lower leg free.

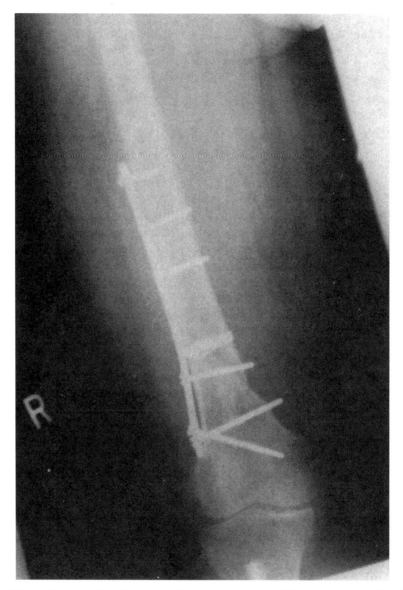

Figure 11.20.   AP radiograph of distal femur, 7 months after fixation. This knee had only 30° of flexion, and caution with active and passive movement was necessary because of the fracture. Soft tissue limitations in the extensor apparatus limited range of motion.

in the patients they treat. Clinical results to date have established the effectiveness of the total knee replacement, thereby suggesting that continued and even more widespread use can be anticipated (13).

The effects of the arthroplasty on the kinematics and kinetics of the joint are of interest to therapists. In some cases the kinematics of the prosthesis is significantly different from the normal knee (111). In general, however, patients and therapists will concede that pain is diminished and functional performance improved. In fact, specific studies evaluating patient performance have been completed. Range of knee motion has been improved, unchanged, or diminished depending on the source cited. The same can be said for the achievement of complete extension, often resulting in the functional difficulties associated with loss of terminal extension (29). According to Ritter and Stringer (128), the total knee arthroplasty can be expected to correct 5–7° of valgus deformity and return the knee to full extension within one year. Furthermore, because less improvement is seen in patients whose preoperative flexion was less than 75°, less ultimate flexion can be anticipated in patients with less initial flexion.

Preoperative function has a definite effect on ultimate functional outcome in patients whose knees have undergone arthroplasty because of arthritis. Osteoarthritic patients generated from 56 to 103 Nm of extension torque before surgery and from 21 to 102 Nm after surgery. Rheumatoid arthritics had an increased range of values, 4–76 Nm preoperatively and 23–109 Nm one year after surgery (29). Not only is the range very large but the values are quite below the values of 191 and 108 Nm

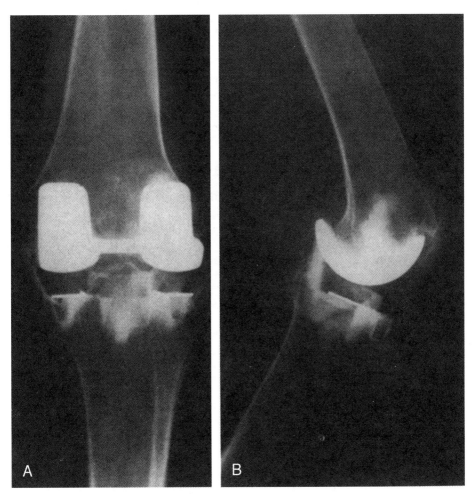

Figure 11.21. AP (**A**) and lateral (**B**) views of total knee replacement. Note shape of new femoral condyles that allow for some rotation and varus and valgus. Tibial plateaus can be discerned by using wire inserts in the components.

for 70-year-old asymptomatic men and women, respectively (4). Since the age range for the operative group is generally comparable with the normative data, significant problems may exist for the therapist in restoring normal torque values to the surgical group.

Other measures post arthroplasty have also been evaluated. In monoarticular degenerative arthritis, the measurements of gait had returned to normal levels within two years of the surgery; specific areas measured were normality of velocity, stride lengths, and kinematics of the hip, knee, and ankle. The data did determine, however, that the patients spent about 30% longer for double stance and had increased cycle times (137). Shorter than normal stride lengths, reduced midstance knee flexion, and uncharacteristic flexion-extension moments at the knee have also been shown (4). That the type of prosthesis can influence the results is also established. Five types of prostheses have been used to analyze the effect of the design on walking and stair climbing. Differences could be discerned from the design. For example, a normal range of motion during stair ascent and descent was achieved with only the least-constrained, cruciate-retaining prosthesis. Although all the implants were considered clinically successful, all patients had abnormalities of gait (4). At least a part of this result may be due to the geometry of the prosthetic components. It is interesting that the mechanics of the cruciate ligaments are altered to varying degrees, depending on the prosthetic design involved. Apparently, components with single radius of curvature geometry cause constraint forces to exist in the posterior cruciate ligament. Such a problem is nonexistent if multicurvature designs simulating the actual configuration of the femoral condyles are used (93). These findings further establish the nature of the interaction between the bony and soft tissue structures. Therapists must be aware of these features to realize effective therapeutic intervention necessary.

SUMMARY

The knee is an interesting joint to study because the anatomical conditions produce a great variety of kinetic and kinematic events. Pathology often alters these events, producing abnormal motion that is often difficult to restore to normal. Factors that alter the normal mechanics of the joint and the surrounding structures will continue to be modified by surgical and other therapeutic interventions. As trauma and degenerative conditions are unlikely to disappear from the human experience, the understanding of normal and abnormal mechanics of the knee will likely remain important to practicing therapists.

References

1. Ahmed AM, Burke DL, Duncan NA, Chan KH. Ligament tension pattern in the flexed knee in combined passive anterior translation and axial rotation. *J Orthop Res.* 1992;10:854–867.
2. Allum R, Jones D, Mowbray MAS, Galway HR. Triaxial electrogoniometric examination of the pivot shift sign for rotatory instability of the knee. *Clin Orthop.* 1984;183:144–146.
3. Andriacchi TP, Birac D. Functional testing in the anterior cruciate ligament-deficient knee. *Clin Orthop.* 1993;288:40–47.
4. Andriacchi TP, Galante JO, Fermier RW. The influence of total knee-replacement design on walking and stair-climbing. *J Bone Joint Surg.* 1982;64:1328–1335.
5. Aniansson A, Grimby G, Rundgren A. Isometric and isokinetic quadriceps muscle strength in 70 year old men and women. *Scand J Rehabil Med.* 1980;12:161–168.
6. Arms SW, Pope MH, Johnson RJ, Fischer RA, Arvidsson I, Eriksson E. The biomechanics of anterior cruciate ligament rehabilitation and reconstruction. *Am J Sports Med.* 1984;12(1):8–18.
7. Aune AK, Nordsletten L, Skjeldal S, et al. Hamstrings and gastrocnemius co-contraction protects the anterior cruciate ligament against failure: an in vivo study in the rat. *J Orthop Res.* 1995;13:147–150.

8. Basmajian JV, Lovejoy JF. Functions of the popliteus muscle in man. *J Bone Joint Surg.* 1971;53:557–562.

9. Beard DJ, Kyberd PJ, O'Connor JJ, et al. Reflex hamstring contraction latency in anterior cruciate ligament deficiency. *J Orthop Res.* 1994;12:219–228.

10. Benum P. Anterolateral rotary instability of the knee joint. *Acta Orthop Scand.* 1982;53:613–617.

11. Berchuk M, Andriacchi TP, Bach BR, Reider B. Gait adaptations by patients who have a deficient anterior cruciate ligament. *J Bone Joint Surg.* 1990;72(A):871–877.

12. Blackburn TA, Craig E. Knee anatomy—a brief review. *Phys Ther.* 1980;60:1556–1560.

13. Blauth W, Hassenpflug J. Are unconstrained components essential in total knee arthroplasty? *Clin Orthop.* 1990;258:86–94.

14. Bohannon RW, Gajdosik RL, LeVeau BF. Isokinetic knee flexion and extension torque in the upright sitting and semireclined sitting positions. *Phys Ther.* 1986;66:1083–1090.

15. Borges O. Isometric and isokinetic knee extension and flexion torque in men and women aged 20–70. *Scand J Rehabil Med.* 1987;21:45–53.

16. Bos RR, Blosser TG. An electromyographic study of vastus medialis and vastus lateralis during selected isometric exercises. *Med Sci Sports.* 1970;2:218–223.

17. Branch TP, Hunter R, Donath M. Dynamic EMG analysis of anterior cruciate deficient legs with and without bracing during cutting. *Am J Sports Med.* 1989;17:35–41.

18. Brask B, Lueke RH, Soderberg GL. Electromyographic analysis of selected muscles during the lateral step-up exercise. *Phys Ther.* 1984;64:324–329.

19. Brown LE, Whitehurst M, Gilbert R. The effect of velocity and gender on load range during knee extension and flexion exercise on an isokinetic device. *J Orthop Sports Phys Ther.* 1995;21:107–112.

20. Butler DL, Noyes FR, Grood ES. Ligamentous restraints to anterior-posterior drawer in the human knee. *J Bone Joint Surg.* 1980;62:259–270.

21. Cabaud HE. Biomechanics of the anterior cruciate ligament. *Clin Orthop.* 1983;172:26–31.

22. Cameron HU, Hunter GA. Failure in total knee arthroplasty. *Clin Orthop.* 1982;170:141–146.

23. Chao EYS, Neluheni EVD, Hsu RWW, Paley D. Biomechanics of malalignment. *Orthop Clinics N Am.* 1994;25:379–386.

24. Chen C, Ost JJ, Salathé EP. Biomechanical analysis of the knee extension exercise. *Arch Phys Med Rehabil.* 1993;74:1336–1342.

25. Cheng C-K, Yao N-K, Liu H-C. Surgery simulation analysis of anterior advancement of the tibial tuberosity. *Clin Biomech.* 1995;10:115–121.

26. Chick RP, Collins HR, Rubin BD, et al. The pes anserinus transfer. *J Bone Joint Surg.* 1981;63:1449–1452.

27. Clancy WG, Nelson DA, Reider B, Narechania RG. Anterior cruciate ligament reconstruction using one-third of the patellar ligament, augmented by extra-articular tendon transfers. *J Bone Joint Surg.* 1982;64:352–359.

28. Close JR. *Motor Function in the Lower Extremity: Analyses by Electronic Instrumentation.* Springfield, IL: Charles C Thomas; 1964.

29. Collopy MC, Murray MP, Gardner GM, et al. Kinesiologic measurements of functional performance before and after geometric total knee replacement: one year follow up of twenty cases. *Clin Orthop.* 1977;126:196–202.

30. D'Arcy J. Pes anserinus transposition for chronic anteromedial rotational instability of the knee. *J Bone Joint Surg.* 1978;60:66–70.

31. DeLee JC, Riley MB, Rockwood CA. Acute posterolateral rotatory instability of the knee. *Am J Sports Med.* 1983;11:199–207.

32. Dibrezzo R, Gench BE, Hinson MM, et al. Peak torque values of the knee extensor and flexor muscles of females. *J Orthop Sports Phys Ther.* 1985;2:65–72.

33. DiStefano V, Nixon JE, O'Neil R, Davis O. Pes anserinus transfer: an in vivo biomechanical analysis. *Am J Sports Med.* 1977;5:204–208.

34. Duarte-Cintra AI, Furlani J. Electromyographic study of quadriceps femoris in man. *Electromyogr Clin Neurophysiol.* 1981;21:539–554.

35. Elftman H. The function of the muscles in locomotion. *Am J Physiol.* 1939;125:357–366.

36. Ellis MI, Seedhom BB, Wright V, Dowson D. An evaluation of the ratio between the tensions along the quadriceps tendon and the patellar ligament. *Eng in Med.* 1980;9:189–194.

37. Ellison AE. Distal iliotibial band transfer for anterolateral rotatory instability of the knee. *J Bone Joint Surg.* 1979;61(A):330–337.

38. Feagin JA, ed. *The Crucial Ligaments.* New York: Churchill-Livingstone; 1994.

39. Ferguson AB. Elevation of the insertion of the patellar ligament for patellofemoral pain. *J Bone Joint Surg.* 1982;64:766–771.

40. Ferguson AB, Brown TD, Fu FH, Rutkowski R. Relief of patellofemoral contact stress by anterior displacement of the tibial tubercle. *J Bone Joint Surg.* 1979;61:159–166.

41. Fillyaw M, Bevins T, Fernandez L. Importance of correcting isokinetic peak torque for the effect of gravity when calculating knee flexor to extensor muscle ratios. *Phys Ther.* 1986;66:23–31.

42. Fisher NM, Pendergast DR, Calkins EC. Maximum isometric torque of knee extension as a function of muscle length in subjects of advancing age. *Arch Phys Med Rehabil.* 1990;71:729–734.

43. Fisk R, Wells J. The quadriceps complex in bipedal man. *J Am Osteopath Assoc.* 1980;80:291–294.

44. Francis K, Hoobler T. Comparison of peak torque values of knee flexor and extensor muscle groups using Cybex II and Lido 2.0 Isokinetic dynamometers. *J Orthop Sports Phys Ther.* 1987;8:480–483.

45. Frankel VH, Burstein AH. *Orthopaedic Biomechanics.* Philadelphia: Lea & Febiger; 1970.

46. Frankel VH, Nordin M. *Basic Biomechanics of the Skeletal System.* Philadelphia: Lea & Febiger; 1980.

47. Freeman BL, Beaty JH, Haynes DB. The pes anserinus transfer. *J Bone Joint Surg.* 1982;64:202–207.

48. Fukubayashi T, Kurosawa H. The contact area and pressure distribution pattern of the knee. *Acta Orthop Scand.* 1980;51:871–879.

49. Fukubayashi T, Torzilli PA, Sherman MF, Warren RF. An in vitro biomechanical evaluation of anterior-posterior motion of the knee. *J Bone Joint Surg.* 1982;64(A):258–264.

50. Fuss FK. Principles and mechanisms of automatic rotation during terminal extension in the human knee joint. *J Anat.* 1992;180:297–304.

51. Fuss FK. The restraining function of the cruciate ligaments on hyperextension and hyperflexion of the human knee joint. *Anat Rec.* 1991;230:283–289.

52. Ghena DR, Kurth AL, Thomas M, Mayhew J. Torque characteristics of the quadriceps and hamstring muscles during concentric and eccentric loading. *J Orthop Sports Phys Ther.* 1991;14:149–154.

53. Goslin BR, Charteris J. Isokinetic dynamometry: normative data for clinical use in lower extremity (knee) cases. *Scand J Rehabil Med.* 1979;11:105–109.

54. Greenberger HB, Wilkwski T, Belyea B. Comparison of quadriceps peak torque using three different isokinetic dynamometers. *Isokin Exerc Sci.* 1994;4:70–75.

55. Griffin JW, Tooms RE, van der Zwaag R, et al. Eccentric muscle performance of elbow and knee muscle groups in untrained men and women. *Med Sci Sports Exerc.* 1993;25:936–944.

56. Grood ES, Noyes FR, Butler DL, Suntay WJ. Ligamentous and capsular restraints preventing straight medial and lateral laxity in intact human cadaver knees. *J Bone Joint Surg.* 1981;63:1257–1269.

57. Grood ES, Suntay WJ, Noyes FR, Butler DL. Biomechanics of the knee-extension exercise. *J Bone Joint Surg.* 1984;66(A):725–734.

58. Gross MT, Credle JK, Hopkins LA, et al. Validity of knee flexion and extension peak torque prediction models. *Phys Ther.* 1990;70:3–10.

59. Gross MT, McGrain P, Demilio N. Relationship between multiple predictor variables and normal knee torque production. *Phys Ther.* 1989;69:54–62.

60. Gough JV, Ladley G. An investigation into the effectiveness of various forms of quadriceps exercises. *Physiotherapy.* 1971;57:356–361.

61. Harding B, Black T, Bruulsema A, et al. Reliability of a reciprocal test protocol performed on the kinetic communicator: an isokinetic test of knee extensor and flexor strength. *J Orthop Sports Phys Ther.* 1991;10:218–223.

62. Heegaard J, Leyvraz P-F, Van Kampen A, et al. Influence of soft structures on patellar three-dimensional tracking. *Clin Orthop.* 1994;299:235–243.

63. Hehne H-J. Biomechanics of the patellofemoral joint and its clinical relevance. *Clin Orthop.* 1990;258:73–85.

64. Helgeson K, Gajdosik RL. The stretch-shortening cycle of the quadriceps femoris muscle group measured by isokinetic dynamometry. *J Orthop Sports Phys Ther* 1993;17:17–23.

65. Herzog W, Read LJ. Lines of action and moment arms of the major force-carrying structures crossing the human knee joint. *J Anat.* 1993;182:213–230.

66. Hobbel SL, Rose DJ. The relative effectiveness of three forms of visual knowledge of results on peak torque output. *J Orthop Sports Phys Ther.* 1993;18:601–608.

67. Hollister AM, Jatana S, Singh AK, et al. The axes of rotation of the knee. *Clin Orthop.* 1993;290:259–268.

68. Holm I, Ludvigsen P, Steen H, et al. Isokinetic hamstrings/quadriceps ratios: normal values and reproducibility in sport students. *Isokin Exerc Sci.* 1994;4:141–145.

69. Howell SM. Anterior tibial translation during a maximum quadriceps contraction: is it clinically significant? *Am J Sports Med.* 1990;18:573–578.
70. Hungerford DS, Barry M. Biomechanics of the patellofemoral joint. *Clin Orthop.* 1979;144:9–15.
71. Imwold CH, Rider RA, Haymes EM, Green KD. Isokinetic torque differences between college female varsity basketball and track athletes. *J Sports Med Phys Fitness.* 1983;23:67–73.
72. Jackson RT, Merrifield HH. Electromyographic assessment of quadriceps muscle group during knee extension with weighted boot. *Med Sci Sports.* 1972;4:116–119.
73. James SL. Biomechanics of knee ligament reconstruction. *Clin Orthop.* 1980;146:90–101.
74. Johnson D. Controlling anterior shear during isokinetic knee extension exercise. *J Orthop Sports Phys Ther.* 1982;4:23–31.
75. Johnson RJ, Eriksson E, Haggmark T, Pope MH. Five- to ten-year follow-up evaluation after reconstruction of the anterior cruciate ligament. *Clin Orthop.* 1984;183:122–140.
76. Jonsson H, Kärrholm J. Three-dimensional knee joint movements during a step-up: evaluation after anterior cruciate ligament rupture. *J Orthop Res.* 1994;12:769–779.
77. Kålund S, Sinkjaer T, Arendt-Nielsen L, Simonsen O. Altered timing of hamstring muscle action in anterior cruciate ligament deficient patients. *Am J Sports Med.* 1990;18:245–248.
78. Kannus P. Hamstring/quadriceps strength ratios in knees with medial collateral ligament insufficiency. *J Sports Med Phys Fitness.* 1989;29:194–198.
79. Kannus P. Knee flexor and extensor strength ratios with deficiency of the lateral collateral ligament. *Arch Phys Med Rehabil.* 1988;69:928–931.
80. Kannus P. Relationship between peak torque and angle-specific torques in an isokinetic contraction of normal and laterally unstable knees. *J Orthop Sports Phys Ther.* 1991;13:89–94.
81. Kapandji, IA. *The Physiology of the Joints.* New York: Churchill-Livingstone; 1970;2.
82. Kaufman KR, An K, Litchy WJ, et al. Dynamic joint forces during knee isokinetic exercise. *Am J Sports Med.* 1991;19:305–316.
83. Kessler R, Hertling D. *Management of Common Musculoskeletal Disorders.* Philadelphia: Harper & Row; 1983.
84. Kettelkamp DB, Jacobs AW. Tibiofemoral contact area-determination and implications. *J Bone Joint Surg.* 1972;54:349–356.
85. Knight KL, Martin JA, Londeree BR. EMG comparison of quadriceps femoris activity during knee extension and straight leg raises. *Am J Phys Med.* 1979;58:57–69.
86. Krebs DE, Staples WH, Cuttita D, Zickel RE. Knee joint angle: its relationship to quadriceps femoris activity in normal and postarthrotomy limbs. *Arch Phys Med Rehabil.* 1983;64:441–447.
87. Kurosawa H, Yamakoshi K-I, Yasuda K, Sasaki T. Simultaneous measurement of changes in length of the cruciate ligaments during knee motion. *Clin Orthop.* 1991;265:233–240.
88. Lane JG, Irby SE, Kaufman K, et al. The anterior cruciate ligament in controlling axial rotation: an evaluation of its effect. *Am J Sports Med.* 1994;22:289–293.
89. Lass P, Kaalund S, leFevre S, et al. Muscle coordination following rupture of the anterior cruciate ligament. *Acta Orthop Scand.* 1991;62:9–14.
90. Laubenthal KN, Smidt GL, Kettelkamp DB. A quantitative analysis of knee motion during activities of daily living. *Phys Ther.* 1972;52:34–42.
91. Lehmkuhl LD, Smith LK. *Brunnstrom's Clinical Kinesiology.* 5th ed. Philadelphia: FA Davis; 1996.
92. Levy IM, Torzilli PA, Warren RF. The effect of medial meniscectomy on anterior-posterior motion of the knee. *J Bone Joint Surg.* 1982;64:883–888.
93. Lew WD, Lewis JL. The effect of knee-prosthesis geometry on ligament mechanics during flexion. *J Bone Joint Surg.* 1982;64:734–739.
94. Lieb FJ, Perry J. Quadriceps function—an electromyographic study under isometric conditions. *J Bone Joint Surg.* 1971;53:749–758.
95. Lieb FJ, Perry J. Quadriceps function—an anatomical and mechanical study using amputated limbs. *J Bone Joint Surg.* 1968;50:1535–1548.
96. Lindahl O, Movin A, Ringqvist I. Knee extension: measurement of the isometric force in different positions of the knee joint. *Acta Orthop Scand.* 1969;40:79–85.
97. Lipke JM, Janecke CJ, Nelson CL, et al. The role of incompetence of the anterior cruciate and lateral ligaments in anterolateral and anteromedial instability. *J Bone Joint Surg.* 1981;63:954–960.
98. Losee RE. Concepts of the pivot shift. *Clin Orthop.* 1983;172:45–51.
99. Lunnen JD, Yack J, LeVeau BF. Relationship between muscle length, muscle activity, and torque of the hamstring muscles. *Phys Ther.* 1981;61:190–195.
100. Lutz GE, Palmitier RA, An KN, et al. Comparison of tibiofemoral joint forces during open-kinetic-chain and closed-kinetic-chain exercises. *J Bone Joint Surg.* 1993;75(A):732–739.

101. Mann RA, Hagy JL. The popliteus muscle. *J Bone Joint Surg.* 1977;59:924–927.

102. Maquet P. Mechanics and osteoarthritis of the patellofemoral joint. *Clin Orthop.* 1979;144:70–73.

103. Markolf KL, Bargar WL, Shoemaker SC, Amstutz HC. The role of joint load in knee stability. *J Bone Joint Surg.* 1981;63:570–585.

104. Markolf KL, Mensch JS, Amstutz HC. Stiffness and laxity of the knee—the contributions of the supporting structures. *J Bone Joint Surg.* 1976;58:583–594.

105. Matthews LS, Sonstegard DA, Henke JA. Load bearing characteristics of the patello-femoral joint. *Acta Orthop Scand.* 1977;48:511–516.

106. More RC, Karras BT, Neiman R, et al. Hamstrings—an anterior cruciate ligament protagonist. *Am J Sports Med.* 1993;21:231–237.

107. Morrison JB. The mechanics of the knee joint in relation to normal walking. *J Biomech.* 1970;3:51–61.

108. Muller W. *The Knee: Form, Function and Ligament Reconstruction.* Berlin: Springer-Verlag; 1983.

109. Murray MP, Duthie EH, Gambert SR. Age-related differences in knee muscle strength in normal women. *J Gerontol.* 1985;40:275–280.

110. Nicholas JJ, Robinson LR, Logan A, et al. Isokinetic testing in young nonathletic able-bodied subjects. *Arch Phys Med Rehabil.* 1989;70:210–213.

111. Nilsson KG, Kärrholm J, Ekelund L. Knee motion in total knee arthroplasty. *Clin Orthop.* 1990;256:147–161.

112. Noyes FR, Grood ES, Suntay WJ, Butler DL. The three dimensional laxity of the anterior cruciate deficient knee as determined by clinical laxity tests. *Iowa Orthop J.* 1983;3:32–44.

113. Noyes FR, Sonstegrad DA. Biomechanical function of the pes anserinus at the knee and the effect of its transplantation. *J Bone Joint Surg.* 1973;55:1225–1241.

114. Odenstein M, Lysholm J, Gillquist J. Long-term follow up study of a distal iliotibial band transfer (DIT) for anterolateral knee instability. *Clin Orthop.* 1983;176:129–135.

115. Ogden JA. The anatomy and function of the proximal tibiofibular joint. *Clin Orthop.* 1974;101:186–191.

116. Okamoto T. Electromyographic study of the function of muscle rectus femoris. *Research J of Phys Educ.* 1968;12:175–182.

117. Osternig LR, Bates BT, Tseng YL, James SL. Relationship between tibial rotary torque and knee flexion/extension after tendon transplant surgery. *Arch Phys Med Rehabil.* 1981;62:381–385.

118. Osternig LR, Bates BT, James SL. Patterns of tibial rotary torque in knees of healthy subjects. *Med Sci Sports Exerc.* 1980;12:195–199.

119. Otis JC, Gould JD. The effect of external load on torque production by knee extensors. *J Bone Joint Surg.* 1986;68:65–70.

120. Pavone E, Moffat M. Isometric torque of the quadriceps femoris after concentric, eccentric and isometric training. *Arch Phys Med Rehabil.* 1985;66:168–170.

121. Peeples RE, Margo MK. Function after patellectomy. *Clin Orthop.* 1978;132:180–186.

122. Peterson SR, Bagnall KM, Wenger HA, et al. The influence of velocity-specific resistance training on the in vivo torque-velocity relationship and the cross-sectional area of quadriceps femoris. *J Orthop Sports Phys Ther.* 1989;11:456–462.

123. Perry J, Fox JM, Boitano MA, et al. Functional evaluation of the pes anserinus transfer by electromyography and gait analysis. *J Bone Joint Surg.* 1980;62:973–980.

124. Pocock GS. Electromyographic study of the quadriceps during resistive exercise. *J Am Phys Ther Assoc.* 1963;43:427–434.

125. Radin EL, Simon SR, Rose RM, Paul IL. *Practical Biomechanics for the Orthopedic Surgeon.* New York: John Wiley & Sons; 1979.

126. Reilly DT, Martens M. Experimental analysis of the quadriceps muscle force and patello-femoral joint reaction force for various activities. *Acta Orthop Scand.* 1972;43:126–137.

127. Reynolds L, Levin TA, Medeiros JM, et al. EMG activity of the vastus medialis oblique and the vastus lateralis in their role in patellar alignment. *Am J Phys Med.* 1983;62:61–70.

128. Ritter MA, Stringer EA. Predictive range of motion after total knee replacement. *Clin Orthop.* 1979;143:115–119.

129. Rovere GD, Adair DM. Anterior cruciate-deficient knees: a review of the literature. *Am J Sports Med.* 1983;11:412–419.

130. Sailors ME, Keskula DR, Perrin DH. Effect of running on anterior knee laxity in collegiate-level female athletes after anterior cruciate ligament reconstruction. *J Orthop Sports Phys Ther.* 1995;21:233–239.

131. Salzman A, Torburn L, Perry J. Contribution of rectus femoris and vasti to knee extension. *Clin Orthop.* 1993;290:236–243.

132. Scudder GN. Torque curves produced at the knee during isometric and isokinetic exercise. *Arch Phys Med Rehabil.* 1980;61:68–72.

133. Seebacher JR, Inglis AE, Marshall JL, Warren RF. The structure of the posterolateral aspect of the knee. *J Bone Joint Surg.* 1982;64:536–541.

134. Shirakura K, Kato K, Udagawa E. Characteristics of the isokinetic performance of patients with injured cruciate ligaments. *Am J Sports Med.* 1992;20:754–760.

135. Shoemaker SC, Markolf KL. In vivo rotatory knee stability. *J Bone Joint Surg.* 1982;64:208–216.

136. Shrive NG, O'Connor JJ, Goodfellow JW. Load-bearing in the knee joint. *Clin Orthop.* 1978;131:279–287.

137. Simon SR, Trieshmann HW, Burdett RG, et al. Quantitative gait analysis after total knee arthroplasty for monarticular degenerative arthritis. *J Bone Joint Surg.* 1983;65:605–613.

138. Singerman R, Davy DT, Goldberg VM. Effects of patella alta and patella infera on patellofemoral contact forces. *J Biomech.* 1994;27:1059–1065.

139. Smidt GL. Biomechanical analysis of knee flexion and extension. *J Biomech.* 1973;6:79–92.

140. Snow CJ, Cooper J, Quanbury AO, Anderson JE. Antagonist cocontraction of knee flexors during constant velocity muscle shortening and lengthening. *J Electromyogr Kines.* 1993;3:78–86.

141. Soderberg GL, Cook TM. An electromyographic analysis of quadriceps femoris muscle setting and straight leg raising. *Phys Ther.* 1983;63:1434–1438.

142. Soderberg GL, Minor SD, Arnold K, et al. An EMG analysis of quadriceps exercises for patients with knee pathology. *Phys Ther.* 1987;67:1691–1696.

143. Soudan K, Van Audekercke R. Methods, difficulties and inaccuracies in the study of human joint kinematics and pathokinematics by the instant axis concept. Example: the knee joint. *J Biomech.* 1979;12:27–33.

144. Steindler A. *Kinesiology of the Human Body under Normal and Pathological Conditions.* Springfield, IL: Charles C Thomas; 1955.

145. Stratford P. Electromyography of the quadriceps femoris muscles in subjects with normal knees and acutely effused knees. *Phys Ther.* 1982;62:279–283.

146. Sutton FS, Thompson CH, Lipke J, Kettelkamp DB. The effect of patellectomy on knee function. *J Bone Joint Surg.* 1976;58:537–540.

147. Svensson OK, Weidenhielm L. Variability of knee moment arms in the frontal and sagittal planes during normal gait. *Clin Biomech.* 1993;8:59–65.

148. Tamea CD, Henning CE. Pathomechanics of the pivot shift maneuver—an instant center analysis. *Am J Sports Med.* 1981;9:31–37.

149. Thomeé R. *Patellofemoral Pain Syndrome in Young Women.* Göteborg, Sweden: Göteborg University; 1995. Thesis.

150. Thomeé R, Renström P, Karlsson J, Grimby G. Patellofemoral pain syndrome in young women—I. A clinical analysis of alignment, pain parameters, common symptoms and functional activity level. *Scand J Med Sci Sports.* 1995;5:237–244.

151. Thomeé R, Renström P, Karlsson J, Grimby G. Patellofemoral pain syndrome in young women—II. Muscle function in patients and health controls. *Scand J Med Sci Sports.* 1995;5:245–251.

152. Tibone JE, Antich TJ. Electromyographic analysis of the anterior cruciate ligament-deficient knee. *Clin Orthop.* 1993;288:35–39.

153. Torzilli PA, Deng X, Warren RF. The effect of joint-compressive load and quadriceps muscle force on knee motion in the intact and anterior cruciate ligament-sectioned knee. *Am J Sports Med.* 1994;22:105–112.

154. Trudelle-Jackson E, Meske N, Highgenboten C, et al. Eccentric/concentric torque deficits in the quadriceps muscle. *J Orthop Sports Phys Ther.* 1989;11:142–145.

155. van der Leeuw GHF, Stam HJ, van Nieuwenhuyzen JF. Correction for gravity in isokinetic dynamometry of knee extensors in below knee amputees. *Scand J Rehabil Med.* 1989;21:141–145.

156. Vandervoort AA, Kramer JF, Wharram ER. Eccentric knee strength of elderly females. *J Gerontol.* 1990;45:B125–128.

157. van Eijden TMGJ, de Boer W, Verburg J. A dynamometer for the measurement of the extension torque of the lower leg during static and dynamic contractions of the quadriceps femoris muscle. *J Biomech.* 1983;16:1019–1024.

158. Wahrenberg H, Lindbeck L, Ekholm J. Knee muscular moment, tendon tension force and EMG during a vigorous movement in man. *Scand J Rehabil Med.* 1978;10:99–106.

159. Walla DJ, Albright JP, McAuley E, et al. Hamstring control and the unstable anterior cruciate ligament-deficient knee. *Am J Sports Med.* 1985;13:34–39.

160. Wang CJ, Walker PS. Rotatory laxity of the human knee joint. *J Bone Joint Surg.* 1974;56:161–170.

161. Wang CJ, Walker PS, Wolf B. The effects of flexion and rotation on the length patterns of the ligaments of the knee. *J Biomech.* 1973;6:587–596.
162. Warwick R, Williams PL, eds. *Gray's Anatomy.* 35th British ed. Philadelphia: WB Saunders; 1973.
163. Wigerstad-Lossing I, Grimby G, Jonsson T. Effects of electrical muscular stimulation combined with voluntary contraction after knee ligament surgery. *Med Sci Sports Exerc.* 1988;20:93–98.
164. Wild JJ, Franklin TD, Woods GW. Patellar pain and quadriceps rehabilitation: an emg study. *Am J Sports Med.* 1982;10:12–15.
165. Woo SL-Y, Livesay GA, Engle C. Biomechanics of the human anterior cruciate ligament—ACL structure and role in knee motion. *Orthop Rev.* 1992;21:835–842.
166. Wyatt MP, Edwards AM. Comparison of quadriceps and hamstring torque values during isokinetic exercise. *J Orthop Sports Phys Ther.* 1981;3:48–56.
167. Yack HJ, Riley LM, Whieldon TR. Anterior tibial translation during progressive loading of the ACL-deficient knee during weight-bearing and nonweight-bearing isometric exercise. *J Orthop Sports Phys Ther.* 1994;20:247–253.
168. Yost JG, Chekofsky K, Schoscheim P, et al. Intra-articular iliotibial band reconstruction for anterior cruciate ligament insufficiency. *Am J Sports Med.* 1981;9:220–224.
169. Zaricznyj B. Reconstruction of the anterior cruciate ligament using free tendon graft. *Am J Sports Med.* 1983;11:164–176.

12

Ankle and Foot

The ankle and foot are a complex series of joints whose integrity is maintained primarily by an expansive ligamentous network. Yet, these joints and their interactions are responsible for activities such as jumping (propulsion and the rapid elevation of the body into space). Compared with the knee, little is known about the ankle and foot. In fact, much of what is known comes from studies of gait. However, pathologies of the ankle and foot are just as incapacitating as knee problems. This chapter will focus first on normal function, then on biomechanics, and finally on pathokinesiology.

TERMINOLOGY

Because of the multiplicity of joints and variety of terms concerning the ankle and foot, it is necessary to define the commonly used descriptors of ankle and foot motion. The ankle is the joint formed by the tibia, fibula, and talus. The foot includes all the joints distal to the ankle; in general, the five metatarsals and the phalanges comprise the forefoot. The midfoot consists of the cuneiform, navicular, and cuboid bones while the hindfoot (rearfoot) includes the talus and calcaneus (51). Plantarflexion and dorsiflexion will be considered the motion about a horizontal axis through the ankle that lies in the frontal plane. Subtalar joint motion occurs about an axis oblique to the three axes around which the usual flexion-extension, abduction-adduction, and rotation occur. Pronation consists of dorsiflexion, eversion, and abduction. Eversion occurs about an axis running in the anteroposterior direction of the foot. Abduction, in the special case of the foot, occurs around a vertical axis. Supination, in contrast, is the result of combined inversion, adduction, and plantarflexion. Note that eversion and inversion are components of pronation and supination, respectively. Reference is also commonly made to forefoot adduction and abduction, but realize that these movements take place about a vertical axis. Similarly, hindfoot "valgus" and "eversion" are synonymous. Some have attempted to standardize the descriptors, yet no one system is universally accepted. Although the most common systems will be presented here, the reader should be prepared to interpret and apply other systems that may appear in the literature.

MUSCULAR ACTIONS

The actions of the muscles affecting the ankle and foot complex defy simple interpretation for several reasons. First, the muscles originate from an area ranging from the posterior, distal aspect of the femur to the small bones of the distal foot. In addition, most muscles cross many joints, therefore giving the potential actions great diversity. The multiple joint crossings also have implications for length-tension considerations. Finally, whether the foot is fixed (closed kinetic chain) or free (open chain) will determine if the leg will move about the foot, as in gait, or the foot about the leg. Although some early work on muscle function was hampered by little positional

311

information on the axes of the ankle and foot joints, some determinations have been made as to muscle function.

Ankle

Any muscle attached to the femur or to any structures in the lower leg and projecting to the foot will affect the ankle. Often considered of primary interest are the gastrocnemius and the soleus muscles, collectively labeled as the **triceps surae.** Due to the femoral attachment of the gastrocnemius, this muscle can more profoundly affect plantarflexion of the ankle when the knee is in an extended (muscle lengthened) position. In essence, quadriceps contraction facilitates an increased plantarflexion moment by virtue of stretch applied to the gastrocnemius muscle. Many manual muscle tests and clinical tests used for assessing the force exerted by the gastrocnemius and soleus muscles offer knee flexion as a means to differentiate the abilities of the two muscles. Whether the 44 mm shortening of the soleus versus the 39 mm shortening of the gastrocnemius affects the tension generated is unclear (35). The importance of the triceps surae can be realized from data derived in 1911. That work identified cross sections of 23 and 20 cm² for the gastrocnemius and soleus, respectively. These values compare with the total value of 21 cm² for the flexors hallucis and digitorum longus, the tibialis posterior, and the peroneus longus and brevis (41). Because these muscles all pass relatively close to the axis for plantarflexion, clearly the most important musculature for propulsive activities is the triceps surae. It may be significant that the triceps surae concurrently supinates the foot during plantarflexion (35). Even this is in dispute since it has been reported that the medial soleus is active during foot eversion. That this muscle was more active during eversion than inversion was perhaps due to the muscle acting as a restraint to hyperversion by the peroneals (8). This eversion may be because the axis for subtalar motion lies lateral to the insertion of the Achilles tendon on the posterior aspect of the calcaneus. Electromyographic evidence that the gastrocnemius muscle is active in inversion also exists (22).

During standing posture, the gastrocnemius and soleus play different roles. Although both muscles would be in an anatomically advantageous position to generate tension, considerable EMG and histochemical data indicate that the soleus muscle is primarily responsible for producing the plantarflexion moment at the ankle. During support of the body by the foot, the leg is moving over the fixed distal segments that are usually considered the muscle insertion. Whether this reversal has any specific meaning for muscle function is not clear, but the literature shows that the plantarflexors play a role in maintaining the knee in extension during the stance phase of gait (85). More complex analyses have suggested that calf muscle activity be used to restrain forward momentum rather than to propel the body farther (75). More specific attention will be given to this matter in Chapter 15 (Posture, Balance, and Gait).

The roles other muscles play in plantarflexion and their additional motions also raise some interesting points. In plantarflexion, although muscles other than the triceps surae make a minimal contribution, of the five remaining muscles, the peroneals contribute about one-half of the remaining torque (35). Further evidence for the necessity of effective plantarflexion is the stiffness of the sagittal plane motion of the subtalar joint, allowing for transfer of torque to the ankle (20).

Foot

The **peronei** are given credit as the primary producers of forefoot eversion. Yet, the longus reaches all the way to the inner aspect of the foot, demonstrating its capacity to pull the medial aspect of the foot down into the supporting surface. Other explanations for muscle function in arch control can be offered. The peroneus longus tendon passes under the "keystone" or apex of the lateral longitudinal arch and thereby provides a supportive function. The peroneus longus also bowstrings across the transverse arch as the tendon projects to the medial border of the foot. By pulling the medial border toward the lateral border it supports the transverse arch that bridges between the two longitudinal arches. Furthermore, the tibialis posterior inserts at the apex of the medial longitudinal arch and also serves a supportive role. The peroneus longus and posterior tibialis together form a sling.

In the functional closed-kinetic chain, however, body weight passively produces pronation, rather than requiring muscle activity to pull the bones down. This action, combined with the motions of the triceps surae, provides an excellent example of the synergistic action of muscles in producing more effective plantarflexion. This is probably true though plantarflexion was a secondary function of the peroneus longus and the posterior tibialis muscles (1).

Supinator muscles include the group on the medial aspect of the ankle mortise. The posterior tibialis is clearly important to this function. Although the anterior tibialis is still regarded as responsible for inversion, its line of action lies almost precisely along the subtalar axis, thereby negating motion around this axis. The anterior tibialis and the extensors digitorum and hallucis longus together provide an excellent balance for dorsiflexion of the foot. Generally, small cross sections are observed in these muscles because of the low torques required in this direction of motion. Returning to the medial aspect of the ankle, the role of these muscles in supporting the longitudinal arch has been long debated. EMG data show that the muscles potentially responsible are active only at low levels and over very short intervals (4). The attachment of the posterior tibialis, by means of a sling arrangement spanning several tarsal bones, is in an anatomically advantageous position to support the longitudinal arch (87). Evidence that loss of this muscle leads to a collapse of the arch provides support for the role of this muscle (20). Perhaps the muscle, tendon, and other soft tissues are also elongated if direct and/or aperiodic muscle support is lost. Other muscular actions of these extrinsic muscles are specific to the locus of attachment. For example, a long toe extensor serves to extend the toes, whether the muscle is attached to the hallux or the remaining digits.

The other muscles affecting the function of the foot are the **intrinsic** muscles. Found predominantly on the plantar aspect of the foot, these muscles assist in propulsion and potentially affect the position of the arch. Although the structure of the interossei and lumbrical differs from the hand, their positions and functions are very similar. An imbalance of forces among these muscles can lead to decreased function and abnormal joint position; however, when this occurs in the hand it is much more incapacitating than in the foot, where gross movements often suffice. Some attention should, however, be given to the influence of the plantar fascia and ligaments, because attachments spanning the tarsals allow the structures to act much like a truss (Fig. 12.1). The extremely high tensile strength of the fascia, coupled with its tensile stiffness, makes the fascia an ideal structure for the receipt of repetitive loads such as occur during walking. In such dynamic cases the toes are brought, by either an active or passive process, into dorsiflexion. Because the fascia inserts distally at the metatarsophalangeal joints, the fascia becomes tighter as the toes are dorsiflexed. Thus, as body weight passes forward over the foot the fascia tightens and raises the longitudinal arch (20, 87).

Others have considered supination to occur simultaneously with this **windlass**

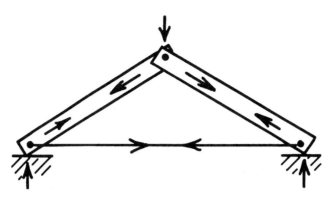

Figure 12.1. Schematic representation of a truss. Here, the two bony segments are pinned together at each end. The tie across the bottom functions like the plantar fascia.

effect of the plantar fascia. Supination is responsible for the close-packed position of the tarsals and produces a "rigid lever" for propulsion (15). By this mechanism the foot provides a stable segment about which the rest of the body may move. Without such a rigid system in the most distal segment, motion in the more proximal segments could not be carried out as effectively. Static conditions produce a similar effect in that tarsal bones have relatively tight interfaces that assist in constraining motion. Although motion can occur in many joints, the ligaments of the foot also are partly responsible for limiting motion, thus providing a rigid structure under static and dynamic conditions (20).

ARTHROLOGY AND ARTHROKINEMATICS
Ankle

The ankle mortise, also known as the **talocrural joint,** is composed of three bones: the tibia, fibula, and talus. The distal end of the tibia is expanded in both anteroposterior and mediolateral directions. Matching the inferior aspect of the tibia is the convex surface of the talus. Often called the dome of the talus or the trochlear region, the articular surface is wider anteriorly than posteriorly. Perhaps most important is that the radius of curvature of the medial segment is smaller anteriorly than posteriorly compared with the lateral trochlea whose radius seems constant from anterior to posterior (29). This mediolateral difference in radius is responsible for the ankle kinematics described later. The articulations of the talus with the medial and lateral malleoli and of the inferior tibiofibular joint are perhaps unimportant except for stability. Another fact pertinent to pathologies is that the lateral malleolus is smaller and projects more distally than does the medial.

Stability of the joint, primarily in medial and lateral directions, is maintained by the expansive medial and the smaller, more specific lateral ligaments. By connecting specific bony structures, each set of ligaments normalizes joint kinematics and prevents abnormal ranges of movement. Detailed presentation of these ligaments is available (35), but is outside the scope of this text. Reference to several of these structures is included in the section on pathokinesiology.

Understanding the kinematics of the ankle depends on knowledge of the bony shapes previously described. The tapering of the trochlea from anterior to posterior and the different radii of curvature of the medial and lateral aspects account for asymmetry and thus the conjunct rotation seen with ankle dorsiflexion and plan-tarflexion. The greater length of the trochlear surface in the posterior direction also determines that plantarflexion has a greater range of motion than does dorsiflexion. Extremes of motion in either direction are limited either by bony impingement, capsular or ligamentous constraints, or available length of muscles and tendons antagonistic to the attempted motion (35).

Other principles of joint motion, such as the movement of convex on concave surfaces (or vice versa), also apply to the ankle and should not need restatement. The close-packed position of the ankle is considered the position of extreme dorsi-flexion (14). According to Kapandji, the slight spreading of the malleoli and rotation of the fibula occurring upon extreme dorsiflexion become important only if such spreading is severely restricted (35). Conversely, excess spread can lead to a widened mortise and an unstable ankle.

Subtalar

The subtalar joint is complicated: two or three talar facets, depending on how they are considered, articulate with the calcaneus. In essence, both the posterior and anterior facets (perhaps further divided into anterior and middle) are complex, slightly curved surfaces. The posterior articulation of the calcaneus on the talus is convex on concave, respectively (66). The anteromedial facet surfaces also are convex on concave (37). The latter surface, or surfaces, are supported by the bony shelf of the calcaneus: the sustentaculum tali. Using the principles of motion behavior of articulating curved surfaces (Chapter 4) movement of these articulating surfaces rapidly becomes complicated. How the surfaces interact to produce the motions about the subtalar axis has been described in detail, but essentially, motions of the subtalar joint are produced by the combined action of all the articulating surfaces (14, 17, 66). Recall from the opening paragraphs of this chapter that the orientation of the axis of subtalar motion (Fig. 12.2) requires a three-plane description of the resulting movement. Therefore, during supination the calcaneus moves distally (plan-tarflexion), medially (adduction), and rotates around the longitudinal axis of the foot to lie on the lateral surface (inversion). Pronation creates the opposite motions (Fig. 12.3).

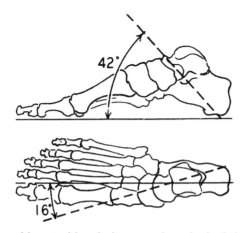

Figure 12.2.   The position of the axis of the subtalar joint is shown by the dashed line in each projection.

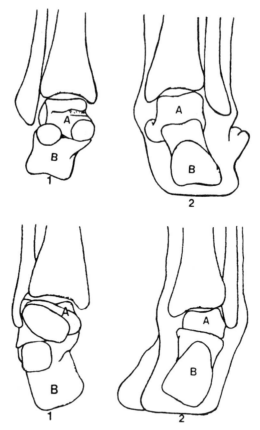

Figure 12.3.   Closed kinetic chain pronation (*upper*) and supination (*lower*) for anterior (*1*) and posterior (*2*) views of the ankle and foot. *Legend: A,* talus; *B,* calcaneus.

The ligaments also influence motion. Detailed accounts of their role have been presented in the literature (66) but are probably not of specific concern to the therapist. Kapandji maintains that the essential ligament of this joint is the interosseus talocalcaneal ligament consisting of anterior and posterior segments (35). This structure passes from the sulcus tali to the sulcus calcanei and becomes tight during the motion of eversion (90). It also has been identified as playing a role in stabilizing this joint during both static and dynamic activities (35).

Transverse Tarsal

This joint, also called the midtarsal joint, is composed of two articulations, the talus with the navicular and the calcaneus with the cuboid bone (58). Commonly the two joints are considered together because they are functionally similar. The **talonavicular** joint is unremarkable as the rounded head of the talus matches the concavity of the posterior surface of the navicular bone. The **calcaneocuboid** joint is relatively complex, and like the talonavicular joint is tightly bound with multiple ligaments (14).

Motion at the midtarsal joint is constrained by means of ligaments and the matching of articular surfaces. Although the talonavicular joint is considered to have three degrees of freedom, the adjacent calcaneocuboid joint (with only two degrees of freedom) and the tightness of the joint between the calcaneus and navicular restrict midtarsal movement. As described later, the axis for motion is similar in location and orientation to the axis of the subtalar joint. Because of the interaction of these two joints, the motions of most relevance are inversion and eversion (37).

General Considerations for Ankle and Foot Arthrokinematics

The motions of many bones of the ankle and foot are difficult to describe because of most bones' multiple articular surfaces, the locations of the axes of rotation, and interactions among the joints when moved. To understand that gliding and rotation occur among all surfaces is fundamental. If, for example, one attempts to elevate the medial border of the foot so that the sole faces medially, these gliding and rotary motions occur. The greater part of supination is in the mechanism of the subtalar joint. However, the motion of the calcaneus around the talus facilitates movement at the transverse tarsal joint, the net effect of which is to increase the overall range of inversion. The latter is accomplished by rotation in the talonavicular joint and the downward gliding of the cuboid on the calcaneus. Finally, recall that in plantarflexion the dome of the talus is narrower, allowing for additional inversion range through talar tilt within the ankle mortise (90).

Thus, motions of the ankle and foot are composites, meaning that isolated movements of individual segments cannot occur without interacting with other joints and causing changes in the amount of surface congruity. A complete description of foot arthrokinematics would also include the other joints not addressed in earlier sections. However, most motion in the tarsal and metatarsal joints and the phalanges is planar and probably much less important than the motions in the three joints described. More detailed accounts are available (14, 35, 36). At any rate, effective management of the patient with involvement of the ankle and foot will surely depend on the knowledge of their normal arthrokinematics.

The complexity of joint structure and function has important implications for the measurements the clinician can make. Reliable measurements can apparently be made by one therapist for ankle range of motion but the coefficient deteriorates when evaluating between therapist data (95). Most measurements have focused on the ability to measure subtalar joint motion. While one study assessed reliability of measuring rearfoot motion, the work was not designed to examine within or between therapist measures, but rather the reliability of reducing motion analysis data (52). While some have called for measurements in both weight-bearing and non-weight-bearing positions (40), several studies have shown that measurements from either position are not acceptably reliable (16, 61, 78). The only exception is for the interrater measurements for weight bearing in one study (78). These results have probably led to the development and evaluation of other techniques for assessing subtalar joint position, such as the navicular height and the calcaneal position measured with an inclinometer. In this instance the weight-bearing measures were judged to have acceptable intertherapist and intratherapist reliability (70).

BIOMECHANICS
Kinematics

Angular displacements of the ankle and foot have been extensively described. Sagittal plane motion in the ankle appears to total about 80°, 50° of which is available in plantarflexion (35). Lesser values have been reported, particularly if the limb is bearing weight. Less range is also required in the ankle during functional activities such as gait. Functionally, a greater range is available due to the contribution of the forefoot, as in the ability of an adept ballerina. Motion at the subtalar joint is more difficult to isolate and quantify. Total range of values is generally reported to be from 17 to 24°, but Kapandji states that supination range is 52° while pronation is limited to 25–30° (35). Of the total range, 25–30° is likely due to inversion with 5–10° accountable to eversion (66). Subotnick, however, suggests that a minimum of 18° of supination is necessary for subtalar joint function (83). Transverse tarsal joint motion has also been determined, specifying that midtarsal range was 8° about the longitudinal foot axis and 22° about an oblique axis (described later in the section on axes and instant centers of rotation) (27).

Arches of the Foot

Most descriptions of the foot include a discussion of three **arches:** transverse, medial longitudinal, and lateral longitudinal. The medial is seemingly the most important because of the consequences for alterations in total foot mechanics should the medial longitudinal arch undergo significant change. MacConaill and Basmajian (45) describe the foot as a twisted plate that generates what most call the longitudinal arches. For the lateral arch the posterior support is the calcaneus, the keystone is the cuboid, and the fourth and fifth metatarsal heads the anterior support. Further twisting or untwisting of the arches can be accomplished by muscular actions and/ or by combined motions of the ankle and foot. These mechanisms will be discussed in subsequent paragraphs.

The longitudinal arches of the foot have been extensively discussed in relation to the ability to bear weight. Three potential mechanisms exist in the foot for this purpose. First, note that the metatarsals form a bony transverse bow that is convex superiorly. This arrangement allows the bones to act as beams to support body weight effectively. Although the middle three metatarsals may appear to be too small to resist loading effectively, the collective ability of these bones shows them capable of supporting at least three or four times body weight. A second mechanism capable of load bearing is the truss-like configuration of the foot. In this situation the longitudinal bony configuration is supported by ligaments and the plantar aponeurosis. If in fact the bones were not constrained by these soft tissues, the bones could spread apart, leading to the demise of the longitudinal arches. Recall also that the configuration of the longitudinal arches can be altered by means of changes in tension in the plantar aponeurosis as detailed in previous sections of this chapter. The third possible mechanism for arch control, muscular tension, has been discussed previously. In any event, if muscles such as the peroneus longus and tibialis posterior were active, about 15–20% of the body weight could be supported (34). In summary, several mechanisms manage the load created by body weight. Probably no single factor accounts for the ability of the foot to manage the repetitive, high loads that must be tolerated. The suggestion has even been made that management may be in combination, for example, 25% by beam and 50–75% by arch (28).

Axes and Instant Centers of Rotation

The analyses of the ankle, subtalar, and midtarsal joints all have included study of the axes of rotation of the respective joints. Compared with the ankle, the axes have been specified for the transverse and frontal planes (Fig. 12.4) (46), with only minor deviations appearing in the literature (88). Although the ankle axis is 20–30° displaced compared with the axis of the knee, this has few implications for the arthrokinematics

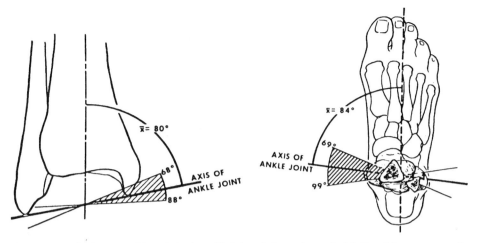

Figure 12.4.   The location of the axis for the ankle joint relative to the vertical (*left*) and the anteroposterior (*right*) directions. Both the means and the extreme locations of the axis are shown for both planes.

of the ankle or foot (46). Some years ago rather extensive work was completed on the location of the instant center of rotation of the ankle (65). For the 22 ankles studied from positions of plantar flexion through dorsiflexion, in only 12 ankles did the instant center of rotation remain in the talus throughout the range of motion. Sample determinations for weight-bearing and non-weight-bearing ankles are shown in Figure 12.5. Note that in the weight-bearing ankle an instant center of rotation lies outside the body of the talus. The investigators also remarked that the normal ankle showed distraction tendencies in the early range of plantarflexion, followed by sliding in the midportion, and compression as the close-packed position was reached toward the limit of dorsiflexion.

The position of the subtalar axis has been defined in cadavers since 1941. Both a vertical and a horizontal reference frame were used to define the axis position compared with the foot. The axis was inclined anteriorly by 42° with respect to the plantar surface of the foot. In the other plane it was medially deviated an average of 16° from the plane that bisected the calcaneus and the first web space (see Fig. 12.2). More recent work confirms these axis locations, demonstrating a 37° inclination and an 18° medial deviation (88). Manter (49) further observed that the plane of rotation of the subtalar joint was not at a right angle to the joint axis. Because "sideways slipping" could not occur, the conclusion was reached that subtalar motion was rotational with an average helix of 12°. Thus, the osteokinematics create a screw-like action of the subtalar joint (Fig. 12.6). Many studies have been completed since this original work. One example was a case where only 20 of 58 specimens showed constant increments of linear displacement that would be consistent with a true screw. Although the helix angle was determined to be only 7.9°, the deviation of these data from the original work is considered small (29).

Axes at the transverse tarsal joint have also been defined. This work led to the identification of two composite axes, a longitudinal and an oblique (Fig. 12.7). Forefoot inversion and eversion would be the movements about the former axis while plantarflexion combined with adduction and dorsiflexion combined with abduction would occur about the oblique axis. More extensive work identified two axes each for the calcaneocuboid and the talonavicular joints. Because of the orientation of

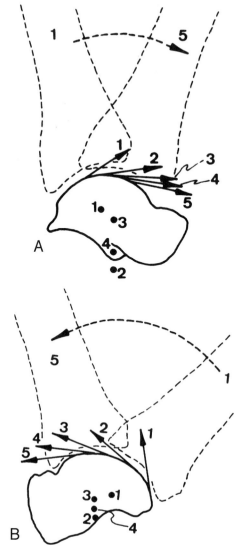

Figure 12.5.   The instant center of rotation for the ankle joint during dorsiflexion in the weight- bearing (**A**) and (**B**) non-weight-bearing ankle. Points numbered 1 through 4 show the location of the instant centers. The vectors represent surface velocities, indicating that primarily shear is taking place.

the axes, pronation of the subtalar joint forced the axes into a parallel position and subsequently allowed free movement of the forefoot. Supination caused a limitation of motion in the forefoot because the movements at the calcaneocuboid and talonavi-cular joints opposed each other (15).

Because the interaction of the tibia and foot is important for control of the body on the foot, i.e., in posture and gait, an understanding of the movements involved may prove helpful. To emphasize that the subtalar joint provides rotation between the foot and tibia, the joint can be described as an oblique hinge. In short, as the tibia is externally rotated the foot assumes a more supinated position. This phenome-non can be easily shown by placing the foot lightly on the floor and rotating the tibia.

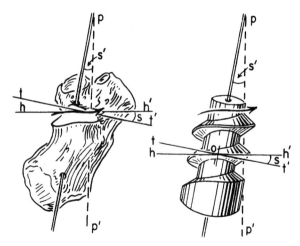

Figure 12.6. Comparative view of the posterior calcaneal facet of the right subtalar joint with a right hand screw. The horizontal plane in which the motion is occurring is indicated with h-h' and t-t' is a plane perpendicular to the screw axis. The angle s' equal to s, the helix angle of the screw. Note that s' is determined by dropping a vertical line from point p to p'. The arrow depicts the path of the body following the screw.

Conversely, internal rotation of the tibia will produce pronation and a subsequent flattening of the medial longitudinal arch (18, 45). The interactions of tibial rotation, subtalar, and midtarsal motion are summarized in Figure 12.8.

Torque

The measurement of torque at the ankle must be interpreted with some caution because multiple joints of the ankle and foot are included in the determinations. If testing conditions are not similar across trials, clinics, or studies, comparisons are difficult or impossible to make. Partly for these reasons a methodological study of

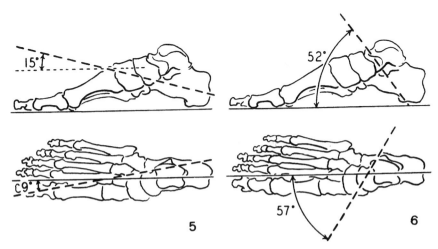

Figure 12.7. Longitudinal (*left*) and oblique (*right*) axes of the transverse tarsal joints for the lateral (*top*) and anteroposterior (*bottom*) views of the foot.

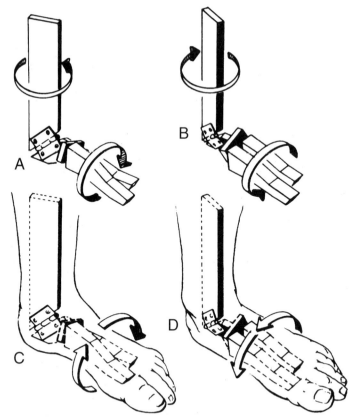

Figure 12.8.   The effects of internal and external rotation on the subtalar and transverse tarsal joints. Consider the external rotation of the tibia in **A** and **C;** concurrently, the subtalar joint supinates. The transverse tarsal joint is made more rigid because the two axes of this joint, shown in Figure 12.7, become less parallel to each other. In **B** and **D** the opposite occurs, including laxity in the transverse tarsal joint because the axes are now more parallel to each other.

ankle torque was completed, finding that errors varied between 5 and 10%. Changes in ankle position caused great differences in the recorded torque values, leading to larger errors when measurements were made of peak torque values (57).

Several data sets are available in the literature that allow for some assessment of ankle plantar flexion torque. One study of 10 adult subjects determined that with the ankle in the neutral position, 113 Nm of isometric torque was produced in an open-kinetic chain arrangement. Plantarflexion of 15° and 30° decreased the values to 83 and 65 Nms, respectively. However, 15° of dorsiflexion caused the torque to increase to 134 Nm (57). Another study provided information on the plantarflexors, showing torque to be greater by 15% when the knee was extended as compared with 90° of knee flexion. Isometric plantarflexion values ranged from 110 to 140 Nm for their group of 30 young men (21). Another study, using various age groups of both sexes, has shown plantarflexion torque values for young men and women to range from 30 to 122 Nm when isometric testing was performed in the neutral position. These investigators concluded that significant torque differences were due to weight and age and not to the subjects' sex or height (19).

Isokinetic dynamometers have also been used to study ankle plantarflexion torque.

A test protocol completed at 30, 90, and 180° per second produced values of 101, 54, and 27 Nm, respectively (57). Another evaluation provided similar results in that torque was about 100 Nm at 30°/sec and diminished to 40 Nm at 180°/sec (21). Falkel (19) tested only at 30°/sec and determined values that ranged from 29 to 106 Nm for young adult men and women (Table 12.1).

Less objective data are available for dorsiflexion, perhaps because of the relatively small torque needed for effective function. Representative findings for dorsiflexion performed isometrically by normal young adult subjects range from 29 to 31 Nm in the neutral position of the ankle. As could be anticipated, data from 60 and 180° per second isokinetic trials were less: 24 and 13 Nm, respectively (5).

Inversion and eversion torques have also been measured in two separate groups of normal subjects (43, 44). Table 12.1 summarizes the results for the variety of conditions tested. In one study, reliability was improved when range of motion targets were improved. No difference was elicited when tests were performed at two angles of plantarflexion (44). The other study concluded that the knee angle influences the test results, the angle of 70° of flexion allowing for participation by the hamstrings and other tibial rotators (43). Finally, how torques at the subtalar joint during single limb stance and just before movement will translate to meaningful information is not yet clear. Applications may be more in the arena of control of balance (24).

KINETICS
Ankle

Information about the kinetics of the ankle and foot is sparse when compared with that available for the knee and hip. The primary reason is that the ankle is less prone to osteoarthritic (osteoarthrotic) changes, therefore creating less joint pathology than encountered in other joints of the lower limb. Considerable attention has been paid, however, to the transmission of loads and the mechanics of the foot during gait. Thus, in most circumstances the kinetics of the ankle and foot have been considered under dynamic conditions.

Under static conditions, such as in the assumption of the symmetrical standing posture, the joint reaction forces are rather easy to determine. The magnitudes of these forces would be one-half body weight plus the force resulting from contraction of musculature that crosses the joint. Because minimal muscle contraction is required during normal standing posture, the joint reaction forces are relatively low. Rising to tiptoe on one leg will increase the force to more than two times body weight for two reasons: the entire body weight is supported by one limb and the plantarflexors are now required to sustain a strong contraction (20). One would expect forces during gait and other dynamic activities to increase the compressive force in the ankle joint. Stauffer and coworkers have shown this in their analytic work on the ankle. Their data showed a compressive force about three times body weight from heel strike to foot flat and a further rise to a peak value of 4.5–5.5 times body weight during heel off when the plantarflexors were undergoing strong contraction (Fig. 12.9) (79). These data agree well with the maximal ankle joint reaction forces of 5.2 times body weight derived from a mathematical model, but differ slightly from the 3.9 times body weight peak found by others (63, 71). Consideration of the ankle cannot ignore the presence of tangential or shear force. This force was in the posterior direction, i.e., the talus tending toward posterior movement on the mortise, during most of the stance phase of gait. Magnitude was just over 0.6 times body weight.

Table 12.1. Normative Ankle Torque Values

Source Reference	Gender	Age Mean	Age SD	Age Range	n	Movement	Concentric (°/sec)	Eccentric (°/sec)	ROM	Testing Position	Peak Torque Nm	Peak Torque SD	Testing Device
44	f			20–33	20	ev	30			sup, ank 0	21	3	Cybex II
						ev	30			sup, ank pf 20	23	4	
						inv	30			sup, ank 0	26	5	
						inv	30			sup, ank pf 20	25	3	
						ev	120			sup, ank 0	12	3	
						ev	120			sup, ank pf 20	13	3	
						inv	120			sup, ank 0	19	4	
						inv	120			sup, ank pf 20	17	3	
26	m			18–35	15	ev	90			sidelying	19	3	Lido
						inv	90			sidelying	23	2	
	f			18–35		ev	90			sidelying	9	2	
						inv	90			sidelying	11	2	
92	m	32	15	20–75	21	inv	30			sup, hip 55, kn 55	32	8	Cybex II
						ev	30			sup, hip 55, kn 55	28	8	
						inv	60			sup, hip 55, kn 55	23	7	
						ev	60			sup, hip 55, kn 55	24	7	
						inv	120			sup, hip 55, kn 55	23	5	
						ev	120			sup, hip 55, kn 55	20	4	
	f	32	15	20–75	23	inv	30			sup, hip 55, kn 55	24	6	Cybex II
						ev	30			sup, hip 55, kn 55	20	3	
						inv	60			sup, hip 55, kn 55	20	4	
						ev	60			sup, hip 55, kn 55	16	2	
						inv	120			sup, hip 55, kn 55	16	4	
						ev	120			sup, hip 55, kn 55	14	2	
19	m	7	1		20	pf	0			sit	17	10	Cybex II
		7	1			pf	30			sit	9	3	
		15	1			pf	0			sit	53	17	
		15	2			pf	30			sit	36	13	
		25	2			pf	0			sit	87	41	
		25	1			pf	30			sit	71	15	
	f	7	1		20	pf	0			sit	15	7	Cybex II
		7	1			pf	30			sit	15	7	
		15	1			pf	0			sit	48	22	
		15	1			pf	30			sit	34	14	
		24	1			pf	0			sit	57	17	
		24				pf	30			sit	45	11	

Legend: ank, ankle; ev, eversion; inv, inversion; kn, knee; pf, plantar flexion; sup, supine.

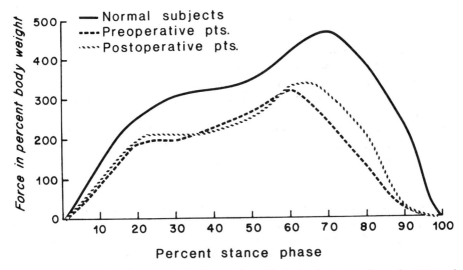

Figure 12.9. Mean values for compressive force at the ankle during the stance phase of gait. Note the similar pattern but smaller forces in the patient groups.

After 80% of stance phase had passed, talocrural shear was anterior and less than 50% of the magnitude produced in the early weight-bearing phases (79).

Also of relevance is the **contact area** available in the ankle. Unpublished data, cited in other work (94), show that the load bearing surface of the ankle is from 11 to 13 cm². This relatively large area can be responsible for the low loads per unit area, potentially offering a sound reason for the low incidence of osteoarthrosis. Of further interest is the demonstration that under small loads achieved during the early stance phase of gait, the contact areas on the talus are two distinct oblong areas on its medial and lateral aspects. As the load is increased the distribution of the pressure changes so that the load is distributed over the entire superior surface of the talus. Thus, the maximal area for load transfer is used, minimizing the force per unit area.

Subtalar

Little information is available on the kinetics of the subtalar or other joints of the foot, probably because of the complexities associated with the joint mechanics. Little truly objective data are available, and the analyses usually result from either clinical evaluations or mathematical models. To describe the events functionally, the mechanisms can be discussed in terms of the gait cycle. Eversion in the subtalar joint is hastened at heel strike by two mechanisms. The first is caused by off-center (eccentric) loading of the foot, that is, when body weight is considered relative to the center of rotation in the subtalar joint (Fig. 12.10). Thus, in such circumstances the calcaneus is forced somewhat anteriorly and also laterally into a valgus position. Simultaneously, the talus is shifting medially and downward. Further, this internal rotation of the talus is responsible for inducing internal rotation of the tibia and thus perpetuating eversion in the subtalar joint (59). Apparently these 10° of motion occurs within the first 8% of the stance phase of the average walking cycle (58). Only during the terminal stance phase does supination reverse the cycle (59). Further discussion of these issues occurs in a later section on gait.

The only objective data that exist on the subtalar joint have been provided by

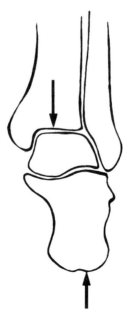

Figure 12.10.   The loading effect on the ankle. Calcaneal floor contact (*bottom arrow*) is lateral to the force due to body weight (*top arrow*), causing potential eversion in the subtalar joint.

mathematical modeling. In this case the peak resultant force in the anterior facet of the talocalcaneonavicular joint was 2.4 times body weight. The average peak force for the posterior facet was 2.8 times body weight and also occurred in the late stance phase of the gait cycle (63).

Soft Tissues

A discussion of the forces in the ankle and foot would be incomplete without the inclusion of **tendinous and ligamentous forces.** Little information is available regarding the forces of such structures. The Stauffer group (79) thought the tibialis anterior tendon force to be of negligible importance in their study of the ankle joint since the magnitude of tensile loading is probably 20% of body weight or less. Further, electromyographic data show that the muscle contracts for a very short time, primarily at the end of the swing phase of the gait cycle. Force in the Achilles tendon is much greater and accounts for a good portion of the compressive force across the ankle.

Analyses of restraining effects and failure in the ligaments of the foot and ankle have also been performed. One of these ligaments, the anterior talofibular ligament, is considered of particular significance because of the control this ligament may have on talar motion. The literature disagrees as to the role of the ligament, primarily in the amount of allowed talar tilt. Johnson and Markolf (33) have studied 30 cadaver ankles in an attempt to more definitively determine the effects of the anterior talofibular ligament section. Overall, they found that ankle laxity depended on position. The least motion was found in the dorsiflexed position, confirming that this is the close-packed position of the joint. Section of the ligament significantly increased anterior-posterior laxity, but greatest increases in motion were seen in inversion-eversion (5.2°) and in internal-external rotation (10.8°) in the position of plantarflexion. Because of the importance of the anterior talofibular ligament in controlling these motions the ligament is felt to be a prime stabilizer of the ankle and an indirect stabilizer of the subtalar joint.

An understanding of the ligaments has also been aided by evaluation of their tensile strength, in that cadaver tests have shown a wide variation in the tensile strength of the anterior talofibular ligament. This ligament has been noted to have the weakest tensile strength (6) as compared with the deltoid ligament, which was shown to be able to sustain the highest load before failure (2). The talofibular load of 206 N was derived from a range of 58 to 556 N, identifying almost a tenfold increase in the difference found among ankles. Midsubstance failures and bony attachment site failures were about equally divided, creating greater difficulty in the ability to account for the variability seen across specimens (82). A low tensile failure level of 3 N was established after anterior talofibular ligament section in some specimens; this may affect some cases of ankle sprains, many of which will injure the anterior tibiofibular ligament (33).

PATHOKINESIOLOGY

Many pathologies produce abnormalities in the foot that lead to disruptions of normal mechanics. Such conditions lead to potentially disabling circumstances, because motion of the proximal segments of the body depends on the most distal segment of the lower limb being adequately related to the supporting surface. Discussed in this section will be common mechanical problems, the influence of muscular function, and the effect of overuse syndromes. Results of arthroplasties and the changes produced by various pathologies on the forces measured under the foot will also be presented.

Mechanical Behavior

Because the foot and ankle are located most distally in the limb, the joints comprising these segments are responsible for allowing effective weight reception and for generating the torque required for propulsion. Thus, as in most other joints, the mechanism must be flexible yet allow for adequate control. Various pathologies, whether in the forefoot or hindfoot, are known to affect most of the population. Although hindfoot varus has been identified, a far more pervasive problem is forefoot varus. This condition contributes to abnormal compensatory pronation in the subtalar joint so that a more equal weight distribution may occur on the metatarsal heads during stance (86). Such pronation, coupled with midtarsal joint unlocking, causes instability of the forefoot and renders this segment of the propulsive device ineffective. Sgarlato states that pronation beyond 50% of stance phase in gait causes foot unlocking and instability at heel lift as well as shearing and subluxation at the subtalar joint (73).

A significant consequence of pronation is the effect on the foot's arches and the implications for arch changes on foot and ankle mechanics. Long-term stress on the soft tissues most likely elongates them and alters the positions of the bony segments relative to each other. Subsequently, pronation can lead to poor positioning, manifested most often as loss of height in the medial longitudinal arch of the foot. Manifestations can be local but are often reported to be more proximal (18, 62). Since there is a reasonable amount of evidence that musculature provides little support of the arch, the maintenance of joint integrity and control would be important. This flatfoot condition can occur in children from alterations in connective tissue composition, bony structure, or inadequate development of muscular mechanisms (3).

In adults the most common etiologies of acquired flatfoot are arthritis, rupture of the posterior tibial tendon, and profound peripheral neuritis conditions (48). According to McPoil and Brocato, five foot types cause subtalar joint compensation as manifested by abnormal pronation: forefoot varus, forefoot valgus, rearfoot varus, tibia vara, and equinus deformity (51).

Management of the pronated foot consists of many methods, including surgery, exercise, and the use of a foot orthosis. In many surgical cases, joint mechanics are significantly altered, and sometimes bones are fused. Exercise has been generally conceded to be ineffective because of the apparent inability of the musculature to support the arch adequately, particularly over extended periods. The most recently developed treatment mode, that of the balanced foot orthosis, achieves forefoot equilibrium by placing a wedge or post under the medial forefoot (73). This technique can thus eliminate the necessity for abnormal compensatory pronation during the stance phase of gait. The effectiveness of this or similar methods, however, is controversial (7, 31). Another investigator has shown that use of an orthosis significantly decreased mean foot pronation during standing immediately after and four weeks after application of the orthosis. Other results showed an orthosis to be ineffective in decreasing mean foot pronation during walking when testing was done immediately after application. However, significant decreases were noted in the midstance and late stance phases of gait after four weeks of use (76). Whether this treatment makes additional changes or has long-term effects is awaiting further research.

Gait

Because of the dependency on the foot and ankle for receipt of load and its distribution up the lower extremity, there has been considerable focus on the mechanics during both running and walking. The literature contains many discussions of both the normal and pathomechanics of the foot and ankle (9, 12, 14, 46, 50, 51, 72, 73). Considerable effort will continue to determine how the mechanics of the ankle and foot affect the dynamics of the lower extremity.

The motion patterns of the subtalar joint were described in the previous section on subtalar kinetics. A more functional summary is provided in Figure 12.11. During the first 15% of the cycle, the foot rapidly adapts to the supporting surface. Note that many changes in motions or levels of muscular activity occur at 15% of the cycle, the point at which foot flat is achieved. Inversion, indicated earlier as part of supination of the subtalar joint, is accompanied by increased stability in the transverse tarsal and the talonavicular joints. Although not shown on the chart, recall that extension of the toes occurs from the natural progression of the body over the foot, leading to elongation of and tension in the plantar fascia. Thus, additional stability is given to the foot. The net effect of the events of late stance is stabilization of the longitudinal arches of the foot at the time of toe off. The remaining events of the cycle are accomplished in the non-weight-bearing position and go on to position the foot for the next contact with the supporting surface (46). The course of the interactive events that take place in the foot and ankle must be understood, because the proper event and the order of occurrence will be the determinants of normal or pathological motion. Realizing the complexity of the events and the fact that the entire cycle is completed in about one second, emphasizes how important both proper arthrokinematics and muscular control is for normal function of the ankle and foot.

With new technologies researchers have determined motions at other foot joints

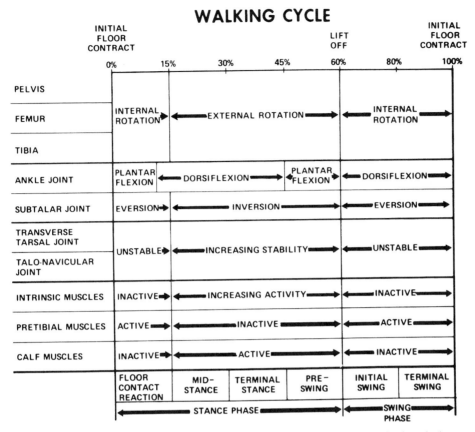

Figure 12.11. Summary diagram for the entire gait cycle that shows the kinematics for the subtalar joint and for other segments. General descriptions of levels of muscle activity are also provided.

besides the ankle during gait. Although assumptions were made that the talocrural and talocalcaneal joints were limited to single degrees of freedom, the motions at these joints were determined for the stance phase (Fig. 12.12). Discrepancies in sagittal plane representations are confounded by the combined rotations of the two joints, which in the figure are pronation and supination. The suggestion is made that these offsetting rotations assist with maintaining the leg in a sagittal plane, or plane of progression, throughout stance (67). Extensions of this work have also been applied to the other joints of the foot but the results are more difficult to interpret with particular meaning (68).

A manifestation of nearly all pathologies is altered gait. Such changes are usually demonstrated in many ways, including but not limited to kinematic and kinetic effects. For example, Katoh and coworkers showed that patients with painful heel pads and plantar fasciitis had altered temporal and distance parameters during gait (36). Others have compared the alterations in patients with plantar fasciitis to deficits in the "strength" and flexibility of supporting posterior calf and foot musculature (38). These same patients also had altered kinetics, manifested in decreased vertical loading components at heel strike and at toe off, and decreased anterior shear at the shoe-force plate interface during early stance. These same investigators evaluated patients with isolated talonavicular fusion and found decreased pronation, especially

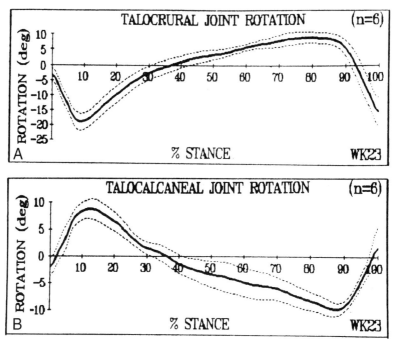

Figure 12.12. Rotations about the (**A**) talocrural and (**B**) talocalcaneal joints for one subject. The solid line represents average rotation from six trials. Dashed line indicates +/− 1SD. Positive rotation defines combined dorsiflexion, eversion, and abduction.

during side-slope walking with the involved foot on the upper side. Their data support the clinical observation that subtalar motion is coupled with motion occurring at the transverse tarsal joint (36).

Alterations in gait are also commonly associated with rheumatoid arthritis. Hindfoot instability may be a factor in other difficulties and may therefore require specific evaluation. Other difficulties that are frequently encountered by these patients include the pronated foot, valgus of the great toe, painful heel, and toe deformities. The pathomechanics associated with pronation have been discussed in earlier sections. Hallux valgus influences gait because of the import of the great toe during push-off. Because of discomfort the patient is likely to attempt to push off with greater loading through the lateral aspect of the foot than is usually required or wanted. Another possibility is that these patients do just not achieve much heel off, but instead propel themselves with the foot flat. Changes in the toes can lead to multiple problems, such as diminished propulsive force during terminal stance (13). Conditions with an etiology of muscular imbalances are the major initiating factor in foot deformities (12).

How loads are transmitted through the foot has received considerable attention. Some debate centers on whether all the metatarsals are loaded during stance. In static postures the load is apparently distributed throughout the foot. Approximately 50% of the load is borne by the heel. The remaining 50% is distributed across the metatarsal heads with twice as much load being taken on the first metatarsal head as on the others.

Transmission of loads during gait has also been evaluated in subjects with normal and pathological feet. Overall, this is the pattern for progression of the center of pressure through the foot: when pressure is received just lateral to the midline of the heel, the path moves forward in virtually a straight line toward the head of the third metatarsal. Toward the end of stance the pressure is directed medially and at toe off it leaves the foot at the first web space (36, 64). More specific data have been provided about the metatarsal heads, showing the highest pressures under the heads of the second and third metatarsals of normal subjects. Patterns for three patients with rheumatoid arthritis showed a wide variance, probably indicative of the differences produced by the total disease process (10). Presumably most of the patients that Stokes et al. (81) studied before and after surgery for hallux valgus also suffered from rheumatoid arthritis. Their predictable results showed significantly reduced loads imposed on the toes and the medial side of the forefoot when compared with healthy feet. Another important factor was metatarsal length, there being a direct relationship between length and receipt of load.

Muscular Dysfunction and Alterations

As noted in the section of this chapter on muscle function, the foot is kinetically balanced by muscle tensions and their respective moment arms in relationship to the joints that the muscles cross. Without disruption of this balance, the foot and ankle can function effectively. Under any circumstances creating changes in this balance, the therapist must be prepared to deal with pathological motion. Some of these potential changes have been discussed concerning imbalances resulting from rheumatoid arthritis. The remainder of this section will discuss other muscular dysfunctions and losses.

The loss of any given muscle or group of muscles can create ankle and foot deformity or dysfunction consistent with the loss. For example, loss of the musculature of the **anterior tibial compartment** resulting from injury to the peroneal nerve will leave no dorsiflexion capability. The foot drifts into a plantarflexed and supinated position due to the unopposed pull of the tibialis posterior and triceps surae muscles. Conversely, tibial nerve injury paralyzes calf musculature and leads to extreme and usually continuous positioning of the foot in dorsiflexion, called the calcaneal foot (93).

The effects of the common **ankle sprain** have received considerable attention. Interest has focused on the muscular control and proprioceptive capabilities. Usually, evaluation of patients has shown that mechanical damage occurs before muscles can be recruited (30, 32, 54). While passive movement sense and stability, as measured by talar tilt, should be greater concerns than "strength" deficits (42), mechanoreceptor impairment may be rehabilitated (32).

A frequent injury affecting the posterior calf muscle group is the **Achilles tendon rupture.** Efforts to manage these patients are geared toward restoration of the ability to exert normal plantarflexion torque. Patients with Achilles tendon rupture can reach comparable levels of torque (57, 77). The Sjostrom study evaluated patients at about 23 months postoperatively and found that static and dynamic mean peak torque for the injured leg was similar to that for the non-injured leg. However, two of the nine subjects showed torque losses greater than 50 Nm (77). The other study compared two groups: patients post surgery and those who were nonsurgically treated. In this case only minor differences were noted between the groups that had a mean follow-up time of 2.5 years. However, patients in both treatment groups generally produced less torque on the injured than on the uninjured side, except for 11 nonsurgical and eight surgically treated patients who generated greater isokinetic torque on the injured side. The surgical treatment group for the uninjured side developed 149 Nm while the nonsurgical group produced 161 Nm of torque in the neutral position. Surgically treated injured legs produced 124 Nm plantarflexion torque as compared with the 127 Nm for the nonsurgical group. One other study evaluated 32 patients, a mean 35 months after injury, and noted mean torques of 63 Nm for the injured leg and 75 Nm for the normal leg (56). Other investigators noted that the closed method of repair resulted in a larger loss of torque (74). In any case, a summary of these data shows that losses of plantarflexion torques can be avoided with adequate care. Therapists that institute appropriate rehabilitation programs can anticipate achieving the torque that can be produced in the uninjured limb. Surgical procedures requiring removal of the triceps surae would also be projected to have a devastating effect. Based on theoretical calculations of the torque contributed by the triceps surae, the loss should be approximately 80%. However, it is interesting that Murray and coworkers have reported such a case showing the loss to be only 62% of the total torque (53). Combined paralysis of the invertors and evertors is unusual. Isolated loss of the tibialis posterior may result in a very pronated foot, while loss of the peroneus longus and brevis would lead to supination.

Often, foot and ankle deformity is caused by conditions such as cerebral palsy or congenital disorders. In these situations it is the most often necessary to reestablish kinetic balance. The most popular procedure to accomplish this is the **tendon transfer** (91). Such a procedure has been successfully used for decades, a sufficient length of time to establish some general principles for its use. Crawford (11) has been among those who have identified the important considerations. First, the transfer should involve a muscle that has good to normal strength. In addition, if the muscle has to work against an existing deformity, the likelihood of an unsuccessful transfer is high. The procedure should always allow the tendon to be directed in a straight line and pass through smoothly gliding tissue without restriction. A further criterion is that a patient should be of sufficient age to participate in a program of therapeutic muscle reeducation effectively. Finally, when function is taken into account, the phase of activity becomes important. That is, if the muscle transfer requires a plantarflexor to become a dorsiflexor during an activity such as gait, the probability is high that the transfer will fail.

Most frequently the disabilities managed by tendon transfer are for lateral instability and loss of active dorsiflexion. An example would be the lateral transfer of the anterior tibial tendon for treatment of extreme equinovarus (clubfoot) deformity. In this procedure the tendon is released from its attachment and surgically transferred to the cuboid and the base of the fifth metatarsal (23). Another example is the use of the posterior tibial tendon in cases of plantarflexion and inversion deformities. In this procedure the tendon was split proximal to the medial malleolus, and passed posteriorly and laterally so that the new insertion would lie next to that of the tendon of the peroneus brevis. Although two patients required osteotomies of the calcaneus for fixed deformities, no varus deformity recurred and the equinus portion occurring during gait was eliminated (25). Many other examples of transfers at the foot and ankle could be cited. The principles of the procedures are similar: the primary focus is to locate the new insertion in such a position that the mechanical effect produces the appropriate kinetic balance.

EMG may also be used effectively in the evaluation and treatment of the inappropriate phasic behavior or muscles that affect the ankle and foot. Monitors that can be applied to specific muscles are available to determine the timing and degree of activity of the musculature. A muscular contraction pattern may be determined to be inconsistent. Therapeutic interventions may be indicated that will modify the muscles' sequence of activity. That there are abnormal patterns of firing in neurological patients has been demonstrated in the premature firing of the triceps surae and prolonged firing of the tibialis anterior during stance phase (60).

Overuse Syndromes

Conditions that appear commonly in the lower leg and foot, mostly due to sports or other high levels of activity, have been known to produce dysfunction. Among the injuries most frequently occurring from improper conditioning, training, or biomechanical faults include **shin splints, tendinitis, bursitis,** and **stress fractures.** Although some of these disorders have been related to muscle imbalances, leg length discrepancies, and lumbosacral disorders, most problems come from the biomechanics of the foot and ankle. Of primary concern are the altered mechanics of the subtalar joint, because changes at this joint may produce changes in patterns of muscular use. For example, consider that the foot cannot move into supination during the latter stage of the support phase. Here, the normal arthrokinematics of the subtalar and transverse tarsal joints are disrupted and the foot will not have become an effective lever to which muscle and passive forces can be applied (84).

A particular overuse syndrome, shin splints, has been analyzed in terms of mechanics of the foot. This condition, characterized by pain in the lower leg, has been variously considered to have its etiology based in bone, vascular, or soft tissues. In an attempt to evaluate the biomechanical aspects of the etiology, lower leg and heel position, the passive range of the subtalar joint, and the angular displacement of the midline of the Achilles tendon was assessed. Results showed significantly greater Achilles tendon angles and subtalar mobility of the shin splint subjects. Other differences between the two groups implicate both structural and functional abnormalities in the feet and ankles of those with the shin splint overuse syndrome (89).

Arthrodesis and Arthroplasty

Surgical fusion of the ankle and joints of the foot has been used for decades, primarily for the treatment of painful feet. These **arthrodeses** have not been limited to any single joint; instead, they have been used according to the location of the pathology. An understanding of the mechanics of the ankle and foot will clarify the significance of fusion of any single joint or collective joints.

Consider arthrodesis of the ankle joint. Any such successful procedure will place additional stress on the subtalar joint, although the amount of this stress can be somewhat controlled by the position of the ankle joint. Excessive deviation in either supination or pronation is thought to cause the patient difficulty when the center of gravity of the body passes over the foot. Increased joint loading can also lead to subtalar and midtarsal pain and to secondary knee and hip pain. Excessive pronation may cause the patient to roll over the medial aspect of the foot, which may in turn lead to hallux valgus deformity or pain on the medial aspect of the knee. Similar considerations can be applied to varus or valgus tilt of the talus and dorsiflexion or plantarflexion of the ankle. For example, in the latter case the ankle should be placed in the plantarflexed position in cases where the limb is comparatively shortened. On the other hand, too much plantarflexion will potentially cause a circumstance where genu recurvatum (hyperextended knee) deformity results.

Similar difficulties can readily arise with fusions of other joints of the foot. Increased stress will occur in surrounding joints, leading to other pathological situations. Disrupted gait patterns have been blamed on an arthrodesis of the subtalar joint. According to some, a valgus (pronation) tilt of 5° in the subtalar joint is preferred because good stability of the ankle is permitted (47).

Ankle **arthroplasties** have also been done, sufficiently so that results from clinical trials have been reported. In a group of 102 patients, more than 90% reported significant postoperative pain relief. Although ankle range of motion increased by only 6°, 75% of the patients had improved gait (80). In another series 50 patients were reviewed (55). In this sample, ankle scores that measured pain, range of motion, and function were improved in patients having osteoarthritis (osteoarthrosis), failed arthroplasties, and rheumatoid arthritis (37). Usually, the best results are in cases with rheumatoid arthritis or in post-traumatic arthritis among patients younger than 60 years old (80). In any case rehabilitation involves the restoration of normal arthrokinematics in the ankle and other joints of the foot. As further investigations of the capabilities of the components used in surgical procedures for the ankle are accomplished, the characteristics associated with each design will become more widely known (39, 69).

SUMMARY

In this chapter the pertinent anatomical and biomechanical factors that affect the ankle and foot have been presented. As the segment that contacts the supporting surface, the foot and ankle must be flexible enough to accommodate different surfaces yet stiff enough to provide the torque required. The foot and ankle meet the criteria necessary for effective function by combining a series of joints and controlling forces that interact so that the requirements of both static and dynamic situations can be met. Disruption of the mechanics of the kinetic chain leads to pathological function. Several alterations that produce these disruptions were presented and discussed.

References

1. Ambagtsheer JBT. The function of the muscles of the lower leg in relation to movements of the tarsus. *Acta Orthop Scand Suppl.* 1978;172:1–196.
2. Attarian DE, McCrackin HJ, DeVito DP. A biomechanical study of human lateral ankle ligaments and autogenous reconstructive grafts. *Foot Ankle.* 1985;13:377–381.
3. Barry RJ, Scranton PE. Flat feet in children. *Clin Orthop.* 1983;181:68–75.
4. Basmajian JV. *Muscles Alive.* Baltimore: Williams & Wilkins; 1979.
5. Black KD, Halverson JL, Majerus KA, et al. Alterations in ankle dorsiflexion torque as a result of continuous ultrasound to the anterior tibial compartment. *Phys Ther.* 1984;64:910–913.
6. Boruta PM, Bishop JO, Braly WG, Tullos HS. Acute lateral ankle ligament injuries: a literature review. *Foot Ankle.* 1990;11:107–113.
7. Brown GP, Donatelli R, Catlin PA, et al. The effect of two types of foot orthoses on rearfoot mechanics. *J Orthop Sports Phys Ther.* 1995;21:258–267.
8. Campbell KM, Biggs NL, Blanton PL, et al. Electromyographic investigation of the relative activity among four components of the triceps surae. *Am J Phys Med.* 1973;52:30–41.
9. Chan CW, Rudins A. Foot biomechanics during walking and running. *Mayo Clin Proc.* 1994;69:448–460.
10. Collis WJMF, Jayson MIV. Measurement of pedal pressures: an illustration of a method. *Ann Rheum Dis.* 1972;31:215–217.
11. Crawford AH. A discussion of tendon transfers in the paralytic foot. *Arch Pod Med Foot Surg.* 1974;II:47–60.
12. D'Amico JC. The pathomechanics of adult rheumatoid arthritis affecting the foot. *J Am Podiatr Assoc.* 1976;66:227–236.
13. DiMonte P, Light H. Pathomechanics, gait deviations, and treatment of the rheumatoid foot: a clinical report. *Phys Ther.* 1982;62:1148–1156.

14. Donatelli R. Abnormal biomechanics of the foot and ankle. *J Orthop Sports Phys Ther.* 1987;9:11–16.
15. Elftman H. The transverse tarsal joint and its control. *Clin Orthop.* 1960;16:41–46.
16. Elveru RA, Rothstein JM, Lamb RL, Riddle DL. Methods for taking subtalar joint measurements: a clinical report. *Phys Ther.* 1988;678–682.
17. Engsberg JR. A biomechanical analysis of the talocalcaneal joint-in vitro. *J Biomech.* 1987:20:429–442.
18. Evans P. Clinical biomechanics of the subtalar joint. *Physiotherapy.* 1990;76:47–51.
19. Falkel J. Plantar flexor strength testing using the Cybex isokinetic dynamometer. *Phys Ther.* 1978;58:847–850.
20. Frankel VH, Nordin M. *Basic Biomechanics of the Skeletal System.* Philadelphia: Lea & Febiger; 1980.
21. Fugl-Meyer AR, Sjostrom M, Wahlby L. Human plantar flexion strength and structure. *Acta Physiol Scand.* 1977;107:47–56.
22. Furlani J, Vitti M, Costacurta L. Electromyographic behavior of the gastrocnemius muscle. *Electromyogr Clin Neurophysiol.* 1978;18:29–34.
23. Garceau GJ, Palmer RM. Transfer of the anterior tibial tendon for recurrent club foot. *J Bone Joint Surg.* 1967;49(A):207–231.
24. Gauffin H, Areblad M, Tropp H. Three-dimensional analysis of the talocrural and subtalar joints in single-limb stance. *Clin Biomech.* 1993;8:307–314.
25. Green NE, Griffin PP, Shiavi R. Split posterior tibial-tendon transfer in spastic cerebral palsy. *J Bone Joint Surg.* 1983;65(A):748–754.
26. Greene TA, Roland C. A comparative isokinetic evaluation of a functional ankle orthosis on talocalcaneal function. *J Orthop Sports Phys Ther.* 1989;11:245–252.
27. Hicks JH. The mechanics of the foot: I. The joints. *J Anat.* 1953;87:345–357.
28. Hicks JH. The three weight-bearing mechanisms of the foot. In: Evans FG, ed. *Biomechanical Studies of the Musculoskeletal System.* Springfield, IL: Charles C Thomas; 1961.
29. Inman VT. *The Joints of the Ankle.* Baltimore: Williams & Wilkins; 1976.
30. Isakov E, Mizrahi J, Solzi P, et al. Response of peroneal muscles to sudden inversion of the ankle during standing. *Int J Sports Biomech.* 1986;2:100–109.
31. Johanson MA, Donatelli R, Wooden MJ, et al. Effects of three different posting methods on controlling abnormal subtalar pronation. *Phys Ther.* 1994;74:149–161.
32. Johnson MB, Johnson CL. Electromyographic response of peroneal muscles in surgical and nonsurgical injured ankles during sudden inversion. *J Orthop Sports Phys Ther.* 1993;18:497–501.
33. Johnson EE, Markolf KL. The contribution of the anterior talofibular ligament to ankle laxity. *J Bone Joint Surg.* 1983;65(A):81–88.
34. Jones RL. The human foot: an experimental study of its mechanics, and the role of its muscle and ligaments in the support of the arch. *Am J Anat.* 1941;68:1–39.
35. Kapandji IA. *The Physiology of the Joints.* New York: Churchill Livingstone; 1970;2.
36. Katoh Y, Chao EYS, Laughman RK, et al. Biomechanical analysis of foot function during gait and clinical applications. *Clin Orthop.* 1983;177:23–33.
37. Kessler RM, Hertling D. *Management of Common Musculoskeletal Disorders.* Philadelphia: Harper & Row; 1983.
38. Kibler WB, Goldberg C, Chandler TJ. Functional biomechanical deficits in running athletes with plantar fasciitis. *Am J Sports Med.* 1991;19:66–71.
39. Lachiewicz PF, Inglis AE, Ranawat CS. Total ankle replacement in rheumatoid arthritis. *J Bone Joint Surg.* 1984;66(A)340–343.
40. Lattanza L, Gray GW, Kantner RM. Closed versus open kinematic chain measurements of subtalar joint eversion: implications for clinical practice. *J Orthop Sports Phys Ther.* 1988;9:310–314.
41. Lehmkuhl LD, Smith LK. *Clinical Kinesiology.* 5th ed. Philadelphia: FA Davis; 1996.
42. Lentell G, Baas B, Lopez D, et al. The contributions of proprioceptive deficits, muscle function, and anatomic laxity to functional instability of the ankle. *J Orthop Sports Phys Ther.* 1995;21:206–215.
43. Lentell GL, Cashman PA, Shiomoto KJ, et al. The effect of knee position on torque output during inversion and eversion movements at the ankle. *J Orthop Sports Phys Ther.* 1988;10:177–183.
44. Leslie M, Zachazewski J, Browne P. Reliability of isokinetic torque values for ankle invertors and evertors. *J Orthop Sports Phys Ther.* 1990;11:612–616.
45. MacConaill MA, Basmajian JV. *Muscles and Movements: A Basis for Human Kinesiology.* Baltimore: Williams & Wilkins; 1969.
46. Mann RA. Biomechanics of the foot. In: American Academy of Orthopedic Surgeons, eds. *Atlas of Orthotics: Biomechanical Principles and Application.* St. Louis: CV Mosby; 1975:257–266.

47. Mann RA. Surgical implications of biomechanics of the foot and ankle. *Clin Orthop.* 1980;146: 111–118.
48. Mann RA. Acquired flatfoot in adults. *Clin Orthop.* 1983;181:46–51.
49. Manter JT. Movements of the subtalar and transverse tarsal joints. *Anat Rec.* 1941;80:397–410.
50. McClay IS. The use of gait analysis to enhance the understanding of running injuries. In: Craik RL, Oatis CA, eds. *Gait Analysis: Theory and Applications.* St. Louis: CV Mosby; 1995.
51. McPoil TG, Brocato RS. The foot and ankle: biomechanical evaluation and treatment. In: Gould JA, Davies GJ, ed. *Orthopaedic and Sports Physical Therapy.* St. Louis: CV Mosby; 1985.
52. Mueller MJ, Norton BJ. Reliability of kinematic measurements of rear-foot motion. *Phys Ther.* 1992;72:731–737.
53. Murray MP, Guten GN, Baldwin JM, et al. A comparison of plantar flexion torque with and without the triceps surae. *Acta Orthop Scand.* 1976;47:122–124.
54. Nawoczenski DA, Owen MG, Ecker ML, et al. Objective evaluation of peroneal response to sudden inversion stress. *J Orthop Sports Phys Ther.* 1985;7:107–109.
55. Newton SE. Total ankle arthroplasty: clinical study of fifty cases. *J Bone Joint Surg.* 1982;64(A): 104–111.
56. Nistor L. Surgical and non-surgical treatment of achilles tendon rupture. *J Bone Joint Surg.* 1981;63(A):394–399.
57. Nistor L, Markhede G, Grimby G. A technique for measurements of plantar flexion torque with the Cybex II dynamometer. *Scand J Rehabil Med.* 1982;14:163–166.
58. Oatis CA. Biomechanics of the foot and ankle under static conditions. *Phys Ther.* 1988;68:1515–1521.
59. Perry J. Anatomy and biomechanics of the hindfoot. *Clin Orthop.* 1983;177:9–15.
60. Perry J, Waters RL, Perrin T. Electromyographic analysis of equinovarus following stroke. *Clin Orthop.* 1978;131:47–53.
61. Picciano AM, Rowlands MS, Worrell T. Reliability of open and closed kinetic chain subtalar joint neutral positions and navicular drop test. *J Orthop Sports Phys Ther.* 1993;18:553–558.
62. Powers CM, Maffucci R, Hampton S. Rearfoot posture in subjects with patellofemoral pain. *J Orthop Sports Phys Ther.* 1995;22:155–160.
63. Procter P, Paul JP. Ankle joint biomechanics. *J Biomech.* 1982;15:627–634.
64. Rodgers MM. Dynamic biomechanics of the normal foot and ankle during walking and running. *Phys Ther.* 1988;68:1822–1830.
65. Sammarco GJ, Burstein AH, Frankel VH. Biomechanics of the ankle: a kinematic study. *Orthop Clin North Am.* 1973;4:75–96.
66. Sarrafian SK. Biomechanics of the subtalar complex. *Clin Orthop.* 1993;290:17–26.
67. Scott SH, Winter DH. Talocrural and talocalcaneal joint kinematics and kinetics during the stance phase of walking. *J Biomech.* 1991;24:743–752.
68. Scott SH, Winter DH. Biomechanical model of the human foot: kinematics and kinetics during the stance phase of walking. *J Biomech.* 1993;26:1091–1104.
69. Scranton PE, Fu FH, Brown TD. Ankle arthrodesis: a comparative clinical and biomechanical evaluation. *Clin Orthop.* 1980;151:234–243.
70. Sell KE, Verity TM, Worrell TW. Two measurement techniques for assessing subtalar joint position: a reliability study. *J Orthop Sports Phys Ther.* 1994;162–167.
71. Seireg A, Arvikar RJ. The prediction of muscular load sharing and joint forces in the lower extremities during walking. *J Biomech.* 1975;8:89–102.
72. Selby-Silverstein L. Gait assessment of children to enhance evaluation of foot and ankle function and treatment efficiency. In: Craik RL, Oatis CA, eds. *Gait Analysis: Theory and Applications.* St. Louis: CV Mosby; 1995.
73. Sgarlato TE. *A Compendium of Podiatric Biomechanics.* San Francisco: California College of Podiatric Medicine; 1971:209–225.
74. Shields CL, Kerlan RK, Jobe FW, et al. The cybex II evaluation of surgically repaired achilles tendon ruptures. *Am J Sports Med.* 1978;6:369–372.
75. Simon SR, Mann RA, Hagy JL, et al. Role of the posterior calf muscles in normal gait. *J Bone Joint Surg.* 1978;60(A):465–472.
76. Sims DS. *The Effect of a Balanced Foot Orthosis on Muscle Function and Foot Pronation in Compensated Forefoot Varus.* Iowa City, IA: University of Iowa; 1983. Masters thesis.
77. Sjostrom M, Fugl-Meyer AR, Wahlby L. Achilles tendon injury: plantar flexion strength and structure of the soleus muscle after surgical repair. *Acta Chir Scand.* 1978;144:219–226.
78. Smith-Oricchio K, Harris BA. Interrater reliability of subtalar neutral, calcaneal inversion and eversion. *J Orthop Sports Phys Ther.* 1990;12:10–15.

79. Stauffer RN, Chao EYS, Brewster RC. Force and motion analysis of the normal, diseased, and prosthetic ankle joint. *Clin Orthop.* 1977;127:189–196.

80. Stauffer RN, Segal NM. Total ankle arthroplasty: four years' experience. *Clin Orthop.* 1981;160: 217–221.

81. Stokes IAF, Hutton WC, Stott JRR, et al. Forces under the hallux valgus foot before and after surgery. *Clin Orthop.* 1977;142:64–72.

82. St. Pierre RK, Rosen J, Whitesides TE, et al. The tensile strength of the anterio talofibular ligament. *Foot Ankle.* 1983;4:83–85.

83. Subotnick SI. Biomechanics of the subtalar and midtarsal joints. *J Am Podiatr Assoc.* 1975;65: 756–764.

84. Subotnick SI. Lower extremity problems in athletes: a biomechanical approach. *Arch Pod Med Foot Surg.* 1978;2:23–29.

85. Sutherland DH. An electromyographic study of the plantar flexors of the ankle in normal walking on the level. *J Bone Joint Surg.* 1966;48(A):66–71.

86. Tiberio D. Pathomechanics of structural foot deformities. *Phys Ther.* 1988;68:1840–1849.

87. Thordarson DV, Schmotzer H, Chon J, et al. Dynamic support of the human longitudinal arch. *Clin Orthop.* 1995;316:165–172.

88. van den Bogert AJ, Smith GD, Nigg BM. In vivo determination of the anatomical axes of the ankle joint complex: an optimization approach. *J Biomech.* 1994;27:1477–1488.

89. Viitasalo JT, Kvist M. Some biomechanical aspects of the foot and ankle in athletes with and without shin splints. *Am J Sports Med.* 1983;11:125–130.

90. Warwick R, Williams PL, eds. *Gray's Anatomy.* 37th British ed. Philadelphia: WB Saunders; 1989.

91. Wiesseman GJ. Tendon transfers for peripheral nerve injuries of the lower extremity. *Orthop Clin North Am.* 1981;12:459–467.

92. Wong DL, Glasheen-Wray M, Andrews WF. Isokinetic evaluation of the ankle invertors and evertors. *J Orthop Sports Phys Ther.* 1984;5:246–252.

93. Wright DG, Desai ME, Henderson BS. Action of the subtalar and ankle joint complex during the stance phase of walking. *J Bone Joint Surg.* 1964;46(A):361–382.

94. Wynarsky GT, Greenwald AS. Mathematical model of the human ankle joint. *J Biomech.* 1983;16:241–252.

95. Youdas JW, Bogard CL, Suman VJ. Reliability of goniometric measurements and visual estimates of ankle joint active range of motion obtained in a clinical setting. *Arch Phys Med Rehabil.* 1993;74:1113–1118.

13

Trunk

The trunk is important to the kinesiology of the body because the arms, legs, and head must often rotate around this segment. This series of intervertebral joints, arranged in a column of anteroposterior deviations, produces an incredible array of movement patterns. Yet, this flexibility must be coupled with the capacity to handle significant loads, either as part of regular or imposed activities. These requirements probably predispose the spine to dysfunctions that are often manifested in postural, gait, or other functional disorders. Although entire volumes have been written about the spine, this chapter will discuss aspects of muscular control, arthrology, arthrokinematics, and biomechanics. The pathokinesiology associated with several common disorders will also be presented. A short discussion of respiration will conclude the chapter.

SPINE
Muscular Actions

We can classify control schemes for the trunk either by flexors versus extensors or by spinal region. The former provides the ability to categorize the musculature functionally while the latter allows for discussion based on some important regional differences. This section ·will combine the two approaches and close with some information on the role of the musculature in various exercises.

The **extensor** musculature is composed of much muscle that is layered both in depth and breadth. Extensive descriptions are available in classic anatomy texts, and it is not the intention of this volume to reiterate anatomical relationships. Instead, we should stress the functional significance of the different portions. In general, the deepest may be considered responsible for finer movements of intervertebral joints because their attachments extend over a few vertebral segments. Certain sections are also larger in a given area of the spine, such as the multifidus in the lumbar and sacral regions. The contributions of these segments to the overall mass of the erector spinae musculature thus account for greatest extensor muscle mass in the lumbar spine. According to some, the deeper portion of the multifidus thins out over the thoracic spine, becoming thicker again in the cervical spine (45). The necessity for increased extensor torque in these two areas may explain their increased mass.

The specific role of each segment of the erector spinae has escaped identification because of the difficulties associated with in vivo studies. Isaacson (45) goes so far as to say that the short deep portions of the erector spinae are responsible for maintaining some degree of rigidity in the vertebral column. Because change in the position of one of any of the motion segments with respect to another can produce stretch, passive tension can certainly exist. Further comments on this topic are found in the section on kinetics. Conversely, the superficial and longest layers can be considered the prime movers for vertebral extension, lateral flexion, and rotation. In fact, the contributions of the different layers have been found to vary by location. For example, thoracic fibers of the lumbar erector spinae contribute 50% of the total extensor moment exerted on L4 and L5, multifidus about 20%, and the remainder by the lumbar fibers. At higher lumbar levels the thoracic fibers contribute between 70 and 86% of the total extensor moment (12).

Other descriptive systems of the posterior musculature of the lumbar spine also exist. For example, the musculature has been described according to three planes: deep, intermediate, and superficial. The deepest is composed of all components of the erector spinae group, the intermediate of the serratus posterior inferior, and the most superficial of the latissimus dorsi. Besides extension of the lumbar spine, these muscles are also effective in increasing lumbar lordosis (52). For a detailed description of the erector spinae in the lumbar spine the work of Bogduk would be of considerable interest (10). In considering the extensors of the thoracic spine no additional comment is necessary because the topography and function of the erector spinae muscle in this area are similar to those of the lumbar segment of the spine.

The posterior muscles of the neck are far more complex because of the increased rotational requirements of this segment of the spine. For purposes of convenience and function, Kapandji (52) has identified four planes. The deepest contains primarily the suboccipital muscles, while the semispinalis plane includes the semispinalis capitis and cervicis and three other small muscles. The splenius and levator scapulae compose the area just deep to the superficial plane, which is made up of the trapezius and the sternocleidomastoid muscles. All but the superficial plane muscles extend, rotate, and laterally flex ipsilaterally. With the trapezius and sternocleidomastoid the fiber direction of the muscles is such that rotation is in the contralateral direction.

With the extensive musculature in the posterior cervical spine, we can cite many examples of synergistic and antagonistic action. For example, contraction of the unilateral suboccipital group causes lateral flexion while bilateral contraction causes extension of the cervical spine. Rotation provides an additional example. Contraction of one splenius capitis muscle causes rotation of the head to the same side. To complement this action the contralateral sternocleidomastoid muscle must be active. Thus, here, these two muscles participate as a force couple in producing rotation of the head and the cervical spine (Fig. 13.1).

The erector spinae muscles unquestionably hold the trunk erect during postures and also make possible the generation of sufficient tension required to lift heavy objects. In cases of standing postures, nonexistent or low levels of activity appear to predominate across subjects and across different levels of the spine (50). They evaluated EMG activity at 12 vertebral levels and subjectively graded according to pre-established voltage ranges. Data show rather high degrees of variability from segment to segment and from subject to subject. Presumably the resulting activity depends on the configuration of the spine and the posture assumed during the test. Placing electrodes at different depths has also obtained similar results from EMG evaluations of the erector spinae at one vertebral level. Although debate will continue about activity of the erector spinae in standing and sitting postures, a fair summary would be that the slight EMG activity of the thoracic levels of the muscles is greater than that recorded from the lumbar and cervical regions (49, 84).

As the trunk goes into flexion from the standing position, the activity of the erector spinae increases commensurate with the flexion moment created; that is, as the trunk is inclined anteriorly, the flexion at each motion segment requires greater tension in the extensors at each respective segment. At around 50° of flexion, however, erector

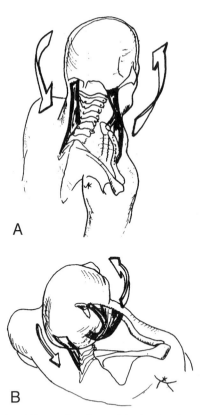

Figure 13.1.   A, posterolateral and **B,** superior views of the head and upper trunk showing how the left splenius capitus and the right sternocleidomastoid muscles act as a force couple for rotation of the head. The approximate location of the axis of rotation is in the cervical spine as shown in Figure 13.11.

spinae activity diminishes until, at full flexion, the muscles are inactive (Fig. 13.2). This progressive decrease in muscular tension is due to the fact that as the erector spinae are elongated, sufficient passive tension is generated in elastic elements of the muscle. In fact, there is an established interaction between erector spinae muscles and the thoracolumbar fascia as these two tissues function to control the trunk (11). Combined with tension arising in the posterior spinal ligaments, and compression of the anterior aspect of the intervertebral disc, support of the trunk in the fully inclined position becomes a passive mechanism (15). In this position the hamstring muscles are active to secure the pelvis and the trunk over the feet and legs. If this were not so, the entire body would fall in an anterior direction.

Lateral flexion and rotation of the trunk also require activity from the back extensors. On lateral flexion muscle activity is contralateral to the side of flexion. Rotation produces a more complex pattern and opinion differs as to the role of each segment. Unilateral loading requires the primary use of the contralateral erector spinae muscles; the response of these muscles was greater when the direction of the bending moment was altered compared with increases in the bending moment (61). Most evidence appears to show that lumbar rotation is produced by ipsilateral longissimus and iliocostalis muscles in combination with contralateral multifidus and rotator muscles.

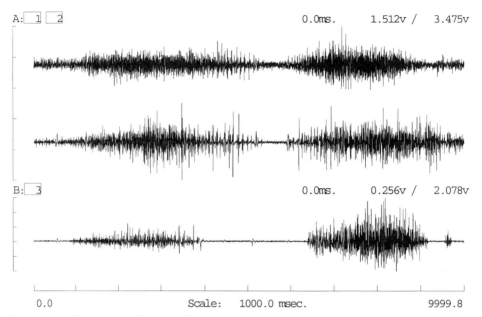

Figure 13.2. Electromyographic record from erector spinae muscles. Cervical spine is on top, thoracic spine in the middle, and the lumbar segment in the lowest trace. Subject bends forward to touch the ground and returns to the upright position. Note that the lumbar erector spinae activity ceases in the completely forward bent position, between 4 and 6.3 seconds.

Because rotation during lifting accounts for many back injuries, one can anticipate continued interest in this area.

Activity of the extensors has been studied during functional activities and exercises. Lifting, often the culprit in low back injury and pain, has been a subject of particular interest. In general, lifting style and load are major determinants in the activity required of the extensors. The former case produced intermittent low activity while the latter caused continuous moderate to maximal activity (30). Resistance also affects the timing of the contractions of the extensors and the abdominal musculature (95), while unilateral loading requires the primary use of the contralateral erector spinae muscles (60). Suffice it to say that most people flex the spine to between 80 and 95% of the total range to achieve the maximum extensor moment (24). Chapter 16 will elaborate on this topic. The properly executed Valsalva maneuver also produces moderate changes in the intensity of muscle contraction (110). Finally, because of interest in the sit-up exercise as a preventive measure for the back patient, researchers have monitored the extensor activity during this movement. Recordings from four paraspinal locations from the cervical to the sacral regions established that the levels respond independently of each other during the performance of Williams' flexion exercises. When minimal activity of the extensors is desirable, the pelvic tilt, curl up, knees to chest, and hamstring stretch with posterior tilt should be used. Conversely, higher levels of activity exist in the standing exercises and anterior pelvic tilt positions (8).

Flexor musculature can also be considered from the viewpoint of contributions to the motion of the lumbar and cervical portions of the spine. In the cervical spine several muscles are responsible for flexion: the scalenes, sternocleidomastoid, longus colli, and longus capitis. Kapandji (52) adds the longus cervicis to the flexor group. As is true for the posterior neck musculature, the flexors can perform multiple functions. Because all the muscles are attached to structures (cervical spine and head) that are mobile in three dimensions, contraction of any single muscle ordinarily produced triplanar motion. Bilateral contraction of muscles results in neutralization of rotation and lateral flexion functions and produces the most effective flexion. Although most authors consider the sternocleidomastoid and scalene muscles to be neck flexors, certain qualifications need to be made regarding their function. For example, if the cervical spine is not held rigid, the bilateral contraction of the sternocleidomastoid muscles will increase the cervical lordosis, in effect causing flexion of the lower cervical spine on the upper thoracic spine and extension of the head. On the other hand, if other prevertebral muscles hold the neck rigid, the sternocleidomastoid and the scalenes can draw the head forward during cervical spine flexion. Therefore, contractions of these muscles have different effects depending on the underlying conditions.

The musculature comprising the abdominal wall is of much interest because of the potential for controlling the lumbar spine. The transversus and rectus abdominis and the internal and external oblique muscles form an effective syncytium that can protect and support the abdominal viscera and produce motions of the lumbar spine. Generally the transversus has been credited with the ability to increase the intra-abdominal pressure. The oblique muscles are productive in rotation, the contralateral components being active together. Clearly the oblique muscles contribute to flexion, as can be seen from the somewhat vertical orientation of the muscle fibers. The rectus abdominis receives credit for the primary responsibility for flexion, however.

Another muscle on the anterior aspect is the **psoas** muscle, extending from the upper lumbar spine to an insertion at the lesser trochanter of the femur. The complex function of the muscle is due to multiple-segment attachments. Furthermore, the muscle is draped over the anterior rim of the pelvis, which provides a mechanism for altering the position of the pelvis. Because upward and downward tilting of the anterior rim of the pelvis is directly related to the degree of respective flexion and hyperextension in the lumbar spine, the effect of this muscle on the lumbar spine can be dramatic. To elucidate, consider the patient to have tightness of the psoas muscles. Here the tension in the muscles will pull the anterior rim inferiorly, called a downward or anterior tilt. Such tilt causes the sacrum to be inclined further forward, which in turn positions the fifth lumbar vertebrae more anteriorly. The result, shown in Figure 13.3, increases the lumbar lordosis.

The **segmental interaction** that occurs is noteworthy. Hip flexion, accomplished by the psoas and other musculature, would shorten the length of the muscle and remove the potential for production of the downward tilt of the pelvis. Hip flexion carried through a full range of motion ultimately requires that the pelvis be tipped posteriorly, altering the sacral angle and reducing the lumbar lordosis. Thus, hip flexion, posterior pelvic tilt, and flexion of the lumbar spine are related, as would be hip extension or hyperextension, anterior pelvic tilt, and extension or hyperextension of the lumbar spine. Besides being a powerful hip flexor, the psoas can strongly influence the lumbar spine indirectly or through the usual functions of lumbar spine flexion, lateral flexion, or rotation. The function of the psoas is so important that an entire book has been written about it (75).

Evaluation of in vivo function has been completed for the abdominal musculature. Of most interest have been activities intended to strengthen the anterior abdominal

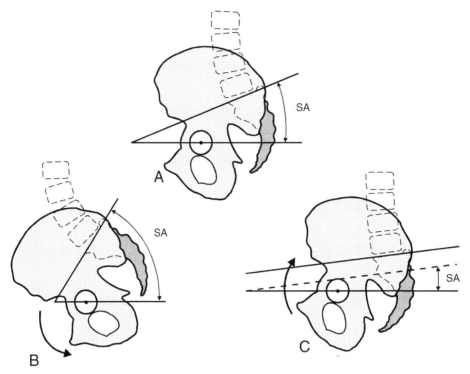

Figure 13.3.   Potential influence of a tight iliopsoas muscle on the sacral angle (*SA*), the position of the pelvis, and the degree of lumbar lordosis. **A,** normal attitude. **B,** the effect of a tight iliopsoas muscle. **C,** the result of contraction of the abdominal-gluteal muscle force couple.

wall. Among these exercises is the straight leg raise, which has been shown to require the greatest contraction in the rectus abdominis and external oblique as judged by subjective grading of muscle activity (16). Yet, when compared to conventional, hooklying, and arched back bilateral leg raises, straight leg raises were judged to be less effective in eliciting motor unit activity in the rectus abdominis (64). Analysis of the pelvic tilt has also produced interesting results. In the supine position this motion was apparently performed primarily by the rectus abdominis and the external oblique muscles. In standing, the internal obliques were more active than the external obliques, with little activity in the rectus.

The sit-up maneuver has been the most commonly assessed, research that is clearly a search for the most effective means of strengthening the anterior abdominal wall. Methodological differences across studies make comparisons difficult if not impossible. We may safely make some generalizations, however. All of the analyses appear to demonstrate that highest levels of rectus abdominis activity occur during the sit-up performed in the hooklying position. Long-lying positions produced activity in the rectus abdominis and the obliques for an average of 19–37% of the total duration of the sit-up maneuver (38), although one investigation states that the sit-up performed quickly in the long-lying position produced the greatest duration of activity (33).

The curl, which is performed until the scapulae clear the floor, is also affected by the abdominals. Compared to EMG produced by maximal voluntary contractions, about 50% of the maximal activity is achieved during a curl to 45° of upper trunk flexion (27). Another comparative study showed the rectus to be active for 93% of the cycle associated with the curl exercise (38). Although suggested that simultaneous plantar flexion of the feet or completion of the exercise with a dorsally extended spine would produce more rectus abdominis activity, results have not supported these arguments (27). Always, the oblique muscles will make a more effective contribution if rotation is added to the trunk flexion motion.

Arthrology and Arthrokinematics

An analysis of motion in the spine shows that the cervical, thoracic, and lumbar segments each function differently. In addition, there exist special segments, such as those found at the atlanto-occipital, atlanto-axial, and lumbosacral joints. In spite of their functional variation, all of the joints are synovial and enjoy relatively common forms of ligamentous support. Usually, the joints of the spine are planar. Available motion, however, can be considered to consist of six degrees of freedom, because rotations and translations can occur in any of the three planes. To consider these joints as less than capable of these motions would not represent an accurate picture. This section of the chapter will describe the arthrology attendant to the motions of the spine and will discuss the influence of passive structures on the achievable range of movement.

Intervertebral Joints

Although the articulation of one vertebral body on an adjacent vertebral body and the interposition of the disc can be considered a joint, most of the significance of this articulation is associated with the mechanical properties of the disc. Some consider that the disc allows relatively unconstrained motion in all six degrees of freedom, while the facets serve to constrain motion. However, here our focus will be on the role of the facet joint in determining the direction and size of the motion in the various spinal segments.

The **facet joints,** so named because of their bony outgrowths from the vertebral arches, are synovial joints made up of the inferior and superior articular facets of the respective vertebrae. The capsules of these joints are thin and loose, being longer and looser in the cervical than in the thoracic or lumbar spine (125). Each is freely movable yet constrained by its own capsule and the ligaments that support the entire vertebral arch. Of primary importance are the ligamenta nuchae, the ligamenta flava, and the supraspinous, interspinous, and intertransverse ligaments. Detailed descriptions can be found in classic anatomy texts, but in essence their names are descriptive of their attachment sites. These ligaments, plus the posterior longitudinal ligament that is inside the vertebral canal and adherent to the posterior surfaces of the vertebrae, compose the posterior elements that are crucial to support of the human spine.

Motion in the spinal segments is easily understood with study of the planes of the facets. Beginning at the occiput, the atlas has bilateral concave superior facets tilted somewhat medially and directed so that the axes are of an oblique nature. Such a combination allows for slight lateral flexion and considerable flexion and extension (125). Researchers have compared this flexion and extension (which occurs with repetitive nodding of the head) to the motion of a ball rolling back and forth. Because these joints exist bilaterally, rotation is extremely limited. The C1–C2 facet joints are almost circular but the superior facet of the axis is flattened posteromedially. The C2 facet is convex, sloping posteriorly and laterally (111). Such a horizontal

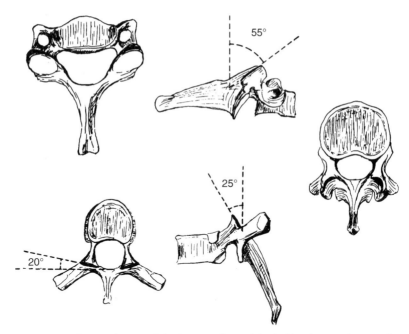

Figure 13.4. Views of cervical (*upper left*), thoracic (*lower left*), and lumbar vertebrae (*right*) to show the plane of the facet joints in each segment of the spine. Note the cupped shape arrangement of the lumbar facets.

joint configuration is conducive to large amounts of rotation. Perhaps as much as 50% of the cervical spine range of motion exists at this joint. Note that lateral bending at this joint would be markedly limited.

From the C2–C3 facet joint to the lumbar-sacral junction the female, or concave surface, is the superior portion of the joint. A gross examination of these joints shows that they follow an orderly change in the transverse and frontal planes. These changes, shown in Figure 13.4, originate in the upper cervical spine, progressing so that in the lower thoracic spine the joints are quite vertical. Then, in the lower thoracic spine the joints begin to rotate to the sagittal plane; throughout the lumbar spine the articulating surfaces have been turned by 90°. We should also note that the lumbar facets are curved so that the anterior portion of the joint is in the frontal plane while the posterior portion is in the sagittal plane. At the termination of the lumbar spine an interesting and significant change occurs: at the articulation of the fifth lumbar vertebra with the sacrum, the facet joints have returned to a frontal plane orientation. We will discuss this feature in the section on pathokinesiology. Of some interest is that modified vertebrae appear at approximately C7–T1, T12–L1, and at L5. In these locations, the joints have superior and inferior facet orientations that allow a transition to a different portion of the spinal column. Clinicians may need to focus specifically on the evaluation and treatment of these joints.

Besides the joint orientation and the role that ligamentous structures may play in restraining movement, we should mention three other factors. First, bony geometry is important because such factors as length of the spinous process may determine the available range of motion. Second, the disc and its mechanical properties provide an important fulcrum upon which the vertebrae can displace. Furthermore, the disc contains a nucleus pulposus that has hydrodynamic properties (57). Third, that the articular height of the superior articular processes, but not the slope of the articular facet, is the factor "perfectly related" to the locations of the axes of rotation. This finding has, to date, been limited to the cervical spine (83), but facet joint orientation in the lumbar spine also creates a "positive stop" to axial rotation. As a result, injury of the intervertebral disc may only be possible after failure at the facet (6). Although the relative importance of each factor involved in spinal motion is unknown, surely each element makes some contribution, particularly if a complete range of motion is attempted.

Kinematics

Prior to considering the range of motion available in the spine, description of the motion of one segment on another may prove helpful. Consider flexion of the trunk that moves the third lumbar vertebra on the fourth. During this movement, the body of the third vertebra slides anteriorly on the intervertebral disc. Simultaneously, tilting of the vertebral body will cause compression of the anterior portion of the disc. At the facet joint, the articular surface of the third vertebra slides superiorly on the surface of the fourth vertebra, causing compression of the facet surfaces face to face while concurrently having a shearing effect. Note also that this movement is potentially unlimited, were it not for restraint imposed by the ligaments of the vertebral arch, the posterior longitudinal ligament, the facet capsules, posterior musculature, thoracolumbar fascia, and the posterior annulus (52). A corollary sequence of events could be described for extension. Now, however, consider lateral flexion. Here, compressive disc forces would occur on the side to which the lateral flexion takes place. At the facet joints the motion is more limited, because with this movement, joint compressive forces are increased due to the tendency for the articular surfaces to move only slightly in this plane of motion. Thus, limited lateral flexion may be anticipated in the lumbar spine.

The possibility of completing the motion of flexion followed by lateral flexion raises another interesting phenomenon associated with spinal kinematics. These two motions require the bending of a flexible rod (the spine) in two planes that are perpendicular to each other. To do so requires that the rod also undergo axial rotation (92). This characteristic is known as **coupling,** which involves the consistent association of axial rotation with movement about another axis (121). This coupling will occur in any segment of the spine, but recall that facet planes restrict rotation in the lumbar spine. The cervical and thoracic facets allow much rotation while the rib cage, with its sternal junctions, restricts rotation. This feature will be important in later discussions of the kinematics and kinetics of scoliosis.

Researchers have summarized the ranges of motion available in each of the spinal segments in a variety of ways (13, 87, 107). Figure 13.5 shows one useful representation. Several key aspects related to joint orientation should be emphasized. Lack of axial rotation in the occiput–C1 joint and in the C1–C2 areas for lateral flexion is entirely consistent with the joint geometry. An example of the complexity of the process exists in that some consider the "true" upper cervical articulation to be between the occiput and C2, with C1 functioning as a "washer" interposed between. Upon lateral flexion to the left, C1 translates to the left to adjust the position of the left lateral mass of C1 which otherwise would prevent the left side flexion. The right alar ligament is pulled tight by the left side flexion, and it then pulls on the dens, rotating C2 to the left. This rotation allows the atlas to approximate the axis, as they

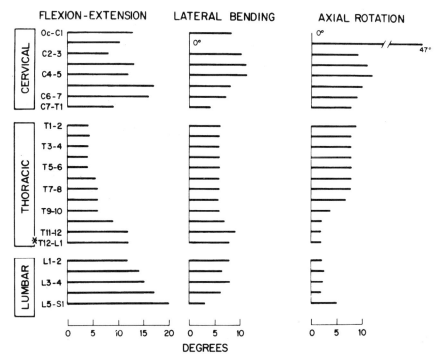

Figure 13.5. Composite of the degrees of rotation in each plane of movement for all regions of the spine.

are no longer riding on the "high point" which occurs in neutral, allowing further slack in the alar ligaments which permit further side flexion. The conjunct right rotation of the occiput relative to C2 also tends to slacken the right alar ligament, allowing further left side flexion to continue. This process continues until the right occipital rotation has taken up all the slack in the left alar ligament (which was slackened by the approximation of C1–2 and the left side flexion). At this point, all components of the mechanism have reached their limits, resulting in side flexion of about 10° (47). Note should also be made of the relatively large total excursion of the cervical spine in all of the planes of motion.

Conversely, motion in the thoracic spine is limited in all planes, mostly due to the ribs. The spinous processes primarily constrain extension. The lumbar spine can be characterized by the large excursions in flexion and extension but by markedly limited range in rotation. The rotation limitation is largely due to the plane of the facet joints, but contributing to the limitation may be the wedge morphology of the joint that permits greater twisting when the joints are flexed (83). Finally, we should call attention to the great degree of flexion-extension available at the articulation of the fifth lumbar vertebra with the sacrum. Figure 13.5 and other resources (57, 122) provide more detailed analyses of the differences between segments.

Researchers have noticed certain coupling patterns. For example, axial rotation accompanies lateral bending from C2 through C7. Specifically, if lateral bending is to the left the rotation in the cervical spine is to the left, frequently observed by viewing the spinous processes deviating to the right. Data on coupling in the thoracic spine is less convincing because the results have been somewhat varied depending on the segments studied (122). Little information exists as to coupling in the lumbar spine (123), but Pearcy and Tibrewal have found no simple mechanical coupling of the rotations in the lumbar spine. The lumbar lordosis and muscular control have been identified as the two primary factors in determining the relation between primary and accompanying rotations (89).

More precise analytic work provides detailed descriptions of spinal segment motion. A study providing one such example evaluated the size of the intervertebral foramen. In the normal spine, as compared to a degenerated cadaver specimen, flexion-extension showed the most change of width in the intervertebral foramen. Figure 13.6 shows an example of the changes. Of significance is that flexion caused an increase in the foramen area of 30% while extension closed the foramen by about 20%. Note in the figure the difference in what is called the neutral zone. This zone, according to Panjabi and coworkers, represents a discontinuity between flexion and extension flexibility curves and implies that within this zone one vertebra may move with minimum effort with respect to the other vertebra. Furthermore, within this zone the ligaments, disc, or facets offer no appreciable resistance to motion. Outside this zone the elasticity of various structures will impede further motion (85). Others consider the anteroposterior dimension of the intervertebral foramen to be critical, rather than the vertical dimension. This is because disc and facet osteophyte trespass usually involve anteroposterior compression rather than vertical. Even in segments having undergone disc thinning and facet overriding, it is the anteroposterior diameter that is affected in much greater proportion than the vertical. Further details of how such motion is restricted follow in the next section.

Vertebral motion on the foramen is of specific interest because of how it may affect the nerve root exiting from the two-compartment foramen. The compartment is divided by a limiting membrane, creating a superior (or conduction) compartment and an inferior (or motion) compartment. Normal motion of the segments does not perturb the superior compartment; however, in pathology, distortion of the limiting

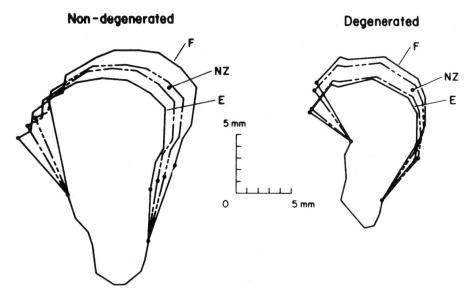

Figure 13.6.   Changes in the intervertebral foramen shape for the boundaries of a defined neutral zone (*NZ*). The extremes of flexion (*F*) and extension (*E*) ranges of motion for a moment of 7.5 Nm are also shown.

Table 13.1.   The Averaged Results

	Supraspinatous/ Interspinous Ligaments	Ligamentum Flavum	Capsular Ligaments	Intervertebral Disc
Bending moment resisted at full flexion (%)	19 (±7)	13 (±6)	39 (±8)	29 (±12)
Bending moment resisted at half flexion (%)	8 (±5)	28 (±10)	25 (±8)	38 (±13)

membrane may affect the roots and vessels entering and leaving the conduction compartment (45).

Detailed analyses of the various segments of the spine also provide insight into normal kinematics. For example, motion in the cervical spine has been analyzed by radiography, cineradiography and stereoradiography (29, 42). These studies allow for more precise identification of the geometric relationships and the angular changes occurring with motion and are likely to contribute to a better understanding of normal and pathological motion of vertebral segments. One specific example should suffice. In full flexion the upper cervical spine was almost straight (lateral view), remaining so until complete extension. At this time occiput–C1 motion recurred. By comparison, the cervical spine's lower half displayed motion throughout, concave anteriorly in full flexion to convex anteriorly in full extension. Furthermore, there was evidence that the motion in the lower cervical spine was greater than in the upper levels, which showed greater variability of motion between segments (23).

Specific data on rotation in the thoracic and lumbar areas are also available via an early study that mounted pins directly into spinous processes of multiple vertebrae. Generalizations are difficult to make because subjects did not have all the spinous processes marked. However, up to 9° of rotation occurred between the lumbar vertebrae while an average of 6° of rotation was available in all joints above the thoracolumbar junction (37). We will discuss implications of this and other information on spinal kinematics in the section on pathokinesiology.

Role of Passive Structures

An understanding of the kinematics of the human spine requires knowledge of the role of supporting structures, which include the intervertebral discs, the joints, and the ligaments. Commonly, the assessment of the role of these structures has been completed in cadaver specimens, because of the inability to study the contribution of each factor in vivo.

In sectioning the various structures that offer spinal support, researchers have analyzed nearly all tissues. Because the **posterior structures** are relied upon to control the flexion moment (74), this motion has been used to evaluate the role of individual structures. For two positions of flexion the average results for each structure are found in Table 13.1. Note that the supraspinous/interspinous ligaments and the ligamentum flavum have reciprocal roles in the two positions while the capsular ligaments and intervertebral disc do likewise (5). In any case these structures likely function in the elastic portion of their stress-strain curve (40). The properties of several tissues have also been reported. In Charzal et al. (18), the spinal ligaments studied exhibited elastic properties, demonstrating a load-deformation response that was sigmoid in shape. The most resistant structures were the intertransverse posterior longitudinal ligament and the ligamentum flavum. These data appear to establish the import of these structures in supporting the spine during the flexed posture.

Others have presented similar data resulting from sectioning of the ligaments of the spine. Facet joint apposition had a greater restraining influence than the ligamentous factors on the sagittal plane range of motion in the lumbar spine. Apparently the restraining influence of the facet joint is greater than for the ligaments, in extension and in flexion. Figure 13.7 summarizes the contribution of each factor. Some caution may need to be used in interpreting these data, however, because the pedicles of the vertebrae were cut, allowing the facet joints to slide anteriorly during the flexion motion (116). Similar analyses have also been completed in the cervical spine. Here the anterior ligaments contributed more to stability of the spine in extension than the posterior ligaments. The converse was true in flexion (122).

Other work has evaluated the role of spinal structures in resisting and limiting torsion. Adams and Hutton, for example, have performed studies that established that primary resistance is from the apophyseal (facet) joint that is in compression. The intervertebral disc also is a primary limiting factor in resisting torsion, but the capsular ligaments and the supraspinous and interspinous ligaments are unimportant (4). Further work will allow other determinations of the contribution of specific structures. In fact, some works have shown progress toward an indepth understanding of the mechanics of the spine (85, 122, 123).

Total motion of the spine is thus the product of the collective kinematics of multiple joints made up of the multiple segments. Forward inclination of the trunk is a classic example of the collective participation of these segments, the sacroiliac joints and the hip. In the forward-bending position perhaps 50–70 total degrees of flexion are available from the sacrum to the first thoracic vertebrae. Recall that most of this

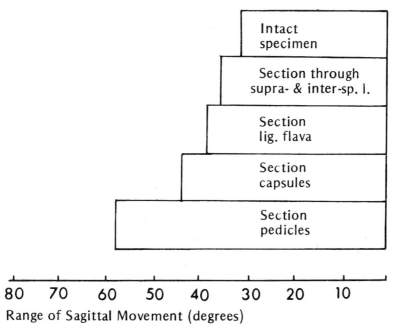

Figure 13.7. Mean ranges of sagittal plane movements of the lumbar spine following progressive release of the identified posterior vertebral elements.

motion occurs in the lumbar spine, with little contribution from the thoracic region. The remaining motion is accounted for by interaction of the pelvis with the hip, a large range of motion being available in this joint. We have discussed the role of the musculature and the passive contribution of the other structures.

Biomechanics

Spinal column biomechanics are of interest to the practitioner because the joints or the soft tissues of the spine seem incapable of tolerating the mechanical requirements of this multiple segmented column. Injuries to the low back have become a primary focus of attention due to the considerable monetary compensation paid to persons suffering from probable mechanical faults of the spine. This segment of the chapter will deal with general considerations, will discuss the mechanical properties of the tissues, and will include information on torque and instant centers of rotation.

General Mechanical Requirements

Discussed in the earlier sections of this chapter have been the anatomical structures that support the spine and the associated kinematics that result during motion. Due to the supporting nature and functional requirements of the spine external loads are imposed in several ways. As has been indicated previously, each of the motion segments is capable of six degrees of freedom: three translational and three rotational. As a result, the soft tissues are subjected to different effects as the loads and resulting motions occur at each segment. In turn, the mechanical properties of these tissues influence the biomechanics of the spine and the individual motion segments. Before discussing the material properties of the pertinent structures, we need to consider the various loads imposed upon the spine.

Axial loading in compression is inherent to the spine by virtue of the weight of the trunk, head, and arms. There have been some accounts that the facet joints can carry 18% of the load in compression (90). Other work shows that these joints in the lumbar spine carry no load in flexion, large loads during extension, torsion, and lateral bending (97). Primarily responsible for withstanding compressive forces in the spine are the intervertebral discs. Another study has established that during axial loading the load is along a direction perpendicular to the facet surfaces. The authors go on to state that this orientation implies that the total load is distributed to share axial loading between intervertebral and facet joints and resist anterior and lateral shear (65). Notably larger in the lumbar segment of the spine, these discs also can respond to motion by resisting shear and adapting to spinal segment rotations.

In contrast with compressive loading, another form of axial force is **tensile loading.** Usually applied only in treatment situations such as traction, tensile loading increases the distance between each segment. The intervertebral disc itself becomes elongated and narrowed as the ligaments become stretched. Because surrounding soft tissues may guide the vertebrae, surgeons often institute elongation because of fractures or fracture/dislocations in the spine (92). No matter the direction of the axial load, factors of stress, strain, and elasticity are all to be considered. The effect is dependent on the direction, size, and rate of application of the load.

Bending, commonly labeled as flexion, extension, and lateral flexion, creates different demands. Here moments produce the respective bending. As has been discussed in the section on kinematics the effects of the soft tissues or the bones may be important limiting factors, the former due primarily to excessive elongation. We should take note that the compressive effect due to bending is entirely dependent upon the locus of the center of rotation of the segments undergoing the motion. Thus, for forward flexion the anterior structures are compressed while the supraspinal ligaments are elongated, if the axis of rotation is in the posterior aspect of the vertebral body-disc-vertebral body (intervertebral) joint. Compressive stress is realized in the anterior structures while tensile stress occurs in the posterior structures. Tissues found along the axis about which the turning is taking place remain relatively unstressed. We will offer further discussion of the effects of various tissues in the kinetics section.

Two other motions of considerable import are **shear** and **torsion**. The former is known to be a problem because the anteroposterior curvatures in the spine, particularly in the lumbar region and at the lumbosacral joint, tend to produce anterior translatory motion of the superior vertebra on the inferior vertebra. Here shear occurs in the intervertebral joint and also in the facet joints. The forward leaning of the body increases the size of the shear, because the effect of gravity on the superior vertebra will be more pronounced. Any effects on soft tissue can be specified by means of a free body diagram and the analysis of the tendencies for motion.

In torsion (rotation) about the longitudinal axis of the spine, the effects of movement depend on the location of the center of rotation (77). Particularly in the lumbar segments is the shear force at a maximum. Recall also that the plane of the lumbar facet joints differs from that of the thoracic, influencing the resulting kinematics. In any case, torsion produces asymmetrical effects. For example, considering the facet joints during rotation, one joint is compressed. Once rotation has progressed to the point that one lumbar facet engages its joint partner, the center of rotation of further movement must move to a point between those facet surfaces. Since the disc is at some distance from this center, it must necessarily experience shear if further rotation occurs. The contralateral facet is simultaneously further distracted. The soft tissues maintaining the integrity of these joints are shortened and elongated, respectively (47).

Mechanical Properties

Of the elements responsible for maintaining the integrity of the spine, the intervertebral discs, ligaments, and vertebrae each have important mechanical properties. Of these, we will not fully discuss the properties of the vertebrae, partly because the general structure and functions of the facet joints have been presented earlier in the chapter. Bone strength is pertinent, however, in cases of large and/or sudden axial loads that may readily result in fractures. Furthermore, the cartilaginous end plate can be considered an interface with the intervertebral disc, yet this structure is subject to failure (e.g., an end plate fracture).

Of greatest interest to students of spinal biomechanics is the intervertebral disc, often because many have seen the structure as a significant factor in low back pain. In general, the disc serves to absorb loads and distribute the forces applied to the spine. Two constituents assume responsibility for these functions. The most centrally located is the nucleus pulposus. This substance contains a relatively high proportion of glycosaminoglycans which can imbibe (or hold) water. As a result, the nucleus is a gelatinous hydrophilic substance that contains as much as 88% water (54). Because of this affinity for water and the contained space in which it resides, the nucleus is always under pressure to expand outwardly. This preexisting tension is known as **preload,** and influences the mechanical behavior of the disc. Except for the lumbar spine, the nucleus can be considered centrally located within the disc. In this case the position is somewhat more posterior (122).

A second structure, the annulus fibrosus, surrounds the nucleus. This fibrocartilaginous structure is composed of fibers arranged in a laminated fashion; that is, the fibers run obliquely to each other at an angle of about 30° to the plane of the disc. Centrally the fibers are attached to the cartilaginous end plates while peripherally the attachments are directly into the osseous tissue of the vertebral body. We should also note that the fibers are thicker and more numerous anteriorly than posteriorly. In addition, the posterior and posterolateral fibers have a more parallel alignment than do the anterior fibers (44, 86).

Because of these anatomical features of the intervertebral disc, the structure can be considered **anisotropic;** that is, the mechanical properties vary with different spatial orientations (122). For example, the elastic properties of the annulus vary with the distance from the center of the disc and with the relative orientation of fibers and the applied load (54). Note that the laminated structure in effect "contains" the preloaded nucleus pulposus while simultaneously resisting tensile and shear forces resulting from movement of the spine.

Because of the role of the discs in spine mechanics, extensive work has been done on behavior during various loading conditions. Axial loading, producing compression of the disc, has been of most interest because of the similarities with the loads imposed on the disc by virtue of the upright posture and lumbar extension (3). In general, compressive loads increase the internal pressure in the disc, stretching the fibers of the annulus and loading the endplates. Therefore, load is transmitted to the adjacent vertebrae and absorbed in the outer layers of the annular fibers (56). With high compressive loads, we would expect herniation of the nucleus through the annulus. However, studies have shown that failure occurs in the body of a vertebra or in the cartilaginous end plates, usually as a fracture (41).

Other tests have evaluated the **rate of loading** of the disc. Results have shown loading properties in that low loads produced little resistance while at higher loads the disc becomes stiffer. Thus, flexibility is provided at low loads and stability at high loads (122). Consider these events with what Kapandji has called the mechanism of self-stabilization. In this situation when an asymmetrical load applies a moment to a vertebra, the pressure increases in the nucleus on the side toward which the bending occurs. As a result, the tendency is for unbending to occur, equilibrating the stretch on the fibers of both sides of the annulus. Thus, the mechanisms associated with spinal motions are contingent on the interaction of both the nucleus and the fibers of the annulus (52).

Resistance to tension and shear produced by spinal movement is another important feature of disc mechanics. Again, the angular orientation of the laminated annular fibers assists to resist excessive motions such as those in the posterior fibers during forward bending. Simultaneously with flexion, the anterior, as well as posterolateral, portions of the disc become remarkably compressed and stretched respectively, and may sustain potentially dangerous injuries. During rotation, both tension and shear are created in the annulus. Shear, of course, takes place in the horizontal plane around which the rotation is occurring. Tension would develop in the fibers oriented in the direction of the rotation and shear would exist between these fibers and the adjacently oriented fibers of the annular laminae. Because motion is greatest in the fibers that are farthest from the center of rotation, we expect the greatest stresses in the peripheral segments of the annular fibers. Figures 13.8 and 13.9 show the effects of these motions (122).

Experimental studies have also evaluated the behavior of the intervertebral joints under conditions of physiological loading. In this type of testing, axial and shear

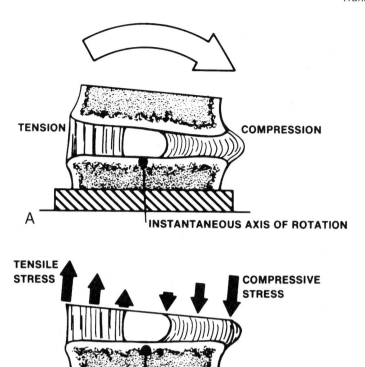

Figure 13.8. Stress in the disc with bending in flexion, extension, and lateral bending. **A,** one portion of the disc is subjected to compression while the opposite side is under tension. **B,** the stresses vary in magnitude in relationship to the location from the instantaneous axis of rotation.

loads have been used in isolation, in combination with each other, and with eccentric (off-center) loading. Such techniques allow the study of disc and annulus behavior and the mechanical analysis of the effects of sectioning various structures. Lin and colleagues (63) produced an exemplary piece of work that established that anterior disc bulging is usually greater than the lateral bulge during axial or eccentric loads. Furthermore, failure occurred in the vertebral body and not in the annulus fibrosus, confirming many other studies offering the same finding. Their study also sectioned the posterior elements. Following testing of the specimens, the researchers reached the conclusion that the posterior elements play a minor role in bearing axial loads. However, during complex loading consisting of compression, bending, and/or shear, a load path through the superior and inferior articular processes is activated. These authors also found that the posterior elements are responsible for increased shear stiffness of the intervertebral joint (63). Other studies have used models of the disc, evaluating the loads that can be tolerated within normal physiological limits. Some of these studies which primarily concern the annulus, have shown that fiber rupture is not likely to occur because of the tendency for endplate failure to be reached first. In fact, bending, shear, or axial rotation does not appear to produce fiber rupture, unless these loads are combined with very high axial loads (14).

Behavior of the disc is typical of a viscoelastic material. This is displayed in the

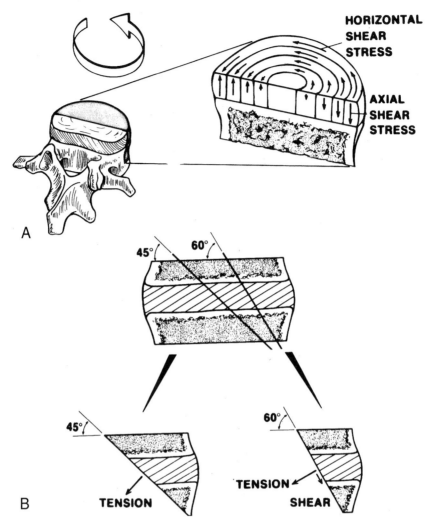

Figure 13.9. Stress in the disc with torsion. **A,** shear is produced in the horizontal plane as well as in the axial direction, both of equal magnitude. The stress varies at different points in the disc in proportion to the distance from the instantaneous axis of rotation. **B,** at 45° to the plane of the disc, there is no shear (because of the orientation of the annular fibers). Note that at 60° both shear and tension stresses would exist.

effects of loading rate on the stiffness of the disc. Recall also that the nucleus has a high percentage of water. Furthermore, because of viscoelastic qualities, **creep, relaxation,** and **hysteresis** are demonstrable. With hysteresis, where energy is lost when a structure is subjected to repetitive loading and unloading cycles, greater loads have been found to produce greater hysteresis. Virgin found that lower lumbar discs had greater hysteresis than the upper lumbar and lower thoracic vertebrae and that younger groups had more than a middle-aged population (118). Each of these factors may eventually play a role in the normal or abnormal mechanics of the spine.

These structures have been evaluated for their material properties because they do appear to play a significant role in both the kinematics and kinetics of the spine. Of most interest are the posterior elements, primarily because of their apparent ability to assist with control or production of extension moments. Recalling the anatomy of the posterior ligamentous system reminds one that some ligamentous structures are posterior to the spinous processes by as much as 1 to 1.5 cm. Two benefits accrue. First, ligamentous tension improves passive extension leverage and reduces the compression at the intervertebral joint due to muscular contraction. The second advantage relates to the orientation of ligament fibers: they are more perpendicular to the spinous processes rather than in a superior-inferior direction as is often depicted. Because of the direction of the supraspinous and interspinous ligaments, this allows flexion to occur up to a point rather than constrain the motion of one vertebra over the others. Note also that the ligaments span only one joint, because if 30% extensibility were allowed, abnormally large rotations would occur at the intervertebral joints (34).

Another interesting finding is that **pre-tension** apparently exists in spinal ligaments. A stress-strain plot based on studies of the ligamentum flavum is shown in Figure 13.10. First, note that the ligament is under 15% pre-tension in the neutral position. This level of tension means that if the ligament were transected, shortening would occur to a new length 15% shorter than the in situ length. If the neck is extended, the strain decreases to 5%, but does not allow the ligament to buckle into the spinal canal. Conversely, flexion allows an increase of 35% strain. If force, stiffness, and energy absorbed were calculated from the curve, relatively small values for these mechanical parameters would result. However, after the full range of flexion is reached, note that the curve has a very steep slope, indicating a high degree of stiffness. Thus, the cervical spine has the capability of operating effectively within the physiological range as the ligament accomplishes supportive functions. Yet, the ligamentum flavum can protect the spine by absorbing large amounts of energy before the failure point is reached (80). Although the ligamentum flavum has a uniquely high elastic fiber constituency, we may apply similar principles to other ligaments. Little specific experimental evidence exists as to the function of these ligaments but different tissue constituency will be responsible for differing degrees of mechanical effect.

Analyses have incorporated the effects of various tissues on and during the move-

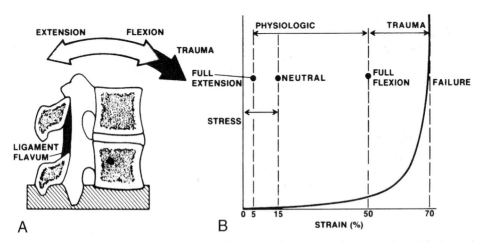

Figure 13.10.   **A,** the functional position of the ligamentum flavum preceding the motions of flexion and extension. **B,** a stress-strain curve showing specific points in the range of motion.

ment of the spine. For example, during flexion the interspinous ligament sustains significant amounts of stress, over 40,000 N, causing in turn large shear components resisted by the facet complex (69). In hyperextension, investigators have determined that the disc can be damaged if high compressive forces are occurring simultaneously (3). Furthermore, models have shown a unique degree of lordosis that minimizes and equalizes the compressive stress within the spine. Although these results stem from a model rather than in vivo Gracovetsky et al. make a case for the benefits of the pelvic tilt exercise in controlling the pelvic attitude (35). Lumbar compressive and shear forces have also been calculated from other models believed to have valid applications to the in vivo situation. These results show that lumbar forces were maximized during the initial position of the long-lying curl-up exercise. In hooklying the compressive forces were reduced by 4–5% and the shear forces by 39–46%, depending on the evaluation of male or female subjects. The bench curl-up (hips and knees flexed 90°) minimized the forces to 17–18% in compression and to 87–97% in shear (46). Should these data be accurate effects on the lumbar spine could be significant. Finally, the wearing of belts has been evaluated, partly in response to their use in many work environments. From assessing the effect of the belt and breath holding on the passive bending properties of the intact human torso in all three planes, the data suggest that stiffness was not increased in flexion and extension movements (73). Further work in all areas of trunk control and stabilization is needed to provide definitive answers as to the best control mechanisms to use. Many variables, difficult to control, will confound the analyses and the subsequent therapeutic implications.

Instant Centers of Rotation

The various motion segments of the spine are of interest to study because of the distinct relationship to kinematics and kinetics and potential impact on pathomechanics. Study of the axes of motion is complicated, however, by the influence of each of the adjacent motion segments and the difficulties associated with study of multiple motion segments, each possessing six degrees of freedom. In spite of these factors, some information is available on the instant centers of rotation.

In the cervical spine the occiput–C1 and C1–C2 joints deserve special consideration. In the former, the sagittal plane (for flexion and extension) is believed to be 2–3 cm above the tip of the dens. For lateral bending the axis appears to be in the midline slightly more distant from the tip of the dens. Although this information was published long ago, little additional information has disputed these findings (122).

In the C1–C2 joint, the axis for sagittal plane motion is believed to be in the middle third of the dens. As may be anticipated, rotation occurs about the axis, and, because lateral flexion at this joint is small or nonexistent, the location of an axis for this motion may be irrelevant. Details associated with this issue were discussed in the previous section on kinematics. The locations of the axes for the remainder of the cervical spine have been identified for the sagittal and the horizontal planes. The latter is less well agreed upon, but the anterior portion of the subjacent vertebra is the likely location. Keep in mind the issue of coupling (see section on kinematics) (122).

The literature has no consensus on lateral bending axes in the cervical spine. For the thoracic spine locations have been identified for all planes. Compared to the other segments of the spine, the centers in the lumbar spine are located more specifically for the motion taking place in the respective plane (122). These are

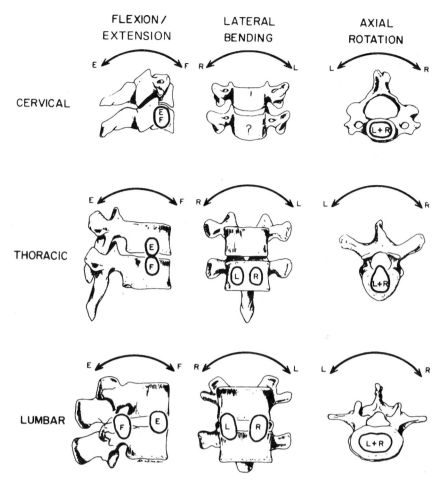

Figure 13.11. The approximate locations of the instantaneous axes of rotation. *Legend*: *F*, flexion; *E*, extension; *L*, left; *R*, right.

shown in Figure 13.11 and is reproduced directly from the cited 1975 source. However, in the 1990 edition of the White and Panjabi book the F and E in the lumbar spine have been reversed (122). Furthermore, question has been raised as to the confidence with which we can regard the instant centers of rotation. For example, only the center for flexion from extension can be plotted with acceptable confidence as there was considerable variation in the measurements (88).

The locations of these instant centers further the understanding of the kinematics of the spine and assist the study of kinetics because forces can then be related to axes of motion about which the turning effect can be determined. In many activities, whether functional or therapeutic, therapists can apply known mechanics to produce desired effects. We will discuss the application of these principles in a subsequent section on pathokinesiology.

Torque

Despite the professed importance of the trunk musculature in the prevention and/or treatment of low back pain and dysfunction, generally little is known about the ability of the flexors or the extensors to exert torque. The problem is confounded by motion occurring at multiple segments simultaneously, making it a methodologically difficult question to answer.

Researchers have attempted to determine flexor and extensor torque but comparisons across studies are difficult at best. One study used the sidelying position to evaluate concentric, isometric, and eccentric torque capabilities. In all cases of dynamic exercise, the velocity was limited to 13°/sec. Peak isometric flexion torque was 194 Nm in the neutral position, increasing to 211 Nm at 20° of trunk extension. Isometric extension torque was 380 Nm at 40° of flexion, diminishing to 312 Nm at 20° of flexion. As anticipated from the force-velocity relationship, the eccentric values were higher than isometric torque and the concentric values were lower. Variation of dynamic torques from the isometric values was relatively small due to the slow velocity used during testing (105).

Many other studies have tested subjects from a variety of age ranges, mostly with constant velocity dynamometers (39, 51, 72, 81, 82, 102, 114). In general, large variation is found in the values in Table 13.2. The differences across these studies can serve as primary examples of the importance of testing technique. Although comparison is made possible because of the use of the torque (rather than force) measurements, the large discrepancies probably are due in large part to the methodologies employed. With the arrival of better, more valid dynamometers, additional data on both normals and subjects with low back pain and dysfunction will be forthcoming.

Among the most important variables may be the position of the lumbar spine during the testing. For example, McGill has shown that a hyperlordotic spine produced significantly smaller axial torques. A hypolordotic spine produced even small values. McGill explained the data saying that tissues other than muscles with a passive component contribute to the torque (71). Other evaluations include those that have shown measurements to be reliable (at least in selected situations) (36), or those whose results from various postures cause us to question the validity of the current lifting recommendations commonly used (112). We may derive the explanation for some of these results from known anatomical relationships. For example, locations of the lines of action of the erector spinae and other muscles have been determined with MRI (117) and with computed tomography (76), establishing variance in the locations of these muscles as the kinematics of the segments is altered. Sometimes extreme postures tended to alter the torque potential of some muscles (70).

Kinetics

For reasons previously cited, the forces associated with motion of individual or collective segments of the spine are difficult to determine. This does not negate the importance of these determinations, because the magnitudes and temporal sequencing of the contributions of both the active and passive structures are critical factors for normal movement. Disruptions in normal kinematics may alter kinetic requirements and subsequently alter the ability of the individual to perform either functional or work-related tasks. This section will address the kinetics of the spine, first concentrating on intradiscal pressure, then focusing on muscular and ligamentous forces, and finally on their interaction as related to trunk movement.

Intradiscal Pressure

Measurement of the pressure within the disc has been completed in vitro and in vivo. Under the former conditions, cadaver specimens were used to demonstrate that pressure was 1.3–1.6 times the vertical load applied per unit area. Pressure increased linearly for loads up to 2000 N. Motion studies on such specimens have become less important since the coming of a special transducer used for direct measurement of the intradiscal pressure. This technique has been used to collect information on intradiscal pressure during various postures, activities, and exercises. Table13.3 provides a summary of the approximate loads in the third lumbar disc of a person with a mass of 70 kg. Note specifically that standing at ease and upright sitting without support both result in considerable intradiscal pressure, the latter being about 40% greater than that of standing. All modifications of posture are seen to influence pressure values. One posture not listed but of potential interest is the standing position with one foot placed in front and elevated by 6–12 inches. In this case the intradiscal pressure is decreased from the standing value. A summary of the technique and results can be found in Nachemson (78).

Lifting Mechanisms

Many functions of the human body, during either work or everyday activities, require flexion of the spine. As implied in earlier sections of this chapter, this task demands the generation of forces in many tissues of the spine, primarily those of the lumbar region. To support the weight of the trunk and any object that may be held in front of the body, the spine has to develop an adequate extension moment. Although the size of this moment is contingent upon the mass and location of the object being held and the mass and position of the trunk, the tissues responsible for the extension moment are the posterior muscles and ligaments, the anteriorly compressed disc, and those other tissues involved in increasing intra-abdominal pressure. Any changes in the former parameters affect the latter forces required to maintain the trunk in equilibrium or alter the dynamic state. The size of such changes is based on the amount of the load variation, the new position assumed, and such factors as the velocity with which the changes occur. Clearly, the greater the loads and/or degree of trunk flexion, the greater the requirements of the structures responsible for the extension moment. In essence, the extension moment required to offset the weight of the trunk would reflect the trigonometric functions (see Appendix A). Any additional load would commensurately increase the size of the flexion moment produced and that must conversely be neutralized by the extension moment so that equilibrium is maintained.

Not to be minimized is the concurrent tendency, in greater angles of forward leaning, for increased **shear forces.** A simple diagram of the pelvis and the lumbar vertebrae (Fig. 13.12) can demonstrate this tendency. In the upright posture, the greatest amount of load is in axial compression. As the fully flexed posture is assumed, each vertebra tends to shift anteriorly due to the weight of the trunk and any load supported by the hands. This shifting tendency becomes an important factor, because it determines what forces are needed to counteract an anterior displacement and maintain appropriate kinematics and/or moments.

Much attention has been paid to the role of the musculature in the control of trunk flexion. Very low levels of erector spinae and lower extremity extensor muscle activity are required during the normal standing posture. As the trunk is inclined forward, activity progressively increases until about 45 to 60° of flexion. At that point, muscle activity rapidly diminishes (Fig. 13.2), although there is a necessity for large extension moments.

Researchers have attempted to determine the force generated in the back extensors to assess the contribution of these muscles to the total extension moment. Calculations

Table 13.2.   Shoulder Torques for Subjects Without Pathology

Source Reference	Gender	Age Mean	Age SD	Age Range	n	Spine Level	Movement	Concentric (°sec)	Eccentric (°sec)	ROM	Testing Position	Peak Torque Nm	Peak Torque SD	Testing Device
72	f	20	2		21	cervical	(R) rot	0		0		60	20	Cybex II
						cervical	(L) rot	0		0		61	19	
						cervical	(R) rot	0		30 (R) rot		37	14	
						cervical	(L) rot	0		30 (L) rot		68	22	
						cervical	(R) rot	0		30 (R) rot		70	24	
						cervical	(L) rot	0		30 (L) rot		40	12	
						cervical	(R) rot	30		full		64	19	
						cervical	(L) rot	30		full		61	15	
						cervical	(R) rot	60		full		56	18	
						cervical	(L) rot	60		full		56	19	
	m	21	9		10	cervical	(R) rot	0		0		94	21	Cybex II
						cervical	(L) rot	0		0		100	16	
						cervical	(R) rot	0		30 (R) rot		71	16	
						cervical	(L) rot	0		30 (L) rot		102	19	
						cervical	(R) rot	0		30 (R) rot		109	17	
						cervical	(L) rot	0		30 (L) rot		74	22	
						cervical	(R) rot	30		full		92	17	
						cervical	(L) rot	30		full		87	15	
						cervical	(R) rot	60		full		83	19	
17	m	39	9		21	lumbar	e	0		0		214	41	Med Ex
						lumbar	e	0		12		266	50	
						lumbar	e	0		24		304	61	
						lumbar	e	0		36		336	60	
						lumbar	e	0		48		381	71	
114	m	43			23	lumbar	f	30			stand, knee 15	267		Cybex II
						lumbar	e	30				244		
						lumbar	f	60				260		
						lumbar	e	60				249		
						lumbar	f	90				249		
						lumbar	e	90				249		
						lumbar	f	120				243		
						lumbar	e	120				254		

n	sex	age		age range		site	motion	vel			position	mean	SD	device
82	f	38			21	lumbar	f	30			stand, knee 15	161	19	Cybex II
						lumbar	e	30				151	23	
						lumbar	f	60				149	28	
						lumbar	e	60				148	40	
						lumbar	f	90				142	38	
						lumbar	e	90				145	41	
						lumbar	f	120				140		
						lumbar	e	120				143		
	f	28		18–48	101	lumbar	f	0			sup	61	9	Cybex II
						lumbar	e	0			prone, resist. @tip of scap	98	9	
						lumbar	f	30			sup	111	9	
						lumbar	e	30			prone, resist. @tip of scap	122	13	
						lumbar	f	60			sup	107	4	
						lumbar	e	60			prone, resist. @tip of scap	108	5	
51	f	31	5		18	lumbar	f	0				59		Cybex II
						lumbar	e	0				95		
						lumbar	f	30				104		
						lumbar	e	30				128		
						lumbar	f	60				116		
						lumbar	e	60				122		
	f	56	7	38–73	61	lumbar	f	0	35			97	23	KinCom
						lumbar	e	0	35			196	54	
						lumbar	f	20		20		84	28	
						lumbar	e	20		20		168	48	
						lumbar	f					95	32	
						lumbar	e					213	78	
81	m	8	10	20–5	35	lumbar	e	60				237	70	Cybex II
						lumbar	e	90				225	70	
						lumbar	e	120				198	70	
						lumbar	f	60				213	47	
						lumbar	f	90				206	46	
						lumbar	f	120				198	42	
						lumbar	(L) rot	60				127	39	
						lumbar	(L) rot	120				118	39	
						lumbar	(L) rot	150				115	35	
						lumbar	(R) rot	60				127	38	
						lumbar	(R) rot	120				119	37	
						lumbar	(R) rot	150				118		

Table 13.2—*continued*

Source Reference	Gender	Age Mean	Age SD	Age Range	n	Spine Level	Movement	Concentric (°sec)	Eccentric (°sec)	ROM	Testing Position	Peak Torque Nm	Peak Torque SD	Testing Device
8	f	8	10	20–5	35	lumbar	e	60				129	42	Cybex II
						lumbar	e	90				126	43	
						lumbar	e	120				104	47	
						lumbar	f	60				126	31	
						lumbar	f	90				122	34	
						lumbar	f	120				108	37	
						lumbar	(L) rot	60				68	26	
						lumbar	(L) rot	120				71	26	
						lumbar	(L) rot	150				71	23	
						lumbar	(R) rot	60				69	26	
						lumbar	(R) rot	120				71	26	
						lumbar	(R) rot	150				73	24	

Legend: e, extension; f, flexion; (L) rot, left rotation; (R) rot, right rotation; scap, scapula.

Table 13.3.   Approximate Load on L3 Disc in a Person Weighing 70 kg

	Newton (N)
Supine, awake	250
Supine, semi-Fowler position	100
Supine, traction 500 N	0
Supine, tilt table 50°	400
Supine, arm exercises	500
Upright sitting, without support	700
Sitting with lumbar support, back rest inclination 110°	400
Standing at ease	500
Coughing	600
Straining	600
Forward bend, 20°	600
Forward bend, 40°	1000
Forward bend, 20° with 20 kg	1200
Forward flexed 20° and rotated 20° with 10 kg	2100
Sit-up exercises	1200
Bilateral leg lift	800
Lifting 10 kg, back straight, knees bent	1700
Lifting 10 kg, back bent	1900
Holding 5 kg, arms extended	1900

From Nachemson AL: Disc pressure measurements. *Spine.* 6:93–97, 1981.

Newton (N) is the force unit of the SI system. N is defined as the force necessary to give a mass of 1 kg the acceleration 1 m/sec². 1 N = 0.102 kp. For practical purposes 10 N = 1 kp = 2.25 lbf.

have shown that the erector spinae group contributes between 37 and 59% of the total extensor moment at the L4–L5 interspace for two different specimens (91). Schultz and coworkers determined that the contraction forces of the extensors ranged from 0 to 890 N, the latter for the case of 30° of trunk flexion with the arms out and holding an 8 kg weight (99). In a separate study the extensor muscle force ranged from 100 to 2270 N (bilaterally), with the highest value required during trunk flexion with a load of 80 N held in the hands (98). These large forces point out the significant contribution of the extensor muscle mass. Yet, as the need for the extension moment

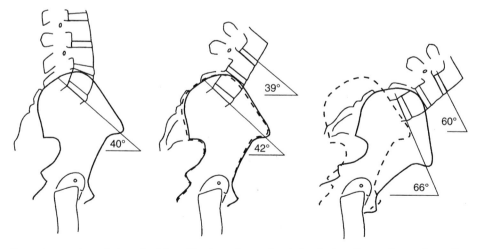

Figure 13.12.   Lateral view of pelvis and lumbar spine motion during flexion. Composite angular motions are shown, but particularly note that with increased flexion the shear of each vertebra on adjacent segments is markedly increased.

increases with forward flexion of the trunk from the standing position, active muscle contributions diminish in favor of reliance upon passive elements. Although elastic tissue in the extensor muscles and tendons can contribute some tension, the ligaments appear to play a major role. How the posterior ligaments can control much of the moment is open to speculation. However, by knowing the cross-sectional area of the midline and facet joint ligaments and the thickness of the lumbodorsal fascia, a determination of the support can be made if individual tensile muscle strengths are known. Following this procedure, Gracovetsky et al. calculated that the posterior structures can support a moment of about 127 kgm (1245 Nm) (34). Others have suggested that the increase in lumber tissue length adds passive tissue strain to the requirements for extensor torque (115).

An alternative would be to adopt another strategy to accomplish the lift. We primarily discuss this matter in Chapter 16, but relative to the moment requirements studies have shown that the stoop lift decreased the peak extensor moment by about 10% compared to squat lifting. However, the bending torque increased by approximately 75%. Consideration should also be given to the speed of the movement, as well as to the size, position, and mass of the object lifted (25).

Pathokinesiology

Many and extensive injuries to the various segments of the spine are responsible for movement abnormalities, and much has been written on pathologies that affect the spine. Rather than attempt an exhaustive survey of the possible causes of pathological motion, only selected but representative problems will be discussed. Several problems disrupting cervical spine motion will first be presented. Following a brief discussion of spondylolisthesis, the problem of low back dysfunction and forms of exercise treatment will be considered. Finally, we will provide more extensive analysis of the mechanical principles of scoliosis treatment.

Cervical Spine Pathomechanics

Within the cervical region of the spine, as with the other regions, **dislocations** can occur between any two motion segments. Such dislocations can be unilateral or bilateral, depending on the type and degree of forces that create the abnormal kinematics. Unilateral dislocation results from a combination of excessive lateral bending and axial rotation such that the superior vertebra is carried anteriorly and superiorly on the inferior surface. Bilateral dislocations cause the unit to lock until reduction is attained. Excessive flexion that forces anterior and superior gliding of the superior surface on the lower vertebra is the most likely cause. In either case, capsular integrity may be totally lost, presenting problems with spine stability across the injured segments. Furthermore, bilateral facet joint dislocation can significantly damage the posterior elements, leading to further loss of stability. Ultimately treatment is directed toward correcting alignment, allowing healing, and restoring normal joint kinematics (122).

Extension injuries usually create more complex problems. Forcible extension, particularly at high velocity, may rupture the anterior longitudinal ligament. Extreme range of motion may even cause the annulus fibrosus to be separated from the upper vertebra. Commonly this hyperextension injury follows some degree of flexion, as seen in the whiplash injury. Often the sixth cervical vertebra is affected more often than adjacent segments because sagittal plane motion is more limited in this portion of the cervical spine. At any rate, the restoration of normal cervical kinematics is difficult because of the apparent myriad of problems associated with this injury. For example, disc narrowing, pain, and muscle spasm are often encountered, leading to compounding of the pathology, although the problem may be limited to small quantities of soft tissue.

Central to the issue of cervical spine pathology are **neck orthoses.** Although they are frequently used to control motion of the spine in both acute and chronic injuries, little assessment of their effects has been completed. One group studied the effectiveness of five different braces, ranging from soft collars to a skeletally fixed halo device. The study showed that increasing the rigidity and length of the orthosis improved ability to limit motion. However, lateral bending and rotation of the entire cervical spine, as well as flexion and extension in the upper levels, were not well controlled with any of the orthoses tested. In general, the best conventional means of bracing controlled 45% of flexion and extension while the skeletally attached device restricted 75% of these motions (48). This study and others point out that even judicious use of bracing may not result in limiting motion at the desired spinal level.

Lumbar Spine Dysfunction

Because studies have reported pain or discomfort in the lower spine in as high as 80% of the population, the question of causative factors has been the subject of frequent study. Specific attempts have been undertaken to identify the risk factors associated with painful conditions. In a sample of over 1200 patients, those with severe pain were found to hold jobs requiring repetitive heavy lifting, the use of jackhammers and machine tools, or the operation of motor vehicles (31). Fatigue-induced failures have been specifically addressed (96). In fact, mechanical fatigue damage has been suggested as a frequent cause of low back pain (2). It is of some interest that those with moderate pain tend to maintain a higher level of sports activity than those with severe pain, but the explanation for this finding could be due to the fact that severe pain limited participation (31). Certainly the low back dysfunction patient is likely to have a diminished range of motion (68).

Included among the potential causes of low back dysfunction is the problem of **spondylolisthesis.** This anterior slipping, usually of the fifth lumbar vertebra on the sacrum, may result from several causes, for example a fracture through the pars interarticularis (92). In effect, the superior vertebra slides anteriorly because of anterior shear force. Natural lumbar hyperextension is partly at fault but flexion of the lumbar spine may worsen the condition because, as discussed earlier, the flexed trunk posture increases the likelihood of anterior shear. Resistance to shear would be available via the facet joints, but such force, applied continuously, leads to plastic deformation of the anterior and posterior ligaments and fibers of the annulus. Restoration of normal biomechanics may require operative intervention to stabilize the joint. Until that time, the joint would be considered unstable from both a clinical and functional standpoint. However, a spondylolisthesis may involve a fixed displacement—one that doesn't alter as seen on stress films. Thus, instability may not be present. In contrast, a spondylolisthesis that involves less total displacement may also very easily displace and reduce: this one is symptomatic, while the former may not be at all (47).

A common opinion as to the cause of low back pain is **degeneration of the disc.** High incidence of narrowing of the intervertebral space has been associated with low back pain. Narrowing also occurs with aging, another factor closely linked to low back pain. However, we should note that symptomatic lumbar spines often become asymptomatic with advanced age, apparently because dehydration of the

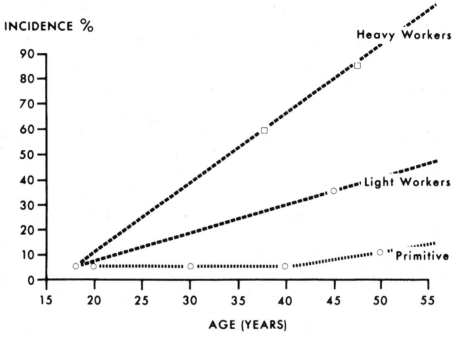

Figure 13.13. Incidence of disc narrowing, determined by radiograph, plotted versus age. Primitive cultures consistently assume a full crouched position as opposed to the lordotic position of workers.

disc and stiffness of the ligaments serve to immobilize the spine and prevent aggravation by movement.

Fahrni has raised an interesting point (28). Because disc lesions and chronic back pain are rare in cultures that frequently adopt the full-squat position, he evaluated the degree of **disc narrowing** in several groups. Perhaps not surprisingly the groups assuming the primitive posture had by far the least incidence of disc narrowing. Note in Figure 13.13 that the incidence for a Swedish group involved in heavy labor was as high as 80%. Caution may be necessary, however, because the study does not state that the primitive people were involved in as heavy labor as the Swedish group. If not, this element could be a very significant confounder because we know that heavy lifting versus light lifting—for groups with consistent postural habits— makes a great difference in the incidence of disc narrowing. Thus, there may still be some question as to the effects of the lordotic posture on disc degeneration. Physiological phenomena such as thinning of the cartilaginous plates, loss of nuclear water content, and changes in the annulus are other factors that demonstrate degeneration of the disc. Thus, as expected, degeneration leads to loss of the intrinsic stability of the spine, predisposing the segments or entire regions to injury and/or dysfunction. Investigations providing data to support this concept have determined that centrodes (instant centers of rotation or ICRs) of spinal motion segments were significantly increased, even in the earliest stages of degenerative disc disease. Centrodes for normal spines were found in the posterior half of the disc space and averaged 21 mm (101). Clearly one way to eliminate the unstable segment is through surgical fusion. Often criticized for relatively high rates of unsatisfactory results, the use and success of fusion have been variable. Often, adjacent stable segments have a postfusion increase in range of motion and added stress on the facet joints. Although all fusions provide increased stiffness the bilateral-lateral fusion may be the best to use, at least at the lumbosacral joint (62). Procedures based on the properties of materials and techniques that include biomechanical principles are important to follow to assure success (55).

Morris and Markolf go so far as to state that disc narrowing and instability tend to cause a posterior displacement of the segment centers of rotation during flexion and extension (77). Further causes of back pain and resulting dysfunction can be related to impingement of a nerve or nerves exiting through the intervertebral foramen (9, 67). Although possibly caused by disc narrowing, pressure on a nerve root could also result from herniation of the nucleus, bulging the posterior portion of the annulus. Because these and other pathologies, such as acute strains and facet syndromes, are also known to produce low back pain, only when more discriminating tests are available will the more precise cause of low back pain be identified (77).

Therapeutically, practitioners are faced with procedures that should enable the patient to have a more stable lumbar spine for the performance of both functional and lifting activities. Based upon previous information in this chapter, the primary objective of treatment then would be to increase the "strength" of the extensors and the flexors. The fact that weakness in both muscle groups has been demonstrated would lend credence to this approach (17, 106).

Strengthening the abdominal musculature as a form of treatment may not be as specific as that for the back extensors. Many exercises have been suggested for abdominal strengthening, but in all cases selection is based on several considerations. Of primary concern is the effect on the lumbar spine while the exercise is being performed. In the hooklying position, for example, lordosis in the lumbar spine is reduced. However, the degree of anterior compression of the disc is probably increased (see earlier sections of this chapter). Longlying may be dangerous from the standpoint of allowing the greatest anterior displacement of the fifth lumbar vertebra on the sacrum. Bilateral straight leg raising also has a potentially undesirable effect in that iliopsoas muscle tension contributes to the elevation of the legs. In the early portion of the range of motion, the weight of the legs produces a large moment in the direction of hip extension. The result is that the tension in the iliopsoas muscle causes the anterior lip of the pelvis to move in an inferior direction. Thus, the indirect effect is to increase lordosis, since the angle of inclination between the top of the sacrum and the fifth lumbar vertebra must increase. Holding down a patient's feet during the exercise may be ill-advised since this maneuver allows the distal attachment of the iliopsoas muscle to be fixed, allowing force to be exerted on the lumbar spine. One alternative that has been commonly used is the hooklying curl exercise. In this exercise, the patient flexes the head, neck, and shoulders forward until the sternum and the crest of the pubis can come no closer together. At the point where the scapulae just clears the supporting surface, the patient stops and then "uncurls" in reverse sequence. Little lumbar spine motion has occurred, but tension in the abdominal musculature is generally required to be at a high level (109). As studies have shown that velocity of muscle contraction had an effect on performance, avoiding high-velocity exercise may be well advised.

Intradiscal pressure measurements made while subjects complete therapeutic exercises are also important. Table 13.3 shows that the sit-up exercise creates pressure over twice the value attained during standing at ease. Bilateral leg lifts do not demonstrate such a pronounced effect, perhaps because the transducer measuring the pressure was in the posterior aspect of the disc. The inference from these data is that patients recovering from back pathology should use forms of isometric training on the basis that these exercise forms produce the least increase in intradiscal pressures (79).

One further consideration in treatment would be instruction in the principles of correct lifting technique. These principles have been presented earlier in the chapter. We also provide more precise guidelines in Chapter 16. As evidence is now surfacing on differences in the muscular and other mechanisms used to function (59), knowing what activities require large moments and what procedures should be followed for control of the kinematics and kinetics of the lumbar spine may effectively prevent further recurrences of injury.

Scoliosis

Abnormal spinal curvatures in the frontal plane have proven difficult to prevent or treat. Because the condition is likely to present in a relatively high percentage of patients, clinically effective treatment must be understood and vigorously pursued. We can directly relate such changes in curvature to the principles associated with the treatment applied. This section will discuss the application of these principles to the management of scoliosis.

Before considering the specifics of the mechanisms available to reduce the scoliotic curve, recall that the spine is similar to a flexible rod. If the rod is bent in two planes perpendicular to each other, rotation must occur. Now consider the case of lateral flexion of the thoracic and lumbar spine. Both portions of the spine have sagittal plane deviations, upon which we impose lateral flexion. In the normal circumstance, the body of a vertebra rotates toward the side of the concavity of the laterally flexing spine. Because of the location of the center of rotation, each spinous process points to the convexity of the curve. However, in scoliosis, the mechanics are altered so that the resulting motion is opposite that of the normal coupled motion, i.e., the axial rotation coupled with the lateral bending is in the wrong direction (124). The result is a clinical presentation in which the spinous processes appear straighter than the vertebrae's real configuration, i.e., the curvature is greater than appears (47).

Now, to apply the principles of treatment, consider the case of the simple lateral curvature known as a C curve. If movement of the spine is possible, two mechanisms can be used to straighten the curve. One mechanism applies **axial loading,** i.e., along the long axis of the spine (Fig. 13.14). Note that the forces must be applied in the opposite direction so that the entire spine is moved in the direction of the force. The tendency to reduce the curve thus depends on two factors: the size of the load and the length of the moment arm between the applied force and the spine.

Consider that the curve is more extreme than that shown in the figure. Given the same axial load, the tendency to reduce the curvature will be increased. The other mechanism of reducing the curve is by means of the application of **transverse load.** Figure 13.15 again demonstrates the three-point principle of force application. The applied force toward the left is equal to the two forces shown directed to the right, the result being a clockwise rotation of the upper portion of the curve and a counter clockwise rotation of the lower portion. Now consider, as for the axial load, that the curve is more extreme than that shown in Figure 13.15. Here the result is a decrease in the tendency of the applied moment to reduce the curve.

The net effect of the two mechanisms provides a third alternative for the management of the patient with scoliosis. This form of treatment is the **combined approach,**

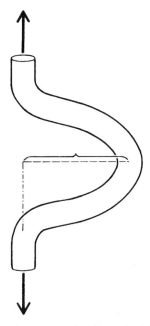

Figure 13.14. A simple C curve to demonstrate the effect of axial loads on scoliosis. The unbending moment would be considered as the force (vectors) multiplied by the distance to the apex of the curve.

used because at all degrees of angular deformity the result is best (Fig. 13.16). As indicated the effect of the axial load increases as the angular deformity increases. For the transverse load technique the maximal corrective moment is for the cases with the mildest degree of curvature. Combining the two techniques of reduction results in a corrective moment that is adequate at any degree of angular deformity. Note, however, that at an angle of 53°, the effects of either load are similar (124).

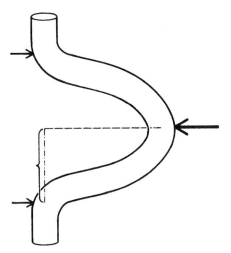

Figure 13.15. Lateral forces applied to a simple C curve. Because the moment arm is less there is less effect on straightening of the curve.

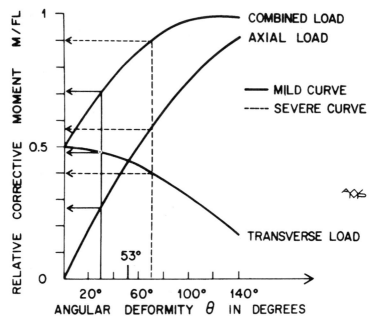

Figure 13.16. The relative corrective moment plotted versus the angular deformity for each of three methods used to control or alter scoliosis. Data for two theoretical patients are shown: one with mild (30°) scoliosis (*solid arrows*), the other with severe (70°) scoliosis (*dashed arrows*).

In managing scoliosis with either technique, the effects of **tissue creep** and **relaxation** are used. The former is realized by additional correction after no additional load is applied. The tissues continue to deform, in this case elongate, without any increase in load. Relaxation, the observed decrease in load with time, is also prevalent since as the deformation remains constant, the tissue accommodates, reducing the load on the supporting device or structure. Manipulation of these factors is responsible for the accommodation seen in the scoliotic curve. As the tissue is loaded elongation allows reduced curvature. As the tissues relax, additional loads can be tolerated that will achieve even further distraction.

Treatment of scoliosis is a classic example of the use of axial and transverse loading systems. Halo-femoral or halo-pelvic traction can apply pure axial load through fixation of the cranium and the femora or pelvis. A body jacket can apply transverse loads, which restrains the curve from further deformation. Serial casting can then modify the position of the spine.

Special comment is reserved for the **Milwaukee brace** and internal means of fixation, particularly the **Harrington rod.** Figure 13.17 shows a patient in a Milwaukee brace. Note that axial forces are applied by means of supports from the occiput and mandible to the upper rims of the pelvis. Transverse loading is accomplished by a pad applied to the lateral aspect of the ribs. Adjustment of the pads and the forces, along with the patient's conscious effort to unload the supports, offers some advantages. On the other hand, the relatively localized application of forces limits the force that can be produced at any one point. Other disadvantages accrue with larger curves; thus, the use of this device is limited to curves of less than 60° (92). There is also evidence that the Milwaukee brace is best for curves in the high thoracic region of the spine, although other body jacket methodologies are starting to produce promising results for cases of scoliosis with the apex of the curve from T7 to T9 (58).

Of several fixation techniques, Harrington rods have been popular. This surgical method uses rods in which tension can be adjusted at the time of the insertion. In effect they apply axial loads through either a compression on the convex side and/ or a tension on the concave side of the curve. Figure 13.18 shows the rods in place after they have been secured to the posterior elements of the spine. Note that the distraction rod (the one on the right side of the spine in Figure 13.18) would be more effective based on greater moment arm, but would become less effective as the curve decreases. The disadvantages, however, are that only a moderate force can be applied through the rods, primarily because of the relative weakness of the bony points of attachment. Of interest are the findings that the recommended force levels are sometimes exceeded during the insertion procedure. Conversely, too little force may explain some results in which less than the desired 40% of minimum correction is achieved (26). Reapplication of the forces after pausing several minutes between distractions, or reoperating 10–14 days later, may also take better advantage of tissue relaxation. Although some desirable changes may occur in the sagittal plane, fusion with the rods below the level of L3 is contraindicated on the basis that low back pain may increase (1, 20). In addition, posture and gait are likely to be altered (120).

Finally, we should consider **muscular effects** on the reduction of scoliosis, some of which may have bearing on the alteration of the seated posture (108). Of at least some relevance is that there are differences in fiber type proportions on the two sides of the scoliotic spine. The convex side of the curve has a higher proportion of type 1 fibers, thus reflecting abilities associated with endurance capabilities (126). To investigate the biomechanics of scoliosis Schultz et al. (100) completed theoretical

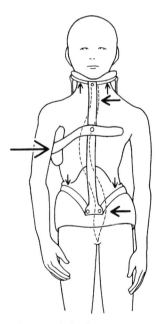

Figure 13.17. A Milwaukee brace, shown with the forces it exerts. Note that this is a combined loading system that should allow for maximum control and alteration of the scoliosis.

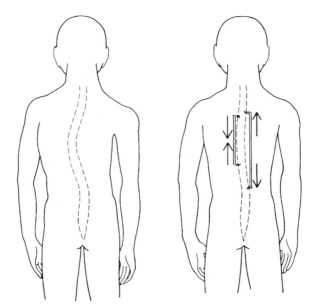

Figure 13.18. Posterior view of uncorrected scoliosis and the same scoliosis following the surgical insertion of Harrington rods. Tensile and compressive forces, in equal and opposite directions, create bending moments to control and alter the scoliosis.

analyses, stating that the muscles on the convex side of a lateral curvature can correct the curve. Their work also showed that the bulkiest, most laterally placed musculature would have the greatest effect. Some muscles included for correction of a left lumbar curve were the left lateral erector spinae, the left internal and external obliques, and the rectus abdominis. Now that asymmetries have been shown to exist in the lumbar multifidus cross-sectional area (smaller opposite to convexity of a primary thoracic curve and on the convex side of a lumbar or thoracolumbar curve) (53), other evaluations of the effect of exercise may be facilitated. Studies have made other potential treatment suggestions, some of which have been tested in an in vivo study (7). This work is of interest because of their confirmation of theoretical work. In this effort, curvature correction was found to be a linear function of the length of the moment arm between the lateral musculature and the vertebral elements of the spinal column. For example, the unbending moment from electrical stimulation of the lateral musculature was three times that from the stimulation of the paravertebral musculature. These results, which demonstrated that compensatory curves were also reduced, provide a promising method for control or correction of scoliosis and reconfirm the ability of the muscles to effect significant torque.

RESPIRATION

Compared with the function of other mechanisms of the body, the mechanics and pathomechanics of respiratory function have received little attention. Their continuous function, required to maintain a respiratory rate, requires some special considerations to maintain the respiratory function we require. Although some may claim that care of patients with abnormal kinematics or kinetics of respiration are not within the purview of the therapist, the clinical responsibilities can be justified because of the kinesiologic requirements and biomechanical considerations. This section will discuss the relevant features of the biomechanics of respiration and will conclude with a discussion of the alterations in some more common clinical conditions that affect respiration.

Muscular Actions

Function of the muscles producing respiration is somewhat difficult to study because of their size and the anatomical relationships to other muscles. Intramuscular electrodes make EMG study technically and methodologically arduous at best, often yielding results that are not definitive. Thus, much of the function has been derived based on nonexperimental data. In any case, the muscular actions can be considered based on function during the distinct motions leading to either inspiration or expiration.

With inspiration, or expansion of the thorax, one muscle thought to be primarily responsible is the **diaphragm.** Upon contraction, this dome-shaped muscle moves downward and somewhat forward, enlarging the thorax in the vertical direction. Wade was able to quantify the movement of the muscle, stating that its movement is about 1.5 cm in quiet respiration. When subjects were placed supine, less reserve diaphragmatic movement was available, perhaps due to pressure exerted by the abdominal contents (119). Other work supports this idea (93). Kapandji describes the diaphragm as descending inferiorly until the central tendon becomes fixed. At this point the muscle can elevate the lower ribs by means of lateral fibers because the origin of these fibers is more superior than their site of attachment to the ribs. In this fashion, the lateral diameter of the thorax is increased (51). In almost any case some have credited the diaphragm with being the principal, although not essential, muscle of inspiration (102).

Other muscles participating in inspiration are the sternocleidomastoid, scalene, serratus posterior superior, and pectoralis minor muscles. Some have made a case that the **scalenes** effectively lift and expand the rib cage and thus should be considered a primary and not an accessory muscle of inspiration (21). As these two primary muscles of inspiration contract and the diaphragm flattens, the compression of the abdominal contents increases intra-abdominal pressure (94). This in turn facilitates lateral pressure on the rib cage, causing expansion that contributes to the intrathoracic pressure changes that pull air into the lungs (22). Acting in concert with the actions of the diaphragm and the scalenes, more passively than actively, is the **abdominal wall.** If "tone" or intentional contraction exists the intra-abdominal pressure will be further increased, resulting in better inspiration.

Accessory muscles of inspiration can be considered the **parasternal** and the **sternocleidomastoid** muscles (94). The latter function by exerting force on the sternum, increasing the anterior-posterior diameter of the upper rib cage during inspiration. Usually the role of the external intercostals during inspiration is questionable (113). Finally, if the glenohumeral joint is abducted to at least 90° and fixed in this position, other thoracoscapulohumeral muscles can assist with elevation of the thorax.

Expiration as a result of muscle action has been debated for some time. Most evidence suggests that the **internal intercostal** muscles have this responsibility, when indeed such activity is required. Under normal, quiet respiration, expiration is thought to be a passive process, controlled by a braking action through eccentric contraction of the diaphragm and the intercostal muscles (93, 94). Under conditions involving forced expiration, as during exertion, the expiratory muscles may play an active role in rib depression and diminution of the size of the thorax. Such motions may also be aided by accessory muscles such as the rectus abdominis, serratus posterior inferior, iliocostalis, and quadratus lumborum. Thus, respiration operates as an efficient system, capable of responding to different demands by altering the contraction intensity and timing of the active muscles while simultaneously using the elastic properties inherent within the lungs.

Arthrology and Arthrokinematics

The motion of the ribs can be described through events that occur between the ribs and the vertebrae, and among the ribs, costal cartilages, and sternum. Beginning at the spine each rib has two articulations. As a rib approaches the vertebra, it contacts each transverse process. This synovial joint has strong ligaments that restrict gross ranges of motion. Each rib articulates proximally with the superior border of the lower vertebra and the inferior border of the upper vertebra, forming the costovertebral joint (52). This is true in all cases except the singular articulations at T1 and T12. Moving anteriorly, each rib (except the eleventh and twelfth) is contiguous with costal cartilage that articulates with the sternum. Although a synchondrosis directly attaches the first costal cartilage to the sternum, the second through seventh cartilages attach through fibrocartilaginous expansions (125).

Ligaments restrain movement at the costovertebral and costotransverse joints. Furthermore, the arrangement of the two joints dictates a mechanical coupling between them, such that rotation occurs about an axis that passes through each. Study of the axes of these two joints for the various levels of the thoracic vertebrae reveals that the axis for the upper vertebrae is more mediolateral in direction. Thus, rotation about this axis produces an anterior elevation of the rib. For the lower ribs, however, the axis through the two joints is more anteroposterior, causing elevation in the lateral direction. The result is an increase in the anteroposterior dimension of the upper ribs and an increase in the mediolateral dimension of the inferior ribs. Concurrently, modest gliding motions occur at the respective costosternal joints (52).

Other descriptions of the motion of the thorax are also possible. Note, for example, that the anterior aspect of each rib is lower than the posterior aspect. Thus, as the shaft of a rib is elevated, it rises in a forward direction. Their anterior attachments influence movement also. In the superior, or vertebrosternal ribs, motion is as described for the upper and lower ribs in the previous section. Starting at the anterior attachment of the seventh rib (vertebrochondral), motion contributes to enlargement of the upper abdominal space to allow expansion of the organs displaced by contraction of the diaphragm muscle. Furthermore, the costal cartilages of ribs 5 through 10 articulate with each other, in effect causing elevation of the rib superior in location and elevation of the distal sternum. Ribs 11 and 12, called vertebral ribs because of their lack of anterior attachment, have limited motion due to fixation by the quadratus lumborum. Such fixation does, however, provide a fixed point of action for the diaphragm, which inserts on their superior aspects.

Studies have evaluated the mechanical characteristics of the ribs to some degree. Stiffness measurements have shown variation between ribs, but generally the individual ribs are highly flexible. Although stiffness in each joint may also be measured, there is little impact of these measures upon the mechanics of the thorax (122). An elastic effect may be related to the costal cartilages. In inspiration, the elevation of the thorax causes rotation of the cartilage. Because the costochondral and the sternochondral joints are both articulations that allow little motion, the cartilage becomes twisted. As inspiration is completed, the elasticity within the cartilage tends to untwist the cartilage, completing the process as expiration follows (52).

We should also note the effect of the ribs on thoracic spinal motions. Generally, flexion-extension range of motion of any of the intervertebral segments does not exceed that of any of the cervical or lumbar motion segments. Lateral bending is limited to less than 10° per segment while rotation is similar to that available in the lower cervical spine. In actuality, were it not for the rib cage, the angulation of the thoracic facets would permit the most motion of any spinal region, except for extension (due to apposition of spinous processes).

Biomechanics and Kinetics

Information about the biomechanics and kinetics of the ribs is scant. We have covered the salient features under the topic of arthrology and arthrokinematics. Further work in this area is likely to continue to be slow in developing because of persistent technical problems that may preclude definitive data as to the mechanics and kinetics of motion of the ribs.

Pathokinesiology

Research has not described the effects of respiratory or thoracic spine pathology in a kinesiologic or biomechanical sense. Most information available concerns chronic respiratory problems and the changes that occur secondary to scoliosis. Earlier in this chapter, discussion focused on the influence of posture as related to the effectiveness of respiratory mechanics. Treatment goals, however, may be to reduce bronchial obstructions and alter the mechanical properties of the chest wall (43). As noted, in the supine position, the abdominal organs push the diaphragm superiorly, making inspiration more difficult but potentially more effective. Furthermore, in the sidelying position the diaphragm is pushed upwards much more on the lower side, making this lung less efficient than the other (52). Although loss of abdominal tone may have further effects, the remainder of this section will concentrate on **chronic obstructive pulmonary disease (COPD)** and scoliosis.

Among the most common COPDs is emphysema. In this case the chest is held in a position of inspiration, partly due to a loss of lung elasticity. As a result, the diaphragm is unable to move superior in an attempt to assume its usual dome shape. To compensate for the decreased effectiveness of the diaphragm, the accessory muscles become primary. The result is that the diaphragm only contributes 30% (compared with its more usual 70–80%) (66) of inspiratory force while the accessory muscles play an increased role (32). To respirate effectively, the patient performs a slow, deep or rapid, uncontrolled inspiration, primarily with the accessory muscles, followed by a forced and usually prolonged expiration. Such a pursed-lip technique may be facilitated in expiration by contraction of the abdominal muscles. The literature details these and other instructions (19, 33).

Evidence exists to support the positioning often employed by therapists in the treatment of COPD. For example, some have shown that although the EMG of the accessory inspiratory muscles was greater in standing and erect sitting than in forward leaning, one patient group reported relief of dyspnea in the latter position. The suggestion was made that this position allowed for better fixation of the accessory muscles, so that synergistic action made respiration more efficient (104). Earlier work had also strongly suggested that, in COPD, the diaphragm was under two mechanical disadvantages. One is related to the geometry of the muscle, and the other relates

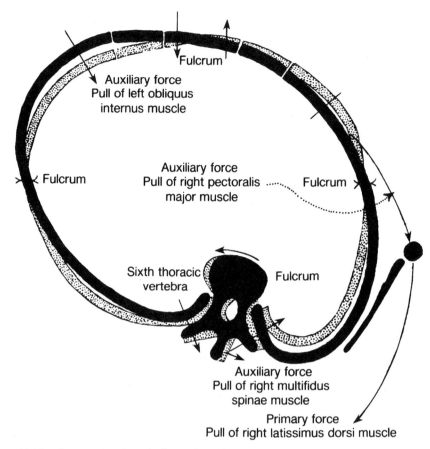

Figure 13.19. Cross section through the trunk to demonstrate the deformity that can be associated with scoliosis.

to the ability of the muscle to exert tension because of the alterations in length. Similar deficiencies are not likely to occur in the intercostal or accessory muscles of respiration (103).

Orthopaedic disorders of the thoracic spine may also influence respiratory mechanics and function. Some of the most acute effects can result from advanced stages of scoliosis. Lateral curvature and rotation can alter the shape and the spatial relationship of the ribs and have the potential to severely retard lung function (122). Figure 13.19 is a graphic depiction of the dimensional alterations that can occur in the thoracic cavity. Obviously chest wall motion will be distorted at all segments, predisposing the patient to symptoms associated with fatigue, shortness of breath, and chronic respiratory problems. The magnitude of the problems in patients with deformities past 90° has been shown, in that almost two-thirds of the vital capacity and one-half of the total lung capacity are lost (127). Therefore, these patients need assurance that respiratory mechanics will not be totally compromised.

Weakness, inefficiency, and increased effort required by changes in the lungs or chest wall due to pathology may result in increases in requirements of the inspiratory muscles. While the therapist may have difficulty in differentiating between muscle weakness and fatigue in patients (94), cognizance of the factors associated with normal and pathological function are important to be able to provide the best quality patient care.

SUMMARY

This chapter has considered normal and pathological mechanics of the trunk. This region of the body has an incredibly complex structure, primarily because of the multiple joints of each of the motion segments of the spine. This region of the body is very important, however, because adequate trunk control is essential for effective use of the upper limbs. Any disruption of normal kinematics or kinetics, particularly of the lumbar spine or the respiratory system, can have the ultimate effect of total incapacitation. Recognition of normal and abnormal states and the location of the pathology often make the difference in restoring normal motion.

References

1. Aaro S, Ohlen G. The effect of Harrington instrumentation on the sagittal configuration and mobility of the spine in scoliosis. *Spine*. 1983;8:570–575.
2. Adams MA, Dolan P. Recent advances in lumbar spinal mechanics and their clinical significance. *Clin Biomech*. 1995;10:3–19.
3. Adams MA, Dolan P, Hutton WC. The lumbar spine in backward bending. *Spine*. 1988;13:1019–1026.
4. Adams MA, Hutton WC. The relevance of torsion to the mechanical derangement of the lumbar spine. *Spine*. 1981;6:241–248.
5. Adams MA, Hutton WC, Stott JRR. The resistance to flexion of the lumbar intervertebral joint. *Spine*. 1980;5:245–253.
6. Ahmed AM, Duncan NA, Burke DL. The effect of facet geometry on the axial torque-rotation response of lumbar motion segments. *Spine*. 1990;15:391–401.
7. Axelgaard J, Nordwall A, Brown JC. Correction of spinal curvatures by transcutaneous electrical muscle stimulation. *Spine*. 1983;8:463–481.
8. Blackburn SE, Portney LG. Electromyographic activity of back musculature during Williams' flexion exercises. *Phys Ther*. 1981;61:878–885.
9. Bogduk N. The anatomy of the lumbar intervertebral disc syndrome. *Med J Australia*. 1976;1: 878–881.
10. Bogduk N. A reappraisal of the anatomy of the human lumbar erector spinae. *J Anat*. 1980;131: 525–540.
11. Bogduk N, MacIntosh JE. The applied anatomy of the thoracolumbar fascia. *Spine*. 1984;9:164–170.
12. Bogduk N, Macintosh JE, Pearcy MJ. A universal model of the lumbar back muscles in the upright position. *Spine*. 1992;17:897–913.
13. Boocock MG, Jackson JA, Burton AK, Tillotson KM. Continuous measurement of lumbar posture using flexible electrogoniometers. *Ergonomics*. 1994;37:175–185.
14. Broberg KB. On the mechanical behavior of intervertebral discs. *Spine*. 1983;8:151–165.
15. Carlsoo S. *How Man Moves*. London: W. Heinemann; 1972:77.
16. Carmon DJ, Blanton PL, Biggs NL. Electromyographic study of the anterolateral musculature utilizing indwelling electrodes. *Am J Phys Med*. 1972;51:113–129.
17. Cassisi JE, Robinson ME, O'Conner P, MacMillan M. Trunk strength and lumbar paraspinal muscle activity during isometric exercise in chronic low-back pain patients and controls. *Spine*. 1993;18:245–251.
18. Chazal J, Tanguy A, Bourges M, Gaurel G, Escande G, Guillot M, Vanneuville G. Biomechanical properties of spinal ligaments and a histological study of the supraspinal ligament in traction. *J Biomech*. 1985;18:167–176.
19. Clanton TL, Diaz PT. Clinical assessment of the respiratory muscles. *Phys Ther*. 1995;75:983–995.
20. Cochran T, Irstam L, Nachemson A. Long-term anatomic and functional changes in patients with adolescent idiopathic scoliosis treated by Harrington rod fusion. *Spine*. 1983;8:576–584.
21. De Troyer A, Estenne M. Coordination between rib cage muscles and diaphragm during quiet breathing. *J Appl Physiol*. 1984;57:899–906.
22. De Troyer A, Sampson M, Sigrist S, Macklem PT. Action of the costal and crural parts of the diaphragm on the rib cage in dog. *J Appl Physiol*. 1982;53:30–39.

23. Dimnet J, Pasquet A, Krag MH, Panjabi MM. Cervical spine motion in the sagittal plane: kinematic and geometric parameters. *J Biomech.* 1982;15:959–969.

24. Dolan P, Earley M, Adams MA. Bending and compressive stresses acting on the lumbar spine during lifting activities. *J Biomech.* 1994;27:1237–1248.

25. Dolan P, Mannion AF, Adams MA. Passive tissues help the back muscles to generate extensor moments during lifting. *J Biomech.* 1994;27:1077–1085.

26. Dunn HK, Daniels AU, McBride GG. Intraoperative force measurements during correction of scoliosis. *Spine.* 1982;7:448–455.

27. Ekholm J, Arborelius U, Fahlcrantz A, et al. Activation of abdominal muscles during some physiotherapeutic exercises. *Scand J Rehabil Med.* 1979;11:75–84.

28. Fahrni WH. Conservative treatment of lumbar disc degeneration: our primary responsibility. *Orthop Clinics N Am.* 1975;6:93–103.

29. Fielding J. Cineroentgenography of the normal cervical spine. *J Bone Joint Surg.* 1957;39(A):1280–1288.

30. Fraser EJ. Extensor muscle of the low back: an electromyographic study. *Phys Ther.* 1967;47:200–207.

31. Frymoyer JW, Pope MH, Clements JH, et al. Risk factors in low back pain—an epidemiological survey. *J Bone Joint Surg.* 1983;65(A):213–218.

32. Garodz Y. Rehabilitation of the patient with chronic obstructive pulmonary disease. *Geisinger Med Bull.* 1971;31:10–16.

33. Godfrey KE, Kindig LE, Windell EJ. Electromyographic study of duration of muscle activity in sit-up variations. *Arch Phys Med Rehabil.* 1977;58:132–135.

34. Gracovetsky S, Farfan HF, Lamy C. The mechanism of the lumbar spine. *Spine.* 1981;6:249–262.

35. Gracovetsky S, Kary M, Pitchen I, et al. The importance of pelvic tilt in reducing compressive stress in the spine during flexion-extension exercises. *Spine.* 1989;14:412–416.

36. Graves JE, Pollock ML, Carpenter DM, et al. Quantitative assessment of full range-of-motion isometric lumbar extension strength. *Spine.* 1990;15:289–294.

37. Gregersen GG, Lucas DB. An in vivo study of the axial rotation of the human thoracolumbar spine. *J Bone Joint Surg.* 1967;49(A):247–262.

38. Halpern AA, Bleck EE. Sit-up exercises: an electromyographic study. *Clin Orthop.* 1979;145:172–178.

39. Hasue M, Fujiwara M, Kikuchi S. A new method of quantitative measurement of abdominal and back muscle strength. *Spine.* 1980;5:143–148.

40. Hedtmann A, Steffen R, Methfessel J. Measurement of human lumbar spine ligaments during loaded and unloaded motion. *Spine.* 1989;14:175–185.

41. Hirsch C. The reaction of intervertebral discs to compression forces. *J Bone Joint Surg.* 1955;37(A):1188–1191.

42. Hohl M. Normal motions in the upper portion of the cervical spine. *J Bone Joint Surg.* 1964;46(A):1777–1779.

43. Housset B, Tetard C, Derenne JP. Kinesitherapie respiratoire et mecanique respiratore des insuffisants respiratoires chroniques. *Rev Fr Mal Resp.* 1983;11:915–921.

44. Inoue H, Takeda T. Three-dimensional observation of the collagen framework of lumbar intervertebral discs. *Acta Orthop Scand.* 1975;46:949–956.

45. Isaacson PR. Living anatomy: an anatomic basis for the osteopathic concept. *J Am Osteopath Assoc.* 1980;79:745–759.

46. Johnson C, Reid JG. Lumbar compressive and shear forces during various trunk curl-up exercises. *Clin Biomech.* 1991;6:97–104.

47. Johnson R. Personal communication. Iowa City, Iowa; 1985.

48. Johnson RM, Hart DL, Simmons EF, et al. Cervical orthoses—a study comparing their effectiveness in restricting cervical motion in normal subjects. *J Bone Joint Surg.* 1977;59(A):332–339.

49. Jonsson B. The function of individual muscles in the lumbar part of the spinae muscle. *Electromyography.* 1970;10:5–21.

50. Joseph J, McColl I. Electromyography of muscles of posture: posterior vertebral muscles in males. *J Physiol (Lond).* 1961;157:33–37.

51. Kahanovitz N, Nordin M, Verderame R, et al. Normal trunk muscle strength and endurance in women and the effect of exercises and electrical stimulation. Part 2: Comparative analysis of electrical stimulation and exercises to increase trunk muscle strength and endurance. *Spine.* 1987;12:112–118.

52. Kapandji IA. *The Physiology of the Joints.* New York: Churchill Livingstone; 1974;3.
53. Kennelly KP, Stokes MJ. Pattern of asymmetry of paraspinal muscle size in adolescent idiopathic scoliosis examined by real-time ultrasound imaging. *Spine.* 1993;18:913–917.
54. Koreska J, Robertson D, Mills RH, Gibson DA, Albisser AM. Biomechanics of the lumbar spine and its clinical significance. *Orthop Clin N Am.* 1977;8:121–133.
55. Krag MH. Biomechanics of thoracolumbar spinal fixation—a review. *Spine.* 1991;16:S84–S99.
56. Kulak RF, Belytschko TB, Schultz AB, et al. Non-linear behavior of the human intervertebral disc under axial load. *J Biomech.* 1976;9:377–386.
57. La Rocca H. Biomechanics of the cervical spine. In: *Atlas of Orthotics: Biomechanical Principles and Application.* St. Louis: CV Mosby; 1975:283–299.
58. Laurnen EL, Tupper JW, Mullen MP. The Boston brace in thoracic scoliosis—a preliminary report. *Spine.* 1983;8:388–395.
59. Lavender S, Marras WS, Miller RA. The development of response strategies in preparation for sudden loading to the torso. *Spine.* 1993;14:2097–2105.
60. Lavender S, Trafimow J, Andersson GBJ, et al. Trunk muscle activation—the effects of torso flexion, moment direction, and moment magnitude. *Spine.* 1994;19:771–778.
61. Lavender S, Tsuang Y-H, Andersson GBJ. Trunk muscle activation and cocontraction while resisting applied moments in a twisted posture. *Ergonomics.* 1993;36:1145–1157.
62. Lee CK, Langrana NA. Lumbosacral spinal fusion: a biomechanical study. *Spine.* 1984;9:574–581.
63. Lin HS, Liu YK, Adams KH. Mechanical response of the lumbar intervertebral joint under physiological (complex) loading. *J Bone Joint Surg.* 1978;60(A):41–55.
64. Lipetz S, Gutin B. An electromyographic study of four abdominal exercises. *Med Sci Sports.* 1970;2:35–38.
65. Lorenz M, Patwardhan A, Vanderby R. Load-bearing characteristics of lumbar facets in normal and surgically altered spinal segments. *Spine.* 1983;8:122–130.
66. Loring SH, De Troyer A. Actions of the respiratory muscles. In: Roussos C, Macklem PT, eds. *The Thorax.* New York: Marcel Dekker; 1985:327–349.
67. Macnab I. Negative disc exploration. *J Bone Joint Surg.* 1971;53(A):891–903.
68. Mayer TG, Tencer AF, Kristoferson S, Mooney V. Use of noninvasive techniques for quantification of spinal range-of-motion in normal subjects and chronic low-back dysfunction patients. *Spine.* 1984;9:588–595.
69. McGill SM. Estimation of force and extensor moment contributions of the disc and ligaments at L4–L5. *Spine.* 1988;13:1395–1402.
70. McGill SM. Kinetic potential of the lumbar trunk musculature about three orthogonal orthopaedic axes in extreme postures. *Spine.* 1991;16:809–815.
71. McGill SM. The influence of lordosis on axial trunk torque and trunk muscle myoelectric activity. *Spine.* 1992;17:1187–1193.
72. McGill SM, Hoodless K. Measured and modelled static and dynamic axial trunk torsion during twisting in males and females. *J Biomed Eng.* 1990;12:403–409.
73. McGill SM, Kippers V. Transfer of loads between lumbar tissues during the flexion-relaxation phenomenon. *Spine.* 1994;19:2190–2196.
74. McGill SM, Seguin J, Bennett G. Passive stiffness of the lumbar torso in flexion, extension, lateral bending, and axial rotation. *Spine.* 1994;19:696–704.
75. Michele AA. *Iliopsoas—Development of Anomalies in Man.* Springfield, IL: Charles C Thomas; 1962.
76. Moga PJ, Erig M, Chaffin DB, Nussbaum MA. Torso muscle moment arms at intervertebral levels T10 through L5 from CT scans on eleven male and eight female subjects. *Spine.* 1993;15:2305–2309.
77. Morris JM, Markolf KL. Biomechanics of the lumbosacral spine. In: *Atlas of Orthotics: Biomechanical Principles and Application.* St. Louis: CV Mosby; 1975:312–331.
78. Nachemson AL. Disc pressure measurements. *Spine.* 1981;6:93–97.
79. Nachemson AL. The lumbar spine—an orthopedic challenge. *Spine.* 1976;1:59–71.
80. Nachemson AL, Evans J. Some mechanical properties of the third human lumbar interlaminar ligament (ligamentum flavum). *J Biomech.* 1968;1:211–220.
81. Newton M, Thow M. Trunk strength testing with iso-machines. *Spine.* 1993;18:812–824.
82. Nordin M, Kahanoritz N, Verderame R, et al. Normal trunk muscle strength and endurance in women and the effect of exercises and electrical stimulation. Part 1: Normal endurance and trunk muscle strength in 101 women. *Spine.* 1987;12:105–111.
83. Nowitzke A, Westaway M, Bogduk N. Cervical zygapophyseal joints: geometric parameters and relationship to cervical kinematics. *Clin Biomech.* 1994;9:342–348.

84. Ortengren R, Andersson GBJ. Electromyographic studies of trunk muscles, with special reference to the functional anatomy of the lumbar spine. *Spine*. 1977;2:44–52.

85. Panjabi MM, Takata K, Goel VK. Kinematics of lumbar intervertebral foramen. *Spine*. 1983;8:348–357.

86. Parke W, Schift D. The applied anatomy of the intervertebral disc. *Orthop Clin N Am*. 1977;2:309–324.

87. Pearcy MJ. Twisting mobility of the human back in flexed postures. *Spine*. 1993;18:114–119.

88. Pearcy MJ, Bogduk N. Instantaneous axes of rotation of the lumbar intervertebral joints. *Spine*. 1988;13:1033–1041.

89. Pearcy MJ, Tibrewal SB. Axial rotation and lateral bending in the normal lumbar spine measured by three-dimensional radiography. *Spine*. 1984;9:582–587.

90. Pope M. Mechanics of the spine. Presented at AAOS Symposium on the Spine, Miami, 1981.

91. Rab GT, Chao EYS, Stauffer RN. Muscle force analysis of the lumbar spine. *Orthop Clin N Am*. 1977;8:193–199.

92. Radin EL, Simon SR, Rose RM, Paul IL. *Practical Biomechanics for the Orthopedic Surgeon*. 2nd ed. New York: John Wiley & Sons; 1992.

93. Reid DC. Electromyographic studies of respiration: a review of current concepts. *Physiotherapy*. 1970;56:534–540.

94. Reid WD, Deckman G. Considerations when testing and training the respiratory muscles. *Phys Ther*. 1995;75:971–980.

95. Ross EC, Parnianpour M, Martin D. The effects of resistance level on muscle coordination patterns and movement profile during trunk extension. *Spine*. 1993;13:1829–1838.

96. Sandover J. Dynamic loading as a possible source of low-back disorders. *Spine*. 1983;8:652–658.

97. Schnedel MJ, Wood, KB, Buttermann GR, et al. Experimental measurement of ligament force, facet force, and segment motion in the human lumbar spine. *J Biomech*. 1993;26:427–438.

98. Schultz A, Andersson G, Ortengren R, et al. Analysis and quantitative myoelectric measurements of loads on the lumbar spine when holding weights in standing postures. *Spine*. 1982;7:390–397.

99. Schultz A, Andersson G, Ortengren R, et al. Loads on the lumbar spine: validation of a biomechanical analysis by measurements of intradiscal pressures and myoelectric signals. *J Bone Joint Surg*. 1982;64(A):713–720.

100. Schultz A, Haderspeck K, Takashima S. Correction of scoliosis by muscle stimulation—biomechanical analyses. *Spine*. 1981;6:468–476.

101. Seligman JV, Gertzbein SD, Kapasouri A. Computer analysis of spinal segment motion in degenerative disc disease with and without axial loading. *Spine*. 1984;9:566–573.

102. Shaffer TH, Wolfson MR, Bhutani VK. Respiratory muscle function, assessment, and training. *Phys Ther*. 1981;61:1711–1723.

103. Sharp JT, Danon J, Druz WAS, et al. Respiratory muscle function in patients with chronic obstructive pulmonary disease: its relationship to disability and to respiratory therapy. *Am Rev Respir Dis*. 1974;110:154–161.

104. Sharp JT, Druz WAS, Moisan T, et al. Postural relief of dyspnea in severe chronic obstructive pulmonary disease. *Am Rev Respir Dis*. 1980;122:201–211.

105. Smidt GL, Amundsen LR, Dostal WF. Muscle strength at the trunk. *J Orthop Sports Phys Ther*. 1980;1:165–170.

106. Smidt GL, Herring T, Amundsen L, et al. Assessment of abdominal and back extensor function: a quantitative approach and results for chronic low-back patients. *Spine*. 1983;8:211–219.

107. Smidt GL, Van Meter SE, Hartman MD, et al. Spine configuration and range of motion in normals and scoliotics. *Clin Biomech*. 1994;9:303–309.

108. Smith RM, Emans JB. Sitting balance in spinal deformity. *Spine*. 1992;17:1103–1109.

109. Soderberg GL. Exercises for the abdominal muscles. *J Health Phys Ed Rec*. 1966;37:67–70.

110. Soderberg GL, Barr JO. Muscular function in chronic low-back dysfunction. *Spine*. 1983;8:79–85.

111. Stoddard A. *Manual of Osteopathic Technique*. London: Hutchinson & Co; 1980.

112. Tan JC, Parnianpour M, Nordin M, et al. Isometric maximal and submaximal trunk extension at different flexed positions in standing. *Spine*. 1993;18:2480–2490.

113. Taylor A. The contribution of the intercostal muscles to the effort of respiration in man. *J Physiol*. 1960;151:390–402.

114. Thompson N, Gould J. Descriptive measures of isokinetic trunk testing. *J Orthop Sports Phys Ther*. 1985;7:43–49.

115. Toussaint HM, de Winter AF, de Haas Y, et al. Flexion relaxation during lifting; implications

for torque production by muscle activity and tissue strain at the lumbo-sacral joint. *J Biomech.* 1995;28:199–210.

116. Twomey LT, Taylor JR. Sagittal movements of the human lumbar vertebral column: a quantitative study of the role of the posterior vertebral elements. *Arch Phys Med Rehabil.* 1983;64:322–325.

117. Tweit P, Daggfeldt K, Hetland S, Thorstensson A. Erector spinae lever arm length variations with changes in spinal curvature. *Spine.* 1994;19:199–204.

118. Virgin W. Experimental investigations into physical properties of intervertebral disc. *J Bone Joint Surg.* 1951;33B:607–611.

119. Wade OL. Movements of the thoracic cage and diaphragm in respiration. *J Physiol.* 1954;124:193–212.

120. Wasylenko M, Skinner SR, Perry J, Antonelli DJ. An analysis of posture and gait following spinal fusion with Harrington instrumentation. *Spine.* 1983;8:840–845.

121. White AA, Johnson RM, Panjabi MM, Southwick WO. Biomechanical analysis of clinical stability in the cervical spine. *Clin Orthop.* 1975;109:85–96.

122. White AA, Panjabi MM. *Clinical Biomechanics of the Spine.* Philadelphia: JB Lippincott; 1990.

123. White AA, Panjabi MM. The basic kinematics of the human spine: a review of past and current knowledge. *Spine.* 1978;3:12–20.

124. White AA, Panjabi MM. The clinical biomechanics of scoliosis. *Clin Orthop.* 1976;118:100–112.

125. Williams PL, Warwick R, eds. *Gray's Anatomy.* 37th British ed. Edinburgh: Churchill Livingstone; 1989.

126. Zetterberg C, Aniansson A, Brimby G. Morphology of the paravertebral muscles in adolescent idiopathic scoliosis. *Spine.* 1983;8:457–462.

127. Zorab PA. Respiratory function in scoliosis. In: Zorab PA, ed. *Scoliosis.* Springfield, IL: Charles C Thomas; 1969.

14

Special Joints

TEMPOROMANDIBULAR JOINT

The temporomandibular joint (TMJ) has become of more interest to therapists because a significant percentage of the population suffers from disorders associated with dysfunction of this joint. Cooperative evaluative and treatment programs with members of the dental profession usually lead to the most effective management of the problems that can typically arise (39).

Relevant Anatomy

This synovial joint is found just anterior to the external ear and is made up of the mandibular condyle, an articular disc, and the articular eminence of the temporal bone. The mandibular condyle is smooth and convex and approximately twice the size mediolaterally as anteroposteriorly (4). The articular surfaces are lined with fibrocartilage that is somewhat thickened on the articular eminence (Fig. 14.1). The functional advantage of lining the TMJ with fibrocartilage is that it distorts well under compressive forces and spreads the load, thus minimizing damage to the joint (37).

The articulating components of the TMJ are separated and cushioned by the articulating disc (5, 69). Osborn suggests that the disc minimizes excessive wear on the fibrocartilage. If no disc were present, the fibrocartilage on the articular eminence would be squeezed over the edges of the condyle and potentially be damaged as the condyle gouges through the fibrocartilage during grinding movements (37). Insertion of an articular disc overcomes this disadvantage because now the condyle indents the disc but only slightly indents the articular eminence. This also allows the disc to slide freely over the articular eminence when the condyle is loaded during grinding movements (37). The disc is described as a biconcave structure innervated in the anterior and posterior edges but the midportion where the biconcave structures meet are avascular and aneural (4, 24, 47). The inferior surface of the disc relates to the anterior portion of the mandibular condyle while the superior surface faces the middle third of the articular eminence.

The three articular surfaces (anterior mandibular condyle, articular disc, and middle third of articular eminence) are kept together during mandibular rest positions or maximum intercuspation (natural fitting together) of the teeth by **periarticular connective tissue** (PCT) (47). This PCT is made up of ligament, tendon, capsule, and fascia. Its function is to connect tissues, maintain the TMJ joint configuration, and limit the range of motion of the joint (47). The main ligament of the TMJ is the temporomandibular, located lateral to the capsule but not easily distinguishable from it. As shown in Figure 14.2 the fibers pass from a wide origin on the articular tubercle and funnel into a site on the neck of the condyle. Accompanying collateral ligaments are small and probably insignificant except for controlling distal displacement of the condylar head. Other ligaments that affect the TMJ are the sphenomandibular, stylomandibular, and pterygomandibular raphe, each of which is shown in Figure 14.2 (31). The

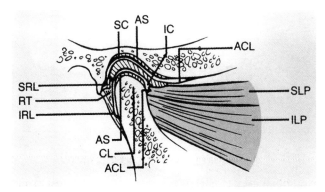

Figure 14.1. Lateral view of right temporomandibular joint with disc. *Legend*: *SC*, superior joint cavity; *AS*, articular surface; *IC*, inferior joint cavity; *ACL*, anterior capsular ligament; *SLP*, superior lateral pterygoid muscle; *ILP*, inferior lateral pterygoid muscle; *CL*, collateral ligament; *IRL*, inferior retrodiscal lamina; *RT*, retrodiscal tissues; *SRL*, superior retrodiscal ligament.

capsule is reinforced laterally by the temporomandibular ligament. However, the capsule is thin and loose posteriorly and on the medial side. The attachment posteriorly is, however, attached to the disk by highly elastic tissue that is innervated and vascularized (5).

The PCT, type I collagen fibers have an intimate relationship with the biomechanics of the TMJ. Irregular arranged collagen fibers, such as those in the joint capsule,

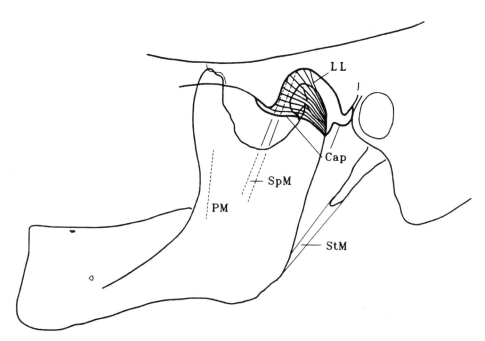

Figure 14.2. Lateral view of left TMJ capsule, outlined with a heavy line, and the joint ligaments. *Legend*: *LL*, lateral or temporomandibular ligament; *Cap*, capsule; *StM*, stylomandibular ligament; *SpM*, sphenomandibular ligament; *PM*, pterygomandibular ligament.

allow for stretching in many directions. Regularly arranged collagen fibers, such as those found in tendon and ligaments, run essentially in the same direction and give excellent tensile strength (47). Another key element to be considered when discussing PCT is proteoglycans, which are found in the matrix of the PCT. Proteoglycans bind with water to form a gel that lubricates the collagen fibers and maintains space between the fibers (critical fiber distance) to allow for free sliding of the collagen fibers (37). The key concept of collagen fiber is one of quasi-elasticity (47). Histological studies reveal that collagen is crimped, giving it a wavy appearance and that elongation of ligament can occur without actual stretching of collagen fibers (see Chapter 5). Rocabado suggests that this crimping of collagen fibers gives TM ligament the ability to lengthen 20–30% more than its actual length (47). If we evaluated the stress-strain curve for the PCT of the TMJ, we would find that in the 70–80% range of actual ligament length, stress and strain are proportional (47). As noted in Chapter 5, anytime within this elastic range of 70–80% of actual length the tissue will return to its original length without elongation being permanent. If the elastic range is exceeded with loading, the connective tissue may elongate and TMJ dysfunction may be manifested (3).

Many muscles are responsible for the motions available at the TMJ. Classification systems depend on labeling of the motions, and what follows is a generalization of the activities based on the description of motion and the potential for six degrees of freedom. Moore includes the digastric, mylohyoid, geniohyoid, sternohyoid, omohyoid, sternothyroid, and thyrohyoid as muscles that can depress the mandible, which result in **opening** the mouth (34). *Gray's Anatomy* lists only the lateral pterygoid muscles, aided when the mouth is widely open or when resistance is encountered, by the digastric, geniohyoid, and mylohyoid muscles (69). Primary elevators, or mouth closers, include the temporalis, masseter, and medial pterygoid muscles (4, 34, 69). While some disagree, **protractors** are considered the lateral pterygoid and perhaps the medial pterygoid (69) and deep portion of the masseter (34), at least partially. **Retraction** is primarily the task of the temporalis muscle (34, 69). The temporalis, pterygoids, and masseter are believed to be responsible for the lateral, or side-to-side, movements of the TMJ (34, 69).

Descriptions of the muscular activity associated with the management of the mandible are not readily available in the literature, in spite of a high incidence of TMJ dysfunction. Usually, however, most of the function of interest to the therapist is the action of mastication. Swallowing and talking also require coordinated movements of the TMJ but most pathology is felt to be related to the forceful closure required during chewing and biting. The muscles identified in the previous paragraph are responsible for the performance of highly integrated activities required in chewing. Opening of the mouth is facilitated by gravity, relaxation of the mouth closers, and mild contraction of the **depressors** when necessary. Additional jaw opening has been credited to the concurrent forward translation of the condyle, caused by the contraction of the lateral pterygoid muscles. Thus, protraction also occurs. Once any food has been placed in the mouth closure is the responsibility of the temporalis, masseter, and medial pterygoid muscles (4, 17). We should note specifically that the muscles responsible for closure are the same muscles responsible for lateral movement of the TMJs. Coordinated actions of these muscles, as they contract or relax on the ipsilateral and contralateral sides, account for both compression of any bolus of food while lateral shifts grind the bolus. Thus, chewing is effectively accomplished.

Arthrology and Arthrokinematics

Given the anatomical configuration and soft tissue arrangements, we should consider the capability for movements available in the TMJ. Its unique motion comes from a high degree of dependence on bilateral joints. This "structural constraint" does not distract from the establishment of three orthogonal axes that can be centered at the locus of motion of the TMJ. While rotations around axes are more limited in some directions as compared, for example, to the rotation required for mouth opening and closing, the rotations still need to exist for the joints to have normal function. Bourban corroborates that there are three axes at the TMJ (4). In addition, as noted in Chapter 4, translational motion can also occur along these axes. Thus, in total, six degrees of freedom of motion are available in each TMJ joint. That the instant center of rotation has been mobile and at a variable distance and direction from the TMJ supports the position that the joint does not function as a simple hinge (32). While, in fact, studies have been completed with six degrees of freedom included, remember that some motions are clearly more limited than others (35, 51).

The two primary movements of the TMJ are rotation about a mediolateral axis and translation along the anterior-posterior and superior-inferior axes. The first motion to occur with mouth opening is rotation and is generally agreed upon by multiple sources (5, 47, 48, 69, 70). Rocabado describes this rotation as a roll movement that takes place between the condyle and inferior joint surface of the disc (47). Throughout the rotation movement, the annulus stabilizes the disc on the condyle, which is thickened anteriorly and posteriorly. Flattening of the disc likely assists with the passage of the mandibular condyle under the eminence (24). Concurrently, according to Rocabado, an inferior joint surface posterior **glide** is completed. The upper lateral pterygoid muscle relaxes as the lower lateral pterygoid contracts (47). As rotation reaches completion (average, 25 mm [5]; maximum 60 mm [69]), the temporomandibular ligament constrains motion due to tightening. Aided possibly by the activity of the lateral pterygoid muscle, the condyle and disc may be moved anteriorly (26, 47). The disc passively follows the condyle anteriorly as the collateral ligaments of the joint tighten and the condyle and disc move together in relationship to the disc's superior surface and the articular eminence to achieve the maximum range of motion (47). The collective effective is that the mandibular condyle has moved anteriorly and inferiorly on the temporal bone (Fig. 14.3). The displacement in each of these directions, according to an MRI evaluation, is about equal (.45 cm versus .47 cm) (7). During opening, the negative pressure created by the space the condyle vacated is thought to cause expansion of the elastic tissue (with its posterior attachment to the disc) and produce a force that moves the disc posteriorly (37). In normal jaw opening, both the rotation and translation are bilaterally synchronous as the mandible opens without deviation to either side.

After maximal opening of the mouth, the closing movement commences with posterior **translation** of the mandible to about two-thirds of maximal opening (48). At this position the condyles are on the posterior slope of the articular eminence. The return to normal resting position is achieved by reversing the combined translatory and rotatory movements that occurred during opening. The position of occlusion, defined as alignment of the mandibular and maxillary teeth when the jaw is closed or in functional contact, is attained by muscular action that causes rotation (48).

From the rest position the mandible can move anteriorly quite extensively, a motion known as protrusion. Hoppenfeld states that in normals, the mandible should protrude far enough so that one can place the bottom teeth in front of the top teeth (23).

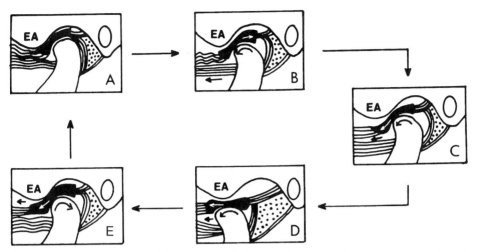

Figure 14.3. Various positions of the mandible with degrees of mouth opening. *EA,* eminentia articularis ossis temporalis. **A,** rest position; **B,** mid mouth open; **C,** mid to full opening; **D,** full opening; **E,** closure.

During this movement the mandible is pulled forward with the articular discs so the movement occurs between the articular disc and the temporal bone. Retrusion, or posterior movement of the mandible, from the occlusal (intercuspal) position is quite limited when compared with protrusion. Sarnat states that it rarely exceeds one millimeter (48). The limitation of the movement of retrusion is due to constraint by the temporomandibular ligament. Concerning protrusion and retrusion some have suggested a functional dominance of the right part of the mandible when transversal condylar shifts are considered (41). The same group of workers has noted and quantified that protrusive movements are greater in the left than the right TMJ in both male and female subjects (40).

The final functional movement to be discussed is the asymmetrical lateral shift. Assuming we want to shift to the right, the left mandibular condyle and its articular disc slide inferiorly, anteriorly, and medially (17). The right mandibular condyle executes limited movement laterally around a vertical axis and moves slightly anteriorly. This latter movement, known as Bennett's movement, is an evasive motion based on limitations of retrusive mandibular movement (48). If one were to try to rotate the mandibular condyle while the right mandibular condyle is rotated in the glenoid (temporal) fossa, the lateral condylar pole would have to move more posteriorly than the temporomandibular ligament would allow. Sarnat states that, under the "guidance" of the stretched temporomandibular ligament, the condyle is forced to move slightly forward, downward, and laterally (48).

The close-packed position (joint maximally congruent, ligaments taut, no further movement in that direction, etc.) of the TMJ is twofold: **posterior close packed** and **anterior close packed.** The posterior close-packed position occurs when the condyle is in its most retruded position compared with the posterior articular eminence or glenoid fossa, and the condyle can go no farther posteriorly and the ligaments are maximally tightened. The anterior close-packed position is one where the anterior position of the condyle is in its most anterior position with the articular eminence (maximal mouth opening). Williams and Warwick state that the joint is maximally stressed in the anterior close-packed position and that this position is an exception for synovial joints (69). The mandibular condyle is not braced in the glenoid fossa (posterior close packed) when loaded but it is balanced by the muscles of mastication on the posterior slope of the articular eminence. This position allows the condyle freedom of movement, which is required while one is grinding food. Freedom of movement would not be allowed if the condyle were braced in the glenoid fossa (37). The loose-packed position can then be described as any position away from the anterior and posterior close-packed positions.

Joint Forces

Historically, some have suggested that the TMJ is a non-weight-bearing joint. This has been shown not to be the case, however, though most of the forces associated with mastication are transmitted through the teeth. The PCT and the arrangement of muscles clearly produce force through the TMJs, the size dependent on the intensity of the biting force (degree of muscular activity) and the structure of the subject's temporal bone and mandible (15). The forces have been calculated to be about 20 to 30 kg(f), being largely dependent on lengths of muscle force moment arms and bite force moment arm. Direction, whether superiorly or inferiorly directed, is determined by the ratio of the length of the bite force moment arm to the muscle force moment arm (55). Of some interest is the symmetry, or lack of it, of the bilateral joint forces, particularly during the action of unilateral clenching. Some have shown that in these conditions the reaction forces, using a model, are not balanced on the two sides (15). The influence of muscle activity level on the balancing of the joint forces across the two sides is yet undetermined (56).

Pathokinesiology

The TMJ is vulnerable to many types of injury. Joint dislocation, improper occlusion, and weight bearing (loading) may traumatize the joint (23). Postural imbalances, muscular insufficiencies, muscle tensions (21), and other factors have also been identified as potential contributors to the dysfunction of this joint (39). As a synovial joint many dysfunctions can occur from changes in the soft tissues. The joint is further imperiled by the imposition of a disk, and when combined with the movements necessary for normal function, a myriad of clinical conditions is possible.

The most common intracapsular dysfunction of the TMJ is internal derangement or **displacement of the articular disk,** characterized by an anterior displacement of the disk and a posterosuperior displacement of the condyle. As supporting connective tissues are concurrently overstretched, lengthened, and weakened, the disk is loose and free to displace further. Often associated with the normal movements of mouth opening and closing is a click. Rocabado states that the most common conditions of internal derangements of the TMJ are (a) the **reciprocal clicking,** (b) **locking,** and (c) degenerative processes such as osteoarthritis (47). Reciprocal clicking is the most common type of click (17, 47) and is so named because it occurs on mouth opening and closing. During opening, the condyle moves beneath the disk and the posterior attachments and "snaps" under the posterior band of the disk. It then falls into its normal relationship on the concave surface. The other part of the click occurs at the end of the closing movement. Then, the condyle slides posteriorly to the posterior band of the disk and the disk becomes displaced anteriorly (47).

Isberg-Holm and Westesson describe a different mechanism for the opening click (25). When the condyle rotates and translates down the articular eminence, the disc is pushed ahead of the condyle but is prevented by the lower anterior fibers of the capsular ligament from moving too far ahead. The disc, being compressed between the condyle and articular eminence plus being prevented from translating too far forward by the lower anterior fibers, stores potential energy as the condyle translates anteriorly. The potential energy reaches a critical level and overcomes the posterior constraint (tension of lower anterior fibers and thickened anterior annulus of the disc) and pops back between the condyle and the articular eminence. As the condyle moves back, the disc is wedged between the condyle and articular eminence into a shape that potentially drives the disc forward. This movement is resisted by the posterior rim of the disc but when the resistance is overcome the disc pops forward, thus making the click associated with the closing movement of the mouth. Even in juvenile chronic arthritis, the click, along with pain, is the most common symptom (36).

When displacement becomes more extreme the disc becomes located anterior to the condyle and the joint "locks." Review Figure 14.3 to note how the disc could be located anteriorly. How often this occurs depends on the mobility of the disc and the laxity of the supporting tissues. Thus, chronicity may become a distinct clinical problem. Further elaborations are associated with the locked position and other manifestations associated with luxation and dislocation that are beyond the scope of this discussion. The student is directed to other sources for further elaboration (4, 5, 17, 19, 24, 39, 47, 52, 62, 68, 71).

In the cases described above, the clinical problem could be generally described as hypermobility. The antithesis, or hypomobility, can also occur, which limits opening, because most of the motion is due to rotation. Limitation can be due to shortening of the PCT. The other scenario causing limitation is created by an anterior displacement of the disc, characterized by a posterosuperior displacement of the condyle with a hard end feel with concurrent limited opening. Treatment of the hypermobile and hypomobile conditions would obviously be dependent on the results of the tissues evaluated during the clinical assessment (47, 59).

SACROILIAC JOINT

The movement of the sacroiliac joint (SIJ) has been of interest for almost 150 years, as noted in the citations in the work of Egund (14). Extensive efforts have been made to explain the kinesiology and mechanics of this joint (18), with special attention paid to the role of joint dysfunction in the creation of disability. Several excellent review articles are available (1, 12, 60). Of primary clinical concern is the magnitude of the motion, how validly and reliably this motion can be assessed, and whether or not variances in joint motion are responsible for producing dysfunction in patients.

Relevant Anatomy

Unique characteristics have been assigned to these synovial joints: the SIJ serves as the mechanism to distribute load either to the spine from the two extremities or to distribute the load of the head, arms, and trunk through the pelvis and into the lower extremities. Asymmetry is the usual case if the two joints of any given subject are compared (2, 50, 54). Wide variations are also found between subjects. Thus, there appears to be little standard for the description of the normal SIJ. It is generally agreed, however, that the cartilage of the sacrum is much thicker than that of the ilium (58, 60). Some have demonstrated variability in SIJ cartilage across the entire joint surface (61).

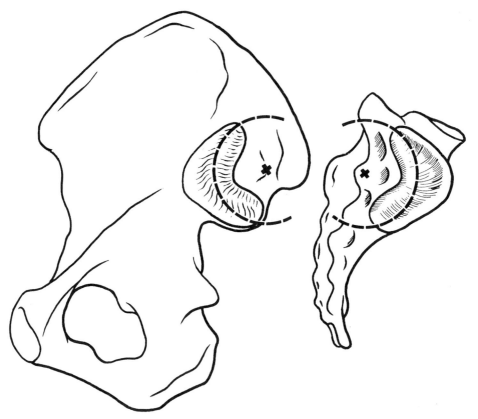

Figure 14.4. Lateral view of the disarticulated pelvis with the sacral segment folded open like a book. Note the crescent shape of the surface of the SIJ.

All sources generally agree that the iliac surface is crescent-shaped and concave posterosuperiorly as it is just posterior to the iliopectineal line (Fig. 14.4) (1, 2, 27, 69). The surface of the ilium is reciprocally shaped but not exactly congruent with the sacral surface (2). In effect, many sections through the joint are required to get an adequate representation of how the two surfaces articulate (27). Adequate representations of the surface topography have been provided, an example of which is shown in Figure 14.5 (53, 58, 63). Weisl has described the sacral surfaces in young adults as two elevations separated by a saddle-shaped depression (63). That there are variations with age is evident. Furthermore, comprehensive data also confirm the existence of **accessory or supernumerary articular facets** in the SIJs. Walker summarizes the data, citing that these joints have been observed in 8–40% of the samples (60). The influence of such findings will be considered when motions at the SIJ are discussed.

The SIJ is not spanned by any muscles, but many adjacent muscles such as the quadratus lumborum, erector spinae, piriformis, iliacus, and gluteal muscles blend fibrous expansions with the pertinent ligaments and joint capsule. Of the ligaments the interosseous has been described as the strongest in the body (53). Beal includes this ligament in the group known as the capsular ligaments, along with the ventral and dorsal sacroiliac ligaments, because they play an "important role in the integrity of the sacroiliac joint'' (2). Those ligaments included in the group known as accessory ligaments are the iliolumbar, sacrotuberous, and sacrospinous, arranged into two groups of fasciculi, one cranial and the other caudal (64). Separation of the iliac bones during movement is resisted by the sacroiliac, iliolumbar, and pubic symphysis ligaments. Forward rotation, known as **nutation** and detailed in the following sections, is purportedly limited by the sacrotuberous, sacrospinous, and anterior sacroiliac ligaments. Dorsal and interosseous ligaments may also resist forward bending while backward bending is limited by tension of both anterior and posterior sacroiliac ligaments (2). Whether or not the surrounding musculature has a direct or indirect influence on the potential movement of the SIJ has been the subject of some speculation (44).

Arthrology and Arthrokinematics

Subscribing to principles previously explained here, the SIJ may be anticipated to have the conventional six degrees of freedom. However, those investigating the motions at the SIJ have yet to be able to agree on the location of axes. Many locations have been proposed (14, 28, 46, 50, 54), as summarized particularly well in the work of Alderink (1). Beal states that axes have been identified at (a) the interosseous ligament, posterior to the auricular joint surface; (b) a bony prominence (Bonnaire's tubercle) on the auricular surface between the cranial and caudal segments of the facet; (c) the second sacral segment; and (d) an anterior sacral position, anterior and

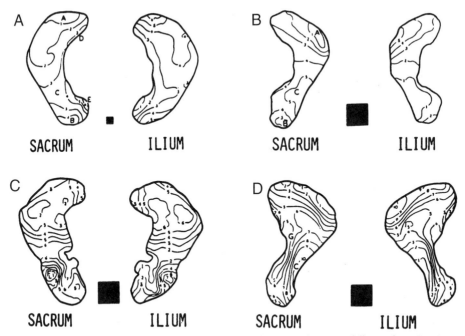

Figure 14.5. Cartographic records of auricular surface changes with age: **A,** full-term fetus; **B,** 20-year-old woman; **C,** 45-year-old man; **D,** 63-year-old man. Note the increase in the frequency and proximity of the contour lines between birth and the sixth decade of life. Cranial (A), caudal (B), and posterocaudal (G) elevations and postcranial (D), posterocaudal (E), and central (C) depressions are shown. The scale is indicated by the black cube; cube sides represent 1 mm in **A** and 1 cm in **B–D**. In **C**, note the prominent elevation on the anterior border (F). Variability is indicated by absence of this in **D**.

Table 14.1.   Reported Values for Rotatory Motion (in Degrees)

Reference	Type	Method	N	Mean	SD	Range	Comment
49	In vitro	Manual pressure	M	4			No method
43	In vivo	Roentgenography/inclinometer		11		3–19	Rotation
10	In vivo	Radiography	M	8	4.9		Pelvic-sacral angle
14	In vivo	Roentgen stereophotogrammetry	S	2			Six movements
46	In vivo	Stereoradiography		2.3			Flexion
28	In vivo	Stereoradiography	S			10–12	Rotation
33	In vitro	Loading	S	1.9			Ilia torsion
50	Model	Computer	S	1			Relative rotation
42	In vivo	Kinematics	M	3	1.5		Gaint, rotation
54	In vivo	Roentgen stereophotogrammetry	M	2.5	0.5		Functional movements

Legend: S, 1–2; M, 13–50.

inferior to the articular surface of the sacrum (2). Other work suggests that the axes show great variation across subjects and accounts for the differences in motions across subjects (27). One study noted that motion could not occur exclusively around the axes as reported and suggested that translatory motion could occur about a "rough axis" if separation of the joint surfaces occurred. Theorized distances were 7.25 mm in the medial plane and 3.43 mm in the frontal plane. This work notes that energy would be required to separate the two surfaces (66).

Despite the lack of agreement on the location of axes, motion has still been determined to exist in the SIJ. Before considering the types and magnitudes, recognize that the superincumbent weight of the trunk, head, and arms provides a force on the sacrum that forces this series of vertebrae between the two respective ilia. While this force is directed from superior to inferior, recall that the sacrum has an inclined position, i.e., the top of the sacrum is not horizontal. As a result the force can be considered as having two components: a vertical force, which creates the wedging between the ilia, and a force that rotates the anterior-superior rim of the sacrum in a counterclockwise direction. While keeping these concepts and the potential effect on the lumbar spine in mind, we can now consider the motions that occur at the SIJ.

The motion that exists at the SIJ has been considered **rotatory** and **translatory**. They may often occur simultaneously. As Walker has pointed out, it may also depend on age: the surface contours vary over the decades (60). Tables 14.1 and 14.2 provide a synopsis of the literature as to the techniques used to report rotatory and translatory motion, respectively. The rotatory motion values are low, with two exceptions. One should also note that the studies of the late 1980s, using what most would consider as more sophisticated techniques, all report values of less than three degrees. However, questions could be raised about the validity of the methods used in any of these studies.

While motion in the sagittal plane is ordinarily called flexion and extension, some sources refer to the motion of the sacrum on the ilia as nutation (27). The literal definition is derived from the word *nutare*, to nod. Considering a lateral view the sacrum rotates about a mediolateral axis so that the promontory moves inferiorly and anteriorly. Simultaneously, the apex of the sacrum and tip of the coccyx move posteriorly (Fig. 14.6). This movement requires that the ischial tuberosities move apart while the iliac bones are approximated, while there is a simultaneous decrease in the anteroposterior diameter from the superior aspect of the sacrum to the pubic symphysis. Counter nutation is considered the return to the original position. Constraints are ligamentous in each of the respective directions (27).

Table 14.2.   Reported Values for Translatory Motion (in Millimeters)

Reference	Type	Method	N	Mean	SD	Range	Comment
				Value			
20	In vitro	Gross observation	M	3			Hip flexion
65	In vivo	Radiology	M	5.6	1.4		Rising from supine position
11	In vivo	Kirschner pins	M	$\not> 5$	1		Functional movements
16	In vivo	Stereoradiography	S	<26	0.3		N = 1
	In vitro		S	2.7		0–15	Movement sacral apex
14	In vivo	Roentgen stereopho- togrammetry	S	~2			Translation
66	In vitro	Topography model	S	7.25	3.7		Median plane
				3.4	1.7		Frontal plane
18	In vivo	Stereophotogrammetry	L			5–8	Pain-free
						1–16	All subjects
28	In vivo	Stereoradiography	S	6			Anterior glide
33	In vitro	Static loading	S	0.5			Ilia torsion
				2.7			Sacral displacement
42	In vivo	Kinematics	M	2.9	1.2		Gait, anterior/posterior
50	Model	Computer	S	<3			"Prime node" translation

Legend: S, 1–12; M, 13–50; L, >50.

For translatory motion the values are again small, except for two reports. Walker discusses the limitations of these works, saying that the results are open to serious question (60). Also of import is the location of the axis along which the translation is occurring, and since there is no agreement as to the location of these axes, the amount of translation will likely vary between the different measurement techniques.

In functional activities there is general agreement that the maximal motion of the

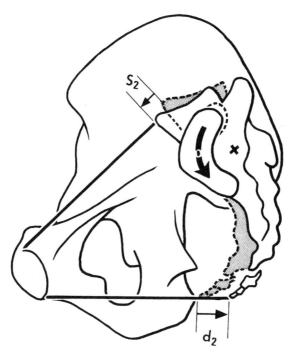

Figure 14.6.   Lateral view of the pelvis showing sacral motion on the ilia during the motion of nutation. Note that in forward movement of the anterior superior portion of the sacrum the distance s_2 decreases and the distance d_2 increases.

sacrum occurs in rising from a supine to a standing or long sitting position (10, 11, 54, 65). As one bends forward the sacrum tends to follow the flexion of the lumbar spine, tightening ligaments as the extreme of the range of motion is reached. With sidebending, the sacrum tends to follow the lumbar spine during early flexion. Rotations and unilateral activities, such as single limb weight bearing, lead to variable results. Contemporary literature on the rotation of the sacrum on the pelvis during gait is difficult to find. We can speculate that the sacrum rotates posteriorly during the lower extremity swing phase, changing to anterior rotation shortly after heel strike. Maximum rotation, not likely to be more than several degrees, appears at terminal stance. The sacrum may rotate forward about a diagonal axis during loading, reaching a maximum at midstance and then reversing itself during terminal stance. As gait is a complex activity involving simultaneous, contralateral trunk rotation, some motions required at the SIJ likely result from both lower extremity motion and weight bearing and the mass and motion of the upper limbs and trunk (1). Patients with bilateral hip disarticulation who choose to ambulate on the cephalad aspects of the pelvis demonstrate the extremes of motions required in the SIJ during gait.

Differences in amount of pelvic motion is related to gender. Morphological studies have shown that a polypeptide hormone, **relaxin,** has an effect. This hormone, produced during pregnancy, alters the state of the collagenolytic system and decreases the intrinsic strength and rigidity of collagen (29). Walker summarizes mixed evidence of measurable changes in mobility of the pubis symphysis and SIJs (60). However, most show increases in mobility at these joints. Whether or not the mobility changes are large enough to create symptoms and dysfunction is an important issue when dealing with patients.

Pathokinesiology

As noted previously in this chapter there appears to be discernible motion in the SIJ. At least some controversy remains over the differentiation of SIJ syndromes from low back pain (38). Serious questions remain about whether or not changes in the magnitudes of motion produce dysfunction, in either the hypomobile or hypermobile state. Most literature seems to indicate that the primary pathology is related to **anterior dysfunction** of the SIJ. DonTigny has completed a thorough review of the topic for the advancement of "theories" about such a dysfunction (13). Cases in which the clinician thought that the patient had involvement of the SIJ have also been reported as successfully treated (8). Summaries of literature regarding treatment can also be found in the works of DonTigny and Walker (12, 60).

Whether or not SIJ movements can be reliably detected is another issue. Probably the most thorough study addressing these issues is from the work of Potter and Rothstein. Thirteen tests for SIJ dysfunction were assessed for intertester reliability between eight physical therapists. When two therapists specializing in orthopaedics independently examined patients the reliability was poor. Eleven of the thirteen tests resulted in less than 70% agreement (45). Similar results have been reported for the palpatory tests for SIJ mobility, such as the standard Piedalu or standing Gillet tests (6, 67). Van Deursen et al. also evaluated several common SIJ orthopaedic tests and concluded that SIJ compression was not helpful in verifying known sacroiliitis patients (57).

One team of investigators assessed the inter- and intraexaminer reliability of a particular technique, the Gillet-motion procedure. Intraexaminer reliability was significant for all agreement scores studied, but the interexaminer values were significant for only some scores. While severity of the low back problem did not appear to influence either agreement score, degree of chiropractic expertise did (22). The application of these results to other test maneuvers can only be open to speculation. In summary, the tests commonly used in the clinic for SIJ dysfunction seem unreliable. Knowledge of these results should help the therapist in developing other techniques or recognizing the limitations of the methods currently used. However, not all results show poor reliability. Pain on resisted external hip rotation or on hip flexion has shown high interexaminer reliability (30, 45). Results on a group of patients with agreed upon SIJ dysfunction have also shown changes in degree of innominate tilt from manipulation of the SIJ (9). Future efforts will help clarify the appropriateness of the techniques purported for use in the evaluation and treatment of dysfunction of this joint.

SUMMARY

This chapter has provided material about the anatomy, kinesiology, and biomechanics of the TMJ and the SIJ. While these synovial joints contain many of the usual synovial features, the structure leads to special considerations when the assessment and treatment of these joints are pursued by therapists. An understanding of these principles is important to effective patient management.

References

1. Alderink GJ. The sacroiliac joint: review of anatomy, mechanics and function. *J Orthop Sports Phys Ther.* 1991;13:71–84.
2. Beal MC. The sacroiliac problem: review of anatomy, mechanics, and diagnosis. *J Am Osteopath Assoc.* 1982;81:667–679.
3. Bell W. Understanding temporomandibular biomechanics. *J Craniomandibular Pract.* 1983;1:27–33.
4. Bourban B. Anatomy and biomechanics of the TMJ. In: SL Kraus, ed. *TMJ Disorders: Management of the Craniomandibular Complex.* New York: Churchill Livingstone; 1988.
5. Bourban B. Musculoskeletal analysis: the temporomandibular joint and cervical spine. In: Scully R, Barnes ML, eds. *Physical Therapy.* Philadelphia: JB Lippincott; 1989.
6. Carmichael JC. Interexaminer and intraexaminer reliability of palpation for SIJD. *J Manipulative Physiol Ther.* 1987;10:164–171.
7. Chen J, Buckwalter K. Displacement analysis of the temporomandibular condyle from magnetic resonance images. *J Biomech.* 1993;1455–1462.
8. Cibulka MT. The treatment of the sacroiliac joint component to low back pain: a case report. *Phys Ther.* 1992;72:917–922.
9. Cibulka MT, Delitto A, Koldehoff RM. Changes in innominate tilt after manipulation of the sacroiliac joint in patients with low back pain. *Phys Ther.* 1988;68:1359–1363.
10. Clayson SJ, Newton IM, Debeucc DF, et al. Evaluation of mobility of hip and lumbar vertebrae in normal young women. *Arch Phys Med Rehabil.* 1962;43:1–8.
11. Colachis SC, Warden RE, Bechtol CO, et al. Movement of the sacroiliac joint in the adult male: a preliminary report. *Arch Phys Med Rehabil.* 1963;44:490–498.
12. DonTigny RL. Function and pathomechanics of the sacroiliac joint. *Phys Ther.* 1985;65:35–44.
13. DonTigny RL. Anterior dysfunction of the sacroiliac joint as a major factor in the etiology of idiopathic low back pain syndrome. *Phys Ther.* 1990;70:250–262.
14. Egund N, Olsson TH, Schmid H, et al. Movements in the sacroiliac joint demonstrated with roentgen stereophotogrammetry. *Acta Radiol.* 1978;19:833–846.
15. Ferrario VF, Sforza C. Biomechanical model of the human mandible in unilateral clench: distribution of temporomandibular joint reaction forces between working and balancing sides. *J Prosthet Dent.* 1994;72:169–176.
16. Figerio NA, Stowe RR, Howe JW. Movement of the sacroiliac joint. *Clin Orthop.* 1974;100:370–377.
17. Friedman MH, Weisberg J. Application of orthopedic principles in evaluation of the temporomandibular joint. *Phys Ther.* 1982;62:597–603.
18. Grieve EFM. Mechanical dysfunction of the sacro-iliac joint. *Int Rehabil Med.* 1983;5:46–52.

19. Goodheart G. Applied kinesiology in dysfunction of the temporomandibular joint. *Dent Clin North Am.* 1983;27:613–630.

20. Goldthwait JE, Osgood RB. A consideration of the pelvic articulations from an anatomical, pathological, and clinical standpoint. *Boston Med Surg J.* 1905;152:593–601.

21. Hendler N, Kozikowski JG, Schlesinger R, et al. Diagnosis and treatment of muscle tension headaches. *Physician Assistant.* 1991;15:72–74.

22. Hezog W, Read LJ, Conway PH, et al. Reliability of motion palpation procedures to detect sacroiliac joint fixations. *J Manipulative Physiol Ther.* 1989;12:86–92.

23. Hoppenfeld S. *Physical Examination of the Spine and Extremities.* Norwalk, CT: Appleton-Century-Crofts; 1976.

24. Iglarsh ZA, Snyder-Mackler L. Temporomandibular joint and the cervical spine. In: Richardson JV, Iglarsh ZA, eds. *Clinical Orthopaedic Physical Therapy.* Philadelphia: WB Saunders; 1994.

25. Isberg-Holm A, Westesson PL. Movement of disc and condyle in temporomandibular joints with clicking. *Acta Odontol Scand.* 1982;40:153–166.

26. Jacobsen, J. *The Temporomandibular Joint.* Iowa City, IA: University of Iowa; 1985. Unpublished paper.

27. Kapandji IA. *The Physiology of the Joints.* 2nd ed. Edinburgh: Churchill Livingstone; 1974.

28. Lavignolle B, Vital JM, Senegas J, et al. An approach to the functional anatomy of the sacroiliac joints in vivo. *Anat Clin.* 1983;5:169–176.

29. MacLennan AH. The role of the hormone relaxin in human reproduction and pelvic girdle relaxation. *Scan J Rheumatol Suppl.* 1991;10(88):7–15.

30. McCombe F, Fairbank JCT, Cockersole BC, et al. Reproducibility of physical signs in low back pain. *Spine.* 1989;908–918.

31. McKay GS, Yemm R. The structure and function of the temporomandibular joint. *Br Dent J.* 1992;173:127–132.

32. McMillan AS, McMillan DR, Darvell BW. Centers of rotation during jaw movements. *Acta Odontol Scand.* 1989;47:323–328.

33. Miller JAA, Schultz AB, Andersson GBJ. Load-displacement behaviour of sacroiliac joints. *J Orthop Res.* 1987;5:92–101.

34. Moore KL. *Clinically Oriented Anatomy.* Baltimore: Williams & Wilkins; 1985.

35. Nagerl H, Kubein-Meesenburg D, Fanghanel J, et al. Elements of a general theory of joints. 6. General kinematical structure of mandibular movements. *Anat Anz.* 1991;173:249–264.

36. Olson L, Eckerdal O, Hallonsten AL, et al. Craniomandibular function in juvenile chronic arthritis. A clinical and radiographic study. *Swed Dent J.* 1991;15:71–83.

37. Osborn JW. The disc of the human temporomandibular joint: design, function, and failure. *J Oral Rehabil.* 1985;12:279–293.

38. Osterbauer PJ, De Boer KF, Widmaier R, et al. Treatment and biomechanical assessment of patients with chronic sacroiliac joint syndrome. *J Manipulative Physiol Ther.* 1993;15:82–90.

39. Passero PL, Wyman BS, Bell JW, et al. Temporomandibular joint dysfunction syndrome. *Phys Ther.* 1985;65:1203–1207.

40. Piehlslinger E, Celar A, Futter K, et al. Orthopedic jaw movement observations. Part I: determination and analysis of the length of protrusion. *Cranio.* 1993;11:113–117.

41. Piehlslinger E, Celar A, Celar RM, et al. Orthopedic jaw movement observations. Part V: transversal condylar shift in protrusive and retrusive movement. *Cranio.* 1994;12:247–251.

42. Pierrynowski MR, Schroeder BC, Garrity CB, et al. Three-dimensional sacroiliac motion during locomotion in asymptomatic male and female subjects. In: Cotton CE, Lamontagne M, Robertson DGE, et al., eds. *Proceedings of the Fifth Biennial Conference and Human Locomotion Symposium.* London, Ontario: Canadian Society for Biomechanics; 1988;132–133.

43. Pitkin HC, Pheasant HC. Sacrathrogenetic telalgia, II: a study of sacral mobility. *J Bone Joint Surg.* 1936;18:365–374.

44. Porterfield JA, Oerosu C. The sacroiliac joint. In: Gould JA, ed. *Orthopaedic and Sports Physical Therapy.* 2nd ed. St. Louis: CV Mosby; 1990:553–559.

45. Potter NA, Rothstein JM. Intertester reliability for selected clinical tests of the sacroiliac joint. *Phys Ther.* 1985;65:1671–1675.

46. Reynolds HM. Three-dimensional kinematics in the pelvic girdle. *J Am Osteopath Assoc.* 1980;80:277–280.

47. Rocabado M. Arthrokinematics of the temporomandibular joint. *Dent Clin North Am.* 1983;27:573–594.

48. Sarnat BG. *The Temporomandibular Joint.* 2nd ed. Springfield, IL: Charles C Thomas; 1965.

49. Sashin D. A critical analysis of the anatomy and pathological changes of the sacroiliac joints. *J Bone Joint Surg.* 1930;12:891–910.

50. Scholten PJM, Schultz AB, Luchies CW, et al. Motions and loads within the human pelvis: a biomechanical model study. *J Orthop Res.* 1988;6:840–850.

51. Siegler S, Hayes R, Nicolella D, et al. A technique to investigate the three-dimensional kinesiology of the human temporomandibular joint. *J Prosthet Dent.* 1991;65:833–839.

52. Solberg WK, Clark GT. *Abnormal Jaw Mechanics: Diagnosis and Treatment.* Chicago: Quintessence Publishing; 1984.

53. Solonen VA. The sacroiliac joint in the light of anatomical, roentgenological and clinical studies. *Acta Orthop Scand Suppl.* 1957;27:1–127.

54. Sturesson B, Selvik G, Uden A. Movements of the sacroiliac joints, a roentgen stereophotogrammetric analysis. *Spine.* 1989;14:162–165.

55. Throckmorton GS, Throckmorton LS. Quantitative calculations of temporomandibular joint reaction forces—I. The importance of the magnitude of the jaw muscle forces. *J Biomech.* 1985;18:445–452.

56. Throckmorton GS, Groshan GJ, Boyd SB. Muscle activity patterns and control of temporomandibular joint loads. *J Prosthet Dent.* 1990;63:685–695.

57. Van Deursen M, Palijn J, Ockhuysen AL, et al. The value of some clinical tests of the sacroiliac joint. *Man Med.* 1990;5:96–99.

58. Vleeming A, Stoeckart R, Volkers ACW, et al. Relation between form and function in the sacroiliac joint, Part I: clinical anatomical aspects. *Spine.* 1990;15:130–132.

59. Waide FL, Bade DM, Lovasko J, et al. Clinical management of a patient following temporomandibular joint arthroscopy. *Phys Ther.* 1992;72:355–364.

60. Walker JM. The sacroiliac joint: a critical review. *Phys Ther.* 1992;72:903–916.

61. Walker JM. Age-related differences in the human sacroiliac joint: a histological study—implications for therapy. *J Orthop Sports Phys Ther.* 1986;7:325–331.

62. Weinberg LA. Role of stress, occlusion, and condyle position in temporomandibular dysfunction. *J Prosthet Dent.* 1983;4:532–544.

63. Weisl H. Articular surfaces of sacro-iliac joint and their relation to movements of sacrum. *Acta Anat (Basel).* 1954;22:1–14.

64. Weisl H. Ligaments of sacro-iliac joint examined with particular reference to their function. *Acta Anat (Basel).* 1954;20:201–213.

65. Weisl H. The movements of the sacroiliac joint. *Acta Anat (Basel).* 1955;23:80–91.

66. Wilder DG, Pope MH, Frymoyer JW. The functional topography of the sacroiliac joint. *Spine.* 1980;5:575–579.

67. Wiles MR. Reproducibility of interexaminer motion palpation findings of the sacroiliac joints. *J Can Chiro Assoc.* 1980;24:59–69.

68. Wilk BR, Stenback JT, McCain JP. Postarthroscopy physical therapy management of a patient with temporomandibular joint dysfunction. *J Orthop Sports Phys Ther.* 1993;18:473–478.

69. Williams PL, Warwick R, Dyson M, et al., eds. *Gray's Anatomy.* 37th British ed. Philadelphia: WB Saunders; 1989.

70. Yustin DC, Rieger MR, McGuckin RS, et al. Determination of the existence of hinge movements of the temporomandibular joint during normal opening by Cine-MRI and computer digital addition. *J Prosthodont.* 1993;2:190–195.

71. Zarb GA, Carlsson GE, eds. *Temporomandibular Joint: Function and Dysfunction.* Copenhagen, Denmark: Munksgaard; 1979.

15

Posture, Balance, and Gait

POSTURE

The arrangement of body segments determines the posture. Although the positions that could be assumed are essentially infinite in number, only a few erect and sitting postures are frequently used by any individual. Any posture demands specific joint positions (kinematics) and forces (kinetics) to maintain it. Many consider posture a static phenomenon and make reasonable assumptions that allow such a description. In fact, even relatively gross analysis has shown that the whole body and individual segments are in motion during these supposed static postures. The influence of body posture on joints and the tissues responsible for maintaining the joints in the desired position has to be considered.

Human postures have largely been derived from our necessity to free the hand for use. Accommodations have been made by bony and soft tissues to enable the performance of tasks now required of a "modern" society. For example, as suspensory postures (hanging by upper limbs) were assumed, the lower limbs became extended in line with the body and the shoulder girdle required greater mobility. Increased supination and pronation also developed and the prehensile hand found even greater use. Other changes were seen in the thorax as flattening developed anteroposteriorly and the scapula moved posteriorly. The lower limb was not free from modification. The foot lost most of its grasping ability, bony articulations were altered, and muscles changed attachment sites. More proximally, the mass of the gluteus maximus developed to a size unique to man, probably forcing a concurrent increase in the size of the quadriceps femoris.

Perhaps most important have been changes in the spine. Because of an approximately 30° anterior-inferior sacral tilt in the upright posture, the lumbar spine has been forced into the commonly known position of hyperextension or lordosis (66). Often blamed, either justly or unjustly, for predisposing human beings to low back pain and dysfunction, the sagittal plane configuration will continue to be of interest to clinicians and scientists alike. Despite these and other effects produced by human postures, dramatic changes are unlikely to occur soon. Therefore, therapists need to understand the implications of the postures that are commonly assumed and how the postures or their determinants can be altered to produce desired results.

Standing Requirements

For maintenance of the upright posture, multiple joints need to be controlled in each of three planes of motion. Usually, such control will be determined by a few factors. One is the relationship of the body's **line of gravity** with respect to the joint. Fortunately, for the sake of efficiency, the vertical line through the body's center of gravity is just anterior to the second sacral level, passing close to or through the sagittal plane axis of most lower limb joints. This line of gravity (force) multiplied by the distance (moment arm) to the center of the joint determines the moment required to control the position of the joint under consideration. Because the distance to any relevant joint axis is usually small in standing, moment requirements are minimal. Another factor is the position of the joint. Often, the posture chosen approximates the close-packed position of the joint. In these cases, with minor modification in the posture assumed, the joints can be placed in positions that require minimal muscle force: ligaments and joint capsules can be used to control joint torque rather than muscle contraction. Because postures are frequently altered and force requirements are modified regularly at all of the joints, events such as venous stasis and fatigue are avoided. Finally, realize that postures such as standing are asymmetric (77). The result is that different requirements exist for different joints. The effects of these and other factors are to produce different joint positions, resultant forces, and torques at the respective joints. The remainder of this section will describe these results for the joints of the lower limb and the spine.

The foot and ankle are important because they provide a foundation for the other joints. As pointed out in Chapter 12, the bony makeup of the foot allows flexibility in conforming to many supporting surfaces. However, the most important consider-ations are the requirements at the ankle as seen in the sagittal plane. In standing, the line of gravity falls anterior to the axis of the ankle. Thus, the muscles of the posterior calf must have active or passive tension so that the body will not fall anteriorly. Although muscles such as the gastrocnemius, tibialis anterior, peroneals, and tibialis posterior all are available to produce the tension required to maintain relative equilibrium, most accounts agree that the soleus muscle is primarily responsible (14, 55). Functionally, this is the most logical selection, because the others either are two-joint muscles or are required for the control of foot motion. Physiologically, as a slow muscle, the soleus is also well prepared to maintain low tensions for long durations. Note that here the moment of the body is taken about the mediolateral axis of the ankle. Conversely, sway in a posterior direction may involve sufficient displacement of the line of gravity such that the musculature of the anterior compartment would contract, pulling the body anteriorly. If this were required, an anterior counteracting moment is produced so that equilibrium can be maintained.

As stated in Chapter 11, the center of rotation of the knee in the sagittal plane is found within the femoral condyles. Because the line of gravity falls anterior to the axis of rotation of the knee, an extended position results, requiring little force from the quadriceps. In fact, during standing, manual movement of the patella is easy because of the lack of tension in the quadriceps muscles. If the knee is allowed to assume full extension, the close-packed position has been achieved and probably diminishes the need for great amounts of muscular tension. Complete hyperextension of the knee, commonly assumed in standing posture for long periods, involves reliance upon the posterior capsule. This practice probably should be avoided, although there is almost no evidence that it has a negative effect.

Carlsöö provides an extensive discussion of the knee during the standing posture, relating events to the principles of a closed kinetic chain. Because the distal segment is fixed and because the pelvis and trunk are carried over the knee and essentially fixed, the knee can be affected by any force that pulls the distal femur or proximal tibia posteriorly. This is the possible action of the hamstring and soleus muscles, both of which are active during standing posture (14, 65). A possible implication of this analysis is that musculature credited with control of the hip or ankle may directly affect the knee. Therefore, as previously explained, therapists should be aware of the functional changes that may occur when a closed kinetic chain is used during the movement.

Posture assumed by the hip has been debated, and no consensus exists on the position most commonly adopted. In fact, the collective line of gravity from the head, arms, and trunk segments fall either directly through, just anterior, or slightly posterior to the center of the hip joint when the upright body is viewed sagittally. As the line of gravity shifts, the moment requirements vary, but in any case the muscular tension requirements are small. This fact appears to have been confirmed with electromyography (3, 65). Mostly, the posture assumed will not place the hip joint in a position of complete extension; about 10 or 15° of motion are allowed (14). If, however, the hyperextended position is assumed, the person can rely on the anteriorly located iliofemoral ligament. Such a condition may be energy efficient, but for reasons cited for the posterior capsule of the knee, the regular assumption of this position may be harmful.

The sacroiliac joints are responsible for transposing the weight transmitted between the spinal column and the two lower limbs. The sacrum, essentially wedged between the two ilia, ordinarily experiences little movement. Upright posture, however, often rotates the sacrum forward and downwards (14). Constraint is provided, however, by the tension produced in the sacrotuberous and sacrospinous ligaments (27). Another important consideration for the sacrum is the role that the pelvic girdle components play in establishing the position of the spine as viewed laterally. This is because the **angle of inclination of the sacrum** (Fig. 15.1) determines the position of the fifth lumbar vertebra relative to the sacrum. The greater the inclination, the greater the tendency for additional lordosis in the whole of the lumbar spine. The effect of large degrees of inclination has been discussed in Chapter 13, but the implications for postural control of the trunk and head segments are also noteworthy.

The posture of the spinal column is thus a matter of balance among the anterior-posterior curvatures of the various segments. That is, greater lumbar lordosis will require greater thoracic kyphosis and perhaps cervical lordosis to balance the vertebrae on each other. Although attempts have been made to specify the respective locations of the lines of gravity for the trunk and the individual vertebrae, the only practical analyses are those that can be formulated from easily accessible body landmarks.

Generally the trunk is well balanced on the line of gravity. Thus, in the upright posture little is required for large muscular tensions and moments. There is clear evidence, however, that low levels of EMG activity exist in most people in the erector spinae muscles (37, 57, 65). The posterior musculature of the neck also is active because of the flexion moment produced by the weight of the head. More detailed descriptions of the postural requirements can be completed by analyzing the motion or potential motion between individual vertebral segments. Such procedures are usually reserved for more sophisticated works, but this type of analytic procedure may soon offer significant information about spinal kinematics.

Forces in the joints are primarily the result of two factors: superincumbent body weight and the contraction of the musculature controlling a specific joint. Only in unusual cases would tightness of structures around a joint be a significant factor in increasing such forces. As discussed previously, when viewed in the sagittal plane, the line of gravity falls through or relatively close to all of the joints about which moments would have to be considered. Subsequently, little need exists for large muscular forces that increase joint forces. In fact, most joints are at or near their

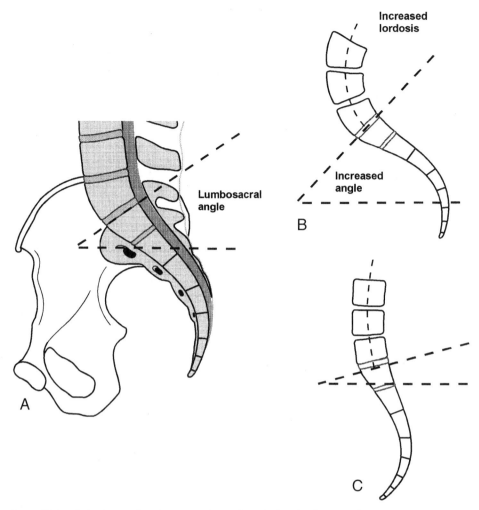

Figure 15.1.   A, lumbosacral angle as seen from a lateral view for the normal posture. An increase (**B**) or decrease (**C**) in the angle of inclination of the sacrum leads to changes in lordosis in the lumbar spine.

close-packed position, which offers maximal surface area over which to disperse force. Thus, the greater the superincumbent weight, the greater the compressive force in the joint. Because the force at the joints is directly dependent on body mass and its distribution, body segment parameter information (see Chapter 1) should determine the relative proportion distributed to each segment, followed by an appropriate mathematical procedure.

Evaluation

Postural evaluations have been widely used, particularly for the young and in situations such as scoliosis, when therapeutic outcome is dependent on proper alignment. Although no one posture is right for everyone, a sagittal view of the line of gravity should probably fall anterior to the ankle and knee and through the hip joint, acromion process, and tragus of the ear. From an anterior or posterior view the body is dissected into two halves: the line of gravity falls through such centrally located landmarks as the spinous processes posteriorly, and the pubic symphysis and nose anteriorly. In either case, the position assumed should have a base of support that compromises neither stability nor mobility. Finally, although evaluation in a third plane may be desirable, deviations noted in the lateral, anterior, or posterior views can adequately describe any abnormalities.

Sitting

Trunk Position

Most volumes addressing kinesiology do not discuss sitting as a posture. This position is extremely relevant, however, since many people spend a great amount of time sitting. Furthermore, there is conflicting evidence that those who assume a sitting posture for work incur an increased risk of low back pain (49, 84). Finally, there is distinct evidence that the mechanics of the pelvis and spine changes when sitting is achieved. For example, Carlsöö states that of the 90° between the trunk and thigh, about 40° are in the posterior tilting of the pelvis and 50° in flexion of the hip (14). Assuming this degree of motion, the angle of sacral inclination is also altered, resulting in a less lordotic posture of the lumbar spine.

Another significant factor is that during sitting, the position of the pelvis can be altered. This change is achieved by positioning of the trunk. Consider the forward leaning posture and the slumped position. Although these postures may produce similar configurations of the lumbar spine, the spinal extensor musculature is required to actively control the forward moment in the former position (assuming the arms are not supporting the weight of the trunk). In contrast, the upright sitting posture demands more lordosis, simulating more closely the lumbosacral position assumed during standing.

That the position of the pelvis and spine is important is partly demonstrated by how much study has been dedicated to alternative postures. One such alternative is a posture that involves direct support of the lumbar spine. Design of office furniture and the manufacture of various sizes and styles of lumbar "support cushions" are ready evidence of the attention paid to this posture. Perhaps at least some of this impetus has been provided by the work of Nachemson, who has stated that unsupported sitting reduces lumbar lordosis and increases the load on the intervertebral discs and posterior structures of the back (54). To combat this criticism of the standard sitting posture there has been some interest in using a seat with a downward inclination of the anterior portion of the supporting surface (Fig. 15.2). To evaluate the orthopaedic considerations associated with this type of seated posture, Keegan used a radiographic approach. Of some interest was that a normal lumbar curve is possible with a thigh-trunk angle of 135° (39). Schlegel also recommended tilting the whole seat forwards (71).

Several works have evaluated various features of sitting posture. Evaluation of an **anteriorly inclined seat** to alter how much EMG is produced by the erector spinae has been done, yielding conflicting findings. In one study, subjects performed a typing task for 15 minutes, with the activity of the musculature evaluated when the angle of the supporting surface was set at 0, 10, and 20° of anterior inclination. Results showed statistically significant differences between postures, such that EMG activity decreased as the inclination of the chair increased (78). Another study, however, found no differences between the inclined position and two other chairs, both with back supports (5). The results may be directly related to changes in the lumbar spine, that is, an increase in extension (lordosis) with the anteriorly inclined

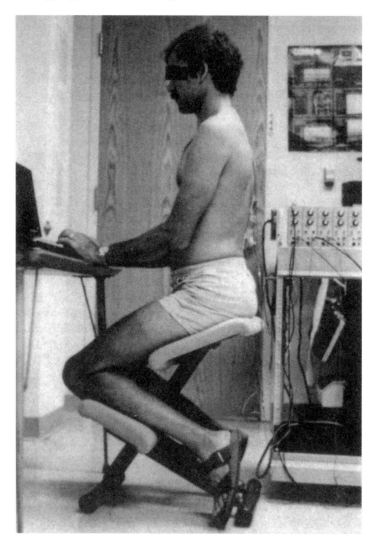

Figure 15.2. Posture of a subject seated on a downwardly inclined supporting surface while EMG data is collected from three levels of erector spinae muscles. Although with this seating device some weight can be borne on the lower leg, the subject also can position the lower limbs so that the feet are flat on the floor.

seating surface (5, 46). In other work, the influence of a lumbar roll on the EMG of the erector spinae has been evaluated. Test conditions were similar to those described in the previous study. Results showed that both a lumbar roll and a lumbar cushion afforded small decreases in EMG activity at the tested erector spinae levels adjacent to T10, L1, and L3 (79). These studies have possible application to patient care, but further data are needed before definitive conclusions can be reached.

The existing information on the seated posture shows significant differences between standing and sitting, and even between the different sitting postures assumed. As the pelvis changes to a configuration different from that of standing, the spine is required to change its configuration. Thus, force requirements of the supporting musculature are altered, as are intradiscal pressure and tension in passive tissues such as ligaments. In fact, how a patient is positioned may significantly influence the intended therapeutic outcome. An upright, unsupported posture is distinctly different from a supported posture with a backward trunk inclination. In the latter case the smallest intradiscal pressures and EMG values have been shown with an inclination of 120°. All other seated postures require larger magnitudes of intradiscal pressure and/or EMG (1).

Specifically, the upright posture produces the highest levels of EMG activity in the erector spinae muscles. Typically, however, these values are only 10% of the maximum activity that can be produced by the greatest effort. Slumping diminishes the activity while more extreme forward bending, even without anterior support mechanisms such as resting the forearms on the thighs, decreases or abolishes the activity. Flexion to approximately 50° eliminates the erector spinae activity in favor of passive tension in the musculature and the posterior elements of the spine.

Pathokinesiology

Many conditions affect posture. Pain and discomfort are frequently causes of the attitude a patient may assume, but the key outcome will be removal of the cause so that normal position and function can be assumed. A classic example is a patient suffering from low back dysfunction. If spinal musculature is in asymmetrical spasm, functional scoliosis can be produced. In addition, the pelvis may be unilaterally elevated, causing discrepancy of leg length and forcing modification of posture. Until the condition resolves, normal kinematics and kinetics will not be available, impeding normal motion.

In discussing how pathologies affect posture, two helpful principles should be remembered. First, recognize that distal involvement may have effects at proximal joints. Consider a patient with cerebral palsy that has developed a plantar flexion contracture of the ankle. Such unilateral plantar flexion requires that the hip and knee of the same limb be placed into flexion so that the pelvis can remain level. Thus, the distal joint has determined the position of two other joints, providing a demonstration of the closed-kinetic chain in a practical situation.

The second principle is that alterations from an ideal postural configuration usually require greater forces in muscles during functional activities because greater moments need to be generated for control of body segments. Returning to the cerebral palsy case cited above, imagine the patient in the sagittal plane. Note that compared with the normal posture and the close approximation of the line of gravity to joint centers, the centers of rotation have been displaced. The greater the distance from the line of gravity the greater the moment required to maintain a joint in the desired position. In fact, studies have determined that, compared to full knee extension, 51% of the maximal quadriceps force is necessary to maintain the body in an upright position (63). Stress resulting from long-term postures in such positions could ultimately lead to altered structure and function.

Lower Limb Injuries

Virtually any injury of the lower limb has the potential for producing alterations in a patient's posture. We previously detailed the **plantar flexion contracture** in this section. Note that similar events would occur if a knee injury resulted in a flexion contracture of this joint. The result would be a concomitant flexion of the hip and dorsiflexion at the ankle assuming that a level pelvis is maintained. Moment requirements at all joints would be increased.

Deviations in the mediolateral direction are less common. Any unilateral involvement would produce asymmetry and distort optimal postural alignment. **Pain,** arising from any number of foot conditions, for example an ankle sprain or degenerative joint disease, can produce such a distortion. The knee is frequently the focus of degeneration and, being at the end of two long levers, may be readily displaced either medially (valgus) or laterally (varus). No matter the direction, stress concentration is likely to develop at one area of the joint while tension is likely to occur in the elongated soft tissue structures. If the deviation is great enough, the limb can be shortened sufficiently to produce a leg-length difference and ultimately a postural discrepancy.

Muscular deficiencies also can produce deficits that have postural implications. Although most muscular involvement can have implications, the most serious deficiencies are those that involve the posterior calf muscles, the quadriceps, and the hip extensors. Fortunately, such losses do not often involve entire groups, resulting only in weakness rather than major loss. If the plantarflexors are lost, however, maintaining balance becomes a problem. Keeping the line of gravity within its anteroposterior limits is more difficult since the primary means of shifting it posteriorly toward the ankle axis has been lost. Frequently patients compensate by adjusting their base of support or shifting their weight to the sounder limb (45).

Quadriceps insufficiency creates little difficulty during standing because, as noted previously, the center of rotation of the knee is posterior to the line of gravity. Precautions may need to be taken against hyperextension of the knee. Hip extensor loss can be difficult for a patient, depending on the location of the axis of rotation relative to the line of gravity. The most common compensation is displayed by the patient with a spinal cord lesion who assumes a position of hip hyperextension. As noted earlier, this allows the load to be borne by the iliofemoral ligament, thus offering sufficient control of the hip extension moment. Maintaining the line of gravity anterior to the hip is extremely important; otherwise, sudden flexion of the trunk on the lower limbs may result in a fall.

We have already stated that the lower limb operates as a closed-kinetic chain. In paralytic cases, remembering the interaction among the three joints of the lower limb is important for the clinician. One example, the above knee amputee, should suffice. In this situation, active control of the knee is lost. Subsequently, to maintain an upright posture the patient must stand with the hip short of complete extension so that postural sway can be controlled at the hip. A backward tilt of the pelvis would create hip flexion and would not allow the upright posture (45).

As previously covered in Chapter 13, the anterior-posterior tilting of the pelvis exerts significant influence on the primary curves of the spinal column. Excessive downward tilting is seen in some cases of contracture of the iliopsoas muscles, creating the need for increased curvature of the thoracic spine as a compensatory mechanism. The other primary deviation of the spine, scoliosis, has also been detailed in Chapter 13.

BALANCE

Maintenance of postures, or balance, is described as the dynamics of body posture to prevent falling (89). Balance is dependent on many factors because of the multiple degrees of freedom available to the systems needing control. For example, each of us depends on the neuromusculoskeletal and sensory systems for the maintenance

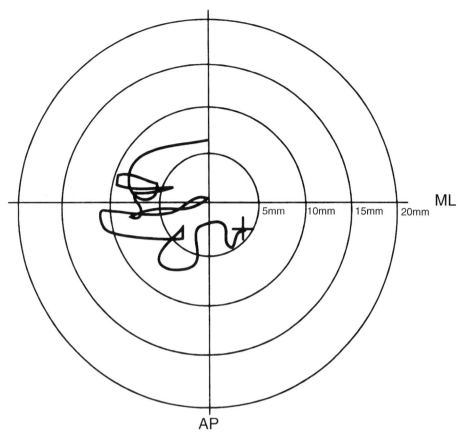

5mm   10mm   15mm   20mm   ML

AP

Figure 15.3. Plot showing the center of pressure during standing posture in which sway was voluntarily controlled by the subject.

and control of routine postures and the assurance of the selected posture. Considering these factors, models for control of postures have been proposed (22, 34). Somatosensory, vestibular, and visual feedback also need to be integrated within the central nervous system (33, 36). If not, the result can be catastrophic falls. Thus, consideration of issues associated with balance is necessary for the understanding of human movement.

Normal

Assessment of balance implies that valid and reliable methods of measuring complex phenomena exist. However, "generalized measures of balance are neither very sensitive nor very specific" (34). Further, these issues are confounded even more when patients are assessed because increased variations occur under these testing conditions. In spite of the limitations, many measurements and scales have been developed that can be helpful in assessing balance. The most common procedure, including those available through commercial devices, is the calculation of the **center of pressure (COP)**. This value, measured in meters, is the point location of the vertical ground reaction force vector. An example of a center of pressure plot during standing is provided in Figure 15.3. In actuality this measure "represents a weighted average of all the pressures over the surface of the area in contact with the ground" (88). The concept and actual measure are often confused with the **center of mass (COM)**, whose vertical projection on the ground is frequently called the **center of gravity (COG)**. The specific, but important, relationship of the COG and the COP is beyond the scope of this volume; the reader is referred to Winter for further explanation (89). In essence, as the COG is varied there will be accompanying shifts in the COP. A summary of the literature has established that COG fluctuations in the anteroposterior and mediolateral directions are smaller than the changes in the COP. The shifts are sometimes called **sway,** which must be controlled to maintain the posture.

Difficulties are encountered because of the many alternatives available for assessing the movement of the COP that results from a test of balance. Choices to consider in the analysis include measures such as duration, displacement, path sway, target sway, and path length and area. More complex statistical analyses have also been performed on the resulting data. Similarly, many different analyses have been completed on the COM to establish appropriate tests and draw relationships to COP measurements. To assist the clinician with the conversion of "postural stability" data to COP location, techniques have now been reported (25).

Control

Because it is recognized that quiet standing is limited as a tool to discriminate among the mechanisms of balance, techniques have been developed that will challenge the controlling systems. To determine the effect of the visual system, most vestibular and somatosensory systems have resorted to **perturbations.** Internal perturbations include activities such as arm raising or trunk bending while external perturbations consist of such things as support platform tilt and pulls or pushes to the arms, legs, shoulders, or pelvis. In the latter, the onset and size of the perturbation are unknown to the subject (88, 89). Thus, we may question whether these perturbations mimic real life experiences. Partly because of this reason others have resorted to gait initiation as a model for the testing sequence (67).

Of interest is how the subject responds to the change in posture. Kinematic, kinetic, and electromyographic data have been the primary sources for evaluation of the changes. Videography of the subject, often while standing on a force plate, is often monitored while EMG data are collected from selected muscles. Responses to the perturbations are dependent on many factors and may be sequenced depending on the perturbation, but according to Horak, three patterns of response are common for correction of anterior-posterior sway in normal adults (34). One, the "ankle strategy," is the most common. Here the center of gravity shifts by rotating the body about the ankle with little movement at the hip or knee joints. An example of the data derived during voluntary flexion-extension adjustments for the ankle and hip strategies is shown in Figure 15.4 (56). As may be suspected, the hip strategy uses hip flexion or extension of the hips. Finally, the stepping (stumbling) strategy occurs when the base of support must necessarily be realigned under the body, such as during a rapid step, hop, or stumble. The strategy adopted depends on the support surface configuration and the size of the perturbation (20, 33). Obviously, the strategy adopted will relate to the onset of EMG activity in the muscles required for control of the strategy. Alterations of these patterns will be apparent in patients, a topic discussed in a later section.

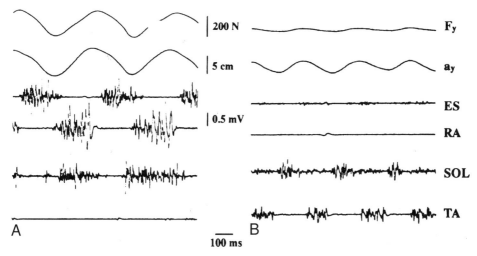

Figure 15.4. Recordings of the horizontal forward-backward reaction force (F_y) and displacement of center of pressure (a_y) with EMG from erector spinae (*ES*), rectus abdominis (*RA*), soleus (*SOL*), and tibialis anterior (*TA*). **A,** voluntary forward-backward movements of the hip (hip strategy). **B,** voluntary flexion-extension movements at the ankle with the feet flat on the ground (ankle strategy).

Changes with Aging

The ability to control posture is known to change with age (94). Typical among the changes are alterations in the temporal organization responses, demonstrated via increases in onset latencies. In addition, antagonist muscles are more often coactivated with agonist muscles. Sensory input reduction also penalizes the elderly when attempting to maintain balance (95). The cause for this is believed to be the deterioration of primary peripheral sensory processes. In addition, the elderly sway more (85) and the functional base of support, defined as the anteroposterior proportion of foot length used in maximal sustained forward and backward leaning, is decreased (40). Some differences in measured parameters have also been found between men and women (97).

Pathokinesiology

Given that postural control is supervised by many systems it is not surprising that a variety of pathologies are represented by deviations from what would be considered normal balance; these include vestibular disorders, visual deficits resulting from cerebral vascular accidents, peripheral vascular disease, Parkinson's disease, and chronic brain syndromes (69). Work has been undertaken to figure out how balance measures differ when subjects with pathology are evaluated (19, 30, 59). Results are variable with the subject's pathology. More important is the relative dearth of literature on the topic of therapeutic benefits of intervention strategies (38).

Balance and Treatment Goals

Balance is an essential component of normal everyday activities. When disruptions alter the capability to respond appropriately the body demonstrates increased sway and, at the extreme, falls occur. The principles that the therapist must apply include an assessment of the patient's ability to control joint torques in the appropriate temporal sequence. Therapeutic goals, however, are confounded by the alterations in the input into the body's systems that modify the appropriate responses required for the maintenance of balance. When the clinician can modify that input or control, the output will likely determine the outcome. Finally, how balance relates to gait initiation has become a topic of considerable interest, both to prevent injuries and to assess the outcomes of our treatment protocols. Some have clearly considered balance and gait initiation and continuation integrally related (67, 89).

GAIT

The act of walking, fundamental to the performance of human movement, has been described as a series of prevented catastrophes. Yet, when analyzed, the activity known also as gait is carried out with remarkable efficiency. Volumes upon volumes have described the movement patterns and mechanics of gait (17, 63, 75). Others have focused on the initiation of gait or the development of gait during childhood (50, 83, 96). Still others have completed more complex analyses of gait through use of the computer and mathematics (16, 32, 98). However, some more useful forms of analysis use systems designed for clinical practice settings (4, 61, 80, 91). Although a normal walking pattern assumes many forms, disruptions in the sequence of actions are easily identified. The clinician must be prepared to recognize these alterations in the normal pattern with knowledge of kinematics and kinetics as applied to the gait pattern. This section will discuss biomechanics as applied to gait and then present the common pathologies that produce changes in the gait pattern.

Definitions

To describe the gait pattern adequately some system of terminology must be adopted. Many attempts have been made to standardize the descriptors, yet no one system is universally accepted. Although some common systems will be presented in this volume the therapist is advised to be prepared to interpret and make applications to other systems that may appear in the literature.

Fundamental to any description of walking is the term **gait cycle,** meaning the beginning of an event by one limb and continuing until the event is repeated with that same limb. Often the cycle is considered from one heel strike until the heel strike of the same extremity. One complete gait cycle is known as a **stride,** while a **step** is considered the beginning of an event by one limb until the beginning of the same event with the contralateral limb (2). Other important terms are **swing, stance,** and **double support,** the latter being the period when both feet are in contact with the supporting surface. Overall, stance accounts for about 60% of the gait cycle for each limb when walking velocity is normal (Fig. 15.5). Methods are available for describing various parts of these phases of the gait cycle, the most useful being shown in Figure 15.6. Note that heel strike is synonymous with initial contact, and that foot flat is part of the loading response. Heel off and toe off are other commonly used events specifying points in the gait cycle. In addition, any of these events can be timed; thus, a temporal sequence can also be ascribed to the events of the gait cycle. Cadence, the number of steps per minute, can also be described.

Caution must be exercised in strict adherence to this system or any proposed terminology, because sometimes all phases are not discernible. This is particularly true when pathology affects the pattern. No matter the system or the terminology, successful locomotion requires the ability to support the body, maintain balance,

0%
RT. HEEL STRIKE
50%
LT. HEEL STRIKE
100%
RT. HEEL STRIKE
RT. STANCE
RT. SWING
LT. SWING
LT. STANCE
DURATION OF TOTAL RT. WALKING CYCLE
(STRIDE TIME)
SINGLE-LIMB SUPPORT
DOUBLE-LIMB SUPPORT
RT. STRIDE LENGTH
RT.-LT. STEP LENGTH
LT.-RT. STEP LENGTH

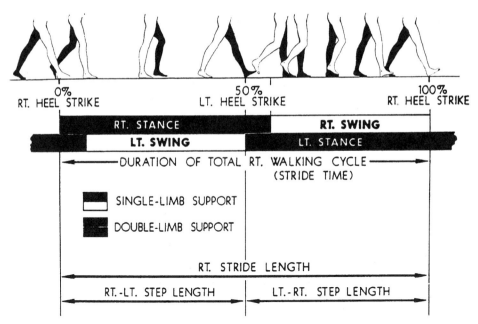

Figure 15.5. The temporal components and the relative step and stride lengths that occur during the gait cycle.

and in some manner execute the stepping movement. As Murray has stated, restraint, support, and propulsion must occur in logical sequence for forward motion to progress (52).

Center of Gravity Displacement

The efficiency of the movement of the total body during gait is produced by the respective kinematics of the segments of the lower limb. One way to describe the efficiency of movement during locomotion is by approximating the location of the center of body mass and plotting its movement during the gait cycle. Although it is possible, and perhaps important, to evaluate the movement of the center of mass in all three planes, a discussion of motion in the sagittal plane will suffice. Here the center essentially moves in a sinusoidal pattern. Three key points are memorable.

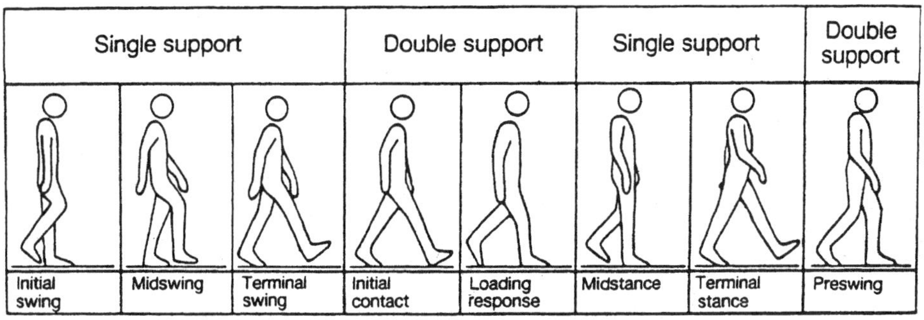

Single support
Double support
Single support
Double support
Initial swing
Midswing
Terminal swing
Initial contact
Loading response
Midstance
Terminal stance
Preswing

Figure 15.6. The endpoints of each phase of the gait cycle. Using this system enables the description of all phases in equal intervals.

First, vertical displacement of the center of mass is minimal over the gait cycle and involves little loss of energy, i.e., little resistance to the desired forward motion. Second, the pattern is repeated ad infinitum as the various cycles recur with forward progression. Finally, the velocity of the center's forward movement varies considerably. For example, following heel strike the forward velocity is decreased. During the propulsive phase in late stance this velocity is increased. All these events, dependent upon the kinematics and kinetics of the joints of the lower limb, occur in a pattern that results in smooth coordinated movement. Similar descriptions of the paths for the centers of mass for the other planes are available, but usually they are more ellipsoid (14).

Kinematics

Angular rotations of each of the lower limb joints occur predominantly in the sagittal plane. A summary of these movements for the entire gait cycle is shown in Figure 15.7 (52). Each of the respective ranges of motion can be correlated with the various phases of the gait cycle. Particularly note the total ranges of motion required for each joint, because the therapist should usually seek to attain these ranges to achieve nonpathological gait.

For the hip, electrogoniometry has been used to analyze triplanar motion during gait. A sample of results is shown in Figure 15.8. Note that only small ranges of motion are required for both abduction-adduction and axial rotation (76). For the knee, virtually no abduction-adduction range would either exist or be desirable. Rotation occurs as part of the screw-home mechanism associated with terminal extension. These features were discussed in Chapter 11. The ankle-foot complex has been more difficult to analyze because of the multiple joints involved in its positioning. Extensive reviews have described the motions at each joint in the foot. In essence, they state that the subtalar joint pronates to allow internal rotation of the leg, while supination allows external rotation. During support phase the foot pronates, and it begins to supinate as the midstance period starts. Supination continues and reaches a maximum shortly before toe off. Similar analyses are available for the midtarsal joint (68). While blame for the creation of clinical syndromes at the knee has been placed on extreme variances in foot mechanics, there is now evidence that such extreme changes produce only slight changes in knee kinematics (44).

Motion of the pelvis is critical to normal locomotion. Movement in the sagittal plane is slight, as depicted in Figure 15.7. In the transverse plane the pelvis has been shown to rotate approximately 11.5°, advancing anteriorly on the side of the limb swinging forward (52). Rotation in the frontal plane (abduction and adduction) is critical. This is a direct application of the abductor mechanism described in Chapter 10. Recall that during stance phase the abductors must be active to prevent the opposite side of the pelvis from dropping. Thus, in effect, the pelvis on the side of the swinging leg is elevated. An average of 8° of motion exists in this plane (21). The upper trunk rotates in the opposite direction of the pelvis. This is apparently a balance mechanism, but the combination of motions requires that rotation occur throughout the spinal column.

Not to be excluded in the kinematics of gait is the motion of the upper limbs. Their motion is correlated with the movement of the upper trunk; therefore, as a lower limb is advanced, the contralateral arm moves forward. Murray has shown that the total amplitude of shoulder flexion and extension is 32°, and that the extension

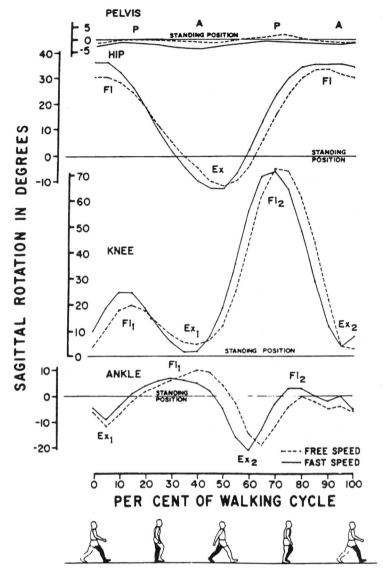

Figure 15.7. Mean sagittal plane kinematics for the pelvis, hip, knee, and ankle for 30 normal men walking at two speeds. The zero was a reference provided by the joint when the subject was standing. For the pelvis an upward deflection represents posterior tilting (*P*) while a downward deflection represents anterior tilting (*A*). For the other joints, flexions are designated with *Fl* and extensions with *Ex*.

range required is much greater than that of flexion. The elbow also participates, and experiences a total flexion-extension range of about 64° (52, 53).

Kinetics

The kinetics associated with gait is an interesting topic because one can integrate and apply most of biomechanics to a functional activity (24, 58). The kinematics just discussed are produced by timely and appropriate levels of muscle contraction required by the interplay of gravitational and inertial forces. These contractions are

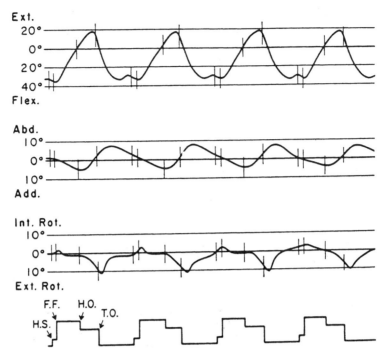

Figure 15.8. Three-dimensional electrogoniometric recording of hip motion during gait. Foot switch patterns are used to locate heel strike (*HS*), foot flat (*FF*), heel off (*HO*), and toe off (*TO*).

responsible for the generation of joint torque and forces. Thus, this section will discuss each of these aspects as applied to human locomotion.

Muscular Actions

Overall, knowing total joint kinematics allows a ready understanding of the musculature involved in producing the motions. For example, a limb in swing or stance phase shows whether a muscle will be required to shorten or lengthen, and at what velocity it will exert tension.

Now, with a review of the sagittal plane motion shown in Figure 15.7, consider the ankle joint throughout the gait cycle. Note that from 5 to 35% of the cycle the ankle is dorsiflexing as the lower leg passes over the foot fixed to the supporting surface. During this time the muscles of the anterior tibial compartment are minimally active or inactive because of little or no moment requirement (Fig. 15.9). Then, the ankle is plantarflexed during the propulsive phase. Note the activity of the plantarflexors in the late support phase. At toe off, dorsiflexion begins so that the foot will clear the ground during the swing phase. The EMG data indicate that activity starts just before the liftoff of the foot from the surface. This activity is probably timed so that sufficient tension is developed before the foot clears the ground.

Similar analyses can be completed for each motion of all the other joints required to participate in the gait cycle. For example, consider how the muscular activity shown in Figure 15.9 for the gluteus maximus, rectus femoris, vastus muscles, and hamstrings acts to control the extension moments required at the hip and knee.

Review of the EMG data would confirm that the muscles affect appropriate moments in each plane for each joint in the temporal sequence required for the normal gait pattern. Correlation of EMG data with moment data will be possible when joint torque data during gait is presented in the next section.

Several other features associated with the muscular control of gait should be discussed. Evaluation of the EMG records shows that muscles not required to control moments are also active during the gait cycle. The adductor group provides a ready

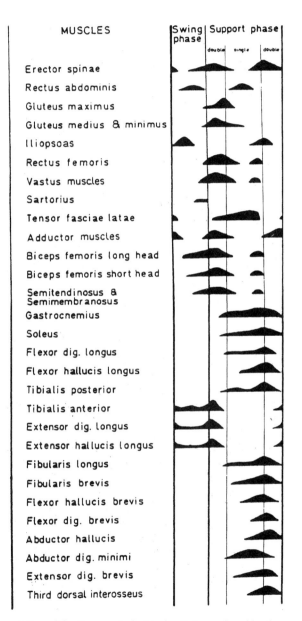

Figure 15.9. Representation of the "average" electrical activity produced by the muscles of the lower limb during gait.

example. Explanation can be offered for activity in early support and early swing phases, in that the former provides stability while the latter assists with flexion at the hip. Based on the anatomical location of the large mass of the adductors, both functions can be postulated. Also, activity in the muscles is initiated before tension is needed. This preliminary tension occurs for two possible reasons. The first is that the muscle may contribute to deceleration of a segment. Second, because of the physiological characteristics of muscle, the contractile component must be activated early to compensate for its elastic properties (see Chapter 2).

Other information about the role of musculature is also of interest. One classic work was completed in which the mechanics of muscle function during locomotion were studied, taking into account active and passive properties and other physiological characteristics. In studying walking at different velocities on both level and ramped surfaces, tension values associated with changes in muscle length were determined. For example, the maximal muscle force, 540 pounds, was generated during a lengthening contraction of the quadriceps muscle. Forces of up to 400 pounds were recorded at contraction rates of up to 6 inches per second. Similar values were achieved for quadriceps lengthening contractions of approximately 9 inches per second. Some import should be ascribed to Morrison's conclusion that the mechanism of muscle function normally contained a period of muscle lengthening as force increased, followed by an interval of concentric contraction under a decreasing load. In observing that the muscles studied had an excursion range of 3–4 inches, the forces were noted to be produced between a mean and maximal operating length. The muscle was normally inactive at shorter lengths (51). That muscle length and type of contraction must be taken into account has frequently been ignored but excellent summaries of these factors and how they relate to gait have now been published (13, 41).

Some work has also evaluated the specific role of certain muscular components during gait. Two corollary studies have assessed the role of the ankle plantarflexors during normal locomotion. The results reinforce the points made earlier regarding the necessity of considering all of the physiological and functional characteristics of muscle. One study evaluated the posterior compartment musculature during the entire support phase of the gait cycle, concluding that the demands in the first half of support are small and not required for normal function. During the second half of support, however, the mechanics of gait are such that the muscles act as a controlling force on the forward momentum of the tibia. Subsequently, the group serves to restrain forward movement of the body (74). Similar findings were independently produced two years later by Sutherland et al. (81). They concluded that the ankle plantarflexors contributed to knee and ankle stability, restrained forward rotation of the tibia on the talus, and minimized vertical oscillations of the body's center of mass, with the latter contributing to energy conservation. A further discussion of the mechanics of the posterior compartment muscles will be presented in the following section of this chapter on applications of mechanics.

Joint Torques

During walking the torques of interest are those in the ankle, knee, and hip. Although swing phase torques are of some interest, they are less important than those during stance phase because they are smaller. This is apparent, as shown in Figure 15.10, for all three joints in all three planes. Of the requirements for extension moments at the three joints during early support, those for the hip are greatest, and those for the

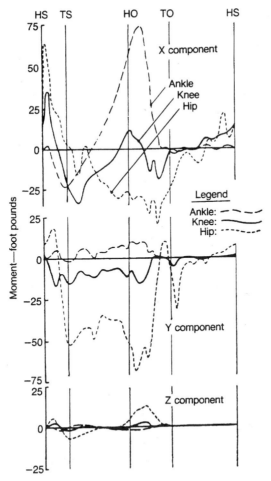

Figure 15.10. Moments at each joint of the lower limb during the gait cycle. The X component is for flexion/extension, the Y for abduction and adduction, and Z for rotations. *Legend: HS,* heel strike; *TS,* toe strike; *HO,* heel off; *TO,* toe off.

ankle the least. All moments progress to flexion moments, but their magnitudes vary considerably. Extension moments for the knee and ankle are produced between heel off and toe off, apparently for propulsion.

For abduction and adduction the most significant moment involves hip abduction, required for almost the entirety of the support phase. This moment is consistent with the contraction of the gluteus medius and minimus muscles in the institution of the abductor mechanism that accomplishes elevation of the contralateral side of the pelvis. The other feature that should be noted from Figure 15.10 is the size of the moments. The hip abduction and ankle extension moments are the greatest: each reaches approximately 70 foot pounds (94.9 Nm) (12). Other work has also generated moment data for the lower limb during gait. Some differences in the magnitudes compared with those shown in the figure exist, but the general configuration of the curves is the same. For example, Winter has reported peak ankle moments of 150 Nm and knee moments of about 140 Nm (92). The data of Crowninshield, however, agree closely with those of Bresler and Frankel (12). Peak values for some trials were reported to be as high as 80 Nm in abduction (18).

Joint Forces

Using engineering methodology in the determination of joint torque, one then may calculate joint forces. Because direct measures of these forces have not generally been possible, **indirect** means such as those discussed in Chapter 6 have been used. Overall, many of these techniques use a force plate to determine the reaction forces at the foot. Kinematic data are collected simultaneously so that segmental velocities and accelerations can be calculated. Body segment parameter information, specifically the mass, mass center locations, and mass moments of inertia, is estimated via mathematical techniques. Solutions to equations of motion provide forces and moments for the prediction of muscle forces that are then used in the determination of joint contact forces (18). These contact forces (bone-on-bone forces) include joint reaction force and the effect of active forces due to muscle contraction (90).

These analyses involve complex data collection and analysis procedures. Therefore, the data on contact forces during gait is not extensive. The earliest of works by Bresler and Frankel established, as expected, that the greatest component of joint force acts vertically. Essentially similar patterns exist for all lower limb joints. Forces in the other two directions are much less and similar in shape over the duration of the gait cycle (12). Later, experiments showed the contact force at the hip to be higher than five times body weight (10, 72). An example of the forces on the femoral head is shown in Figure 15.11. Thus, by using such a complete process, all gravitational, inertial, and muscle forces have been included in the analysis.

These results are remarkably consistent with in vivo information gathered by inserting an instrumented prosthesis into patients to specifically measure hip contact forces (6, 70). In one study, although the subjects walked with significant perturbation in kinetics and kinematics, the contact forces were reported to be from 1.6 to 3.3 times body weight (70). Jogging and very fast walking increased the forces to about 5.5 times body weight (6). Considering that differences occur between the subjects, there is reasonable agreement between in vivo and indirect measurement techniques.

Therapists should realize that forces in the lower limb joints are significant during walking. Only a part of the load is directly due to body weight. Indirectly, however, the factor of body weight influences the mechanics required for function. Major loading is due to the compressive effect of muscle contraction, so in treatment programs an attempt is frequently made to decrease the muscular requirements. The therapist can provide assistive devices so that full weight is not borne on the limb. Peak forces have been diminished to about 60% of usual by using a cane (9). Another method to reduce contact forces would be to decrease the velocity of walking. This distributes the loading over a longer time, avoiding what is known as impulse loading. In addition, decreased velocity lessens the muscular tension requirements, in terms of both the rate of tension development and the total magnitude.

Overall success rates for joint replacements are remarkably high. Not only is loading an important factor, but the number of repetitions required for any semblance of normal function is very high. Thus, considerations related to properties such as material strength and fatigue characteristics must be applied. Surely, further work will help both the surgeon and therapist in the description of the limits that will produce the most effective care.

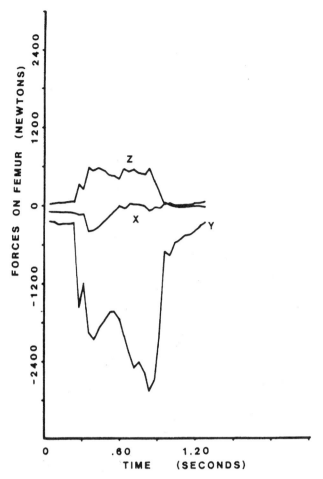

Figure 15.11.   Forces on the femoral head during a cycle of level walking in three orthogonal directions. *Legend*: *Y*, vertical; *X*, anteroposterior; *Z*, mediolateral.

Applications of Mechanics

Analysis of human locomotion provides an excellent opportunity to discuss principles of **mechanical energy.** Defined as the ability to perform work or exert force on another body, mechanical energy is an important measure of the efficiency of human function. Although all of the principles to be discussed can be applied to motion of the individual segments, the example used will be the displacements associated with the body's center of mass during the gait cycle.

Several forms of energy must be considered. **Potential energy** (PE) is the energy due to gravity, as reflected in the formula PE = mgh, where mass and height are the other important factors. **Kinetic energy** can be in two forms, **translational** and **rotational.** The former is the product of one-half the mass and the square of the velocity. In the latter, mass is replaced with inertia and velocity with angular velocity (90). Given these definitions, consider a roller coaster car perched at its track's point of maximal elevation. By virtue of its position the car has PE, but by descending to the bottom it has no more (zero height). Instead, kinetic energy now exists so that the car can be elevated to the next peak.

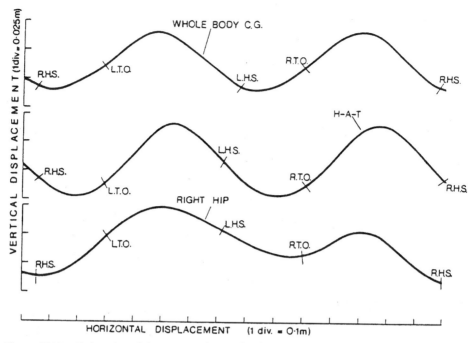

Figure 15.12. Trajectories of the centers of mass for the whole body, the head-arms-trunk (H-A-T) segment and the right hip in the sagittal plane for the gait cycle.

These factors, by which mechanical energy exists either by virtue of position or of motion, allow us to have efficient locomotion. In fact, analysis of the displacement of the center of mass during gait is similar to a roller coaster. Refer to Figure 15.12 and note the displacement of the center of mass. Peaks of displacement are reached during single support, while the lowest points are reached during periods of double support. These alternating events using potential and kinetic energy are responsible for our efficiency. Greater and/or more abrupt changes in the displacement of the center of mass would decrease efficiency because more energy expenditure would be required. Caution must be exerted in generalizing these conditions to the center of mass because, as has been pointed out, energy exchange takes place between body segments. Thus, a more extensive analysis that includes a segment by segment calculation should be done to assess mechanical efficiency accurately (92, 93).

Another application of mechanics to gait can be found in the use of **power.** Winter (92) has effectively used mechanical principles in analyzing the role of the ankle in providing propulsive energy. Figure 15.13 shows power, the product of moment and angular velocity, in the lowest trace. After the foot is flat, a large moment is generated as the leg rotates over the foot, but the product of dorsiflexion velocity and plantarflexion moment is small and negative (A1). Later, however, plantarflexion velocity is rapid and its moment large, resulting in power of 430 watts (A2). These facts, coupled with the position of the limb during the terminal phase of support, provide evidence that the plantarflexors are contributing to the potential (upward) and kinetic (forward) energy of the limbs and the upper part of the body.

Analyses of the **balance** phenomena associated with gait have also been undertaken. For example, consider a high total body moment of inertia and a COG that does not pass forward within the borders of the foot. The nervous system does not attempt to balance mediolaterally until after the foot is on the ground. Instead, the control of the posture appears to relate to the degree of lateral foot placement directly, a function decided during the previous swing phase (89). That subjects with balance disorders use this technique to assist with stabilization may confirm that such a mechanism is important for control of balance during a dynamic activity such as gait. More complex analyses of these control phenomena have been elaborated upon using the whole-body inverted pendulum method to show how interactions occur between the supporting foot and hip musculature (48).

An important clinical note can also be identified by this work. Negative work has been shown to exist throughout the gait cycle, the only exception being when the knee extends slightly during midstance. Because of these findings, the quadriceps may be functioning primarily via eccentric contractions. The therapeutic implications are that perhaps more consideration should be given to eccentric training for the

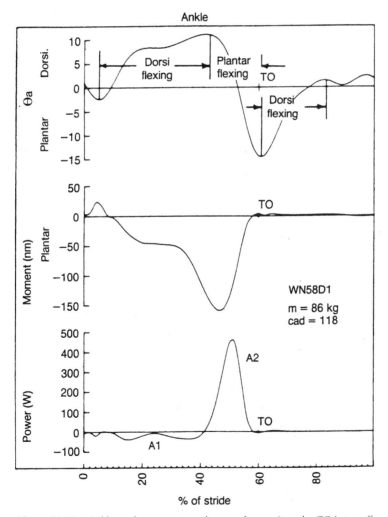

Figure 15.13.   Ankle angle, moment, and power for a gait cycle. *TO* is toe off.

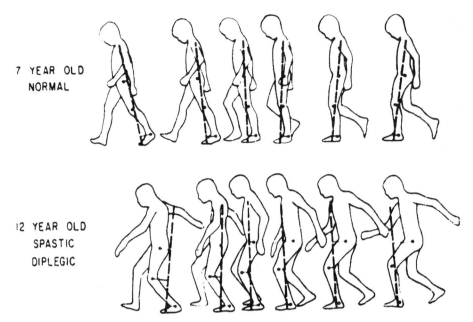

Figure 15.14. The result of the floor reaction force (*dashed line*) and the associated kinematics for two subjects.

quadriceps muscle. Conversely, because of the concentric role of the ankle plantarflexors, attention should be directed to concentric forms of exercise (92).

Pathokinesiology

Virtually any pathology affecting the lower limbs will affect walking. Thus, deviations will be manifested by persons with disorders of neural and musculoskeletal systems. The effects on the kinematics and kinetics can be slightly-to-severely modified, although the former is usually far easier to discern clinically. In a text of this nature all forms of deviation cannot be represented; the reader is instead referred to major volumes that deal with normal and pathological motion (17, 62, 75). This section will discuss representative changes in gait due to pathology.

Neurological Disorders

Central

One condition that has received considerable attention is **cerebral palsy**. Many reports are available in the literature as to the gait abnormalities produced by this condition. The exact perturbation is related to the nature of involvement. For example, the 25 patients evaluated by Bleck showed patterns of either hip flexion–internal rotation with flexed, hyperextended, or normal knees (7). Others reported on the crouch gait of four patients with spastic diplegia. Their kinematic and kinetic analysis showed the effects of exaggerated knee flexion and the requirement of increased dorsiflexion of the ankle. Extensive arm swinging and increased vertical trunk displacements were seen in all subjects. A representation of the patterns of normal and diplegic subjects is shown in Figure 15.14. Note the distinct differences in the line of application of the floor reaction force, such that efficiency of the cerebral palsied individual would be severely hampered. Also, the line of force application is markedly displaced from the centers of rotation of the hip and the knee, particularly early in the stance phase for the hip and late in stance for the knee. An abnormality of knee kinematics is shown in Figure 15.15. For the patients included in this analysis, knee torque was more than six times the value recorded for normals and never approached the normal extension moment occurring during part of the gait cycle (82).

Because of the pathology or the moment requirement, these patients would also produce abnormal EMG patterns. Both level and duration of the pattern of muscle activity are distorted. Frequently, EMG data are a primary focus of gait studies of those with cerebral palsy (23, 24, 60). The foot and ankle complex has drawn much attention, apparently because of the effect on the remainder of the limb and the potential for correction of the kinematics and kinetics of gait. Hoffer and Perry have been very active in pursuing this approach with the cerebral palsied patient, and identified abnormal muscular patterns associated with pes equinus, varus, valgus, and calcaneus. For example, equinus results from premature or prolonged activity of either the gastrocnemius or soleus. Varus can be caused by continuous activity of the anterior or posterior tibialis or phase reversal of the posterior tibialis to swing (31).

Using the information derived from EMG, success can be achieved with modifying the gait pattern by surgical transfer of the distal muscle attachment. The literature supports the use of these transfers, particularly in the ankle and foot, to improve both the temporal and distance factors associated with gait kinematics. For example, a transfer that has been effective for varus is the anterior transposition of the posterior tibialis muscle. However, a key element in the success of a muscle transfer is that

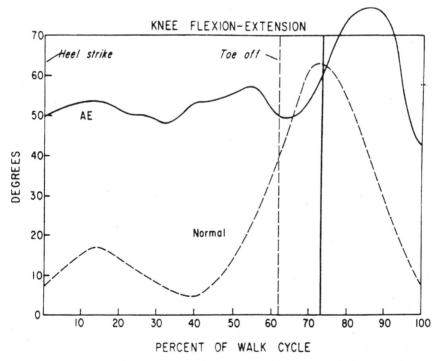

Figure 15.15.   Knee flexion for one normal subject and one subject with spastic diplegia (*AE*). Note that knee flexion of 50–60° is maintained throughout the pathological gait cycle.

the muscle should be active during the appropriate phase of the gait cycle. Otherwise, the muscle has to be retrained to function during a different temporal sequence, and, here, the transfer does not always meet with success (64).

Improved knowledge of the disrupted gait parameters has been and will continue to be of significant assistance in assessing the treatment outcomes for the patient with cerebral palsy. One example is in work on patients who have undergone selective sections of the dorsal root. In this instance at least some work has shown that preoperative to postoperative improvements were made in sagittal plane hip, knee, and ankle motion and that plantargrade foot position in stance occurred with a greater incidence (8). Another study has shown that more upright postures, decreased double stance time, and increased walking velocity results from the use of a posterior versus an anteriorly placed walker (26). As more efficient systems become available to the kinesiologists, investigators, and clinicians, even more improvements in the walking patterns of these patients can be anticipated (23).

Another common pathology that has pronounced effects on gait is **hemiplegia.** As for cerebral palsy, many studies have been made of the alterations in both the kinematics and kinetics of gait. As anticipated, because of the variability associated with the location and size of the lesion, the effects on gait cannot be easily categorized. One of the most thorough analyses, however, included kinematics and multiple channels of EMG for hemiparetic patients. In nine of the patients, the calf muscles were prematurely activated during stance. In another nine, the EMG was absent or extremely low for two or more of the muscles examined. Although in four others no common pattern could be identified, the remaining four showed co-activation of several or all of the muscles (43).

These results point out the difficulty with generalizing changes across patients. Instead, the most appropriate mechanism would be to learn which muscles were involved for each patient and attempt to alter the temporal sequencing and/or level of activation by some therapeutic means. An attempt to do so has been accomplished in that EMG was recorded during gait and used as a criterion measure for determining the appropriateness of muscle transfers in equinus or equinovarus deformities of hemiplegic patients. In their sample of 27 patients, preoperative activation patterns were usually abnormal in the gastrocnemius, soleus, tibialis posterior, flexor hallucis longus, flexor digitorum longus, peroneus brevis, and anterior tibialis. As might have been anticipated, the phase of activity was not altered after the surgery; thus, similar cautions as for cerebral palsied patients are important, i.e., alter only the muscles that are in phase with the desired movement (88).

Other work has evaluated the kinetic and temporal features associated with the gait pattern of the hemiplegic. Findings suggested that the support times of the two limbs was asymmetrical, with those of the affected limb being 10–15% shorter. As measured by the vertical component, floor reaction force patterns were distinctly different across patients. Finding that the magnitudes of the forces for the two legs were different is important because it represents a deviation from the normal pattern (15). Concerning temporal variables, Brandstater et al. have shown that hemiplegic gait is best characterized by the symmetry of single limb support times rather than by the values for each limb. The best indicators of motor recovery are the symmetry of swing phases and walking speed (11).

Further analyses have been applied to those with disturbed motor control, including the **parkinsonian gait.** In patients with Parkinson's disease, the mean velocity and stride length are markedly reduced, while mean cycle time is increased when compared with normals. Stride length is about one-half of that for normals, and velocity only .56 as opposed to 1.36 meters per second for normals. Double stance time is also significantly increased: 25% of the cycle as compared to only 11% for normals. These findings may be expected based on the perceived need for an adequate base of support. Decreased range of motion has also been noted, as may be seen with slower velocities of walking (42).

Peripheral

Injuries to or diseases of **isolated nerves** may also cause a variety of gait deviations. For example, patients with unilateral femoral neuropathies have been shown to have altered kinetics and kinematics: maintenance of full extension of the knee, increasing eccentric plantarflexor control of the tibia, and increasing concentric hip extensor control of the femur (47).

Musculoskeletal Disorders

Other conditions can also clearly and characteristically alter gait. The **gluteus medius gait** has been previously discussed in Chapter 10. Loss of the **gluteus maximus** produces a trunk lurch in a posterior direction during weight bearing. The necessity for such a lurch is due to the patient's insufficient hip extensor power used to control pelvic flexion moment created by trunk weight over the fixed lower limb. To influence mechanics, a patient throws the trunk posteriorly so that the line of gravity, during receipt of body weight by the supporting surface, falls posterior to the hip. As a result, the moment due to trunk weight produces pelvic extension and is controlled by the anterior capsule or flexor musculature of the hip joint.

Complete or partial **quadriceps paralysis** is rare and usually does not affect gait. This is because the knee can be maintained in complete extension or hyperextension during weight bearing, relying on tension in the posterior capsule of the knee. Concurrent loss of both **hip and knee extensors** is a different matter, however, because the line of gravity cannot simultaneously fall posterior to the hip and anterior to the knee. A frequent modification made by patients with combined losses is to press posteriorly on the thigh with the hand during the weight-bearing phase of the gait cycle.

One other important loss is the gait alteration required by paralysis of the **anterior compartment** of the lower leg. Because the only available dorsiflexors of the ankle reside here, paralysis in a patient will result in the inability to clear the foot from the ground during the swing phase. Complete paralysis can be devastating, but functional electrical stimulation or ankle foot orthoses are usually extremely helpful assists.

Orthopaedic and/or musculoskeletal dysfunction can also have a distinct effect in modifying the gait pattern of any given patient. Witness the effect of **pain** in any of the joints of the lower limb, noticing in particular the changes in kinematics as well as in stride parameters and temporal sequences (82). Compare, for example, the sagittal plane motion in Figure 15.16 with the normal pattern shown in Figure 15.8. Other comparisons are available from analyses performed on children with myopathies (Fig. 15.17). In these cases greater disability was associated with gait that was more characteristic of infantile patterns. Changes were also exhibited in muscle onset and magnitudes, particularly in the soleus and tibialis anterior (86).

Generally the severity of the kinematic, kinetic, and temporal sequences of events can be related to involvement of an **individual joint.** Such changes are typical of the patient with degenerative joint disease. Range of motion is usually limited in all

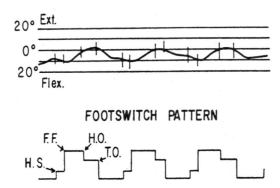

Figure 15.16. Sagittal plane electrogoniogram for a patient with hip pathology. Compared with Figure 15.8 the range of motion is extremely limited. Footswitch events are the same as those for Figure 15.8.

directions. One potentially important finding is that a study of patients with pathological knees revealed no correlation between passive motion available and how much motion was used during gait (29). Others have now published information that shows several atypical patterns in patients with disorders of the anterior cruciate ligament. In these instances there were both time shifts in the peak of major phases of activity and, in some cases, additional phases of activity were added (73).

Rate of loading will also be decreased among patients with limb pain during gait to avoid further discomfort. Assistive devices may also be advocated by both therapist and patient to decrease loading. Assessment of the deviation from the normal pattern will need to be determined individually, and therapeutic recommendations based on a patient's clinical circumstances.

Other clinical entities have been known to alter gait characteristics. Any lower limb **amputee** in the early stages of rehabilitation will display asymmetries and other modifications. Different problems will be associated with each amputation level. Generally, however, a patient must learn to control a new mass (body segment parameter) with appropriate forces (kinetics) in an appropriate temporal sequence to arrive at a pattern (kinematics) perceived to be correct. Walking velocity will also be a factor, as has been shown by Hoy et al. in a study of children with lower limb amputations (35). Although it is encouraging that normal EMG patterns are possible with the use of patellar tendon bearing prostheses, other forms have produced abnormal patterns, such as simultaneous contractions of antagonistic muscles (28).

Finally, **orthoses** can be extremely important in modifying gait characteristics. Those that use a posterior stop at the ankle can compensate for the inability to actively dorsiflex the ankle during swing phase. Mediolateral stability can also be provided by T straps attached to the medial or lateral upright. Other ankle foot orthoses (AFO) are made of plastics or laminates with material properties that can be used to control ankle dorsiflexion and mediolateral shifts in the foot. Furthermore, these materials are appropriate in mass because they provide little change in the total mass of the body segment to which they are applied. No matter the material or the application of the orthosis, the intention is to assist the patient with the control or exertion of appropriate moments during the gait cycle. Design, evaluation, and reevaluation of an orthosis should be based on this intention.

Many other deviations from normal gait will be encountered in the clinic. No matter the cause, the responsibility of the therapist is to find out which characteristics are altered. For example, is decreased stance time due to joint pain, a lack of range of motion, inability of the patient to generate an adequate torque for control of the desired position, or other factors? Finally, logical, scientifically based treatments can be carried out to modify the altered characteristics and return the patient to a more normal pattern. Sufficient attention to all of the factors involved, and their potential interaction, will be necessary to assure the best and most efficient results.

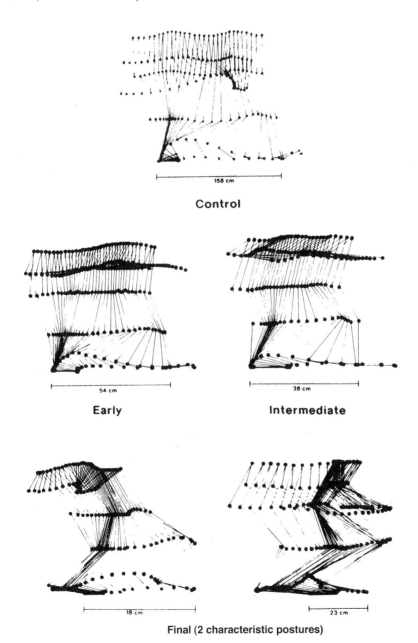

Figure 15.17.   Sagittal plane kinematics for one normal and four subjects with myopathies (hand markers missing for one patient). Forward progression is from left to right.

SUMMARY

This chapter has discussed kinesiological factors associated with posture and gait. Relevant mechanics have been applied while using principles presented earlier in this book. Selected pathologies and their effects on gait have been discussed, and implications for evaluation and treatment reviewed.

References

1. Andersson BJG, Ortengren R, Nachemson AL. The sitting posture: an electromyographic and discometric study. *Orthop Clin North Am.* 1975;6:105–120.
2. Bampton S. *A Guide to the Visual Examination of Pathological Gait.* Temple University Rehabilitation Research and Training Center #8. Philadelphia: Moss Rehabilitation Hospital; 1979.
3. Basmajian JV. *Muscles Alive: Their Functions Revealed by Electromyography.* 4th ed. Baltimore: Williams & Wilkins; 1979.
4. Baumann JU, Hanggi EL. A method of gait analysis for daily orthopaedic practice. *J Med Eng Technol.* 1977;1:86–91.
5. Bennett DL, Gillis DK, Portney LG, et al. Comparison of integrated electromyographic activity and lumbar curvature during standing and during sitting in three chairs. *Phys Ther.* 1989;69:902–913.
6. Bergmann G, Graichen F, Rohlmann A. Hip joint loading during walking and running, measured in two patients. *J Biomech.* 1993;26:969–990.
7. Bleck EE. Postural and gait abnormalities caused by hip-flexion deformity in spastic cerebral palsy. *J Bone Joint Surg.* 1971;53(A):1468–1488.
8. Boscarino LF, Õunpuu MS, Davis RB, et al. Effects of selective dorsal rhizotomy on gait in children with cerebral palsy. *J Ped Orthop.* 1993;13:174–179.
9. Brand RA, Crowninshield RD. The effect of cane use on hip contact force. *Clin Orthop.* 1980;147:181–184.
10. Brand RA, Crowninshield RD, Johnston RC, et al. Forces on the femoral head during activities of daily living. *Iowa Orthop J.* 1982;2:43–49.
11. Brandstater ME, de Bruin H, Gowland C, Clark BM. Hemiplegic gait: analysis of temporal variables. *Arch Phys Med Rehabil.* 1983;64:583–587.
12. Bresler B, Frankel JP. The forces and moments in the leg during level walking. *ASME Trans.* 1950;72:27–36.
13. Cappozzo A, Figura F, Marchetti M. The interplay of muscular and external forces in human ambulation. *J Biomech.* 1976;9:35–43.
14. Carlsöö S. *How Man Moves: Kinesiological Studies and Methods.* London, England: William Heinemann; 1972.
15. Carlsöö S, Dahllof A-G, Holm J. Kinetic analysis of the gait in patients with hemiparesis and in patients with intermittent claudication. *Scand J Rehabil Med.* 1974;6:166–179.
16. Cornwall MW, McPoil TG. Comparison of 2-dimensional and 3-dimensional rearfoot motion during walking. *Clin Biomech.* 1995;10:36–40.
17. Craik RL, Oatis CA. *Gait Analysis: Theory and Application.* St. Louis: CV Mosby; 1995.
18. Crowninshield RD, Johnston RC, Andrews RG, et al. A biomechanical investigation of the human hip. *J Biomech.* 1978;11:75–85.
19. DiFabio RP, Badke MB. Extraneous movement associated with hemiplegic postural sway during dynamic goal-directed weight redistribution. *Arch Phys Med Rehabil.* 1971;71:365–371.
20. Duncan PW, Studenski S, Chandler J, et al. Electromyographic analysis of postural adjustments in two methods of balance testing. *Phys Ther.* 1990;70:88–96.
21. Eberhart H, Inman V, Bresler B. The principal elements in human locomotion. In: Klopsteg P, Wilson PD, et al., eds. *Human Limbs and Their Substitutes.* New York: McGraw-Hill; 1974 (reprinted with bibliography. New York: Hafner Publishing; 1968).
22. Frank JS, Earl M. Coordination of posture and movement. *Phys Ther.* 1990;70:855–863.
23. Gage JR. Gait analysis for decision-making in cerebral palsy. *Bull Hosp Jt Dis Orthop Inst.* 1983;43:147–163.
24. Gage JR. Gait analysis: an essential tool in the treatment of cerebral palsy. *Clin Orthop.* 1993;288:126–134.
25. Grabiner MD, Lundin TM, Feuerbach JW. Converting Chattecx balance system vertical reaction force measurements to center of pressure excursion measurements. *Phys Ther.* 1993;73:316–319.

26. Greiner BM, Czerniecki JM, Deitz JC. Gait parameters of children with spastic diplegia: a comparison of effects of posterior and anterior walkers. *Arch Phys Med Rehabil.* 1993;74:381–385.

27. Grieve GP. The sacroiliac joint. *Physiotherapy.* 1976;62:384–400.

28. Grevsten S, Stalberg E. Electromyographic study of muscular activity in the amputation stump while walking with PTB- and PTB-suction prosthesis. *Upsala J Med Sci.* 1975;80:103–112.

29. Gyory AN, Chao EYS, Stauffer RN. Functional evaluation of normal and pathologic knees during gait. *Arch Phys Med Rehabil.* 1976;57:571–577.

30. Heitmann DK, Gossman MR, Shaddeau SA, et al. Balance performance and step width in noninstitutionalized, elderly, female fallers and nonfallers. *Phys Ther.* 1989;69:923–931.

31. Hoffer MM, Perry J. Pathodynamics of gait alterations in cerebral palsy and the significance of kinetic electromyography in evaluating foot and ankle problems. *Foot Ankle.* 1983;4:128–134.

32. Holzreiter SH, Köhle ME. Assessment of gait patterns using neural networks. *J Biomech.* 1993;26:645–651.

33. Horak FB. Clinical measurement of postural control in adults. *Phys Ther.* 1987;67:1881–1885.

34. Horak FB, Shupert CL, Mirka A. Components of postural dyscontrol in the elderly: a review. *Neurobiol Aging.* 1989;10:727–738.

35. Hoy MG, Whiting WC, Zernicke RF. Stride kinematics and knee joint kinetics of child amputee gait. *Arch Phys Med Rehabil.* 1982;63:74–82.

36. Johaansson R, Magnusson M. Human postural dynamics. *Crit Rev Biomed Eng.* 1991;18:413–437.

37. Joseph J, McColl I. Electromyography of muscles of posture: posterior vertebral muscles in males. *J Physiol.* 1961;157:33–37.

38. Judge JO, Lindsey C, Underwood M, et al. Balance improvements in older women: effects of exercise training. *Phys Ther.* 73:254–265.

39. Keegan JJ. Alterations to the lumbar curve related to posture and seating. *J Bone Joint Surg.* 1953;35(A):567–589.

40. King MB, Judge JO, Wolfson L. Functional base of support decreases with age. *J Gerontol.* 1994;49:M258–M263.

41. Knutson LM, Soderberg GL. EMG: use and interpretation in gait. In: Craik RL, Oatis CA, eds. *Gait Analysis: Theory and Applications.* St. Louis: CV Mosby; 1995.

42. Knutsson E. An analysis of parkinsonian gait. *Brain.* 1972;95:475–486.

43. Knutsson E, Richards C. Different types of disturbed motor control in gait of hemiparetic patients. *Brain.* 1979;102:405–430.

44. Lafortune MA, Cavanagh PR, Sommer HJ, et al. Foot inversion-eversion and knee kinematics during walking. *J Orthop Res.* 1994;12:412–420.

45. Lehmkuhl LD, Smith LK. *Brunnstrom's Clinical Kinesiology.* 5th ed. Philadelphia: FA Davis; 1996.

46. Link CS, Nicholson GG, Shaddeau SA, et al. Lumbar curvature in standing and sitting in two types of chairs: relationship of hamstring and hip flexor muscle length. *Phys Ther.* 1990;70:611–618.

47. Lohmann Siefel K, Stanhope SJ, Caldwell GE. Kinematic and kinetic adaptations in the lower limb during stance in gait of unilateral femoral neuropathy patients. *Clin Biomech.* 1993;8:147–155.

48. MacKinnon CD, Winter DA. Control of whole body balance in the frontal plane during human walking. *J Biomech.* 1993;26:633–644.

49. Magora A. Investigation of the relation between low back pain and occupation. 3. Physical requirements: sitting, standing and weight lifting. *Industr Med Surg.* 1972;41:5–9.

50. Mann RA, Hagy JL, White V, et al. The initiation of gait. *J Bone Joint Surg.* 1979;61(A):232–239.

51. Morrison JB. The mechanics of muscle function in locomotion. *J Biomech.* 1970;3:431–451.

52. Murray MP. Gait as a total pattern of movement. *Am J Phys Med.* 1967;46:290–333.

53. Murray MP, Kory RC, Clarkson BH, et al. A comparison of free and fast speed walking patterns of normal men. *Am J Phys Med.* 1966;45:8–24.

54. Nachemson AL. Lumbar intradiscal pressure. In: Jayson MIV, ed. *The Lumbar Spine and Back Pain.* Kent, England: Pitman; 1980.

55. Norkin CC, Levangie PK. *Joint Structure and Function: A Comprehensive Analysis.* Philadelphia: FA Davis; 1992.

56. Oddsson LIE. Control of voluntary trunk movements in man. *Acta Physiol Scand.* 1990;140;11–60.

57. Okada M. An electromyographic estimation of the relative muscular load in different human postures. *J Hum Ergol.* 1972;1:75–93.

58. Ōunpuu S, DeLuca PA, Davis RB, et al. The application of joint kinetics in clinical gait analysis. Presented at the annual meeting of the American Academy of Cerebral Palsy and Developmental Medicine. Nashville, TN; 1993.

59. Pai Y-C, Rogers MW, Hedman LD, et al. Alterations in weight-transfer capabilities in adults with hemiparesis. *Phys Ther.* 1994;74:647–659.
60. Perry J. Determinants of muscle function in the spastic lower extremity. *Clin Orthop.* 1993;288:10–26.
61. Perry J. The mechanics of walking: a clinical interpretation. *Phys Ther.* 1964;47:778–801.
62. Perry J. *Gait Analysis: Normal and Pathological Function.* Thorofare, NJ: Slack; 1992.
63. Perry J, Antonelli MS, Ford W. Analysis of knee joint forces during flexed-knee stance. *J Bone Joint Surg.* 1975;57(A):961–967.
64. Perry J, Hoffer MM. Preoperative and postoperative dynamic electromyography as an aid in planning tendon transfers in children with cerebral palsy. *J Bone Joint Surg.* 1977;59(A):531–537.
65. Portnoy H, Morin F. Electromyographic study of postural muscles in various positions and movements. *Am J Physiol.* 1956;186:122–126.
66. Rasch PJ, Burke RK. *Kinesiology and Applied Anatomy: The Science of Human Movement.* 6th ed. Philadelphia: Lea & Febiger; 1978.
67. Rogers MW, Hedman LD, Pai Y-C. Kinetic analysis of dynamic transitions in stance support accompanying voluntary leg flexion movements in hemiparetic adults. *Arch Phys Med Rehabil.* 1993; 74:19–25.
68. Root ML, Orien WP, Weed JH. *Normal and Abnormal Function of the Foot.* Los Angeles: Clinical Biomechanics Corp.; 1977.
69. Rubino FA. Gait disorders in the elderly—distinguishing between normal and dysfunctional gaits. *Postgrad Med.* 1993;93:185–190.
70. Rydell N. Biomechanics of the hip joint. *Clin Orthop.* 1973;92:6–15.
71. Schlegel KF. Sitzschaden und deren Vermeidung durch eine neuartig Sitzkonstruction. *Medizinische Klinik.* 1956;51:1940–1942.
72. Seireg A, Arvikar RJ. The prediction of muscular load sharing and joint forces in the lower extremities during walking. *J Biomech.* 1975;8:89–102.
73. Shiavi R, Zhang L-Q, Limbird T, et al. Pattern analysis of electromyographic linear envelopes exhibited by subjects with uninjured and injured knees during free and fast speed walking. *J Orthop Res.* 1992;10:226–236.
74. Simon SR, Mann RA, Hagy JL, et al. Role of the posterior calf muscles in normal gait. *J Bone Joint Surg.* 1978;60(A):465–472.
75. Smidt GL. *Gait in Rehabilitation.* New York: Churchill Livingstone; 1990.
76. Smidt GL. Hip motion and related factors in walking. *Phys Ther.* 1971;51:9–21.
77. Smith JW. The act of standing. *Acta Orthop Scand.* 1953;23:159–168.
78. Soderberg GL, Blanco MK, Cosentino TL, et al. An EMG analysis of posterior trunk musculature during flat and anteriorly inclined sitting. *Human Factors.* 1986;28:483–491.
79. Soderberg GL, Venhuizen JK, Reeves DK, et al. An EMG analysis of the erector spinae muscles during sitting with three lumbar support conditions. Iowa City, IA: University of Iowa; 1984. Unpublished data.
80. Stuberg WA, Colerick VL, Blanke DJ, et al. Comparison of a clinical gait analysis method using videography and temporal-distance measures with 16-mm cinematography. *Phys Ther.* 1988;68: 1221–1225.
81. Sutherland DH, Cooper L, Daniel D. The role of the ankle plantar flexors in normal walking. *J Bone Joint Surg.* 1980;62(A):354–363.
82. Sutherland DH, Cooper L. The pathomechanics of progressive crouch gait in spastic diplegia. *Orthop Clin North Am.* 1978;9:143–154.
83. Sutherland DH, Olshen R, Cooper L, et al. The development of mature gait. *J Bone Joint Surg.* 1980;62(A):336–353.
84. Svensson HO, Andersson GBJ. Low back pain in 40–47 year old men: work history and work environment factors. *Spine.* 1983;8:272–276.
85. Teasdale N, Stelmach GE, Breunig A. Postural sway characteristics of the elderly under normal and altered visual and support surface conditions. *J Gerontol.* 1991;46:B238–B244.
86. Trias D, Gioux M, Cid M, et al. Gait analysis of myopathic children in relation to impairment level and energy cost. *J Electromyogr Kinesiol.* 1994;4:67–81.
87. Wadsworth JB, Smidt GL, Johnston RC. Gait characteristics of subjects with hip disease. *Phys Ther.* 1972;52:829–837.
88. Waters RL, Frazier J, Garland DE, et al. Electro-myographic gait analysis before and after operative treatment for hemiplegic equinus and equinovarus deformity. *J Bone Joint Surg.* 1982;64(A):284–288.
89. Winter DA. *A. B. C. (Anatomy, Biomechanics and Control) of Balance during Standing and Walking.* Waterloo: Waterloo Biomechanics; 1995.

90. Winter DA. *Biomechanics of Human Movement*. New York: John Wiley & Sons; 1979.
91. Winter DA. The locomotion laboratory as a clinical assessment system. *Med Progr Technol.* 1976;4:95–106.
92. Winter DA. Energy generation and absorption at the ankle and knee during fast, natural, and slow cadences. *Clin Orthop.* 1983;175:147–154.
93. Winter DA, Quanbury AO, Reimer GD. Analysis of instantaneous energy of normal gait. *J Biomech.* 1976;9:253–257.
94. Woollacott MH. Age-related changes in posture and movement. *J Gerontol.* 1993;48:56–60.
95. Woollacott MH, Shumway-Cook A. Changes in posture control across the life span—a systems approach. *Phys Ther.* 1990;70:799–807.
96. Woollacott MH, Shumway-Cook A. *Development of Posture and Gait Across the Life Span*. Columbia: University of South Carolina Press; 1990.
97. Wolfson L, Whipple R, Derby CA, et al. Gender differences in the balance of health elderly as demonstrated by dynamic posturography. *J Gerontol.* 1994;49:M160–M167.
98. Zarrugh MY, Radcliffe CW. Computer generation of human gait kinematics. *J Biomech.* 1979;12:99–111.

16

Ergonomics

Some individuals, industries, and countries have long been interested in the effect of the work environment on the individual. Now, agencies such as the National Institute for Occupational Safety and Health (NIOSH) are playing a more active role; ergonomics has begun to receive considerable emphasis. Furthermore, unions and workers have become more aware of the work environment, demanding greater attention to the effects of the workplace on the employees. Physical therapists, as well as industrial psychologists, occupational therapists, occupational mechanists, occupational physicians, and athletic trainers, are becoming increasingly valuable to industry in providing these services. According to Meister the need for human factors should increase in the future (62).

The workplace is important because of the great amount of time spent there. The greatest implications are probably for those persons who are required to handle objects or materials, particularly if lifting is performed. Specific implications exist for therapists in that the focus of treatment should take into account the patient's intention to return to work. In fact, the clinical education of Danish physical therapists has included a training period studying postures and work methods in a factory environment (11). In addition, rehabilitation will probably be considered successful only if work can be adequately performed. This chapter does not intend to discuss all aspects of ergonomics. Instead, selected aspects that have implication for the therapist are presented.

DEFINITIONS AND SCOPE

A certain terminology is associated with the performance of human work. Ergonomics, a term which originated more than 120 years ago, means the laws of work (24). More broadly interpreted as the study of work, this area includes the application of knowledge of the life sciences to well-being and work performance (83). To apply ergonomics, we must take into account the variability associated with human form and function. Some factors to include are height, weight, skills, strength, and age. These factors need to be related to work requirements such as sitting height, arm reach, mass of an object to be moved, visual field, and similar considerations. Thus, the focus of ergonomics is on the interaction of work and people, i.e., physiological and environmental stresses, and such things as complex psychomotor tasks. The primary intent is to establish ways to reduce injuries, accidents, and fatigue and to improve work performance (24).

Human factors and ergonomics are terms often used interchangeably. Both describe the interaction between the operator and the job demands; both attempt to reduce the stress in the workplace. Human factors, however, have sometimes focused more on the human-machine interface. Frequently called human engineering, the primary goal is to reduce human error. For practical purposes, these terms are synonymous.

Others have chosen to use different terminology. For example, we can define the

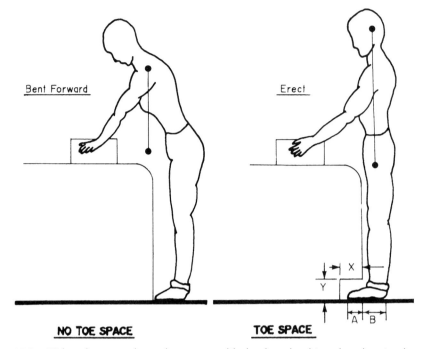

Figure 16.1.   With no foot space the worker must stand farther from the object, thus changing the center of gravity and creating an extension moment in the lumbar spine.

discipline of occupational biomechanics as "the study of the physical interaction of workers with their tools, machines and materials so as to enhance the worker's performance while minimizing the risk of future musculoskeletal disorders." As a part of the general field of biomechanics, this specialized area requires the application of the laws of physics and engineering to the human body when in the work environment. Thus, ergonomics or human factors tend to be a much broader area than occupational biomechanics, yet they are highly complimentary (16). Evidence of this fact is that an entire text is devoted to this topic (81).

WORKSPACE AND ENVIRONMENT

Many approaches are possible when applying design to the workspace. General considerations will be presented here, followed by more specific guidelines.

Usually, **body segment parameters** serve as the basis for defining the needs of the workspace. Therefore, segment length, weight, location of the mass center, moment of inertia, and radius of gyration are of interest. We have discussed these properties and the sources for data about the body segments in Chapter 1. Some have illustrated the effect of a simple modification such as toe space on the control of the center of mass and results this modification has on the lumbar spine (Fig. 16.1) (71). Although few data are available, enough material exists for use in analyses using models of the human body and in estimating the requirements of the workspace.

The **design** of the workspace must take into account many factors. Design should not be based on the average but instead for one extreme or another. Ideally the workspace should adjust to accommodate differences in body height and individual segment length. Most frequent examples are accommodations for short and long legs and allowances necessary for gripping of instruments or tools by individuals with markedly different hand sizes. Reaching should all be ahead of the shoulder and work height should be modified so that the viewing angle is directed slightly downward. Webb suggests that to assess any workspace, determine what the task involves, measure the reach and height conditions, and compare these measurements to existing standards (9, 83). Figure 16.2 displays a sample of the guidelines.

No matter the workplace or workspace the **working height** is important. This is true for both sitting and standing work postures. Concern should be on the position of the head and neck, the lumbar spine, and the shoulder (39). Each of these segments will be considered in the following paragraphs.

For either the standing or the seated work posture the best height for performance of work with the hands is a few centimeters below elbow level. Grandjean is rather specific about the dimensions, stating 5–10 centimeters for standing and a few centimeters for sitting. If possible, work stations that can satisfy individual needs are most desirable. Examples are adjustable chairs and the provision of various sizes of stools or boxes to elevate the standing worker so that the shorter person can reach the working surface (34).

Alterations also need to be made, depending on the task. A typewriter, for example, should be used with the work surface about 10% lower than that used for writing (34). Another modification of the workspace that should be considered is the **inclination** of the work surface towards the subject. This has been purported for centuries but has fallen out of favor in the last several decades (9). For standard postures such as in a school and office, inclinations of 10–30° are recommended. This modification has positive effects on the lumbar spine, brings the line of vision into a better position, and eases tension in the supporting musculature of the cervical spine (60). In support

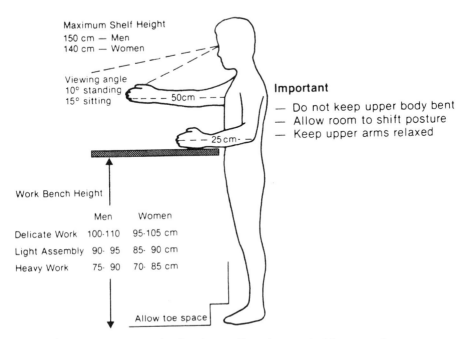

Figure 16.2.   An example of workspace dimensions required for men and women.

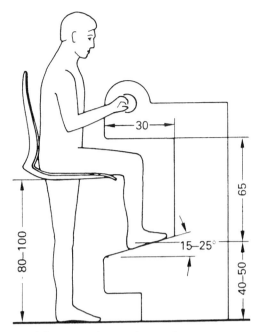

Figure 16.3.   Suggested dimensions for a workspace that allows either sitting or standing.

of this concept Eastman and Kamon also found less fatigue and discomfort when they slanted the surface at angles of 12 and 24°, the latter producing the greatest effect (23). Angles of up to 75° are considered advisable for activities such as technical drawing (34). One other advisable alternative is a workspace that allows either sitting or standing. Such an arrangement is shown in Figure 16.3. Table 16.1 shows 10 principles helpful in designing a workplace that allows varied posture without compromising work efficiency.

Table 16.1.   Ten Considerations in the Design of a Workplace, Listed in Order of Precedence

1. The worker should be able to maintain an upright and forward facing posture during work.
2. Where vision is a requirement of the task, the necessary work points must be adequately visible with the head and trunk upright or with just the head inclined slightly forward.
3. All work activities should permit the worker to adopt several different, but equally healthy and safe, postures without reducing capability to do the work.
4. Work should be arranged so that it may be done, at the worker's choice, in either a seated or standing position. When seated, the worker should be carried equally on both feet, and foot pedals designed accordingly.
5. The weight of the body, when standing, should be carried equally on both feet, and foot pedals designed accordingly.
6. Work activities should be performed with the joints at about the mid-point of their range of movement. This applies particularly to the head, trunk, and upper limbs.
7. Where muscular force has to be exerted it should be by the largest appropriate muscle groups available and in a direction co-linear with the limbs concerned.
8. Work should not be performed consistently at or above the level of the heart; even the occasional performance where force is exerted above heart level should be avoided. Where light hand work must be performed above heart level, rests for the upper arms are a requirement.
9. Where a force has to be exerted repeatedly, it should be possible to exert it with either of the arms, or either of the legs, without adjustment to the equipment.
10. Rest pauses should allow for all loads experienced at work, including environmental and informational loads, and the length of the work period between successive rest periods.

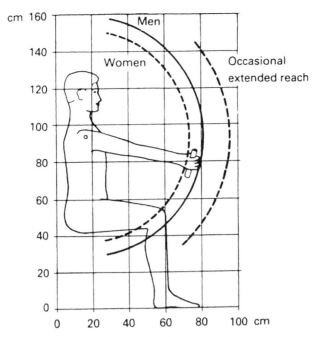

Figure 16.4. Suggested arc for vertical grasp. This figure includes the extreme percentiles and, therefore, the data pertain to even small men and women.

Considerations in design and use of workspace should also take into account the **reach** requirements. Usually, work should be done within a distance of 25 cm of the body. Occasional work is acceptable up to a distance of 50 cm. More comprehensive information is provided if an arc of movement is described that will indicate the positions in which grasp can be capably performed, as shown in Figure 16.4. Note that the average reach is about 7 cm greater for men than for women. As indicated earlier, extension of the shoulders should be avoided, although allowing occasional reaching beyond the normal arc of movement is satisfactory. Other more specific information on height of reach and operating space for the legs is available in the text of Grandjean (34).

In any workspace other factors such as **lighting, noise,** and **air quality** must be appropriate. Because they have little impact on considerations for the therapist, we will not discuss them in this volume. The other issues discussed in this section are, however, well within the purview of the therapist. Yet, they are frequently not considered in either the plan of patient management or the treatment. Effective discharge planning should include inquiries as to the work environment and, as necessary, recommendations should be developed and forwarded to the person or agency responsible. If workspace is inappropriately designed the positive effects garnered from therapy may be reversed in a very short time.

POSTURES AND SEATING
Work Position

The most common positions for work are standing and sitting. Many jobs require, however, some degree of movement, either of a periodic or repetitive nature. **Standing** postures that require movement should follow the guidelines in the previous section

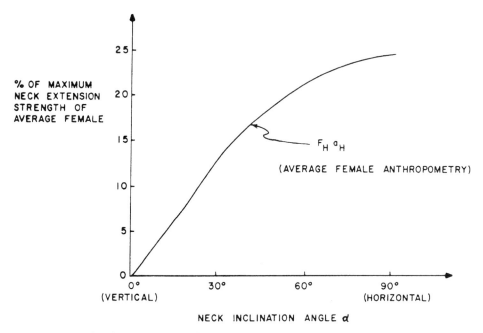

Figure 16.5.   Predicted proportion of neck muscle strength to support the head of an average female at varied inclination angles.

and in the materials handling section later in this chapter. When standing is more static, fatigue can be a potential problem, particularly in the lower extremity. Allowing for movement but avoiding stressful situations for body parts is a common recommendation. Other suggestions are to provide armrests and/or provide for sitting, at least occasionally. Efficiency will be increased and awkward or fatiguing postures will be avoided if properly designed tools are used.

Specific joints are especially susceptible to injury because of work postures. The most commonly affected are the cervical and lumbar spines and the shoulder. The cervical spine is often subjected to poor positioning because of improper workspace design. The location of the work surface is most commonly too low, requiring a flexion moment of the head and cervical spine. Seat height and distance from the work surface are also influencing factors, as is a table that is too low.

Chaffin and Andersson have determined the effect of the angle of forward inclination on the force required in the neck extensors. Considering this force in relation to the neck extension "strength" they have determined that for 30° of flexion the muscle force is at 50% of that necessary to hold the neck at an inclination of 90° (Figure 16.5) (16). The tension required to support the head and neck at any inclination thus may be a major factor in subjective reports of discomfort. Surely, therapists frequently encounter these problems when evaluating and treating musculoskeletal disorders.

The low back is probably the area of the body most frequently subjected to disorders, many of which arise from improper work positions or job requirements. Any posture requiring the maintenance of a trunk flexion moment should be modified. Elevating the work height can usually accomplish this. However, most men and women should be capable of tolerating, without adverse effects, forward flexion of the trunk to 20° (16). Further flexion to 30° increases the moment markedly, in turn increasing the tension requirement and affecting the potential endurance time. Thus, the time workers can hold the posture is dramatically decreased from about 13 minutes at 25% of their exertion level to less than 4 minutes at approximately 35% of their exertion level (46).

Another area subjected to musculoskeletal dysfunction is the shoulder. Degenerative tendinitis in biceps brachii and supraspinatus muscles has been reported in subjects in which arm elevation is required (41). Acute tendinitis is also a possibility. Neck and shoulder pain is frequently reported in jobs that require extended hours working at a desk or computer work station. Kamwendo et al. studied 420 secretaries and found that working with office machines for greater than five hours per day significantly increased their incidence of neck and shoulder pain. Poor psychosocial conditions also indicated a greater occurrence of neck and shoulder pain (47). Furthermore, fatigue has been shown to be significant when elevated arm work is required. For example, at 30° of abduction more than an hour of work can be performed without significant fatigue. At 90° only about 10 minutes is tolerable before the onset of severe pain (15). An additional factor is the reach requirement of the task. The greater the mass to be manipulated and the greater the frequency of the task the more difficulty the shoulder is likely to encounter. One mechanism to counteract potentially harmful effects is to allow support at the elbow, reducing the moment requirement at the shoulder. This procedure usually drastically limits the mobility of the total arm, making this a potentially unacceptable alternative. The specific task may necessitate other adjustments in the work posture. For example, it may require rotation of the forearm. Here elbow flexion may be used to facilitate the ability of the subject to exert a rotational moment. Another example of a modification may be during push-pull operations, when trunk fixation may be helpful.

Seating

Assumption of a **seated** posture has been thought to be desirable in the work situation because of the ability of this posture to reduce fatigue and improve efficiency. Surely the physiological demands are less when compared to standing. Thus the question arose as to the best sitting posture to assume while performing work. Several advantages, besides energy considerations, have been attached to the sitting posture. First, load bearing is removed from the joints of the lower limb. Simultaneously, greater stability is provided, particularly while performing tasks requiring greater degrees of visual and motor control. Furthermore, fewer demands are made on the vascular system because the lower limbs are placed in a more favorable position (16). Conversely, prolonged slackening of the abdominal musculature and the purported ill effect of flexion of the lumbar spine, affecting digestion and breathing, could be considered disadvantages (34).

In comparison with standing, the other most frequent posture assumed, the primary impact may be on the changes in the lumbar spine. Sitting with the back unsupported causes kyphosis of the lumbar spine, placing stress on the posterior structures of the back (63). Evidence exists that changes do occur in the kinematics of the lumbar spine. In one study the lumbar lordosis decreased by an average of 38°. Although some changes did occur intervertebrally, the majority were due to a posterior rotation of the pelvis (3). As a result, several techniques have been used to alter the spine configuration so that lordosis is maintained during sitting. One of these is the addition of a lumbar support, which tilts the pelvis anteriorly and the trunk posteriorly (59).

Thus, the lumbar spine moves from a position of lesser lordosis toward one of greater lordosis. The lumbar spine curve resembled the standing curve when a support of four centimeters thickness was added between the spine and the supporting surface (3).

Keegan also evaluated changes in the lumbar curve in relationship to sitting postures. Using radiographs, he could establish the interactions of the thigh and pelvic segments and study the effects on the lumbar spine. Of some interest was that the normal curve of the lumbar spine is at thigh-trunk and knee angles of 135° (48). Others have also recommended tilting the whole seat forwards (9, 13). Developing a unique solution, Kroemer suggested that the posterior most portion of the seat be wedged up by 30°, tilting the pelvis forwards and allowing maintenance of lumbar lordosis (53). Further research has reinforced these concepts, showing that the sitting posture in which reading and writing is done causes 4.8 cm of "extension of the back muscles." Tilting the chair surface 15° anteriorly and inclining the work surface diminishes this extension to only .7 cm (60). However, many subjects have found comfort, entry, and egress from a particular chair brand less than optimal (21). In yet another study evaluating the posture of the trunk when subjects sat on forward inclining seats, changes in landmarks were evaluated at inclinations of 5, 10, and 15°. With increased seat angles the lumbar spine moved toward more lordosis, one-third of the change occurring in the spine and two-thirds in the hip joints. However, the posture of the cervical spine appeared unaffected by the changes in seat angles and no systematic changes in the back occurred over the one-hour test interval (10). Brunswic analyzed the impact of seat design during unsupported sitting. In essence, a linear relationship between the percentage of lumbar flexion and the angles of the hip and knees was established (13).

Two results from the changes in the kinematics of the lumbar spine deserve comment. The first is the effect of sitting postures on interdiscal pressure. We have discussed these pressures to some degree in Chapter 13. Among the most interesting work is that of Andersson et al. Figure 16.6 shows a graphic depiction of their results. Note that all of the sitting posture pressures exceed those recorded during standing. The results are most probably due to an increase in the trunk moment as the pelvis is rotated posteriorly and the lumbar spine and trunk are rotated forward, and by deformation in the disc due to the decrease in lordosis. Although not shown in the figure, the use of a backrest can markedly decrease pressures, particularly if the backrest is posteriorly inclined 10° or more from the vertical (5). The use of armrests and, as mentioned earlier, lumbar support cushions also decrease interdiscal pressures (4).

The other primary effect of the change in spine kinematics induced by sitting is manifested in changes in the EMG activity of the erector spinae musculature. EMG studies have evaluated specific segments of the musculature or evaluated EMG activity when subjects were performing in the work environment (27, 58). It was shown that extensor activity continued to increase up to the maximum test time of one-half hour. The study also established that with angular changes of the knee the activity stopped if the foot was flat on the floor (58). In general, however, muscle activity, as measured by EMG, is similar when standing is compared to sitting. Compared with activity produced by maximal isometric contraction the levels are between 2 and 10%. Although relatively low, the long durations of activity required to maintain postures show that the levels are somewhat important when considering efficiency and energy. Any method that will decrease the flexion moment will de-

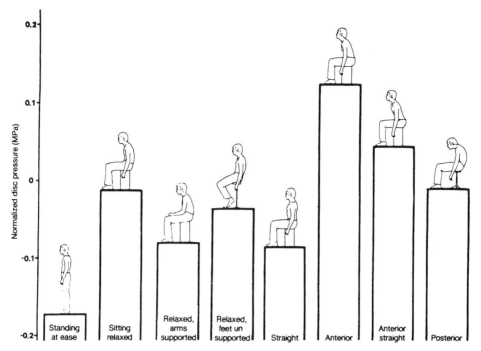

Figure 16.6. Mean values for normalized interdiscal pressure for various postures.

crease the need for active muscle tension. Included would be "slumping," so that passive posterior elements or the discs would assume a supportive role. Anterior arm support or backrests would be two other means of minimizing the flexion moment.

Researchers have derived most EMG data during studies of the influence of a lumbar support and/or degree of backrest inclination. Knutsson et al. analyzed the mechanics and collected intramuscular EMG data from the T12–L1 erector spinae. In asymptomatic subjects 20–46 years old a backrest angle at 110° with the seat was found to give lower EMG than backrests at either 90 or 100° (52). Overall, the optimal parameters for sitting posture in a car driver's seat, using EMG criteria, are achieved when the backrest inclination, the lumbar support, and the seat inclination are all as large as possible (5).

Based on the mechanics explained earlier, sitting on an anteriorly inclined surface should reduce activity levels in the erector spinae. Such was the result of work done by Soderberg and coworkers in evaluating level and 10 and 20° of inclination of the sitting surface. We show a summary of the results in Figure 16.7 (77).

Other considerations applied to the sitting posture are related to the upper and lower limbs. We have already discussed the height of the work surface relative to implications for the shoulders, head, and neck. Height of the chair is also important because too low a chair places inordinate loads on the ischial tuberosities. Too high a chair does not equitably distribute load under the thigh, potentially causing discomfort in the posterior thigh. Seat area is also a factor, suggesting that movement should be allowed to relieve pressure. Figure 16.8 shows suggested dimensions. More detailed figures for specific work circumstances can be found elsewhere (16, 34, 83).

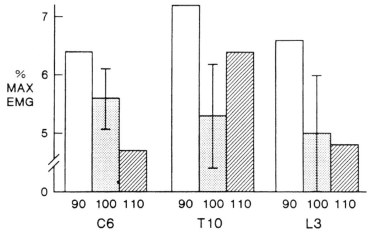

Figure 16.7. Percentage of maximum EMG produced at each of three levels of erector spinae for three different positions of anterior seat angulation. Note the decrease in level of activity as the angulation increased, except for T10 at 110°. Standard error, pooled for all positions, is given in 100° bar.

MATERIALS HANDLING

Most jobs require the direct handling of materials or the manipulation of objects. Approximately one-third of all industrial jobs in the United States involve some form of manual materials handling, usually **lifting, holding, carrying,** or **pushing.** These tasks result in 20–25% of all compensable industrial injuries and illnesses (7, 29). Thus, there are implications for the therapist, particularly in the management of the low back dysfunction patient. This section of the chapter will discuss the most important considerations associated with the manual handling of materials and focus on the implications for the patient with real or potential lumbar spine pathology or dysfunction.

Object

Although guidelines for objects to be handled exist, we often encounter circumstances when compliance has been ignored. Witness, for example, someone lifting an 80-pound (356 N) bag of water softener salt from a pallet lying on the ground, into and out of a car trunk, and then transported to the softener. The weight exceeds the "acceptable lifting conditions" discussed in section "Implications for the Lumbar Spine" later in this chapter. Neither are there any handles nor handholds, as are recommended. Drury et al. studied the effect of nonsagittal plane movements on the lumbar spine. The objects lifted had handles placed laterally and near the top. The results were similar to earlier studies analyzing sagittal plane tasks except that the handles proved more effective than anticipated, reinforcing the need to provide handles on objects whenever possible (20). Unbalanced and loose contents are a condition that should always be avoided. The weight should be clearly marked and the load should be a size that can be carried close to the body. The latter does not offset the need for the former. Whenever any object is to be handled make sure that an accurate assessment of the object's characteristics has been performed. Particularly dangerous are those objects that are likely to produce a sudden change in the body's torque generating requirements, such as object movement or failure of the container holding the object (83). Many occupations require interaction with various sizes, weights, and shapes of objects. One such example is a supermarket checker. In a unique study, Harber et al. videotaped 50 checkers while they checked eight products representative of the most frequently purchased supermarket goods. The researchers then ranked certain object characteristics in order of risk for injury to the checker. Possible modifications to the task and environment that would decrease risk to injury became apparent during the study: very specific education considering objects of greatest risk, a change in the placement of UPC symbols by the manufacturer, selection of products by the grocer regarding worker health, and improved positioning of the worker in the work station (38).

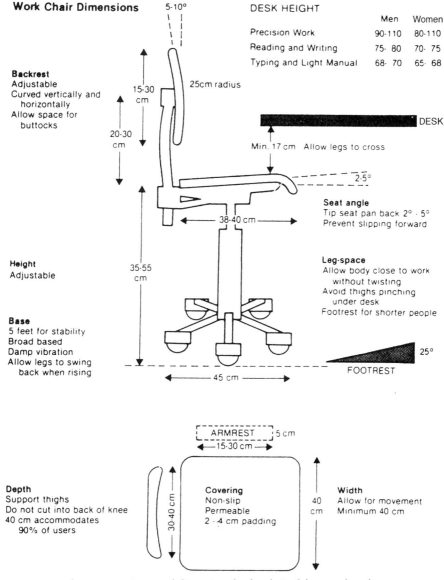

Figure 16.8. Suggested dimensions for the chair of the seated worker.

Task and Environment

Other requirements exist for the task and the environment. Specifically, all **repetitive lifting** should be kept between the height of the knuckle and the shoulder of the standing subject. Adjustable platforms may be the easiest way to ensure that condition. Limitations imposed on rate should depend on the load handled and other factors. Carrying should be minimized, as should upper body movement. As we are aware, the need for accuracy will probably increase muscular effort and perhaps be a significant precursor to the early onset of fatigue. A comprehensive review of ergonomic literature has yielded a preliminary set of guidelines for the analysis of repetition, force, and posture at various joints in the body. Although complete, a significant limitation of the review is that the data are obtained from a wide variety of industries and studies, thus making it difficult to apply the values to unique industrial settings. However, the review is complete and quite valuable because it brings together some "ball park" figures for comparison. It also provides a basis for future studies to develop more universal guidelines (30).

Environmental factors such as avoidance of constricting spaces and inadequate space for foot location are also important. The surface should also be uniform throughout the work area. A sticky or slippery surface, especially if only periodically encountered, is a significant hazard. An adequate visual field is also critical: say a worker is carrying a large object anteriorly. The size of the object may block the view of the supporting surface or where it is intended to be placed (83). We should also make note that temperature and humidity are compounding environmental factors (45).

Operator/Patient

Often neglected are the **worker characteristics.** Nordin and Frankel suggest that when selecting a worker a battery of tests determining the worker's physical, psychological, and physiological capacities should be administered (65). The dilemma is whether to select the worker based on the job requirements, to ergonomically manipulate the job to fit the worker, or both. One example of this situation is the participation of women in noncustomary jobs. Although women are more flexible than men, they differ in muscle cross-sectional area, body composition, and overall size, thus predisposing them to injury under certain circumstances. One study concluded that with attention to ergonomic principles and physical fitness women could significantly decrease their risk of musculoskeletal injury (12). Other practices that have shown significant utility are test batteries used for pre-employment screening or a functional capacity evaluation. Work assessment, physical capacity assessment and functional capacity assessment are other terms applied to similar procedures. Occasionally, some practitioners will define objectives or establish specific criteria for returning to work. These assessments provide objective data to be used in decisions based on the worker's ability to perform certain tasks or return to work after rehabilitation from injury. Further description of this topic is beyond the scope of this text. However, texts have been written with this objective (44, 49).

Anthropomorphic measures as compared to the work requirements are necessary, as are considerations of the postures assumed. For example, would a therapist recommend or expect that a patient with low back dysfunction stand all day during work, even without the option to elevate one foot onto a stool at least periodically? Certainly some avoidance of work conditions that could result in re-injury would be appropriate. Education of the subject should also be required. The importance of this area is now manifested by the formation of "schools" for the patient with low back pain or dysfunction (85). Finally, be sure that all modifications have been made that will make the job the safest and least demanding. This factor, when combined with proper instruction in technique, should minimize the risk of original or recurring injury (83).

Implications for the Lumbar Spine

By far, the most important applications of manual material handling are to the lumbar spine. This is evidenced by the high rate of injury associated with materials handling. Several approaches have been used to address the problem of low back injuries and impairments (14). Stevenson and cohorts have shown evidence of the beneficial effects of ergonomic intervention on lifting mechanics (78). In 1974 the National Institute of Occupational Safety and Health (NIOSH) convened a panel of experts who reviewed all the available information on the hazards of manual materials handling, establishing a taxonomy to catalog relevant literature (42). In 1981, NIOSH published a document entitled "Work Practices Guide for Manual Lifting" that synthesized the available research on overexertion injuries in manual materials handling (86).

This guide, although somewhat limited, does define six variables, such as location of object center of mass and frequency of lifting, that best define hazardous lifts. Furthermore, in developing the guide, epidemiological, psychophysical, physiological, and biomechanical criteria were used. Using these criteria, two levels of hazard were established. The first, called the action limit, is based on facts associated with the four criteria listed above. The second is a maximal permissible limit, based on other known facts associated with the same four criteria. One example is extracted from the biomechanical criteria: that L5/S1 disc compression force over the 6400 N level cannot be tolerated in most workers. As a result, lifting tasks could be categorized. The categories are shown in Figure 16.9 for occasional lifting of objects. Three distinct areas are established. In the upper right hand portion the maximal permissible limit is exceeded and the lifting conditions in this area are intolerable, requiring redesign of the task. The stippled section labeled with administrative controls required indicates that appropriate employee selection, placement and training should exist and/or job redesign should take place. The area to the lower left is considered to contain the conditions in which nominal risk exists for most workers. It is important to realize that muscle strength and compression forces at L5/S1 define the limits and that fatigue is not an issue in these occasional lifts.

The 1981 equation, discussed above, can only be applied to sagittal plane lifts. In 1991 NIOSH published a revised equation, which revises and expands the 1981 edition to cover more lifting tasks (82). Essentially three criteria are analyzed: (a) biomechanical criterion limits the lumbosacral stress, which is most important in infrequent, heavy load lifting; (b) physiological criterion determines metabolic stress and fatigue, which are most important in repetitive lifting tasks (i.e., >6 lifts per hour); (c) psychophysical criterion limits the stress based on the worker's perception of the task's difficulty. These NIOSH guidelines are intended for use by health professionals in assessing the risk factors associated with lifting in certain occupations. A practical appendix is provided in the 1991 NIOSH document which allows quantitative analysis of the three criteria listed above. The NIOSH equation for recommended weight limits (RWL) is as follows:

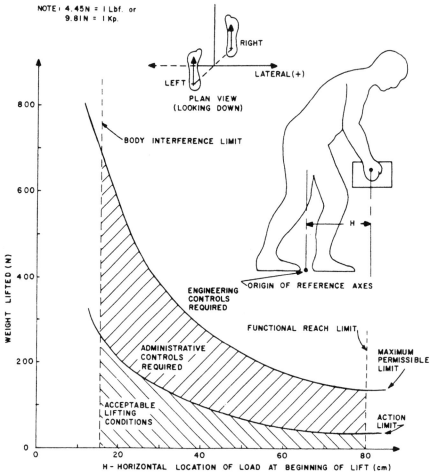

Figure 16.9. The action and permissible limits for different horizontal location of loads lifted from the floor to knuckle height.

$$\text{RWL} = \text{LC} \times \text{HM} \times \text{VM} \times \text{DM} \times \text{AM} \times \text{FM} \times \text{CM}$$

Table 16.2 shows how to calculate the first five values, Table 16.3 the frequency multipler (FM), and Table 16.4 the coupling multipler (CM).

Understanding the load constant (LC) is important in using this equation. The LC refers to the maximum weight that can be lifted under optimal conditions (i.e., where all the other factors are equal to 1). Seventy-five percent of female workers and 90% of male workers could lift this weight without exceeding the disc compression force of 3400 N, which has been shown to increase the risk of back injury (82). Applying this equation to the lifting of the bag of water softener salt discussed earlier, if H = 40.0 cm, V = 0.0 cm, D = 90.0 cm, and A = 0.0 cm, then the RWL = 10.7 kg (23.6 lbs). These data would indicate that most men and women should never lift a bag of water softener salt off the floor in a grocery store. Consider interventions that could be made in this scenario to improve the lifting conditions (e.g., increasing V above 75 cm).

Table 16.2. NIOSH Equation: Calculation of Load Constant (LC), Horizontal Multiplier (HM), Vertical Multiplier (VM), Distance Multiplier (DM), and Asymmetric Multiplier (AM)

Component	Metric	US Customary
LC	23 kg	51 lbs
HM	25/H	10/H
VM	$(1 - (0.003|V - 75|))$	$(1 - (0.0075|V - 30|))$
DM	$(0.82 + (4.5/D))$	$(0.82 + (1.8/D))$
AM	$(1 - 0.0032A)$	$(1 - (0.0032A))$

Legend: H, horizontal distance of hands from midpoint between the ankles. Measure at the origin and the destination of the lift.

V, vertical distance of the hands from the floor. Measure at the origin and destination of the lift.

D, vertical travel distance between the origin and the destination of the lift.

A, angle of asymmetry—angular displacement of the load from the sagittal plane. Measure at the origin and destination of the lift.

Table 16.3. NIOSH Equation: Calculation of the Coupling Multiplier (CM)

Coupling Effectiveness	V < 75 cm (30 in)	V > 75 cm (30 in)
Good	1.00	1.00
Fair	0.95	1.00
Poor	0.90	.90

The quality of the coupling or handles of the object is rated according to the vertical height (V) of the object.

Table 16.4. NIOSH Equation: Calculation of the Frequency Multiplier (FM)

Frequency (lifts/min)	Work Duration					
	< 1h		< 2h		< 8h	
	V < 75	V > 75	V < 75	V > 75	V < 75	V > 75
0.2	1.00	1.00	0.95	0.95	0.85	0.85
0.5	0.97	0.97	0.92	0.92	0.81	0.81
1	0.94	0.94	0.88	0.88	0.75	0.75
2	0.91	0.91	0.84	0.84	0.65	0.65
3	0.88	0.88	0.79	0.79	0.55	0.55
4	0.84	0.84	0.72	0.72	0.45	0.45
5	0.80	0.80	0.60	0.60	0.35	0.35
6	0.75	0.75	0.50	0.50	0.27	0.27
7	0.70	0.70	0.42	0.42	0.22	0.22
8	0.60	0.60	0.35	0.35	0.18	0.18
9	0.52	0.52	0.30	0.30	0.00	0.15
10	0.45	0.45	0.26	0.26	0.00	0.13
11	0.41	0.41	0.00	0.23	0.00	0.00
12	0.37	0.37	0.00	0.21	0.00	0.00
13	0.00	0.34	0.00	0.00	0.00	0.00
14	0.00	0.31	0.00	0.00	0.00	0.00
15	0.00	0.28	0.00	0.00	0.00	0.00
>15	0.00	0.00	0.00	0.00	0.00	0.00

Legend: V, vertical height of object to be lifted.

Holmstrom, consistent with NIOSH, states that musculoskeletal pain occurring in industry is not simply a result of biomechanical stress, but is multifactorial in nature. Her book includes research in biomechanical and psychosocial stressors and their relationship to work injury (43).

A maximum and repetitive limit of compression forces placed upon the spine has been the subject of extensive research (84). As stated, NIOSH placed the limit of spinal compression (i.e., "maximum permissible limit") at the L5/S1 segment as 6400 N, concluding that compression forces above 3400 N (i.e., "action limit") indicated an increased risk for injury. Several authors have argued that these guidelines are not representative of the working population. Chaffin and Page cite literature stating a much higher safe lifting limit than 3400 N for young males, but for older males the safe limit may be much lower (17). Genaidy's group has proposed the use of a regression equation which will subjectively establish compression limits (31). This equation incorporates the variables of gender and age; neither are novel inclusions. Their article presents a rather complete compilation of 10 other regression equations developed predominantly in the past 15 years. Judging from the number of equations, there is apparently much disagreement in this area. In a related issue, Genaidy argues that spinal compression limits should not be established based on the load to fracture, instead the load to injury or "damage load." Damage was defined as the point where the first gross signs of tissue damage occur, such as blood, tissue, fluid, and then bony change. It is suggested that the risk of injury load be established at 60% of the subjects' maximum load limit. Apparently, at best the compression load limits established by NIOSH are just guidelines to aid in the establishment of more subjective load limits.

Others have evaluated the **maximum load** that can be lifted. Poulsen produced data from 50 male and 50 female subjects, proposing that the maximum loads for men should be 1.1 times the isometric erector spinae muscle "strength." For women the formula is .95 times the erector spinae "strength" minus 8 kg (69). It may be interesting to compare Figure 16.9 with Grandjean's data. He establishes a 50 kp (110 lbf) limit for adult men and 20 kp (40 lbf) for women for occasional lifts during a day; the upper limits of permissible weight are shown as 18 (40 lbf) and 12 kp (27 lbf), respectively, when manual lifts are performed frequently (34). It is important to note that each author presents different maximum and repetitive lifting load values; therefore, these values can only be used as a rough guide. The equation generated by NIOSH may provide greater utility when establishing subjective load limits.

Because either the muscular force or the tensile capabilities of the passive structures can support the trunk in any position of forward inclination, knowing how these mechanisms interact is important, particularly in the lowering and lifting of loads. In the lowering phase the muscles can control the movement, as is shown by EMG studies. In the early phases of this movement the posterior ligaments are not able to exert any control since they are not in a position of elongation. However, as trunk flexion proceeds, the ligaments are progressively stretched, assuming a position of tension. Thus, it appears that muscle force increases as the requirement for an extensor moment increases until the ligament tension is sufficient to assume control. However, some postulate that tension in ligaments should always be under active control of muscle, so as to prevent ligamentous injury (33). In a related study, the effects on the lumbar spine of lifting in two separate postures were analyzed. Both postures tested assumed the same lifting positions except at the lumbar spine where one maintained the normal lordotic curve and the other allowed some "bowing" of the lumbar spine. It was concluded that when maintaining the normal lordotic curve the supporting musculature could provide greater stability to the lumbar spine. It is also notable that the "bowing" of the lumbar spine provided additional stability due to the stretch of the passive and elastic elements, but this was considered an increased risk for injury (19).

Now consider the converse, the lift of the load. This movement requires concentric action of the muscles; based on the known force-velocity relationship for the two types of contraction, less tension is available in the contractile unit than during the lowering or eccentric phase of the motion (see also Figure 13.2). Some investigators state that the lumbar spine remains flexed so that the tension in the ligaments and the muscles is maintained. Thus the pelvis must be rotated posteriorly on the hips, at least initially, by the strong hip extensors that can act through a large moment arm (25). As the pelvis rotates, the trunk is lifted, helping to reduce the moment that the extensor musculature has to overcome to return the trunk to the upright position. Because the entire maneuver must be completed with muscle shortening, passive structures such as the ligaments make no contribution. If in fact muscular contributions are not used to protect the ligaments, by way of controlling the motion, soft tissue damage can result.

The most common recommendation given for limiting the need for high extensor moments is that the lift is carried out with the knees bent. Tacit approval of this procedure can only be made if the load can be lifted between the knees; only in this posture can the moment through the lumbar spine be sufficiently reduced to warrant this procedure. Research has verified these fundamental rules. In one example, comparative forward bending moments were calculated for three conditions. In forward bending with the knees straight the moment was 191.5 Nm. Lifting the same load to the same position with the knees bent and the load between the knees decreased the forward bending moment to 151 Nm. However, if the bent knee lift was used but the object was large enough to require lifting in front of the knees the moment increased to just over 212 Nm (57).

Other work has analyzed four different lifting methods relative to the effect on spinal compression. The conventional bent and straight knee lifts were compared to a trunk kinetic lift and a "load kinetic lift." In the former, the hips were first extended, followed by the shoulders and the load. In the latter the load was pulled toward the trunk and swung upwards. Results showed that bent knee lifts produced the least peak compression at L5/S1. The trunk kinetic lift was decisively the most stressful. The authors specifically caution that the bent knee lift is of value only for the lumbar spine if one can avoid lifting the load in front of or beside the knees. Assurance should also be provided that the knee extensors are of sufficient strength to generate the necessary moment (55). These data reinforce the need to consider not only the posture of the spine, but also the size, mass, and location of the object being manipulated. As stated earlier, those are all elements of the revised NIOSH equation.

An additional factor to consider is the effects of contraction of other musculature during the lift. The psoas and multifidus are responsible for producing considerable anterior shear in the lumbar spine. Resistance to this shear probably arises in the facet joints (see Chapter 13), but further contribution to control probably results from the contraction of the internal oblique muscles. This may offer at least a partial explanation as to the activity from this muscle with the lifting of loads greater than body weight (25).

Another factor that contributes to trunk stability during lifting is the increase in

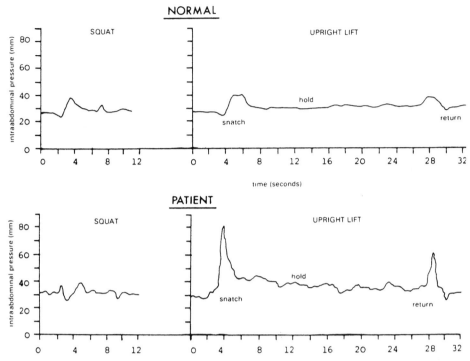

Figure 16.10.   Intra-abdominal pressures measured during lifting of a 15 kilogram mass by a normal subject and a patient.

intra-abdominal pressure. Such pressurization is thought to be reflexive and caused by contraction of the internal and external oblique and transversus muscles. The effect is a distending force between the diaphragm and the rib cage and the pelvic floor, producing an extensor moment for the spine. Studies have shown definitive increases in the intra-abdominal pressures during lifting. We show a sample of typical results in Figure 16.10 (35). Note that the very large increase occurs at the moment of the lift, returning to levels just over the pre-lift value for the static condition. Thus, the amount of the load and the degree of acceleration applied are critical factors in determining the degree of increase in the intra-abdominal pressure. How important this factor is to the reduction of the extensor moment and the load on the spine has yet to be precisely determined. However, it has been shown that intra-abdominal pressure in athletes reduced the loads on the spine by up to 40% (57). Goldish and coworkers studied the effects of twisting the spine while performing a maximal Valsalva maneuver. They showed that maximum intra-abdominal pressure (IAP max) was significantly lower during rotation of the spine in an upright posture. They also showed that the IAP maximum decreased significantly during forward flexion and rotation of the spine compared to forward flexion only. They attributed the decrease in pressure to the biomechanical disadvantage placed upon the contributing muscula-ture. This study concluded that the inability to maintain IAP max during twisting may be contributing to twisting-type back injuries (32). It is well documented that twisting is a significant mechanism of injury to the lumbar spine (26). However, performing a Valsalva maneuver (i.e., contraction of the abdominal musculature against a closed epiglottis) is not recommended because of the strain this pressure places on the cardiovascular system. Also, we must caution against full contraction of the abdominal muscles on the basis that the flexor moment created by such a contraction would potentially cancel any extension effect produced by the increase in the intra-abdominal pressure (70). In summary, some contraction of the abdominal muscles during lifting can provide added stability to the lumbar spine.

Perhaps the important element in the ability of the human to effectively lift loads is the **interaction of the active and passive** elements of the abdomen and spine, along with the motion of the pelvis on the femur. Clearly, for loads to be lifted, considerable extensor moments of the spine must be generated. Using mechanisms that can ensure the accomplishment of these feats while minimizing the risk of injury to the lumbar spine should be invoked for all persons, no matter whether or not low back dysfunction exists. To generalize, as lifting follows, intra-abdominal pressure increases by contraction of the abdominal musculature. Movement of the pelvis on the femur is initiated and finally the active muscle contraction of the back extensors contributes to elevation of the trunk to the upright position. Farfan stated that extensor muscle power is not needed for larger lifts or high rates of acceleration. This is difficult to believe based on the fact that these muscle forces must be required at some point in the effort. Although the contraction of the abdominal muscles may prevent potential shear in the spine while concurrently increasing intra-abdominal pressure, sufficient extensor moments still need to be produced to elevate the trunk to neutral (25). Even then, there is some evidence that activity in the obliques is not a decisive factor in increasing the intra-abdominal pressure (40).

Another factor that we cannot ignore is the effect of the lift on **interdiscal pressure.** Many demonstrations of the effects of different styles of lift and load lifted have been provided. Larger increases associated with lifts performed in the straight leg position essentially confirm that activity in the extensor musculature contributes to the increased interdiscal pressure (67). During slight anterior inclination of the trunk while standing, the pressure in the third lumbar disc increases to more than twice the pressure recorded in erect standing. The same degree of load and inclination while sitting increases the pressure to almost three times the standing measurement (64).

Concerning the vertebral disc the other feature to consider is the **asymmetric loading** that occurs with forward bending. Instead of the relatively equal distribution of the load as in standing, trunk flexion significantly increases the pressure on the anterior aspect of the disc. Some have thought these asymmetries to cause a posterior avulsion, hence the "ruptured disc" in a posterolateral direction. The magnitude of these forces that Chaffin and Andersson have described is a multisegment link model of the body. Their calculations show that for the lift of a 450 N load the compressive force at the L5/S1 disc is 4319 N. Shear force reaches a peak value of 400 N (16). Other procedures to determine the amount of load on the lumbar spine have been advocated (73). In fact, nearly all of the mechanisms associated with lifting increase the compression on the disc and the vertebrae. The remarkable ability of these structures to manage these loads probably enables the lumbar spine to avoid many injuries.

A free-body diagram is often used to determine the loads placed on various segments during lifting tasks. Some have argued that it is improper to use this "static model" for analysis of dynamic lifting because it assumes that the inertia of various segments is negligible. They propose that a thorough analysis include the calculation of both linear and angular accelerations. Various methods for incorporating these measurements are included in the research of Lindbeck and Arborelius (56).

We may make several generalizations regarding lifting and the lumbar spine. Based on mechanics and the literature, the spine should be as straight as possible, maintaining the body in an upright position. With the knees bent the load should be as close to the body as possible. Further, the load should be 40–50 cm above the ground level, which may require the use of ramps and/or elevating pallets. Then, if the load is to be transferred to a new location the spine should be maintained in as straight a posture as possible (34). However, some still say that rules regarding the posture of the lumbar spine to be used in lifting can only be "speculative" (16). Some would say that the lordotic position should be maintained, although lifting "with the legs" does not preclude this event. Maintenance of lordosis by the back extensors, for example, would allow a stronger contraction of the abdominals so that intra-abdominal pressure could be increased. Surely the debate as to the most advised form of lifting will continue until convincing evidence has been presented (19, 68, 80).

Other implications for the lumbar spine arise from tasks requiring **carrying, pushing,** and **pulling.** The best solution for carrying is a yoke across the shoulders; the load is closest to the body's center of gravity, minimizing moments. Little information is present in the literature regarding pushing and pulling. It has been reported that for men the limit in either direction is between 200 and 400 N. In either of the activities, a key factor is foot placement and support. Having a firm base of support allowed by advancement of one foot and a surface that will not allow slipping are the two factors that should receive most attention (16). Males and females can pull loads at greater forces than they can push loads. Also, the low back compressive forces during pushing are 129–627% of the corresponding pulled loads. These data would indicate that loads should be pulled whenever possible (54).

Although little data exist to support recommendations against **asymmetric load handling,** enough information is available that shows that these techniques are more hazardous. A major change in the revised NIOSH equation was the addition of the "asymmetric multiplier," a variable added to convert the equation from the mere sagittal plane assessment provided in the 1981 NIOSH equation. In addition, research has found torsion to increase loads on the lumbar spine significantly (74). The lumbar spine, designed to support compression force, may incur injury with as little as 2° of axial rotation (26). Because completion of dynamic tasks loads the lumbar spine up to 40% more than static loads (28) and because muscles have been reported to respond differently under isometric and isokinetic conditions (61), Bell and coworkers monitored EMG activity of the L3–L4 erector spinae muscles during dynamic execution of sagittal plane symmetric and asymmetric lifting tasks. Results showed that EMG activity was significantly greater for asymmetric than symmetric lifting tasks. Activity was also greater on the side away from the rotation as compared to the side toward the rotation (8). Also note the Goldish study, discussed earlier, that indicated a decreased ability to maintain intra-abdominal pressure during rotation of the spine (32). Relating these findings to loading of the lumbar spine is indirect at best. However, in view of the Drury finding that more than 80% of industrial lifting tasks include a twisting motion at the start of the task, the implications for therapeutic recommendations for patients are becoming more clear (22).

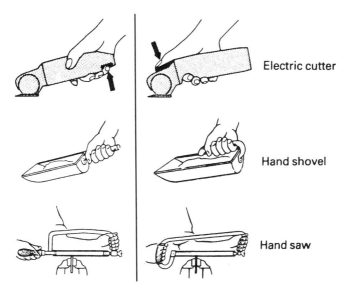

Figure 16.11. Shaping of handgrips should be according to anatomy and function. Poor designs are on the left, good on the right.

MANIPULATION

In most work situations the management of objects is required. In these situations the object itself and the position of the arm and hand are important because of the potential influence on fatigue and musculoskeletal injuries. Usually, mechanizing any repetitive task is best. If not possible, high rates of repetition and extremes of ranges of motion are to be avoided. Another factor that may precipitate fatigue or injury is long duration static contractions that require isometric contractions. For example, one volume on industrial ergonomics recommends a rest-contraction ratio of 10:1 and an avoidance of all contractions in excess of 50% of maximum. Another recommendation is never to exceed 20% of the operator's maximal force in positions requiring prolonged or repetitive work (83).

Because of the attention given to the manipulation of objects, **hand tools** have undergone considerable design changes. This principle has been coined "bending the tool and not the wrist" (72). Several factors are of specific concern. The first is that static positioning and/or muscle loading will lead to fatigue and soreness. To prevent these occurrences the shoulders should be at the sides and the hand and wrist should be positioned in front of the elbow that is in 90° of flexion. The device being manipulated should allow for easy gripping, perhaps through the provision of an angulated handle. The grip surface should also be of a material that will reduce the likelihood of slippage (83).

Another critical factor is the position of the wrist. The neutral position is highly recommended and is shown in the correct positions in Figure 16.11. Specific examples can be provided by noting that standard pliers and cutting knives have been redesigned to match the neutral position of the wrist. In the former the handle of the pliers was bent to conform to the hand. In the latter case the handle was modified to include a wrap-around restraint with a pistol grip configuration. Decreased incidences of both trauma and chronic problems resulted (16).

A final consideration in use of hand tools is that design should avoid pressures on nerves and blood vessels susceptible to injury. Of specific interest is the area on the palmar surface of the wrist known as the carpal tunnel. To avoid chronic pressures wrist positions should be monitored. Hand tools should also be manufactured so that the handles for tools do not end in the palm (24).

To avoid problems caused by the manipulation of objects, extensive information is available as to handle length, diameter, and span. Shapes, such as the commonly recommended oval and circular grips, also have a set of criteria that can be applied to work settings. Factors such as weight and suspension are important because the operator should not be required to resist a large moment caused by the distribution of the mass within the object. Even the location of any triggering mechanism should be given forethought (24). Grip triggers rather than thumb or finger triggers are thought to be the better designs. These and other considerations should allow the worker to perform with maximum efficiency (34).

WORKSITE ANALYSIS

Analysis of the worksite is appropriate for the therapist to perform. It makes no sense to treat a worker for deQuervain's disease (i.e., tenosynovitis of the extensor pollicus brevis and abductor pollicis longus tendons) and send him or her back to work, if the etiology of the injury is an improperly placed button on an iron. The injury will only return in a matter of time. A therapist must be acquainted with the demands of the workplace: the motions required to complete a task, the range of motion necessary in associated joints, the loads imposed upon bones and joints, the degree of "strength" required, and the physiological demands on the body. Answers to these questions and a knowledge of the worker's capabilities will allow the therapist to make proper decisions (65). A variety of methods and data forms for use during worksite assessment are available (36, 50, 51). Much attention has also been given to the analysis of lifting (37). In these cases the weight, position of load, frequency, and duration of lift are all factors that are taken into account. For more details, refer to Chaffin and Andersson or to the reports of the original research (16).

Certainly in all **site analyses** the postures required to perform the task, and the force, duration, and required repetitions are all important factors. Swat has developed an assessment method which allows an estimate of preexisting loads placed on various segments before a worksite is designed. This provides the designer data that will aid in making decisions that will decrease postural loads (79). Tools, particularly those that require manipulative skills, should be viewed with consideration given to joint positioning and fatigue. Analysis of injury records may also reveal areas in which improvements in work conditions can be suggested. Grandjean has developed a comprehensive checklist that is applicable to the analysis of the workplace (34).

APPLICATIONS TO PATIENTS

There is a great deal of evidence that conditions of the work environment can precurse or exacerbate injuries. Direct relationships have been shown for at least the shoulder and wrist, as well as for the joints of the lumbar spine. The role of the therapist could be a preventive one, but more practically the function will be to advise and attempt to control the work situation so that rehabilitation will not be hampered. This section will focus on considerations as they apply to the shoulder, wrist, and spine.

Regarding the **shoulder,** the position required for work is important. As pointed out in previous sections, work height above the position of the elbow creates the necessity for elevation of the shoulder, increasing the likelihood for injury. Fatigue occurs three times faster in 60° of abduction and six times faster in 90° of abduction when compared to the advised angle of 30° (29). Other shoulder injuries can occur because of work requirements. Particularly conducive to producing tendinitis, either acute, chronic, or degenerative, is overhead work that requires repetitive and/or high forces. The biceps brachii and supraspinatus tendons are most susceptible. Therapists should carefully evaluate patients that have had histories of injury and/or pathology of the shoulder complex for deficiencies in strength and range of motion before they return to work in jobs that may demand stress levels that are too high. Our ability to decide is predicated on the collection of additional information so that we know which of the clinical cases are most likely to succeed with rehabilitative efforts.

The most common predisposing mechanism for injury to the **wrist** is repetitive exertion by the hand. Usually improper tool design or tool use can be directly implicated in the onset of impingement of the median nerve in the carpal tunnel. The primary result is manifested in the hand, commonly as pain into the thenar eminence. Losses may also include sensory deficits over the thumb following the distribution of the median nerve. Although surgical relief is usually easily accomplished, the cost and lost time from work make prevention the most desirable means of managing this form of disability.

Other **hand** problems usually focus on tenosynovitis of the long tendons. Again the primary cause is a high repetition rate, often by an individual unaccustomed to that work. Unusual or extreme positions may also account for the pathology. Armstrong suggests the predominant risk factors are repetition, forcefulness, certain postures, mechanical stresses, exposure to vibration, and exposure to low temperatures (6). The goal of rehabilitation is to return the patient to the same kind of work. Although transfers to different jobs are sometimes practical, the relief of the patient's complaints is the immediate goal of effective treatment. Many of these original complaints become chronic, making the circumstances more difficult for the patient, the employer, and the therapist involved. Effective long-term treatment of these cases is probably contingent on consideration given to the work to be resumed by the patient.

Injuries of the **lumbar spine** are so prevalent that the clinical conditions manifested by these patients demand inquiry by the therapist as to working conditions. Those persons in environments that require either repetitive and/or high load lifting are definitely more prone to original or recurring injury. Muscular strains, ligamentous sprains, disc pathology, or other bony or soft tissue injuries have all claimed a significant toll in patient dysfunction and inability to perform at work. Controlling for the conditions to be encountered demands that the therapist take into account many factors before the suggestion can be made that return to work is plausible.

One consideration for the therapist is the overall status of the lumbar spine. Many believe that instability, whether in single or multiple segments, may be critical to the effective function of the lumbar spine. If any patient is found to have instability from any possible cause, treatment should address that cause. Strengthening of the extensor musculature may be indicated, although definitive data is yet lacking. There are questions as to the capabilities for trunk control by the low back dysfunction patient (2, 75). It has been established that the chronic low back dysfunction patient has erector spinae muscle activity that differs from normal when postural and other functional activities are compared (76).

Much clinical debate has also focused on the role of the abdominal musculature in the control of the lumbar spine. Although it is not the role of this book to discuss the merit or the necessity for large tensions in the abdominal muscles, they would, at least empirically, seem desirable. Certainly one advantage of contraction of this muscle group, initiated just prior to the lift, is that the intra-abdominal pressure would be increased. Subsequently, "stabilization" of the trunk should be aided, thus assisting with the production of an effective extensor moment.

Training may also have to follow to ensure that patients perform functional activities and lifting tasks while using the proper mechanics. We have discussed the lifting techniques and their effect on the lumbar spine in previous sections of this chapter. Specific recommendations may need to be made to the patient as to the frequency and duration of the lifting to be performed. The load will also have to be closely monitored.

That the lifting requirements and work postures are important can be verified through the literature. One study evaluated the amount of trunk motion during work by dentists, nurses, and warehouse employees. Although the dentists performed mostly in a semiflexed posture and the nurses in the upright position the dentists performed only 8 flexions requiring more than 73°, while the nurses completed 70 deep flexions in the same one-hour period. The expectation of the warehouse workers was clearly shown in the study. In their case less than half the time was spent in the upright position while 153 deep flexions were required that, in most cases, included lifting (66). This study points out the importance of recognizing the patient's unique work demands. Similar importance may be attached to the sitting or standing posture to be assumed by these patients because prolonged positioning in one posture may have negative effects on the lower back.

Great amounts of information need to be gathered on not only the effect of various therapeutic regimens, but also on the torque generating requirements of both the flexor and extensor musculature. Only after gathering these data, connected with epidemiological studies, will we have a sufficiently clear picture as to the most effective procedures to follow for the successful management of the patient with low back dysfunction. The pathologies, clearly identifiable or nondescript, simply point out the need for the therapist to consider ergonomics in the total rehabilitation of the patient.

SUMMARY

This chapter has discussed relevant portions of the field of ergonomics. Therapists must take into account the various principles presented in this chapter because often the success of treatment, as judged by the patient and by society, will be the ability of the patient to return to work. Intervention has shown optimistic success. Aaras reports a decrease of sick-leave due to musculoskeletal illness from 5.3% to 3.1% and a reduction of job turnover from 30.1% to 7.6% in women employees at various workplaces. There was a savings ratio for the company of 9:1 for every dollar invested in physical therapy intervention (1). These data show the short-term savings possible with ergonomic intervention. We should note that the savings over time are not generally as pronounced as when the initial ergonomic manipulations are in place. In the Potlach Corporation, 70 workers hired before the use of job placement assessments (JPA) were compared to 70 hired after the use of JPAs. Over a two-year period those who did not have a JPA experienced 520 lost work days and 3 million dollars in worker's compensation costs. Those who had JPAs had 26 lost work days and $880,000 in worker's compensation costs (49).

Several textbooks have addressed strategies for incorporating physical therapist intervention in the workplace (44, 49). In this context, the last section of this chapter discussed the ergonomic implications for patients with shoulder, wrist, and low back injuries.

References

1. Aaras A. The impact of ergonomic intervention on individual health and corporate prosperity in a telecommunications environment. *Ergonomics.* 1994;37:1679–1696.
2. Addison R, Schultz A. Trunk strength in patients seeking hospitalization for chronic low back disorders. *Spine.* 1980;5:539–544.
3. Andersson GBJ, Murphy RW, Ortengren R, Nachemson AL. The influence of backrest inclination and lumbar support on the lumbar lordosis in sitting. *Spine.* 1979;4:52–58.
4. Andersson GBJ, Ortengren R. Lumbar disc pressure and myoelectric back muscle activity during sitting. III. Studies on a wheelchair. *Scand J Rehabil Med.* 1974;6:122–127.
5. Andersson GBJ, Ortengren R, Nachemson A, Elfstrom G. Lumbar disc pressure and myoelectric back muscle activity during sitting. I. Studies on an experimental chair. *Scand J Rehabil Med.* 1974;6:104–114.
6. Armstrong TJ. Ergonomics and cumulative trauma disorders. *Hand Clin.* 1986;2:553–565.
7. Automakes J. Claims cost of back pain. *Best's Review.* September 1981.
8. Bell SA, Koester JA, Wilking BJ, Cook TM. *Erector Spinae EMG during Asymmetric and Symmetric Lifting.* Iowa City: University of Iowa. Unpublished data.
9. Bendix T. Adjustment of the seated workplace—with special reference to heights and inclinations of seat and table. *Dan Med Bull.* 1987;34:125–139.
10. Bendix T, Biering-Sorenson F. Posture of the trunk when sitting on forward inclining seats. *Scand J Rehabil Med.* 1983;15:197–203.
11. Blom L, Hauch A. Physiotherapists in ergonomics. *Appl Ergonomics.* 1982;13:289–292.
12. Blue CL. Women in nontraditional jobs: is there a risk for musculoskeletal injury? *Am Assoc Occup Health Nurs J.* 1993;41:235–240.
13. Brunswic M. Seat design in unsupported sitting. Paper presented at the International Conference on Occupational Ergonomics; 1984; Toronto, Ontario.
14. Buckle PW, Kember PA, Wood AD, Wood SN. Factors influencing occupational back pain in Bedfordshire. *Spine.* 1980;5:254–258.
15. Chaffin DB. Localized muscle fatigue—definition and measurement. *J Occup Med.* 1973;15:346–354.
16. Chaffin DB, Andersson GBJ. *Occupational Biomechanics.* 2nd ed. New York: John Wiley & Sons; 1991.
17. Chaffin DB, Page GB. Postural effects on biomechanical and psychophysical weight-lifting limits. *Ergonomics.* 1994;37:663–676.
18. Corlett EN. Analysis and evaluation of working posture. In: Kvalseth TO, ed. *Ergonomics of Workstation Design.* Guildford: Butterworths; 1983.
19. DeLitto RS, Rose SJ, Apts DW. Electromyographic analysis of two techniques for squat lifting. *Phys Ther.* 1987;67:1329–1334.
20. Drury CG, Deeb JM, Hartman B, Woolley S, Drury CE, Gallagher S. Symmetric and asymmetric manual materials handling, part 2: biomechanics. *Ergonomics.* 1989;32:565–583.
21. Drury CG, Francher M. Evaluation of a forward-sloping chair. *Appl Ergonomics.* 1985;16:41–47.
22. Drury CG, Law C, Pawenski CS. A survey of industrial box handling. *Hum Factors.* 1982;24:553–565.
23. Eastman MC, Kamon E. Posture and subjective evaluation at flat and slanted desks. *Hum Factors.* 1976;18:15–26.
24. Eggleton EM, ed. *Ergonomic Design for People at Work.* Belmont, CA: Lifetime Learning Publications; 1983:1.
25. Farfan HF. Muscular mechanism of the lumbar spine and the position of power and efficiency. *Orthop Clin N Am.* 1975;6:135–144.
26. Farfan HF. The torsional injury of the lumbar spine. *Spine.* 1984;9:53.
27. Fountain FP, Minear WL, Allison RD. Function of longus colli and longissimus cervicis muscles in man. *Arch Phys Med Rehabil.* 1966;47:665–669.
28. Frievalds A, Chaffin DB, Garg A, Lee KS. A dynamic biomechanical evaluation of lifting maximum acceptable loads. *J Biomech.* 1984;17:251–262.

29. Garg A. Lifting and back injuries. *Plant Eng.* 1982;36:89–93.

30. Genaidy AM, Al-Shedi AA, Shell RL. Ergonomic risk assessment: preliminary guidelines for analysis of repetition, force, and posture. *J Hum Ergol Tokyo.* 1993:22:45–55.

31. Genaidy AM, Waly SM, Khalil TM, Hidalgo J. Spinal compression tolerance limits for the design of manual material handling operations in the workplace. *Ergonomics.* 1993;36:415–434.

32. Goldish GD, Quast JE, Blow JJ, Kuskowski MA. Postural effects on intra-abdominal pressure during valsalva maneuver. *Arch Phys Med Rehabil.* 1994;74:324–327.

33. Gracovetsky S, Farfan HF, Lamy C. The mechanism of the lumbar spine. *Spine.* 1981;6:249–262.

34. Grandjean E. *Fitting the Task to the Man: An Ergonomic Approach.* London: Taylor & Francis; 1982.

35. Grew ND. Intra-abdominal pressure response to loads applied to the torso in normal subjects. *Spine.* 1980;5:149–154.

36. Gross CM. Ergonomic workplace assessments are first step in injury treatment. *Occup Health Saf.* 1988;57:16–19.

37. Halpern M. Prevention of low back pain: basic ergonomics in the workplace and the clinic. *Baillieres Clin Rheumatol.* 1992;6:705–730.

38. Harber P, Bloswick D, Pena L, Beck J, Lee J, Baker D. The ergonomic challenge of repetitive motion with varying ergonomic stresses: characterizing supermarket checking work. *J Occup Med.* 1992;34:518–528.

39. Haslegrave CM. What do we mean by a 'working posture'? *Ergonomics.* 1994;37:781–789.

40. Hemborg B, Moritz U, Hamberg J, et al. Intra-abdominal pressure and trunk muscle activity during lifting—effect of abdominal muscle training in healthy subjects. *Scand J Rehabil Med.* 1983;15: 183–196.

41. Herberts P, Kadefors R, Andersson G, Peterson I. Shoulder pain in industry: an epidemiological study on welders. *Acta Orthop Scand.* 1981;52:299–306.

42. Herrin G, Chaffin D, Mach R. *Criteria for Research on the Hazards of Manual Materials Handling.* Cincinnati, OH: National Institute of Occupational Safety and Health Contract Report; 1974; CDC publication 99-74-118.

43. Holmstrom E. *Musculoskeletal Disorders in Construction Workers.* Lund, Sweden: Studentlitteratur; 1992.

44. Isernhagen SJ. *The Comprehensive Guide to Work Injury Management.* Gaithersburg, MD: Aspen Publishers; 1995.

45. Jokl MV. The effect of the environment on human performance. *Appl Ergonomics.* 1982;13:269–280.

46. Jorgensen K. Back muscle strength and body weight as limiting factors for work in standing slightly-stooped position. *Scand J Rehabil Med.* 1970;2:149–153.

47. Kamwendo K, Linton SJ, Mortiz U. Neck and shoulder disorders in medical secretaries: part 1. Pain prevalence and risk factors. *Scand J Rehabil Med.* 1991;23:127–133.

48. Keegan JJ. Alterations to the lumbar curve related to posture and seating. *J Bone Joint Surg.* 1953;35(A):589–603.

49. Key GL. *Industrial Therapy.* St. Louis: CV Mosby; 1994.

50. Keyserling WM, Chaffin DB. Occupational ergonomics—methods to evaluate physical stress on the job. *Annu Rev Public Health.* 1986;7:77–104.

51. Keyserling WM, Stetson DS, Silverstein BA, Brouwer ML. A checklist for evaluating ergonomic risk factors associated with upper extremity cumulative trauma disorders. *Ergonomics.* 1993;36:807–831.

52. Knutsson B, Lindh K, Telhag H. Sitting—an electromyographic and mechanical study. *Acta Orthop Scand.* 1966;37:415–428.

53. Kroemer KHE. Seating in plant and office. *Am Ind Hyg Assoc J.* 1971;32:633–652.

54. Kumar S. The back compressive forces during maximal push-pull activities in the sagittal plane. *J Hum Ergol Tokyo.* 1994;23:133–150.

55. Leskinen TPJ, Stalhammar HR, Kuorinka IAA. A dynamic analysis of spinal compression with different lifting techniques. *Ergonomics.* 1983;26:595–604.

56. Lindbeck L, Arborelius UP. Inertial effects from single body segments in dynamic analysis of lifting. *Ergonomics.* 1991;34:421–433.

57. Lindh M. Biomechanics of the lumbar spine. In: Frankel FH, Nordin M, eds. *Basic Biomechanics of the Skeletal Spine.* Philadelphia: Lea & Febiger; 1980.

58. Lundervold A. Electromyographic investigations during sedentary work, especially typewriting. *Br J Phys Med.* 1951;14:32–36.

59. Majeske C, Buchanan C. Quantitative description of two sitting postures: with and without a lumbar support pillow. *Phys Ther.* 1984;64:1531–1533.

60. Mandal AC. The seated man (Homo Sedens): the seated work position: theory and practice. *Appl Ergonomics.* 1981;12:19–26.

61. Marras WS, King AI, Joynt RL. Measurements of loads on the lumbar spine under isometric and isokinetic conditions. *Spine.* 1984;9:176–187.

62. Meister D. The present and future of human factors. *Appl Ergonomics.* 1982;13:281–287.

63. Nachemson AL. Lumbar interdiscal pressure. In: Jayson MIV, ed. *The Lumbar Spine and Back Pain.* Kent, England: Pitman Medical; 1980.

64. Nachemson AL. The lumbar spine: an orthopaedic challenge. *Spine.* 1976;1:59–71.

65. Nordin M, Frankel VH. Evaluation of the workplace: an introduction. *Clin Orthop.* 1987;221:85–88.

66. Nordin M, Ortengren R, Andersson GBJ. Measurements of trunk movements during work. *Spine.* 1984;9:465–469.

67. Ortengren R, Andersson GBJ, Nachemson AL. Studies of relationships between lumbar disc pressure, myoelectric back muscle activity, and intra-abdominal (intra-gastric) pressure. *Spine.* 1981;6:98–103.

68. Parnianpour M, Bejjani FJ, Pavlidis L. Worker training: the fallacy of a single, correct lifting technique. *Ergonomics.* 1987;30:331–334.

69. Poulsen E. Back muscle strength and weight limits in lifting burdens. *Spine.* 1981;6:73–75.

70. Rab GT, Chao EYS, Stauffer RN. Muscle force analysis of the lumbar spine. *Orthop Clin N Am.* 1977;8:193–199.

71. Rys M, Konz S. Standing. *Ergonomics.* 1994;37:677–687.

72. Schoenmarklin RW, Marras WS. Effects of handle angle and work orientation on hammering: I. Wrist motion and hammering performance. *Hum Factors.* 1989;31:397–411.

73. Schultz AB, Andersson GBJ. Analysis of loads on the lumbar spine. *Spine.* 1981;6:76–82.

74. Schultz AB, Andersson GBJ, Haderspeck K, Ortengren R, Nordin M, Bjork R. Analysis and measurement of lumbar trunk loads in tasks involving bends and twists. *J Biomech.* 1982;15:669–675.

75. Smidt G, Herring T, Amundsen L, Rogers M, Russell A, Lehmann T. Assessment of abdominal and back extensor function: a quantitative approach and results for chronic low-back patients. *Spine.* 1983;8:211–219.

76. Soderberg GL, Barr JO. Muscular function in chronic low-back dysfunction. *Spine.* 1983;8:79–85.

77. Soderberg GL, Blanco MK, Cosentino TL, Kurdelmeier KA. An EMG analysis of posterior trunk musculature during flat and anteriorly inclined sitting. *Hum Factors.* 1986;28:483–491.

78. Stevenson J, Bryant T, Greenhorn D, Smith T, Deakin J, Surgenor B. The effect of lifting protocol on comparisons with isoinertial lifting performance. *Ergonomics.* 1990;33:1455–1469.

79. Swat K. An ergonomic system for assessing postural stress in workplaces. *Pol J Occup Med Environ Health.* 1992;5:315–321.

80. Tak-sun Y, Roht LH, Wise RA, Kilian DJ, Wier FW. Low-back pain in industry. An old problem revisited. *J Occup Med.* 1984;26:517–523.

81. Tichauer ER. *The Biomechanical Basis of Ergonomics.* New York: Wiley-Interscience; 1978.

82. Waters TR, Putz-Anderson V, Garg A, Fine LJ. Revised NIOSH equation for the design and evaluation of manual lifting tasks. *Ergonomics.* 1993;36:749–776.

83. Webb RDG. *Industrial Ergonomics.* Toronto, Ontario: The Industrial Accident Prevention Association; 1982.

84. White AW III, Panjabi MM. *Clinical Biomechanics of the Spine.* 2nd ed. Philadelphia: JB Lippincott; 1990.

85. White LA. Back school. In: Isernhagen SJ, ed. *The Comprehensive Guide to Work Injury Management.* Rockville, MD: Aspen Publishers; 1995.

86. *Work Practices Guide for Manual Lifting.* Cincinnati, OH: National Institute of Occupational Safety and Health; 1981; DHHS (NIOSH) publication 81-122.

APPENDIX A

Trigonometry Review

It is possible to solve many force and velocity problems by use of vector diagrams. However, the degree of accuracy is dependent upon the exactness of the person doing the drawing and measuring. In addition, this approach is time consuming when compared to the quicker more accurate method using trigonometry. The word trigonometry means, literally, the measurement of triangles. Most problems in motion analysis involve the use of right triangles. A right triangle is one containing an internal right angle (90°). Recall that the sum of the three internal angles of a triangle always equal 180°. Also, an angle less than 90° is called an acute angle and greater than 90° an obtuse angle. Two angles are said to be *complementary* if their sum equals 90°. Thus, in a right triangle it is apparent that the two acute angles are complementary. If the sum of two angles equals 180°, they are said to be *supplementary*.

In order to understand the trigonometry functions, one must first be able to identify the parts of a right triangle. The following diagram (Fig. A.1) of a right triangle will be used for the purpose of explanation.

The six component parts of the triangle consist of three angles and three sides. (The symbol "∠" is used to denote the word angle.) It should be noted that the longest of the three sides (c) is opposite the right angle (C). This longest side is called the *hypotenuse*. Because the hypotenuse is always opposite the right angle, it is very easy to identify. The other two sides are referred to as the legs of the right triangle. The second notation used for the sides is called the side *opposite*. Which side this is depends upon the angle in question. Referring to the diagram, the side opposite angle A (∠A) is side "a," On the other hand, the side opposite ∠B is side "b." The *adjacent* side is the third term used in identifying the sides. The side adjacent (or next to) refers to the side which along with the hypotenuse forms the given angle. Thus, the side adjacent to ∠A would be side *b*. Likewise, the side adjacent ∠B is side a. Thus, understand that the sides opposite and adjacent depend upon which of the two angles is being considered, whereas the hypotenuse is fixed.

Now that each of the parts of the triangle has been named, the trig functions can be introduced. Although there are six functions, only four will be included. These functions are based upon the relationship that exists between the angles and sides of the triangle.

The first of these is called the sine, abbreviated "sin." The sine of an angle is defined as the ratio (one number divided by another) of the side opposite over the hypotenuse. Thus, the sine of angle A (sin A) = a/c, that is, the length of side a is divided by the length of the hypotenuse. Note that the sine of angle B = b/c.

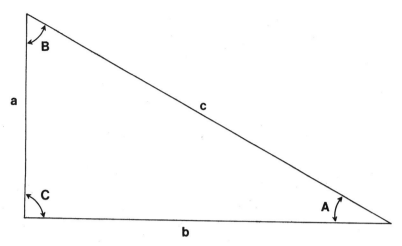

Figure A.1. The right triangle and descriptors of sides and angles.

The second trig function is called the cosine, abbreviated *cos*, and is defined as the ratio of the side adjacent over the hypotenuse. For angle A the cosine is b/c; and for angle B it is a/c.

The third function is called the tangent (tan) and is defined as the ratio of the side *opposite* over the side adjacent. Thus, the tangent of angle A (tan A) = a/b while the tan B = b/a.

The last function is termed the cotangent (cot) and is defined as the ratio of the side adjacent over the side opposite; hence, the cotangent of angle A (cot A) = b/a and the cot B = a/b.

Now that the trig functions have been defined, their use will be discussed. It has been shown that the trig functions have a specific value for a given angle, regardless of the size of the triangle. Since the trig functions are constants for any given angle, it is possible to include these functions in table form for the various angles. This type of table has been included for reference.

Since the one angle is fixed (90°) in a right triangle, only five parts can vary (three sides and two angles). If either one angle and the length of one side or the length of two sides are known, the remaining parts can be determined. The sides can be used to represent distance, magnitude of force, velocity, or some other physical property.

EXAMPLE

Referring to the diagram, assume that the hypotenuse is 6 inches in length and angle A = 40°. Find the following: (1) angle B; (2) side a; (3) side b.

Angle B can be determined very readily since it is complementary to angle A (40°). So, angle B is found by 90° − 40° = 50°.

To find side a, we must select the trig function that involves side a (which is unknown) and side c, the hypotenuse (which is known). It can be seen that sin A equals side a (opposite) over c (hypotenuse).

In equation form:

$$\sin A = a/c$$

Since c is known to be 6 inches and the sin A (40°) can be secured from the table, the only unknown is side a. Thus, the formula appears as follows:

$$\sin 40° = a/6 \text{ inches}$$

Multiplying both sides of the equation by 6 yields: $6 \times 0.6428 = a$, $a = 3.84$ inches.

The same procedure is followed in solving for side b.

The following problems are included as practice exercises. Answers are at the end of the review.

1. 20 feet = 80 units   1 foot = _____ units   1 unit = _____ feet

2. sine 25 = _____   3. cos 57 = _____   4. tan 80 = _____

5.

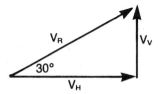

$B =$ _____ degrees

side c = _____

6.

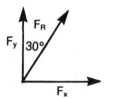

$V_R = 30$ ft/sec

$V_H =$ _____

$V_V =$ _____

7.

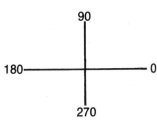

$F_x = 10\#$

$F_y =$ _____

$F_R =$ _____

8. Using a ruler and protractor, devise an appropriate scale factor and sketch the path of a hiker who walks 1 mile at 30°, 3 miles at 120°, 5 miles at 230° and 2 miles at 340°. Measure the resultant displacement of the hiker (magnitude and direction). Use the following coordinate reference system:

```
                    90
                    |
                    |
        180 --------+-------- 0
                    |
                    |
                   270
```

Answers

1. 4 units, .25 feet   5. 22.5°, 13

2. .4226   6. 25.98, 15

3. .5446   7. 17.32, 20

4. 5.6713

CIRCULAR (TRIGONOMETRIC) FUNCTIONS

Degrees	Sines	Cosines	Tangets	Cotangents	
0°00′	.0000	1.0000	.0000		90°00′
1°00′	.0175	.9998	.0175	57.290	89°00′
2°00′	.0349	.9994	.0349	28.636	88°00′
3°00′	.0523	.9986	.0524	19.081	87°00′
4°00′	.0698	.9976	.0699	14.301	86°00′
5°00′	.0872	.9962	.0875	11.430	85°00′
6°00′	.1045	.9945	.1051	9.5144	84°00′
7°00′	.1219	.9925	.1228	8.1443	83°00′
8°00′	.1392	.9903	.1405	7.1154	82°00′
9°00′	.1564	.9877	.1584	6.3138	81°00′
10°00′	.1736	.9848	.1763	5.6713	80°00′
11°00′	.1908	.9816	.1944	5.1446	79°00′
12°00′	.2079	.9781	.2126	4.7046	78°00′
13°00′	.2250	.9744	.2309	4.3315	77°00′
14°00′	.2419	.9703	.2493	4.0108	76°00′
15°00′	.2588	.9659	.2679	3.7321	75°00′
16°00′	.2756	.9613	.2867	3.4874	74°00′
17°00′	.2924	.9563	.3057	3.2709	73°00′
18°00′	.3090	.9511	.3249	3.0777	72°00′
19°00′	.3256	.9455	.3443	2.9042	71°00′
20°00′	.3420	.9397	.3640	2.7475	70°00′
21°00′	.3584	.9336	.3839	2.6051	69°00′
22°00′	.3746	.9272	.4040	2.4751	68°00′
23°00′	.3907	.9205	.4245	2.3559	67°00′
24°00′	.4067	.9135	.4452	2.2460	66°00′
25°00′	.4226	.9063	.4663	2.1445	65°00′
26°00′	.4384	.8988	.4877	2.0503	64°00′
27°00′	.4540	.8910	.5095	1.9626	63°00′
28°00′	.4695	.8829	.5317	1.8807	62°00′
29°00′	.4848	.8746	.5543	1.8040	61°00′
30°00′	.5000	.8660	.5774	1.7321	60°00′
31°00′	.5150	.8572	.6009	1.6643	59°00′
32°00′	.5299	.8480	.6249	1.6003	58°00′
33°00′	.5446	.8387	.6494	1.5399	57°00′
34°00′	.5592	.8290	.6745	1.4826	56°00′
35°00′	.5736	.8192	.7002	1.4281	55°00′
36°00′	.5878	.8090	.7265	1.3764	54°00′
37°00′	.6018	.7986	.7536	1.3270	53°00′
38°00′	.6157	.7880	.7813	1.2799	52°00′
39°00′	.6293	.7771	.8098	1.2349	51°00′
40°00′	.6428	.7660	.8391	1.1918	50°00′
41°00′	.6561	.7547	.8693	1.1504	49°00′
42°00′	.6691	.7431	.9004	1.1106	48°00′
43°00′	.6820	.7314	.9325	1.0724	47°00′
44°00′	.6947	.7193	.9657	1.0355	46°00′
45°00′	.7071	.7071	1.0000	1.0000	45°00′
	Cosines	Sines	Cotangents	Tangents	Degrees

APPENDIX B

*Elements of Vector Algebra**

Detailed analysis of noncoplanar biomechanical systems requires a basic understanding of the elements of vector algebra.

RIGHT HAND RULE

It is customary to use a right-handed coordinate system in most mechanical analyses (Fig. B.1). If the fingers of the right hand are curled in the direction necessary to rotate the positive X axis toward the positive Y axis through the 90° angle between them, the thumb will point in the direction of the positive Z axis. Such a coordinate reference frame is termed right-handed.

UNIT VECTORS

Vectors, one unit in length, are utilized to indicate specific directions. The notations **i, j,** and **k** indicate unit vectors directed along the positive X, Y, and Z axes, respectively (Fig. B.2).

VECTOR NOTATION

A vector is often specified in terms of unit vectors **i, j,** and **k,** with each being multiplied by the appropriate magnitude. The vector notation for a line directed from M(Mx,My,Mz) to N(Nx,Ny,Nz) is:

$$\mathbf{MN} = (Nx - Mx)\mathbf{i} + (Ny - My)\mathbf{j} + (Nz - Mz)\mathbf{k}$$

If the vector were directed from N to M, then it would be designated:

$$\mathbf{NM} = (Mx - Nx)\mathbf{i} + (My - Ny)\mathbf{j} + (Mz - Nz)\mathbf{k}$$

Assuming that the coordinates of M and N were (2,1,−2) and (5,−3,10), respectively, the vector directed from M to N would be:

$$\mathbf{MN} = (5 - 2)\mathbf{i} + (-3 - 1)\mathbf{j} + (10 + 2)\mathbf{k}$$
$$= 3\mathbf{i} - 4\mathbf{j} + 12\mathbf{k}$$

The magnitude of **MN** can be calculated using the three dimensional version of the Pythagorean theorem:

$$MN = \sqrt{3^2 + 4^2 + 12^2} = \sqrt{169} = 13$$

---

* Modified from Miller DI, Nelson RC: *Biomechanics of Sport.* Philadelphia, Lea & Febiger, 1973, pp 241–242.

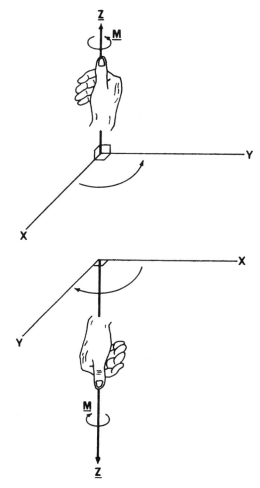

Figure B.1.   Right-handed coordinate reference frames.

MN can be expressed as a unit vector, **u,** by dividing each of its components by the magnitude of the vector. Thus,

$$\mathbf{u} = \frac{\mathbf{MN}}{MN} = \frac{3\mathbf{i} - 4\mathbf{j} + 12\mathbf{k}}{13}.$$

ADDITION AND SUBTRACTION

Vectors can be combined by the addition or subtraction of each of the three orthogonal components. For example, if

$$\mathbf{F} = Fx\mathbf{i} + Fy\mathbf{j} + Fz\mathbf{k} \qquad \text{and}$$
$$\mathbf{G} = Gx\mathbf{i} + Gy\mathbf{j} + Gz\mathbf{k}$$

then $\qquad \mathbf{F} + \mathbf{G} = (Fx + Gx)\mathbf{i} + (Fy + Gy)\mathbf{j} + (Fz + Gz)\mathbf{k}.$

DOT OR SCALAR PRODUCT

The dot product of two vectors is, by definition, a scalar equal to the product of the magnitudes of the two vectors multiplied by the cosine of the smaller angle between them. Thus,

$$\mathbf{M} \cdot \mathbf{N} = MN \cos \theta \text{ (Fig. B.3)}.$$

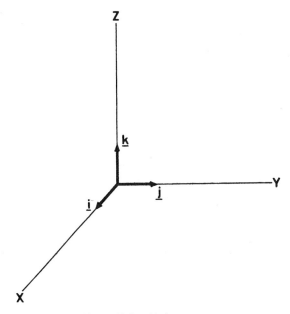

Figure B.2. Unit vectors.

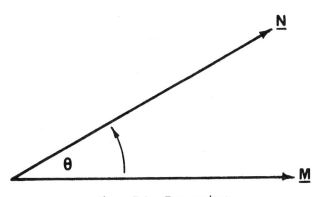

Figure B.3. Dot product.

This gives the component of **M** directed along **N** multiplied by the magnitude of **N**. It is therefore a suitable vector operation for determining work which is equal to the component of force in the direction of the displacement multiplied by the displacement.

The dot products of unit vectors **i, j,** and **k** are:

$$\mathbf{i} \cdot \mathbf{i} = (1)(1)\cos 0 = 1$$

Similarly, $\mathbf{j} \cdot \mathbf{j} = \mathbf{k} \cdot \mathbf{k} = 1$.

Then, $\mathbf{j} \cdot \mathbf{k} = (1)(1)\cos 90 = 0$ and likewise

$$\mathbf{i} \cdot \mathbf{j} = \mathbf{k} \cdot \mathbf{i} = \mathbf{j} \cdot \mathbf{i} = \mathbf{i} \cdot \mathbf{k} = \mathbf{k} \cdot \mathbf{j} = 0.$$

Using these identities to expand **M·N,**

$$\mathbf{M} \cdot \mathbf{N} = (Mx\mathbf{i} + My\mathbf{j} + Mz\mathbf{k}) \cdot (Nx\mathbf{i} + Ny\mathbf{j} + Nz\mathbf{k})$$
$$= MxNx + MyNy + MzNz.$$

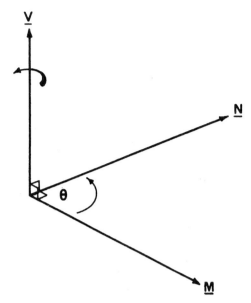

Figure B.4.   Cross product.

VECTOR OR CROSS PRODUCT

By definition, the cross product of two vectors **M** and **N** is a vector **V** acting in a direction perpendicular to the plane of the two original vectors in accordance with the right hand rule (Fig. B.4). The magnitude of **V** is equal to the product of the magnitudes of **M** and **N** multiplied by the sine of the smaller angle between them. The cross products of the unit vectors **i**, **j**, and **k** are:

$$
\begin{aligned}
&\mathbf{i} \times \mathbf{i} = (1)(1)\sin 0 = 0 \quad &\mathbf{j} \times \mathbf{j} = 0 \quad &\mathbf{k} \times \mathbf{k} = 0 \\
&\mathbf{i} \times \mathbf{j} = \mathbf{k} &\mathbf{j} \times \mathbf{k} = \mathbf{i} \quad &\mathbf{k} \times \mathbf{i} = \mathbf{j} \\
&\mathbf{j} \times \mathbf{i} = -\mathbf{k} &\mathbf{k} \times \mathbf{j} = -\mathbf{i} \quad &\mathbf{i} \times \mathbf{k} = -\mathbf{j}.
\end{aligned}
$$

Using these identities, the cross product **M** × **N** can be expanded:

$$
\begin{aligned}
\mathbf{M} \times \mathbf{N} &= (M_x\mathbf{i} + M_y\mathbf{j} + M_z\mathbf{k}) \times (N_x\mathbf{i} + N_y\mathbf{j} + N_z\mathbf{k}) \\
&= M_xN_y\mathbf{k} - M_xN_z\mathbf{j} - M_yN_x\mathbf{k} + M_yN_z\mathbf{i} + M_zN_x\mathbf{j} - M_zN_y\mathbf{i} \\
&= (M_yN_z - M_zN_y)\mathbf{i} + (M_zN_x - M_xN_z)\mathbf{j} + (M_xN_y - M_yN_x)\mathbf{k}
\end{aligned}
$$

This relationship can be more easily expressed in the form of a 3 × 3 determinant:

$$
\mathbf{M} \times \mathbf{N} = \begin{vmatrix} \mathbf{i} & \mathbf{j} & \mathbf{k} \\ M_x & M_y & M_z \\ N_x & N_y & N_z \end{vmatrix}
$$

MOMENT OF A FORCE ABOUT A POINT

The vector product **r** × **F** represents the moment of force **F** about a point, where **r** is any position vector directed from the point to the line of action of **F**. Both magnitude and direction of the moment can be obtained by expanding the determinant:

$$
\mathbf{r} \times \mathbf{F} = \begin{vmatrix} \mathbf{i} & \mathbf{j} & \mathbf{k} \\ r_x & r_y & r_z \\ F_x & F_y & F_z \end{vmatrix}
$$

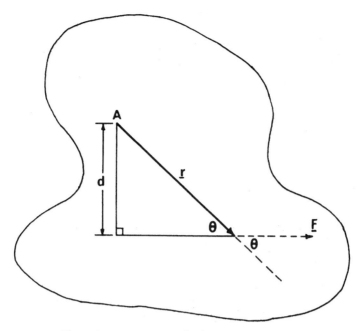

Figure B.5. Moment of a force about a point.

In the planar example shown in Figure B.5, the magnitude of the moment of **F** about point A is equal to the magnitude of the force multiplied by the perpendicular distance d. By trigonometry, it can be seen that

$$d = r \sin \theta$$

It will be recalled that the magnitude of $\mathbf{r} \times \mathbf{F} = rF \sin \theta = Fr \sin \theta$.

MOMENT OF A FORCE ABOUT AN AXIS

The triple scalar product is utilized to determine the moment of force **(F)** about a particular axis **(N)**. The axis must first be expressed in unit vector form. Then, the moment of force **F** about axis **N** is $\mathbf{r} \times \mathbf{F} \cdot \mathbf{N}$, where **r** is any position vector joining **N** and **F**, directed toward **F**. In determinant form, the triple scalar product is

$$\mathbf{r} \times \mathbf{F} \cdot \mathbf{N} = \begin{vmatrix} r_x & r_y & r_z \\ F_x & F_y & F_z \\ N_x & N_y & N_z \end{vmatrix}$$

The triple scalar product is the dot product of two vectors, one of which is the cross product of two other vectors. In computing the moment of force about an axis, the triple scalar product gives the component of rotation in the direction of the specified axis.

Example

The following example illustrates some of the basic concepts of vector algebra which are required in biomechanical analysis.

Given

A 20-N force passes through points D(1,3,5) and E(10,10,12), and is directed from D to E. The coordinates are specified in meters.

Find

The moment of the force with respect to an axis through G(−1,−6,−12) and H(−3,−10,−20). The axis is directed from G to H.

Solution

(1) Express the force in vector form.
   (a) Direction of the force

$$\mathbf{DE} = (10 - 1)\mathbf{i} + (10 - 3)\mathbf{j} + (12 - 5)\mathbf{k}$$
$$= 9\mathbf{i} + 7\mathbf{j} + 7\mathbf{k}$$

   (b) Express the direction as a unit vector.

$$\mathbf{U} = \frac{9\mathbf{i} + 7\mathbf{j} + 7\mathbf{k}}{\sqrt{9^2 + 7^2 + 7^2}}$$
$$= \frac{1}{\sqrt{179}} (9\mathbf{i} + 7\mathbf{j} = 7\mathbf{k})$$

   (c) Multiply the unit vector by the magnitude of the force to determine the force vector.

$$\mathbf{F} = (20)\frac{1}{\sqrt{179}} (9\mathbf{i} + 7\mathbf{j} + 7\mathbf{k}) \text{ Newtons}$$

Thus the components of force in the three orthogonal directions are:

$$\mathbf{F_x} = \frac{180}{\sqrt{179}} \quad \mathbf{F_y} = \frac{140}{\sqrt{179}} \quad \mathbf{F_z} = \frac{140}{\sqrt{179}} \text{ Newtons}$$

(2) Calculate a position vector, **r**, joining the axis to the line of action, **F.**
   (a) Of the several possibilities available, namely, **GD, GE, HD,** and **HE,** vector **GD** is arbitrarily chosen:

$$\mathbf{r} = [(1) - (-1)]\mathbf{i} + [(3) - (-6)]\mathbf{j} + [(5) - (-12)]\mathbf{k}$$
$$= 2\mathbf{i} + 9\mathbf{j} + 17\mathbf{k}$$

(3) Express the axis in unit vector form.
   (a) $\mathbf{GH} = [(-3) - (-1)]\mathbf{i} + [(-10) - (-6)]\mathbf{j} + [(-20) - (-12)]\mathbf{k}$
   $= -2\mathbf{i} - 4\mathbf{j} - 8\mathbf{k}$

   (b) As a unit vector **N,**

$$\mathbf{N} = \frac{-2\mathbf{i} - 4\mathbf{j} - 8\mathbf{k}}{\sqrt{2^2 + 4^2 + 8^2}}$$
$$= \frac{1}{\sqrt{84}} (-2\mathbf{i} - 4\mathbf{j} - 8\mathbf{k}).$$

(4) Use the triple scalar product to determine the moment of the force about the axis.

$$M = \mathbf{r} \times \mathbf{F} \cdot \mathbf{N}$$
$$= [(\mathbf{r} \times \mathbf{F}) \cdot \mathbf{N}]$$
$$= [\mathbf{r} \cdot (\mathbf{F} \times \mathbf{N})]$$
$$= \frac{1}{\sqrt{84}} \cdot \frac{20}{\sqrt{179}} \begin{vmatrix} 2 & 9 & 17 \\ 9 & 7 & 7 \\ -2 & -4 & -8 \end{vmatrix}$$
$$= \frac{20}{\sqrt{84}\sqrt{179}} 2[(7)(-8) - (7)(-4)]$$
$$\qquad - 9[(9)(-8) - (7)(-2)] + 17[(9)(-4) - (7)(-2)]$$
$$= \frac{20}{(9.165)(13.379)} (2)(-28) - (9)(-58) + (17)(-22)$$
$$= \frac{1840}{122.62}$$
$$= 15.01 \text{N} \cdot \text{m}$$

Figure and Table Credits

Figure 1.1. Nordin M, Frankel VH. *Basic Biomechanics of the Musculoskeletal System.* Philadelphia: Lea & Febiger; 1989:xix.

Figure 1.6. Kulig K, Andrews JG, Hay JG. Human strength curves. In: Terjung RL, ed. *Exercise and Sport Sciences Review.* Lexington: Columbia Press; 1984;12:417–466.

Figure 1.15. LeVeau B. *Williams and Lissner's Biomechanics of Human Motion.* Philadelphia: WB Saunders; 1962:108.

Figure 1.18. Richards C, Knutsson E. Evaluation of abnormal gait patterns by intermittent light photography and electromyography. *Scand J Rehabil Med Suppl.* 1984;3:61–68.

Figure 2.1. Tricker RAR, Tricker BJK. *The Science of Human Movement.* New York: Elsevier; 1967:266.

Figure 2.2. Sacks RD, Roy RR. Architecture of the hind limb muscle of cats: functional significance. *J Morphology.* 1982;173:185–195.

Figure 2.3. Edgerton VR, Roy RR, Gregor RJ, et al. Morphological basis of skeletal muscle power output. In: Jones NL, McCartney N, McComas AJ, eds. *Human Muscle Power.* Champaign, IL: Human Kinetics; 1986.

Figure 2.4. Sacks RD, Roy RR. Architecture of the hind limb muscle of cats: functional significance. *J Morphology.* 1982;173:185–195.

Figure 2.5. Phillips CA, Petrofsky JS. The passive elastic force-velocity relationship of cat skeletal muscle: Influence upon the maximal contractile element velocity. *J Biomech.* 1981;14:400.

Figure 2.6. Wilkie DR. *Muscle.* New York: St. Martins Press; 1968:30.

Figure 2.7. Alexander R McN, Goldspink G. *Mechanics and Energetics of Animal Locomotion.* New York: John Wiley & Sons; 1977:7.

Figure 2.8. Alexander R McN, Goldspink G. *Mechanics and Energetics of Animal Locomotion.* New York: John Wiley & Sons; 1977:40.

Figure 2.9. Yamada H. Mechanical properties of locomotor organs and tissues. In: Evans FG, ed. *Strength of Biological Materials.* Baltimore: Williams & Wilkins; 1970:95.

Figure 2.10. Gordon AM, Huxley AF, Julian FT. The variation in isometric tension with sarcomere length in vertebrate muscle fibers. *J Physiol.* 1966;284:185–186.

Figure 2.12. Wilkie DR. *Muscle.* New York: St. Martins Press; 1968:33.

Figure 2.13. Komi PV. Measurement of the force-velocity relationship in human muscle under concentric and eccentric contractions. In: Cerquiglini S, ed. *Biomechanics III.* Basel, Switzerland: Karger; 1973:227.

Figure 2.14. Stothart JP. Relationship between selected biomechanical parameters of static and dynamic muscle performance. In: Cerquiglini S, ed. *Biomechanics III.* Basel, Switzerland: Karger; 1973:212.

Figure 2.16. Engel AG, Franzini-Armstrong C. *Myology: Basic and Clinical.* 2nd ed. New York: McGraw-Hill, 1994.

Figure 2.17. Baker JH, Matsumoto DE. Adaptation of skeletal muscle to immobilization in a shortened position. *Muscle Nerve.* 1988;11:231–244.

Figure 2.18. Cooper RR. Alterations during immobilization and regeneration of skeletal muscle in cats. *J Bone Joint Surg.* 1972;54(A):919–953.

Figure 2.19. Tabary JC, Tabary C, Tardieu C, et al. Physiological and structural changes in the cat's soleus muscle due to immobilization at different lengths by plaster casts. *J Physiol (Lond).* 1972;224:231–244.

Figure 2.20. Woo SL-Y, Maynard J, Butler D. Ligament, tendon, and joint capsule insertions to bone. In: Woo SL-Y, Buckwalter, JA. *Injury and Repair of the Musculoskeletal Soft Tissues.* Park Ridge, IL: American Academy of Orthopaedic Surgeons; 1987.

Figure 2.21. Garrett W, Tidball J. Myotendinous junction: structure, function, and failure. In: Woo SL-Y, Buckwalter, JA. *Injury and Repair of the Musculoskeletal Soft Tissues.* Park Ridge, IL: American Academy of Orthopaedic Surgeons; 1987.

Figure 2.22. Newham DJ. Ultrastructural changes after concentric and eccentric contractions of human muscle. *J Neurosci.* 1983;61:109–122.

Figure 2.23. Gelberman RH, Siegel DB, Woo SL-Y, et al. Healing of digital flexor tendons: importance of the interval from injury to repair. *J Bone Joint Surg.* 1991;73(A):66–75.

Figure 3.2. Nelson RM, Soderberg GL, Urbscheit NL. Alteration of motor-unit discharge characteristics in aged humans. *Phys Ther.* 1984;64:29–34.

Figures 3.3–3.4. Kandel ER, Schwartz JH, Jessell TM, eds. *Principles of Neural Science.* 3rd ed. Norwalk, CT: Appleton and Lange; 1991.

Figure 3.6. Binder MD, Houk JC, Nichols TR, et al. Properties and segmental actions of mammalian muscle receptors: an update. *Fed Proc.* 1981;41:2915.

Figure 3.7. Basmajian JV. *Muscles Alive: Their Function Revealed by Electromyography.* Baltimore: Williams & Wilkins; 1979:55.

Figure 3.9. Winter DA. *Biomechanics of Human Movement.* New York: John Wiley & Sons; 1979:140.

Figure 3.10. Inman VT, Ralston HJ, Saunders JB, et al. Relation of human electromyogram to muscular tension. *Electroencephalogr Clin Neurophysiol.* 1952;4:193.

Figure 3.11. Winter DA. *Biomechanics of Human Movement.* New York: John Wiley & Sons; 1979:143.

Figure 3.12. Bigland B, Lippold OCJ. The relation between force, velocity and integrated electrical activity in human muscles. *J Physiol.* 1954;123:218, 219.

Figure 4.1. Kessler RM, Hertling D. *Management of Musculoskeletal Disorders.* Philadelphia: Harper & Row; 1983:13.

Figure 4.2. Alexander RM. Mechanics of skeleton and tendons. In: Brooks VB, ed. *Handbook of Physiology. Section 1: The Nervous System.* Bethesda, MD: American Physiological Society; 1981;2:19.

Figure 4.3. Moore KL. *Clinically Oriented Anatomy.* Baltimore: Williams & Wilkins; 1985.

Figure 4.4. Clark, JM. The organisation of collagen fibrils in the superficial zones of articular cartilage. *J Anat.* 1990;171:117–130.

Figure 4.5. Warwick R, Williams PL, Dyson M, et al. *Gray's Anatomy.* 37th British ed. Philadelphia: WB Saunders; 1989.

Figure 4.6. Brand RA. Joint lubrication. In: Albright JA, Brand RA, eds. *The Scientific Basis of Orthopedics.* New York: Appleton-Century-Crofts; 1987:374.

Figures 4.7–4.8. Mow VC, Rosenwasser M. Articular cartilage: biomechanics. In: Woo SL-Y, Buckwalter, JA. *Injury and Repair of the Musculoskeletal Soft Tissues.* Park Ridge, IL: American Academy of Orthopaedic Surgeons; 1987.

Figure 4.12. Gowitzke BA, Milner M. *Understanding the Scientific Bases of Human Movement.* Baltimore: Williams & Wilkins; 1980:2.

Figure 4.13. White AA, Panjabi MM. *Clinical Biomechanics of the Spine.* Philadelphia: JB Lippincott; 1990;660.

Figure 4.14. Frankel VH, Burstein AH. *Orthopedic Biomechanics.* Philadelphia: Lea & Febiger; 1970:138.

Figure 5.1. Frankel VH, Nordin M. *Basic Biomechanics of the Skeletal System.* Philadelphia: Lea & Febiger; 1980:23.

Figure 5.2. Frankel VH, Nordin M. *Basic Biomechanics of the Skeletal System.* Philadelphia: Lea & Febiger; 1980:28.

Figure 5.4. Frankel VH, Nordin M. *Basic Biomechanics of the Skeletal System.* Philadelphia: Lea & Febiger; 1980:29.

Figure 5.5. Frankel VH, Nordin M. *Basic Biomechanics of the Skeletal System.* Philadelphia: Lea & Febiger; 1980:35.

Figure 5.6. Carlstedt, CA. Mechanical and chemical factors in tendon healing. *Acta Orthop Scand Suppl.* 1987;58:224.

Figure 5.7. Frankel VH, Nordin M. *Basic Biomechanics of the Skeletal System.* Philadelphia: Lea & Febiger; 1980:19.

Figure 5.8. White AA, Panjabi MM. *Clinical Biomechanics of the Spine.* Philadelphia: JB Lippincott; 1978:495.

Figure 5.9. Burstein AH, Wright TM. *Fundamentals of Orthopedic Biomechanics.* Baltimore: Williams & Wilkins; 1994.

Figure 5.10. Barbenel JC, Evans JH, Jordan MM. Tissue mechanics. *Engineering in Medicine.* 1978;7:5.

Figure 5.11. Yamada H. Locomotor System. In: Evans FG, ed. *Strength of Biological Materials.* Baltimore: Williams & Wilkins; 1970:95.

Figure 5.12. Frankel VH, Nordin M. *Basic Biomechanics of the Skeletal System.* Philadelphia: Lea & Febiger; 1980:88.

Figure 5.13. Frankel VH, Nordin M. *Basic Biomechanics of the Skeletal System.* Philadelphia: Lea & Febiger; 1980:91.

Figure 5.14. Frankel VH, Nordin M. *Basic Biomechanics of the Skeletal System.* Philadelphia: Lea & Febiger; 1980:96.

Figure 5.15. Noyes FR. Biomechanics of ligament failure: II. An analysis of immobilization, exercise, and reconditioning effects in primates. *J Bone Joint Surg.* 1974;56(A):1413.

Figure 6.1. Morrey BF, Askew LJ, An KN, et al. A biomechanical study of normal functional elbow motion. *J Bone Joint Surg.* 1981;63(A):872.

Figure 6.2. Johnston RC, Smidt GL. Measurement of hip joint motion during walking. *J Bone Joint Surg.* 1969;51(A):1087.

Figure 6.3. Johnston RC, Smidt GL. Measurement of hip joint motion during walking. *J Bone Joint Surg.* 1969;51(A):1090.

Figure 6.4. Grieve DW, Miller DI, Mitchelson D, et al. *Techniques for the Analysis of Human Movement.* Princeton: Princeton Book Company; 1976:59.

Figure 6.5. Smidt GL, Arora JS, Johnston RC. Accelerographic analysis of several types of walking. *Am J Phys Med.* 1971;50:297.

Figure 6.6. Richards C, Knutsson E. Evaluation of abnormal gait patterns by intermittent-light photography and electromyography. *Scand J Rehabil Med Suppl.* 1974;3:63.

Figure 6.7. Peak Performance Technologies. Colorado Springs, CO.

Figure 6.10. Mueller MJ. Etiology, evaluation, and treatment of the neuropathic foot. *Crit Rev Phys Rehabil Med.* 1992;3:289–309.

Figure 6.11. FW Kraemer. Remscheid, Germany.

Figure 6.14. Grieve DW, Miller DI, Mitchelson D, et al. *Techniques for the Analysis of Human Movement.* Princeton: Princeton Book Company; 1976:169.

Figure 6.16. Stauffer RN, Smidt GL, Wadsworth JB. Clinical and biomechanical analysis of gait following charnley total hip replacement. *Clin Orthop.* 1974;99:73.

Figure 6.17. Cook TM. Iowa City, IA: University of Iowa.

Figure 7.1. MacConaill MA, Basmajian JV. *Muscles and Movements: A Basis for Human Kinesiology.* Baltimore: Williams & Wilkins; 1969:189.

Figure 7.3. Norkin CC, Levangie PK. *Joint Structure and Function: A Comprehensive Analysis.* Philadelphia: FA Davis; 1983:174.

Figure 7.4. Bechtol CO. Biomechanics of the shoulder. *Clin Orthop.* 1980;146:38.

Figure 7.5. Inman V, Saunders M, Abbott LC. Observations on the function of the shoulder joint. *J Bone Joint Surg.* 1944;26(A):2, 3.

Figure 7.6. Shands AR. *Handbook of Orthopedic Surgery.* 5th ed. St. Louis: CV Mosby; 1971:63.

Figure 7.7. Inman V, Saunders M, Abbott LC. Observations on the function of the shoulder joint. *J Bone Joint Surg.* 1944;26(A):4.

Figure 7.8. Lippitt S, Matsen F. Mechanisms of glenohumeral joint stability. *Clin Orthop.* 1993;291:20–28.

Figure 7.9. Courtesy of RC Skovly. Miami Beach, FL.

Figure 7.10. Poppen NK, Walker PS. Normal and abnormal motion of the shoulder. *J Bone Joint Surg.* 1976;58(A):198.

Figure 7.11. Kronberg M, Németh G, Broström L-Å. Muscle activity and coordination in the normal shoulder. *Clin Orthop.* 1990;257:76–85.

Figure 7.12. Walker PS, Poppen NK. Biomechanics of the shoulder joint in the plane of the scapula. *Bull Hosp Jt Dis.* 1977;38:109, 110.

Figure 7.13. Walker PS, Poppen NK. Biomechanics of the shoulder joint in the plane of the scapula. *Bull Hosp Jt Dis.* 1977;38:110.

Figure 7.18. Bechtol CO. Biomechanics of the shoulder. *Clin Orthop.* 1980;146:39.

Figures 8.1–8.2. Basmajian JV, Griffin WR. Function of anconeus muscle: An electromyographic study. *J Bone Joint Surg.* 1972;54(A):1713.

Figure 8.3. An KN, Hui FC, Morrey BF, et al. Muscles across the elbow joint: A biomechanical analysis. *J Biomech.* 1981;14:660.

Figure 8.4. Kapandji AI. *The Physiology of the Joints.* 5th ed. New York: Churchill Livingstone; 1982:79.

Figure 8.5. Youm Y, Dryer RF, Thanbyrajah K, et al. Biomechanical analyses of forearm pronation-supination and elbow flexion-extension. *J Biomech.* 1979;12:254.

Figure 8.6. Chao EY, Morrey BF. Three dimensional rotation of the elbow. *J Biomech.* 1978;11:67.

Figure 8.7. Morrey BF, Askew LJ, An KN, et al. A biomechanical study of normal functional elbow motion. *J Bone Joint Surg.* 1981;63(A):874.

Figure 8.8. Morrey BF, Askew LJ, An KN, et al. A biomechanical study of normal functional elbow motion. *J Bone Joint Surg.* 1981;63(A):875.

Figure 8.9. An KN, Hui FC, Morrey BF, et al. Muscles across the elbow joint: A biomechanical analysis. *J Biomech.* 1981;14:668.

Figure 8.10. Winters JM, Kleweno DG. Effect of initial upper-limb alignment on muscle contributions to isometric strength curves. *J Biomech.* 1993;26:143–153.

Figure 8.11. vanZuylen EJ, van Velzen A, van der Gon, JJD. A biomechanical model for flexion torques of human arm muscles as a function of elbow angle. *J Biomech.* 1988; 21:183–190.

Figure 8.12. Amis AA, Dowson D, Wright V. Elbow joint force predictions for some strenuous isometric actions. *J Biomech.* 1980;13:772.

Figure 8.13. Amis AA, Dowson D, Wright V. Elbow joint force predictions for some strenuous isometric actions. *J Biomech.* 1980;13:773.

Figure 9.1. Brand PW. Biomechanics of tendon transfer. *Orthop Clin N Am.* 1984; 5:205–230.

Figure 9.2. Flatt AE. *The Care of Minor Hand Injuries.* St. Louis: CV Mosby; 1959:27.

Figure 9.3. Smith RJ. Balance and kinetics of the fingers under normal and pathological conditions. *Clin Orthop.* 1974;104:92–111.

Figure 9.4. Sarrafian SH, Melamed JL, Goshgarian GM. Study of wrist motion in flexion and extension. *Clin Orthop.* 1977;126:153–159.

Figure 9.5. Youm Y, McMurtry RY, Flatt AE, et al. Kinematics of the wrist. *J Bone Joint Surg.* 1978;60(A):423–431.

Figure 9.6. An KN, Ubea Y, Chao EY, et al. Tendon excursion and moment arm of index finger muscles. *J Biomech.* 1983;16:419–425.

Figure 9.7. An KN, Ubea Y, Chao EY, et al. Tendon excursion and moment arm of index finger muscles. *J Biomech.* 1983;16:419–425.

Figure 9.9. Conolly WB. *Color Atlas of Hand Conditions.* Chicago: Year Book; 1980:89.

Figure 9.16. Redrawn from Wadsworth CT. Clinical anatomy and mechanics of the wrist and hand. *J Orthop Sports Phys Ther.* 1983;4:206–216.

Figure 9.18B. Redrawn from Wadsworth CT. Clinical anatomy and mechanics of the wrist and hand. *J Orthop Sports Phys Ther.* 1983;4:206–216.

Figure 9.19. Conolly WB. *Color Atlas of Hand Conditions.* Chicago: Year Book; 1980:281.

Figure 9.20. Brand PW, Cranor KC, Ellis JC. Tendon and pulleys at the metacarpophalangeal joint of a finger. *J Bone Joint Surg.* 1975;57(A):779–784.

Figure 10.1. Dostal WF, Andrews JG. A three dimensional biomechanical model of hip musculature. *J Biomech.* 1981;14:803–812.

Figure 10.2. Radin EL. Biomechanics of the human hip. *Clin Orthop.* 1980;152:28–34.

Figure 10.3. Rydell N. Biomechanics of the hip joint. *Clin Orthop.* 1973;92:6–15.

Figure 10.4. Kessler R, Hertling D. *Management of Common Musculoskeletal Disorders.* New York: Harper & Row; 1983.

Figure 10.5. Pauwels F. *Biomechanics of the Normal and Diseased Hip.* Berlin: Springer-Verlag; 1976.

Figure 10.6. Neumann DA, Cook TM. The effect of load and carry position on the electromyographic activity of the gluteus medius during walking. *Phys Ther.* 1985;65:305–311.

Figure 10.7. Neumann DA, Soderberg GL, Cook TM. Comparison of maximal isometric hip abductor muscle torques between hip sides. *Phys Ther.* 1988;68:496–502.

Figure 10.8. Nemeth G, Ekholm J, Arborelius UP, et al. Influence of knee flexion on isometric hip extensor strength. *Scand J Rehabil Med.* 1983;15:97–101.

Figure 10.9. Olson VL, Smidt GL, Johnston RC. The maximum torque generated by the eccentric, isometric, and concentric contractions of the hip abductor muscles. *Phys Ther.* 1972;52:149–157.

Figure 10.10. Brand RA, Crowninshield RD, Johnston RC, Pedersen DR. Forces on the femoral head during activities of daily living. *Iowa Orthop J.* 1982;2:43–49.

Figure 10.11. Neumann DA, Cook TM. The effect of load and carry position on the electromyographic activity of the gluteus medius during walking. *Phys Ther.* 1985;65:305–311.

Figure 10.13. Redrawn from Radin EL, Simon SR, Rose RM, et al. *Practical Biomechanics for the Orthopedic Surgeon.* New York: John Wiley & Sons; 1979.

Figure 10.14. Redrawn from Radin EL, Simon SR, Rose RM, et al. *Practical Biomechanics for the Orthopedic Surgeon.* New York: John Wiley & Sons; 1979.

Figure 10.16. Stauffer RN. Ten-year follow-up study of total hip replacement. *J Bone Joint Surg.* 1982;64(A):983–990.

Figure 10.18. Delp SL, Bleck EE, Zajac FE, et al. Biomechanical analysis of the chiari pelvic osteotomy-preserving hip abductor strength. *Clin Orthop.* 1990;254:189–198.

Figure 11.1. Hehne H-J. Biomechanics of the patellofemoral joint and its clinical relevance. *Clin Orthop.* 1990;258:73–85.

Figure 11.2. Fuss FK. Principles and mechanisms of automatic rotation during terminal extension in the human knee joint. *J Anat.* 1992;180:297–304.

Figures 11.4–11.5. Kapandji IA. *The Physiology of the Joints.* New York: Churchill Livingstone; 1970;2.

Figure 11.6. Frankel VH, Burstein AH. *Orthopedic Biomechanics.* Philadelphia: Lea & Febiger; 1970.

Figure 11.7. Kapandji IA. *The Physiology of the Joints.* New York: Churchill Livingstone; 1970;2.

Figure 11.8. Fukubayashi T, Torzilli PA, Sherman MF, Warren RF. An in vitro biomechanical evaluation of anterior-posterior motion of the knee. *J Bone Joint Surg.* 1981;64:258–264.

Figure 11.9. Noyes FR, Grood ES, Suntay WJ, Butler DL. The three dimensional laxity of the anterior cruciate deficient knee as determined by clinical laxity tests. *Iowa Orthop J.* 1983;3:32–44.

Figure 11.10. Redrawn from Paulos L, Rusche K, Johnson C, Noyes FR. Patellar malalignment: a treatment rationale. *Phys Ther.* 1980;60:1624–1632.

Figure 11.13. Fukubayashi T, Kurosawa H. The contact area and pressure distribution pattern of the knee. *Acta Orthop Scand.* 1980;51:871–879.

Figure 11.14. Noyes FR, Sonstegrad DA. Biomechanical function of the pes anserinus at the knee and the effect of its transplantation. *J Bone Joint Surg.* 1973;55:1225–1241.

Figure 11.17. Redrawn from Maquet P. Mechanics and osteoarthritis of the patellofemoral joint. *Clin Orthop.* 1979;133:70–73.

Figure 11.19. Frankel VH, Nordin M. *Basic Biomechanics of the Skeletal System.* Philadelphia: Lea & Febiger; 1980.

Figure 12.1. Hicks JH. The three weight-bearing mechanisms of the foot. In: Evans FG, ed. *Biomechanical Studies of the Musculoskeletal System.* Springfield, IL: Charles C Thomas; 1961.

Figure 12.2. Manter JT. Movements of the subtalar and transverse tarsal joints. *Anat Rec.* 1941;80:397–410.

Figure 12.3. Donatelli R. *The Biomechanics of the Foot and Ankle.* Philadelphia: FA Davis; 1990.

Figure 12.4. Mann RA. Biomechanics of the foot. In: American Academy of Orthopedic Surgeons, eds. *Atlas of Orthotics: Biomechanical Principles and Application.* St. Louis: CV Mosby; 1975:257–266.

Figure 12.5. Sammarco GJ, Burstein AH, Frankel VH. Biomechanics of the ankle: a kinematic study. *Orthop Clin North Am.* 1973;4:75–96.

Figures 12.6–12.7. Manter JT. Movements of the subtalar and transverse tarsal joints. *Anat Rec.* 1941;80:397–410.

Figure 12.8. Mann RA. Biomechanics of the foot. In: American Academy of Orthopedic Surgeons, eds. *Atlas of Orthotics: Biomechanical Principles and Application.* St. Louis: CV Mosby; 1975:257–266.

Figure 12.9. Stauffer RN, Chao EYS, Brewster RC. Force and motion analysis of the normal, diseased, and prosthetic ankle joint. *Clin Orthop.* 1977;127:189–196.

Figure 12.10. Perry J. Anatomy and biomechanics of the hindfoot. *Clin Orthop.* 1983; 177:9–15.

Figure 12.11. Mann RA. Biomechanics of the foot. In: American Academy of Orthopedic Surgeons, eds. *Atlas of Orthotics: Biomechanical Principles and Application.* St. Louis: CV Mosby; 1975:257–266.

Figure 12.12. Scott SH, Winter DH. Talocrural and talocalcaneal joint kinematics and kinetics during the stance phase of walking. *J Biomech.* 1991;24:743–752.

Figure 13.3. Calliet R. *Low Back Pain Syndrome.* Philadelphia: FA Davis; 1968.

Figure 13.4. Stoddard A. *Manual of Osteopathic Technique.* London: Hutchinson & Co.; 1980.

Figure 13.5. White AA, Panjabi MM. The basic kinematics of the human spine. *Spine.* 1978;3:12–20.

Figure 13.6. Panjabi MM, Takata K, Goel VK. Kinematics of lumbar intervertebral foramen. *Spine.* 1983;8:348–357.

Figure 13.7. Twomey LT, Taylor JR. Sagittal movements of the human lumbar vertebral column: a quantitative study of the role of the posterior vertebral elements. *Arch Phys Med Rehabil.* 1983;64:322–325.

Figures 13.8–13.10. White AA, Panjabi MM. *Clinical Biomechanics of the Spine.* Philadelphia: JB Lippincott; 1978.

Figure 13.11. White AA, Panjabi MM. *Spinal Kinematics. The Research Status of Spinal Manipulative Therapy.* NINCDS Monograph (No. 15). p 93. Washington, DC: U.S. Department of Health, Education and Welfare; 1975.

Figure 13.12. Farfan HF. Muscular mechanism of the lumbar spine and the position of power and efficiency. *Orthop Clin N Am.* 1975;6:135–144.

Figure 13.13. Fahrni WH. Conservative treatment of lumbar disc degeneration: our primary responsibility. *Orthop Clin N Am.* 1975;6:93–103.

Figures 13.14–13.15. Radin EL, Simon SR, Rose RM, Paul IL. *Practical Biomechanics for the Orthopedic Surgeon.* New York: J. Wiley & Sons; 1979.

Figure 13.16. White AA, Panjabi MM. The clinical biomechanics of scoliosis. *Clin Orthop.* 1976;118:100–112.

Figures 13.17–13.18. Radin EL, Simon SR, Rose RM, Paul IL. *Practical Biomechanics for the Orthopedic Surgeon.* New York: J. Wiley & Sons; 1979.

Figure 13.19. Michele AA. *Iliopsoas: Development of Anomalies in Man.* Springfield, IL: Charles C Thomas; 1982.

Figure 14.1. Iglarsh ZA, Snyder-Mackler L. Temporomandibular joint and the cervical spine. In: Richardson JK, Iglarsh ZA, eds. *Clinical Orthopaedic Physical Therapy.* Philadelphia: WB Saunders; 1994:1–72.

Figure 14.2. McKay GS, Yemm R. The structure and function of the temporomandibular joint. *Br Dent J.* 1992;173:127–132.

Figure 14.3. Rocabado M. Arthrokinematics of the temporomandibular joint. *Dent Clin North Am.* 1983;27:573–594.

Figure 14.4. Kapandji IA. *The Physiology of the Joints.* 2nd ed. Edinburgh: Churchill Livingstone; 1974.

Figure 14.5. Weisl H. Articular surfaces of sacro-iliac joint and their relation to movements of sacrum. *Acta Anat.* 1954;22:1–14.

Figure 14.6. Kapandji IA. *The Physiology of the Joints.* 2nd ed. Edinburgh: Churchill Livingstone; 1974.

Figure 15.1. Cailliet R. *Soft Tissue Pain and Disability.* Philadelphia: FA Davis; 1977.

Figure 15.4. Oddson LIE. Control of voluntary trunk movements in man. *Acta Physiol Scand.* 1990;140:11–60.

Figure 15.5. Murray MP. Gait as a total pattern of movement. *Am J Phys Med.* 1967; 46:290–333.

Figure 15.6. Bampton S. *A Guide to the Visual Examination of Pathological Gait.* Temple University Rehabilitation and Research Training Center #8. Philadelphia: Moss Rehabilitation Hospital; 1979.

Figure 15.7. Murray MP. Gait as a total pattern of movement. *Am J Phys Med.* 1967; 46:290–333.

Figure 15.8. Smidt GL. Hip motion and related factors in walking. *Phys Ther.* 1971;51:9–21.

Figure 15.9. Carsöö S. *How Man Moves: Kinesiological Studies and Methods.* London, England: William Heinemann; 1972.

Figure 15.10. Bresler B, Frankel JP. The forces and moments in the leg during level walking. *ASME Trans.* 1950;72:27–36.

Figure 15.11. Brand RA, Crowninshield RD, Johnston RC, Pedersen DR. Forces on the femoral head during activities of daily living. *Iowa Orthop J.* 1982;2:43–49.

Figure 15.12. Cappozzo A, Figura F, Marchetti M. The interplay of muscular and external forces in human ambulation. *J Biomech.* 1976;9:35–43.

Figure 15.13. Winter DA. Energy generation and absorption at the ankle and knee during fast, natural, and slow cadences. *Clin Orthop.* 1983;175:147–154.

Figures 15.14–15.15. Sutherland DH, Cooper L. The pathomechanics of progressive crouch gait in spastic diplegia. *Orthop Clin North Am.* 1978;9:143–154.

Figure 15.16. Wadsworth JB, Smidt GL, Johnston RC. Gait characteristics of subjects with hip disease. *Phys Ther.* 1972;52:829–837.

Figure 15.17. Trias D, Gioux M, Cid M, Bensch C. Gait analysis of myopathic children in relation to impairment level and energy cost. *J Electromyogr Kinesiol.* 1994;4:67–81.

Figure 16.1. Rys M, Konz S. Standing. *Ergonomics.* 1994;37:677–687.

Figure 16.2. Webb RDG. *Industrial Ergonomics.* Toronto, Ontario: The Industrial Accident Prevention Association; 1982.

Figures 16.3–16.4. Grandjean E. *Fitting the Task to the Man: An Ergonomic Approach.* London: Taylor and Francis; 1982.

Figure 16.5. Chaffin DB, Andersson GBJ. *Occupational Biomechanics.* 2nd ed. New York: J. Wiley & Sons; 1991.

Figure 16.6. Andersson GBJ, Ortengren R, Nachemson A, Elfstrom G. Lumbar disc pressure and myoelectric back muscle activity during sitting. I. Studies on an experimental chair. *Scand J Rehabil Med.* 1974;3:104–114.

Figure 16.7. Soderberg GL, Blanco MK, Cosentino TL, Kurdelmeier KA. An EMG analysis of posterior trunk musculature during flat and anteriorly inclined sitting. *Human Factors.* 1986;28:483–449.

Figure 16.8. Webb RDG. *Industrial Ergonomics.* Toronto, Ontario: The Industrial Accident Prevention Association; 1982.

Figure 16.9. Chaffin DB, Andersson GBJ. *Occupational Biomechanics.* 2nd ed. New York: J. Wiley & Sons; 1991.

Figure 16.10. Grew ND. Intra-abdominal pressure response to loads applied to the torso in normal subjects. *Spine.* 1980;5:149–154.

Figure 16.11. Grandjean E. *Fitting the Task to the Man: An Ergonomic Approach.* London: Taylor and Francis; 1982.

Table 1.3. Winter DA. *Biomechanics of Human Movement.* New York: John Wiley & Sons; 1979.

Table 5.1. Modified from Henshaw JT. The design of orthotic appliances. In: Murdoch G, ed. *The Advance in Orthotics.* Baltimore: Williams & Wilkins; 1976.

Table 9.1. Favill J. *Outline of the Spine Nerves.* Springfield, IL: Charles C Thomas; 1946.

Table 13.1. Adams MA, Hutton WC. The resistance to flexion of the lumbar intervertebral joint. *Spine.* 1980;5:245–253.

Table 13.3. Nachemson AL. Disc pressure measurements. *Spine.* 1981;6:93–97.

Tables 14.1–14.2. Modified from Walker JM. The sacroiliac joint: a critical review. *Phys Ther.* 1992;72:903–916.

Table 16.1. Corlett EN. Analysis and evaluation of working posture. In: Kvalseth TO, ed. *Ergonomics of Workstation Design.* Guildford, England: Butterworths; 1983.

Tables 16.2–4. Modified from Waters TR, Putz-Anderson V, Garg A, Fine LJ. Revised NIOSH equation for the design and evaluation of manual lifting tasks. *Ergonomics.* 1993;36:749–776.

Index

Note: Page numbers followed by a "t" denote tables; those followed by "f" denote figures.

Abdominal musculature
  evaluation of, 343–344
  in inspiration, 375
  in lifting, 453
  in lumbar spine control, 343, 457–458
  strengthening of, 369
Abductor digiti minimi muscle, 202
Abductor pollicis brevis, 200–201
Abductor pollicis longus muscle, 200
Abrasion
  in joint wear, 95
Acceleration
  equation for, 24–25
Accelerometry, 125, 128f
Acetabulum, 233, 233f
Achilles tendon
  angle of
    in shin splints, 333
  rupture of
    plantar flexion torques after, 331–332
Acromioclavicular joint
  degrees of freedom of, 151–152
  motion at, 150
  rotation of, 154
Acromion
  evolution of, 146, 148f
  in shoulder motion, 152–153
Active insufficiency, 12, 264
Adductor magnus muscle, 229
Adhesion
  in joint wear, 95
Aging
  balance in, 411
Amphiarthrosis, 78
Amputation
  lower limb
    gait disorder from, 428
Anconeus muscle
  extensor function of, 178f, 178–179
Ankle, 311–334
  anterior tibial compartment
    injury to, 331
  arthrodesis of, 333–334
  arthrokinematics of, 314–315, 317
  arthrology of, 314–315
  arthroplasty of, 334
  axis for, 318–319, 319f
  biomechanics of, 317–323
  bones of, 311
  bursitis of, 333
  compressive force at
    in stance phase, 323, 325f
  contact area in, 325

  deformity of
    tendon transfer for, 332–333
  dorsiflexion of
    close-packed position in, 314
    torque of, 323
  eversion of
    torque of, 323, 324t
  in gait, 328–331
  instant centers of rotation for, 319, 320f
  inversion of
    torque of, 323, 324t
  kinematics of, 317–318
    bony shapes in, 314
  kinetics of, 323, 325, 325f
    in gait, 414
  ligamentous forces in, 326–327
  load bearing surface of, 325
  moments of
    in gait, 419
  muscular actions of, 311, 312
    dysfunction of, 331–333
    in gait, 416, 417f
  overuse syndromes of, 333
  pathokinesiology of, 327–334
  plantar flexion of
    torque of, 322–323, 324t
  in postural changes, 410, 411f
  propulsive energy of
    in gait, 422, 423f
  reaction forces in, 323
  shear force at, 323, 325
  sprain of, 331
  stability of
    anterior talofibular ligament in, 326–327
  stress fractures of, 333
  tangential force at, 323
  tendinitis of, 333
  tendinous forces in, 326–327
  terminology for, 311
  torques of, 321–323, 324t
    in gait, 418, 419f
    in upright posture, 402
Annulus fibrosus, 353–354
  physiological loading of, 355
Anthropometric data, 20t
Arcuate ligament
  in knee capsule reinforcement, 269
Arms
  elevation of
    serratus anterior paralysis and, 168–169
    shoulder motion in, 153f, 153–154, 155f
    in spinal cord injury, 170–171, 171f
    trapezius paralysis and, 168–169